This book is a remarkable and ambitious enterprise: the presentation of more th__
years-worth of drawings, sketches and finished paintings. The__ __
laborious and painful process of self-exploration throu__
eventually, art therapy as such. The book offers an unu__
excavation of an individual's imaginative world through a__
from serious manic-depressive episodes is traced throug__
which are variations and permutations of the same theme, __ __ is conveyed is not
just moments of insight or breakthrough, but also the feeling of going round in circles or of being stuck. This is true both to the experience of depression and to the artist's steadfast determination.

The book enables us to raise some important questions about the translation of dreams and fantasies through art and art-making, and about the capacity of art-making itself to be therapeutic. We should be grateful to Chris Hoggett for providing us with such a rich store of material with which to begin to attempt some answers.

David Maclagan
Writer, artist and art therapist

I find this book fascinating and varied, and am kept interested by the change in the style of the art work as it progresses and transforms itself. The section in Part One on Chris's mother is both amusing and also poignant. I am sure anyone who has experienced the ageing parent can identify with it. This and the breakdown/breakout theme are very moving. The book [will be] of interest to art therapists but I think it has a wider potential readership.

Professor Joy Schaverien
Professional Member, Society of Analytical Psychology

It is highly unusual to be admitted to such a close encounter with someone's dream life and mental states, rendered vividly and richly by an experienced artist . . . Chris Hoggett has been assailed by demons, but he has been able systematically to look at them and even in some way to train them, if training them means training himself to transform the demons into art . . . He also draws on daydreams, to perform a different imaginative act of visionary metamorphosis. On long, frequent walks to different beloved spots, he has fallen into waking reveries that have gradually disclosed to him hidden figures and meanings in the scene before him . . . This mental discipline brought great rewards: the goddess of the spring and a sleeping magna mater in the secret fall and fold of hill and valley, guardian heroes in the cliff-faces of a limestone quarry and even the Joker himself in the random patterns of a cork tile.

Marina Warner
Author, novelist and critic

THE JOKER

THE JOKER

SELF-TRANSFORMATION THROUGH ART & DREAM

Chris Hoggett

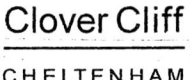

Clover Cliff
CHELTENHAM

FOREWORD
Marina Warner

When Chris Hoggett first showed me his notebooks for *The Joker*, his vividness and skill in rendering the fugitive and broken elements of dreams took me somewhere I wanted to know but had not experienced: another person's dream world.

I had looked at some dream material in the Wellcome Library, where they have several manuscripts bequeathed to them by patients and psychiatrists: an indexed ledger of motifs from one subject, kept in the 1950s, and a box containing an astonishing sequence of hundreds of watercolours done on tissue paper, from the same time. The psychiatrist Marion Milner, who wrote eloquently about art and therapy in her book *The Hands of the Living God*, reproduces drawings and searches their contents for keys to her patients' minds. But the intrinsic properties of dreams - their dissolving, changing, fleeting transformations, their sudden intense moods which can pierce the dreamer with pain, terror, or bliss, their ways of looming and receding, their enhanced colour, scale, and drama - had defeated these analysands' skills, and though their images were sometimes expressive, the unintelligibility and repetitiveness were off-putting, even estranging. (We all know about the boringness of dreams retold!) By contrast, Chris Hoggett does not suffer from their practical limitations; he can communicate his dreams to us with drama and emotion, hold our attention and involve us deeply because he has the practical expertise necessary.

He was trained as a technical draughtsman and can unfold a scene in space on the page: when he paints a self-portrait during a rare phase of expansiveness and confidence ('Hello, Everybody!', fig. 178), he compares the efflorescing figure to an axial perspective cut-away drawing of an engine. His techniques range from rapid notation done at night, immediately after waking, in writings and sketches that capture the scene of the dream before it fades, to fully developed formal picture-making which communicates the narrative, temper, and feel of a dream. The nightmare 'Witch and the Mannikin' (fig. 234), in which the terrifying ogress clutches her tiny victim in one fist, and has meanwhile stuck a knife through her own head, inspires the raw terror of the deepest fairytales about the power of adults and the vulnerability of children. Sometimes, the image has the perfect simplicity of a true symbol: 'The Dark Pool' (fig. 270), for example, shows the dreamer contemplating his own body in a black watery abyss, stirred by a mysterious ominous hand while he looks on apathetically, powerlessly.

The English poetic pastoralism of the New Romantics suffuses Chris Hoggett's art. John Minton was one of his tutors, and he too evokes in passionate reverie the English countryside, as it glows in the visionary paintings of Samuel Palmer, Stanley Spencer, and Eric Ravilious, as well as in the Surrealism of Grace Pailthorpe and Paul Nash. At times, as in the sequence on the Spring Goddess of the landscape near Cleeve Common, Chris elaborates biomorphic blooms of form which resonate with the paintings of the Armenian-American, Arshile Gorky. The ancient rocks and valleys of the Cotswolds, where he lives, have engaged his imagination profoundly for many decades, as the section on Five Visionary Landscapes reveals so powerfully. Furthermore, as a portraitist, Chris Hoggett also has the kind of practised command of features and expression that makes it possible for him to communicate the particular look of a nightmare spectre, the moods cast by a night visitor - of terror or despair, and sometimes, the comic delight of a happier apparition. The 'Zany Prancer', for example, closes this Pictorial Journal on a high note, with a smile and a caper.

It is highly unusual to be admitted to such a close encounter with someone's dream life and mental states, rendered vividly and richly by an experienced artist. Chris's artistic precursors did not usually keep a systematic record, but more often depicted a single, intense dream only now and then, as in the case of the Florentine Cecco Bravo (d.1661), who made a series of dream drawings with scenes of desolation and strange rituals, or Albrecht Dürer, who painted a famous watercolour of an ominous deluge. Francisco Goya chronicled a period of terrible depression, when he was also beset by monsters, cannibal giants, and murderous hags, in the visionary Black Paintings on the walls of his farmhouse. The German symbolist Max Klinger created a haunting fable of sexual longing in the dream sequence, 'Story of a Glove'. Chris himself has referred to the monster images of Odilon Redon, which share some of his mood swings, for Redon's fantasies range in feeling between terror and pain to more sprightly, funnier and even cheering figures. But the closest example I know to Chris's enterprise is exclusively verbal: J W Dunne's classic book, *An Experiment with Time* (1929), in which he argued for the prophetic character of dreams, and for dreamers' visionary voyaging in different temporal dimensions. With this approach, Dunne was following in a long tradition, shaped by Romantics like Coleridge and by Victorian psychic researchers, like Frederic Myers and the Theosophists. Chris Hoggett's work, integrating the chaotic dream world into his conscious life, and searching out retrospectively secret premonitions and annunciations in the record he has kept, claims this occult approach to dreams for psychology and for healing work of self-analysis.

Chris Hoggett has been assailed by demons, but he has also been able to systematically look at them and even in some way to train them, if training them means training himself to transform the demons into art. He responded to a suggestion from his therapist Claire Skailes and, over a long, intense period, he pressed the dream material through different metamorphoses, from rendering the first impact, towards elucidating its meaning in the overall pattern of his psyche and the history of his 'breakdown-breakout'. As an artist, he develops the imagery itself from a rough sketch in pen and ink or wash, to the richly textured and worked oils or pots, meditating on the motifs and the forms, until he condenses the symbols. In this way, his mask and alter ego, his guardian and his dissimulator, the Joker himself took shape and then revealed himself, as Chris writes, to have been there all along.

Chris Hoggett also draws on daydreams, to perform a different imaginative act of visionary metamorphosis. On long, frequent walks to different beloved spots, he has fallen into waking reveries that have gradually disclosed to him hidden figures and meanings in the scene before him. In this activity, he has some notable predecessors: in the *Notebooks*, Leonardo famously advocated the method as 'aid to reflection', recommending the contemplation of 'the stains on walls, or the ashes of a fire, or clouds, or mud, or like things . . . the mind is stimulated to new inventions by obscure things.' They provide a 'way of nourishing and stirring up the "ingegnio" to various inventions': 'if you consider them well, you will find really marvellous ideas.' Interestingly, Leonardo also included the method's acoustic equivalent, and likened it to hearing 'the sound of bells, in whose pealing you can find every name and every word you can imagine'. Such experiences often occurred in the lives of saints such as Joan of Arc, who did indeed hear her voices sometimes in the carillon of her local church. But Leonardo was an empiricist, and imagination was a material organ and he did not associate this faculty with either supernatural causes or extreme psychological states - melancholia or madness. For Chris Hoggett, this mental discipline brought great rewards: the goddess of the spring and a sleeping magna mater in the secret fall and fold of hill and valley, guardian heroes in the cliff-faces of the limestone quarry north of Cleeve Common, and even the Joker himself in the random patterns of a cork tile.

Dreams and their counterpart, visions, used to predict the future, often on behalf of others: Cassandra foresaw all the disasters that would overtake the Trojans but was cursed never to be believed; Caesar's wife Calpurnia has a nightmare that he will be murdered and tries to prevent him going to the Forum on that fateful day. But he waves aside her fears, and goes. Augurs in ancient Greece and Rome scried dream material as they watched and read the flights of ravens or the entrails of sacrificial animals: all of these apparently haphazard and chance convergences of matter in time and space could mean something, if you had the gift of deciphering them, and that mostly fell to others, not to the dreamer. Dreams were prognostications, encrypted in visions in order to reveal the truth to chosen emissaries - in the classical tradition, seers like the sibyls, as at Delphic oracle or Dodona, in the Bible, prophets like Daniel or founder patriarchs like Jacob. Within this long Western history, dreams have played a public role, their meanings generated in group, for its own order and identity; they have helped institute laws and define matters of faith; sometimes, they have revealed a course of action, and designated the site of a new city or a new temple. Ghosts often walk in such dreams, and call sleeping sinners to remember their duties to the dead, and to fear hell. As with Aboriginals in Australia, or many of the Indian nations in North America, dreamwork was highly valued, fulfilled a social and ethical regulatory function, and through the interpretations of dreams, warnings were issued and promises made. In the nineteenth century, the fascination with states of mind changed ideas about dreams and dreaming in profound ways: a dream became unique to the dreamer, a personal creation, grounded in a confluence of memories and emotions that only he - or she - has experienced. Sigmund Freud, in his famous book at the very end of the century, *The Interpretation of Dreams* gathered up many of the strands in his colleagues' psychology to present dreams as the retrospective palimpsest communicating repressed desires; C G Jung, whose influence runs deep in Chris Hoggett's work, saw dreams as fields of possibility, where the dreamer entered the pool of the collective unconscious, and found elements in its water of personal significance and potential healing and well-being. Jung wrote that a dream is 'a spontaneous self-portrayal, in symbolic form, of the actual situation in the unconscious.'

Chris Hoggett's dream journals open his unconscious to us, and invite us to follow his remarkable process of self-scrutiny, self-portraiture and self-fashioning. The journey on which he takes us in *The Joker* conveys with memorable expressiveness the pain and horror of his despair, but it also carries us with him to the places where he found a kind of comfort, and sometimes plenitude, through the work of dreaming, through the art of representing his dreams.

January 2004

CONTENTS

Foreword by Marina Warner   iv - v
Acknowledgments   viii
Illustrations   ix - xx
Preface   xxi - xxii

PART ONE

Breakdown: the Pre-Therapy Years 1979-1990   1

    An introduction to first intimations of a manic-depressive breakdown and the subsequent series of artworks, grouped into chronological order over a period of approximately eleven years.

Clover Cliff 1979-1981	3
Freefall, Autumn 1980	15
Peripheral Visions 1981-1983	31
Figure on a Swivel-Chair 1984-1986	37
Skeletons 1984-1986	47
Drawing, Painting and Nursing Mother 1986-1989	57
Mirrors and Reflections 1988-1990	69

PART TWO

Dream Dominions 1990-1992   79

    This part deals with a selection of dreams extracted from *An Illustrated Dream Journal 1990-1992*, the companion book to *The Joker*. A number of dream themes emerged from the journal and became the seeds for further development in free-style artwork.

Themes and Variations

	The Dream as the Theme, the Artwork as Variations	81
1	Breath and Breathlessness - Asphyxia and Claustrophobia	83
2	A Tumultuous Rush - Confusion, Excess of Feeling	85
3	Automotons - Institutions and Conformity	91
4	A Prophetic Dream - Clay as Therapy	101
5	Unmasking the Monster - Facing the Fear	123
6	An Absence of Light - The Shadow Side	145
7	Metamorphosis - Growth and Transformation	153
8	Confrontation - Conflict and Reconciliation	171

9 Masquerading - Hiding and Seeking	183
10 Decapitation - Death and Regeneration	191
11 Victims and Sacrifices - Acceptance	195

PART THREE
The Volcanic Zone: Breaking out, Bursting forth — 199

Opening up, breaking out and bursting forth: later therapy, 1994-1996, and the post-therapy years, 1997-2000. This part is in two sections expressing the feeling of emotional release, of a 'breakout' - the obverse of breakdown. Breakout in this context denotes a position away from anything thought of as enclosing, hiding or obscuring from others.

1 Thinking the Unthinkable	201
2 Stretching the Wings	215

PART FOUR
Finding One's Own Way - Tour of New Zealand — 241

Land of the Long White Cloud	243

PART FIVE
Five Visionary Landscapes — 285

Cleeve Common and Uffington Ridgeway	287
1 Uffington White Horse	289
2 Belas Knap Long Barrow	297
3 Jurassic Westwood	307
4 The Stone Pit	315
5 Postlip Warren	325

POSTSCRIPT
The Joker's Domain — 331

The Joker, the subject and progenitor of this book, who, like a Jack-in-the-box, shot forth to reveal himself as performer, actor, clown and acrobat; a 'tailor' for my protective costumes; his 'birth', recognition (on my part), his seeking for recognition, his demise and reappearance in a postscript.

ACKNOWLEDGMENTS

I have amassed many debts during the preparation of this book. The first to my friend Michael Henry. He first saw the potential for bringing together the many pictures, jottings, dream notebooks and sketches, and suggested that I assemble them into a book.

Special mention and thanks must go to Claire Skailes who, through many years of therapeutic sessions, helped me through a manic-depressive illness and introduced me to the idea of writing down and sketching my dreams. I am also most grateful that she has chosen to write the analyses for 'A Dream Journal', companion to *The Joker* and now in manuscript.

I have been greatly helped over many years by Professor Patrick Dillon who visited my first exhibition of pictures. His enthusiasm at that time was most supportive and encouraging and he has continued to support me in many ways: in chairing meetings to promote the project, in seeking sponsorship to meet large financial costs and also for looking towards foundations that might assist the venture. I am grateful for his continued support.

Caroline Davis has been of enormous help throughout, giving me faith in the book's future existence when my confidence seemed to be flagging. She has acted as agent, as hostess to various committee meetings and has helped contact professionals in the field of Art Therapy.

I am indebted to Marina Warner for her support over many years and for her perceptive insights into the dream notebooks and images - also for her brilliant Foreword to *The Joker* which was such valuable help in encouraging me to persevere towards the final stages of printing and publication.

I wish to thank Professor Joy Schaverien for finding time to read the early mock-up of the book, for allowing me to add her commentary to the cover and for her advice in seeking out publishers.

Also to David Maclagan, many, many thanks for reading through a large part of the book and for giving such a valuable critique, and also for allowing me to quote part of this as comment on the cover.

To my editor Anne Watts I owe enormous thanks for reading, correcting and offering advice on my text and for being so generous with her time, shaping the project into something structured and coherent. I must thank my son Michael for his work on layouts and for selecting the display typeface. I also thank Charmian Mocatta who organised the complex typography of the preliminary pages.

I have greatly benefited from the advice of a large number of friends and many kind helpers who have so generously given their time, writing letters, holding often long conversations and offering ideas and suggestions. To Jane Bywater, James Biggs, Nick Capaldi, Paul Davis, Laura Gascoigne, Tony and Oonagh Godfrey, Maggie Guilliband, Tricia Henry, Rod Hollom, Ian James, Angela Lord, Paul Newman, Annabel Other, Carmen Reynal, Annabel Rooker and Stephen Stewart-Smith, many and grateful thanks.

ILLUSTRATIONS

Frontispiece **1 Childhood of the Joker**
watercolour and gouache

PART ONE Breakdown: The Pre-Therapy Years 1979-1990

Clover Cliff 1979 - 1981

2 **Surfers** 3
watercolour

3 **High Tide, Paviland, Gower** 4
pen and ink

4 **Surf Lines, towards Worm's Head** 5
watercolour

5 **Mewslade Surf** 6
watercolour

6 **Wave Creature** 6
watercolour

7 **Gower Surf – Night** 6
watercolour

8 **Reflection in a Cracked Mirror** 7
pencil

9 **A Face in the Water** 7
pen and wash

10 **Face in the Surf** 8
pen and ink

11 **A Surf Portrait sketch** 8
pen and wash

12 **Surf Man - Earth Woman** 9
watercolour

13 **Wave Figure** 9
oil on board

14 **Surf Portrait** 10
watercolour

15 **Sacrificial Head** 10
watercolour

16 **A Sea Portrait** 10
acrylic on board

17 **Fragmented Portrait** 11
torn and glued drawing

18 **Artist and his Double** 11
watercolour, cut and reassembled

19 **Figures on the Beach** 12
watercolour

20 **Mirrored Image** 13
gouache

21 **Indecision** 13
relief

22 **Aphrodite** 13
watercolour

23 **Stone Serpent** 14
pencil and crayon

Freefall, Autumn 1980

24 **Dizzy Spell** 15
mixed media

25 **Untitled Drawing** 16
pen and pencil

26 **Freefall - Original Colour Sketch** 16
mixed media

27 **Untitled** 17
mixed media

28 **Untitled - Original Sketch** 17
gouache

29 **Spillage (of coffee, of self, of Halley's Comet)** 17
pencil

30 **Freefall – Turning** 18
acrylic

31 **Freefall – Falling** 18
acrylic

32 **Freefall - Passing Through** 19
acrylic

33 **Freefall - Breakout** 19
acrylic

34 **Freefall: a Diptych (final version of figs 30 and 31)** 18
gouache and acrylic paste

35 **Out of the Black Hole** 19
watercolour

36 **Freefall (the final statement)** 19
relief

37 **Passing Through - Original Sketch** 20
crayon

38 **Passing Through - Nude Version** 20
watercolour

39 **Figure Falling through Doorframe** 20
relief

40 **Passing Through** 20
mixed media

41 **Passing Through - final version** 21
acrylic relief

42 **Threshold** 21
pencil and watercolour

43 **Figure passing through Three Environments** 22
pencil and watercolour

44 **A Psychic Journey** 22
watercolour

45 **Figure in a Garden** 23
watercolour

46 **Figure falling into a Chair** 24
pencil and watercolour

47 **A walk along a Pavement** 25
acrylic paste

48 **In the Garden** 25
mixed media

49 A walk across the Road 25 mixed media	52 Foetal Curved 27 mixed media	55 Celestial Freefall 29 acrylic on board
50 Escaping the Wall 26 pen and ink	53 Two Sketches 27 coloured inks	56 Fallen Angel 30 watercolour and gouache
51 The Trailing Jacket 26 watercolour	54 Re-working of Fig. 31 (unfinished) 28 oil on board	

Peripheral Visions 1981 - 1983

57 The Basic Stuff (discarded clothing) 31 pen and wash	62 Pensive Head 33 pencil	68 Bovine Form 35 pen and ink
58 Slumped 1 32 pen and wash	63 Bandaged Clown Face 33 chalk	69 Bird of Prey 35 pencil
59 Slumped 2 32 chalk	64 Water Turbulence 34 pen and ink	70 Owl 35 pen and pencil
60 Slumped 3 32 chalk	65 Fall of Water 34 pen and ink	71 Figure in a Duvet 36 pencil
60A Untitled 32 chalk	66 Canine - or Vampire 34 chalk	72 Sleeping Figure under Quilt 36 pencil
61 Melancholic Face 33 pen and ink	67 A Mystery Figure 34 ink and chalk	73 Lake surrounded by mountains 36 coloured crayons

Figure on a Swivel-Chair 1984 - 1986

74 Stationary Figure on Swivel Chair 37 pen and watercolour	81 Seated Figure 6 41 gouache	88 Seated Figure - Spinning 43 ink and gouache
75 Untitled 38 pen and wash	82 Seated Figure 7 41 gouache	89 The Dancer 44 pencil
76 Seated Figure 1 38 watercolour	83 Seated Figure 8 41 pen and ink	90 The Draughtsman 44 watercolour
77 Seated Figure 2 39 photo and pencil	84 Seated Figure 9 42 mixed media and acrylic	91 The Cyclist 45 pen and wash
78 Seated Figure 3 39 photo	85 Seated Figure 10 42 acrylic paste and paint	92 Seated Figure - Nude Version 45 gouache
79 Seated Figure 4 40 watercolour	86 Seated Figure 11 42 mixed media and acrylic	93 Dancing with One's Shadow 46 gouache
80 Seated Figure 5 40 pen and ink	87 Seated Figure 12 43 mixed media and acrylic	94 Tightrope Walker 46 gouache

Skeletons 1984 - 1986

95 On the Beach 47 watercolour	99 A Skeletal Landscape 50 watercolour	102 Bone Chalice 1 52 watercolour
96 Clifftop Find 48 ink and watercolour	100 A Sheep's Carcass 51 pen and gouache on toned paper	103 Tree and Tree-root Chalices 53 acrylic
97 Skeletal Form - Gower 49 watercolour	101 Chalice in a barren landscape 52 watercolour	104 Tree-Root Chalice 53 gouache
98 Skeletal Sketch 49 pen and wash		

105 **Bone Chalice 2** 53 gouache	107 **Three Skull Landscapes** 54 watercolour	109 **Claustrophobic Burial** 56 watercolour
106 **Three Skulls** 54 watercolour	108 **Bone Spectre** 55 ink and watercolour	110 **Half Human, Half Skeleton** 56 watercolour

Drawing, Painting and Nursing Mother 1986 - 1989

111 **Communing with Beethoven** 57 poster paint	121 **'Yes, yes, my son will let her in'** 61 pen and ink	132 **'You may leave us now'** 65 pen and ink
112 **'Chris, I'd rather you didn't'** 58 pen and ink	122 **'Well, if you must know'** 61 pen and ink	133 **'That's enough of that!'** 65 pen and ink
113 **'Well of course, Bach's my God'** 58 pen and ink	123 **Tea with the Queen** 61 pencil and crayons	134 **'I am extremely annoyed'** 65 pen and ink
114 **'I never did like Rachmaninoff'** 58 pen and ink	124 **Phobias** 62 gouache	135 **'There's an awful lot of wickedness . . .'** 65 pen and ink
115 **'Play a little Poulenc please'** 59 pen and ink	125 **'There's something nasty . . .'** 62 pen and ink	136 **'We are not amused'** 65 pen and ink
116 **'Somebody's stolen the Moonlight again'** 59 pen and ink	126 **The Cats Disease** 62 pen and ink	137 **'Let's change the subject - shall we?'** 65 pen and ink
117 **'Doing the Hoovering before She comes'** 60 pen and ink	127 **'Do you suppose that they're digging?'** 63 pen and ink	138 **Clouds - and Finger exercises** 66 pencil
118 **'Perhaps I never told you'** 60 pen and ink	128 **Good Friday 1988** 63 ink and gouache	139 **Talking to the Clouds** 67 watercolour
119 **'Come quickly, Chris'** 60 pen and ink	129 **Hunt-the-Handbag** 64 pen and ink	140 **Friendly with the Clouds** 67 oil on board
120 **'You may leave us now'** 60 pen and ink	130 **'I think we'd all better SHUT UP!'** 65 pen and ink	141 **Mother in Bed - sheet of portrait studies** 68 pen and ink
	131 **'Perhaps you'd better leave the room'** 65 pen and ink	

Mirrors and Reflections 1988 – 1990

142 **Peter paints himself** 69 acrylic	148 **Mirrored Self Portrait** 72 acrylic	155 **Pete, Looking Down** 75 pen and ink
143 **Self Portrait in an Ovoid Mirror** 70 photo	149 **The Company of One** 73 acrylic caulk	156 **Dismantling the Head** 75 pen and ink
144 **Multiple Viewpoints on a Swivel Chair** 71 acrylic	150 **Passing Through** 73 acrylic caulk	157 **Pete painting himself 1** 76 gouache
145 **Faces in motion** 71 pen and ink	151 **Pete - Looking Up, Looking Down** 74 pencil	158 **Pete painting himself 2** 76 acrylic relief
146 **Mirrored reflections** 72 oil on canvas	152 **Pete - Mirror Image** 74 acrylic	159 **Three Studies for a Portrait - A Triptych** 77 gouache
147 **Multiple viewpoints sketch** 72 pen and ink	153 **Pete - Multiple View 1** 75 pen and ink	160 **The Armchair - a double portrait** 78 oil on board
	154 **Pete - Multiple View 2** 75 gouache	

PART TWO Dream Dominions 1990 - 1992

161 Dream 102: Duality of the Psyche 81
pen and wash

161A A Session with my Therapist 82
watercolour

1 Breath and Breathlessness

162 Claustrophobic Journeying 83
pen and watercolour

162A Dream 2 83
pencil

163 The Pot-Holer 84
ink and wash

164 Gallows Humour 84
ink

2 A Tumultuous Rush

165 Dream 5 85
pen and ink

166 Untitled 85
pencil and chalk

167 Dream 14 86
gouache

168 Night at the Opera 86
watercolour

169 Opera - A Theatrical Dream 87
watercolour

170 Development of Fig. 169 87
gouache

171 The Dance 88
gouache

172 Falling Figure 89
pen, ink and watercolour

173 Figure Ascending a Staircase 89
gouache

174 Dancing on Stage 90
cardboard comb, dragged paint

3 Automatons

175 Dream 7: Boxed-in Figures 91
pen and ink

176 Exploded view of Gearbox 92
ruling pen

177 Detail from a perspective projection of a Gearbox 83
pen and ink

178 'Hello, Everybody!' 94
oil on board

179 Perspective 'cutaway' drawing of Gearbox 95
ruling pen

180 Doodle sketches of 'Machine Men' 95
pencil

181 Dream 20 96
pencil

182 Dream 27 96
pen and ink

183 Dream 33 97
pen and ink

184 Dream 80 97
pen and ink

185 The Muckspreader 98
pen, brush and ink

186 The Quarryman 99
pen, brush and ink

187 X-Ray Self Portrait 100
pastel

188 Cutaway Section of a Gearbox Arm – technical drawing 100
ruling pen

4 A Prophetic Dream

189 Dream 17 The Stroud Kilns 101
pencil and watercolour

190 Sheet of Studies - 'Wavelets' and Wave Shapes 102
pencil and wash

191 Set of five Wavelets 103
biscuit-fired clay

192 'Coiled Surflines' Pots 103
'Cranks' clay

193 The Nude as approaching wave 104
pen and pencil

194 Slab-building for wave movement 105
ceramic

195 Page of sketches - Waves and Neptune Form 105
pen and pencil

196 Neptune - Theatre Costume 106
photo

197 Neptune - Rear View 106
pencil and wash

197A Neptune - Side View 106
pencil and wash

198 Sheet of studies for Neptune 107
pencil and watercolour

199 Sheet of studies for an Eagle Pot 108
gouache on a toned ground

200 Spreading Wings platter 109
ceramic

201 **Eagle Pot** 109 ceramic	210 **One Portrait - Five View-points** 114 ceramic	219 **Rotting Down - Growing Up. Sheet of Studies** 118 pencil, pen and ink
202 **Winged Planter** 110 ceramic	211 **Self Portrait 1** 115 ceramic	220 **Breakdown - Breakout - top view** 119 ceramic
203 **Four Pecking Birds** 110 ceramic	212 **Self Portrait 2** 115 ceramic	220A **Breakdown- Breakout – front view** 119 ceramic
204 **Little Owl** 111 ceramic	213 **Self Portrait 3** 115 ceramic - biscuit-fired	221 **Potter and his Pots (from a dream in 1993)** 120 calligraphic brush
205 **Bird Bath** 111 ceramic	214 **Sheet of Studies for a Frog Pot** 116 pencil, chalk and paint	222 **Close to Clay** 121 watercolour
206 **Bird Vase** 111 ceramic	215 **Birdbath Lady** 117 ceramic	223 **Looking at Pots** 121 watercolour
207 **Bird Round-a-Bout** 111 ceramic	216 **Little Horse** 117 ceramic	224 **Biscuit-fired Bird Pots** 122 photo
208 **Sleeping Angel** 112 gouache and wax resist	217 **Yoga Posture** 117 ceramic	
209 **Life Vessel - Design for a Large Bowl** 113 pastel drawing	218 **Frog Prince (aka Joker)** 117 ceramic	

5 Unmasking the Monster

225 **A Smile in the Dark** 123 pen, brush, ink, paint	236 **Design for the Giant Typhon** 130 gouache	248 **Rage against the Dark** 135 gouache
226 **Dream 23: Little Bristled Monster** 124 watercolour	237 **Giant Sea Dragon** 130 photo	249 **The Gentle Giant** 135 watercolour
227 **Dream 46: Plant-tailed Monster** 124 watercolour	238 **Design for the Giant Briareus** 131 gouache	250 **Tittle-Tattle or The Censors** 136 chalk, watercolour and gouache
228 **Dream 30: A Spider Dream** 125 pencil and watercolour	239 **Lobster Monster Costume** 131 photo	251 **A little woodland creature** 137 gouache
229 **Self-portrait as a Spider** 125 gouache	240 **Design for an Alien Creature** 131 watercolour	252 **A Dragon Dog's Plea** 137 gouache
230 **Goya'esque Fantasy - Striding Figure** 126 oil on board	241 **The Plea (Variation on Uffington White Horse)** 132 ink chalk, paint	253 **Monsters: Long Ears** 138 pen, brush and ink
230A **Goya'esque Fantasy – a Carnivorous Monster** 126 oil on board	242 **Snake Woman** 132 acrylic	254 **Monsters: Long Trunk - thinking** 138 pen, brush and ink
231 **Dream 108** 127 watercolour, pen and pencil	243 **Gale Force Twelve** 133 watercolour and gouache	255 **Monsters: Little Worrier** 139 pen, brush and ink
232 **Flesh Eater with Sun Glasses** 127 watercolour and gouache	244 **The Un-nerving Creature** 133 brush and wash	256 **Monsters: Hangdog** 139 pen, brush and ink
233 **Untitled Fairy Tale** 128 pen, ink and gouache	245 **Skeletal Figure** 133 watercolour	257 **Monsters: Untitled** 139 pen, brush and ink
234 **The Witch and the Manikin** 129 gouache	246 **Pregnant Dinosaur and friend (two viewpoints)** 134 ash-glazed ceramics	258 **Cock-a-Snook** 140 calligraphic brush, pen and wash
235 **Sketch for a Carnival Dragon** 130 pen and brush	247 **Dinosaur Family - Seven-piece Group** 134 iron-glazed ceramics	259 **Flower Face** 141 calligraphic brush, pen and sponge

260 **Dragon and Serpent** 141
calligraphic brush and pen

261 **Pantomime Bull** 142
brush, pen and ink

262 **Pipe Player** 142
gouache

263 **Old Man with a Quiff** 143
calligraphic brush,
pen and wash

264 **The Guardian** 144
mixed media

265 **Sea Rescue** 144
finger paint and brush

6 An Absence of Light

266 **Darkness at Noon** 145
chalk and gouache

267 **The Abyss** 146
pen, brush and ink

268 **Dream 38: The Black Swimming Pool** 146
pen and wash

269 **Dream 161: The Dark Pit** 147
aquarelle pencil, pen and ink

270 **The Dark Pool 1** 147
etching

271 **The Dark Pool 2** 148
gouache

272 **Floating with the Tide** 148
chalk and watercolour

273 **The Watery Abyss** 149
gouache

274 **Untitled** 149
coloured chalk

275 **The Cavern** 150
pen, brush and ink

276 **Antipodean Dive** 151
acrylic

277 **Entrance to 'Collins Drive'** 152
pen and wash

278 **Healing Place for Birdman** 152
brush and black paint

7 Metamorphosis

279 **Dream 64: Self-Portrait out of Paving Slabs** 153
pen and ink

280 **Dream 67: Part One** 154
crayons

281 **Dream 67: Parts Two and Three** 155
crayons

282 **Fragments before Assembly** 156
pen, brush and ink

283 **'Reaching Out'** 157
charcoal pencil

284 **Woman with a little Monster** 157
pen, brush and ink

285 **Large Self-Portrait (Divided Image)** 158
pastel

286 **New Zealand Self-Portrait** 159
aquarelle pencil

287 **Mugshot** 160
gouache

288 **Nude (cut-up)** 161
watercolour, gouache & ink

289 **A Question of Gender** 162
gouache

290 **Tendencies towards Fragmentation** 162
pen and watercolour

291 **'Metamorphosis'** 163
mixed media

292 **Dream 83: Untitled** 164
pen, ink and chalk

293 **Dream 134: The Escalator - Part One** 165
pencil and watercolour

294 **Dream 134: The Escalator - Part Two** 166
aquarelle pencil

295 **Percussion, Strings, Brass and Woodwind** 167
gouache

296 **Design for a Ceramic Platter** 167
gouache

297 **Impotence** 168
graphite powder and pencil

298 **Woodland Scene** 169
coloured felt-tip pens on tracing paper

299 **Millennium Dog** 170
gouache

8 Confrontation

300 **Dream 65: Parts One and Two** 171
pen and ink

301 **Dream 65: Part Three** 172
pen and ink

302 **The Great Plain** 172
gouache

303 **Encounter with the Ape Boy Cripple** 173
gouache

304 **Rapprochement** 174
gouache

305 **An Ambiguous Moment** 175
gouache

306 **Reconciliation** 175
gouache

307 **Psychic Invasion 1** 176
pen and wash

308 **Psychic Invasion 2** 177
pen and wash

309 **The Watery Cavern** 178
mixed media

310 **Boxed-In** 179
pen, brush, ink

311 **Two Heads** 180
gouache

312 **Animal Fight** 181
gouache and pencil

313 **The Combatants** 182
gouache

9 Masquerading

314 **Dream 88: Removing the Mask** 183
gouache

315 **Design for Swamp Creature** 184
pen and ink

316 **Design for Green Android** 184
gouache

317 **Design for Blue Android** 184
gouache

318 **Design for 'Elephanus' Creature** 184
gouache

319 **Making an Alien Headpiece** 184
photo

320 **Alien on stage** 184
photo

321 **Fish Masks and Batik-treated tights (left)** 185
photo

322 **Portuguese Man-of-War** 185
photo

323 **Lobster Monster on stage** 185
photo

324 **Persephone - Costume for the Titan Briareus and Demeter Headpiece** 186
photo

325 **Costume for Zeus** 187
photo

326 **Design for Enceladus** 187
gouache

327 **Design for Typhon** 187
gouache

328 **Headpiece for Persephone** 187
photo

329 **Design for Demeter** 187
gouache

330 **Design for Zeus** 187
watercolour and gouache

331 **Dream 157: The Music Examiner** 188
gouache

332 **Dream 168: The Child, the Woman and the Old Man Mask** 188
pen and ink

333 **The Maskmaker** 189
pen and ink

334 **Pantomime Lion** 189
gouache

335 **Dream 170: The Birth** 190
pen and wash

10 Decapitation

336 **Dream 94: Pig's Head Surgery** 191
pen and ink

337 **Decapitation from the Heart** 192
pen and gouache

338 **Revolution!** 192
gouache

339 **Warrior Head** 193
pen, brush and ink

340 **Black Tuesday** 194
oil transfer, pen and ink

341 **Dream 96: Dream Vision** 195
aquarelle pencil

342 **Sacrificial Victim** 196
aquarelle pencil and gouache

343 **Writhing Horse** 196
gouache

344 **Sheet of sketches based on Dream 96** 197
pen and ink, crayon

345 **In the Garden** 198
oil on board

PART THREE   The Volcanic Zone: Breaking out, Bursting forth

1 Thinking the Unthinkable

346 **Bursting Forth - Regeneration** 200
gouache

347 **Fragmentation** 201
gouache

348 **Self Hate** 202
gouache

349 **Untitled** 202
brush and black paint

350 **Alter Ego** 203
graphite powder and pencil

351 **Monsters of Rage** 204
brush and ink

352 **Bile** 205
brush and ink

353 **Serpent of Rage** 205
brush and ink

354 **Hospitalisation - a page of sketches** 206
pencil

355 **Hospitalisation** 207
gouache

356 **The Prisoner** 207
gouache

357 **Enraged Boy** 208
gouache and pen

358 **Rage** 208
brush and ink

359 **'I'll knock your head off, you little Sod!'** 209
ink transfer, pen and brush

360 **Kick Boxing** 209
pen, brush and blots

361 **The Mask of Rage** 210
paint, pen and ink

362 The Actor 210 graphite powder, brush, paint	**365 East of Eden** 212 gouache	**367 White Hot Frenzy** 214 chalk and ink
363 Painter and his Easel 211 pen, ink, brush and stippling	**366 'Ride 'em Cowboy!'** 213 ink and wash	**368 Ravished Face** 214 gouache
364 Mother and Child 212 pastel		

2 Stretching the Wings

369 Peace Sculpture 215 photo (glass fibre and cellulose spray)	**382 Learning to Fly** 224 brush and wash	**396 The Dancing Bird Tree** 234 pen, brush and ink
370 Stretching One's Wings 216 pen and gouache	**383 The Fledgling** 225 brush, pen and ink	**397 Invaded by Birds** 235 pen and wash
371 Mother's Lap – Bird's Nest 217 pen, brush and ink	**384 Lift-Off from a desert place** 226 brush, pen and ink	**398 Self-Portrait** 235 pen, brush and ink
372 Fledgling about to leave the nest 218 gouache on toned paper	**385 Origin of the World** 227 pencil	**399 The Fall of Icarus 1** 236 watercolour
373 Coastal Scene 218 pastel and gouache	**386 Wings** 228 pen, brush, ink and chalk	**400 The Fall of Icarus 2** 236 watercolour
374 The Drowning Youth 219 pen and wash	**387 Surprised Angel** 228 gouache	**401 The Fall of Icarus 3** 236 watercolour
375 Death on the Washing Line 220 pencil	**388 Death Wish** 229 ink and gouache	**402 Man with No Sense of Proportion** 237 pen and watercolour
376 Metamorphosis 1 221 finger paint	**389 A Desert Gathering** 229 gouache, pencil and pen	**403 Bird Portrait** 237 pen, brush and ink
377 Metamorphosis 2 221 finger paint	**390 'The Embrace'** 230 watercolour	**404 Birdman Finds a Waterhole** 237 pen, brush and ink
378 The Migration 222 finger paint	**391 Enigmatic Creature** 231 black paint and chalk	**405 The Owl** 237 pen and wash
379 Bird Theatre 1 223 finger paint	**392 Detail from an 'Eruptive Landscape' (see fig. 439)** 231 pen, brush and ink	**406 Confrontation between two birds** 238 ink and wash
380 Bird Theatre 2 223 pencil	**393 Moon Goddess** 232 gouache	**407 Birdman Flying** 238 pen, brush and paint
381 A Strenuous Effort 224 ink and wash	**394 A Possible Revival** 232 oil on board	**408 A Mirrored Image** 239 brush and paint
	395 Gaia with Birds and Animals 233 chalk, gouache and ink	**409 Birdman** 240 finger paints and pencil

PART FOUR Finding One's Own Way – Tour of New Zealand

410 The Southern Alps 243 watercolour	**413 Site of the Buried Village of Te Wairoa, near Rotorua** 246 black aquarelle pencil	**415 Towards White Island Crater** 247 photo
411 Map and Maori Legend of New Zealand 244 pen and ink	**414 'Photorealist' painting of White Island** 247 photo overpainted with gouache	**416 Watching the Volcano (freestyle painting)** 247 oil on board
412 Entering the Abyss 245 pen and wash		**417 The Napier Earthquake of 1931** 248 gouache

#	Title	Medium	Page
418	Charles' boat 'Candida'	watercolour	249
419	Yacht in a Storm off Napier	pastel	249
420	Two illustrations from 'New Year's Day' Dream 96	pen and ink	251
421	A Bach, surrounded by Cabbage Trees, Cable Bay, near Nelson	pen and watercolour	252
422	Estuary, towards Delaware Bay	watercolour	253
423	Roots of Kahikatea Trees	pencil and wash	253
424	Cicadas	pencil	253
425	Dun Mountain Clouds, Nelson (two small sketches)	pencil	254
426	Line of Willows	pencil	254
427	Cabbage Trees, Cable Bay, near Nelson	pen and wash	254
428	Palms, Nelson	pencil	254
429	Fur Seal Colony, Kaikoura	aquarelle pencil	255
430	Sea, Rocks, Waves, Shells and colour notes	pen and ink	255
431	'Rhino Horns': cliff formations	gouache	256
432	'Rhino Horns': cliff formations, with seal colony	gouache	256
433	Beach 'Sculptures', Kaikoura	photo	256
434	Kaikoura Peninsula	watercolour	257
435	Kaikoura Harbour – Purple Sky and Opal Sea	watercolour	257
436	Boy on a Whale	pencil and wash	258
437	The Old Man and the Sea	pencil and finger paint	258
438	Two Studies of Botanical Gardens, Christchurch	aquarelle pencil	259
439	Birdman in an Eruptive Landscape	brush and ink	260
440	Hicks Bay - Maori Carving	pencil	261
441	'Roaring Bravado' Sea Spirit, from South Solomon Islands	pen and ink	261
442	Clay and Skull Mask	pen and ink	261
443	New Ireland Ceremonial Mask	pencil	261
444	A Fernery with native Rimu Trees	aquarelle pencil	262
445	'The Retreat', Horseshoe Bay, Stewart Island	pen and ink	263
446	Shell Collection from Horseshoe Bay	pencil	263
447	Horseshoe Bay and the Muttonbird Islands	photo	264
448	Horseshoe Bay and the Muttonbird Islands, later Christmas card	ink and watercolour	264
449	Sunset over Horseshoe Bay	watercolour	265
450	Evening at Horseshoe Bay	gouache	265
451	Blue Gums on Lonnekers Beach, Oban	ink and watercolour	266
452	Map to show tour of Stewart Island	ink and wash	266
453	Lake Te Anau	coloured crayons	267
454	Paragliding at Queenstown	pen and ink	267
455	Schist Plain, viewed from Mount Iron	pencil	268
456	Mount Aspiring from Matukituki Valley, with cabbage trees	watercolour	268
457	Backpacker in Hilly Country	pen, brush and ink	269
458	'Smoke Signals' from Mount Aspiring	coloured chalks	269
459	Haast Pass Renaissance	gouache	270
460	Fragmentation	gouache	270
461	Nikan Palms on the Haast	gouache	271
462	Uprooted Trees on a Haast Beach	watercolour	271
463	Tasman Sea, Evening	watercolour	272
464	Fox Glacier	pencil and ink	272
465	The Mountainous City	brush and ink	273
466	Inchbonnie Flat	watercolour	274
467	Grant's Catholic Church	watercolour	274
468	Willows near Lake Poerua, Inchbonnie Flat	watercolour	275
469	Lake Poerua and Mountains	watercolour and chalk	275
470	Kahikatea Trees, Inchbonnie	watercolour	275
471	Old Hillman on road to Nelson Lakes	photo	276
472	Forest plantation patterns (from air)	photo	276

473 Lake Rotoiti, the Nelson Lakes 277 photo	**477 Broken Hills district, near Tairua** 280 photo	**480 Near the Southern Alps** 283 gouache
474 The Helping Hand 278 pen and wash	**478 Kava de Hine Aligi - carved wood Goddess from Caroline Islands** 281 photo of silhouette	**481 Otago Journey** 283 oil on board
475 Paku Mount, Tairua 279 watercolour		**482 Antipodian Memories** 284 gouache and collage
476 Entrance to Golden Hills Mine, Coromandel 280 pen, ink and wash	**479 Maps to show Tour of New Zealand** 282 line and wash	**483 The Orchard** 284 gouache

PART FIVE Five Visionary Landscapes

484 A Mythological Map - Cleeve Common 287
gouache, pen and ink

485 The Kissing Stone 288
pen and ink

1 Uffington White Horse

486 Abstract Gliphs of Horse 289 pen and ink	**490 Interpretation of Manger Forms, Uffington** 291 pastel	**494 Little Monkey with a Sleeping Creature** 294 gouache
487 Aerial view of horse gliphs 289 brush and ink	**491 The Sleeping Goddess, Uffington** 292 gouache	**495 Sleeping Earth Mother as Artist's Model** 294 gouache
488 Ridgeway and Manger 289 watercolour	**492 The Sleeping Goddess, Eye of the Sun – Uffington** 292 brush and ink	**496 The Blue Pony - Uffington** 295 oil on board
489 Eight-part photo of Uffington White Horse area 290-291 photos	**493 A Womb-Tomb Place** 293 pen, brush and ink	**497 Artemis of Ephesus** 295 pen and ink
		498 Untitled 296 pen, brush, ink and chalk

2 Belas Knap Long Barrow

499 Belas Knap Long Barrow, Gloucestershire 297 pen and ink	**504 Angel-Bird rejuvenates Elderly Man** 300 watercolour	**509 Reflections on Belas Knap 1** 304 pen and ink
500 Gilgamesh and Enkidu visit Ishtar, the Temple Goddess 298 pastel	**505 Raising the Dead** 301 chalk, wash, pen and ink	**510 Reflections on Belas Knap 2** 304 gouache
501 Humbaba, Guardian of the Cedar Forest 298 graphite powder, pen and wash	**506 Awakening the Dead** 301 pen and wash	**511 The Trumpet Call - A Fairytale** 305 oil on paper
502 The Cedar Forest 299 oil on board	**507 The Dreamer Seeks his child** 302 pen and chalk	**512 Life Vessel** 305 pastel
503 Gilgamesh and Enkidu become friends 299 watercolour and chalk	**508 Sculpture in a Cemetery** 303 pen, brush and ink	**513 Day dream of a Poet** 306 pen and ink

3 Jurassic Westwood

514 **Towards Westwood, Charlton Abbots** 307
oil on board

515 **View towards Westwood - Summer** 308
watercolour and gouache

516 **Rough Sketch of Westwood** 308
pen and ink

517 **General view of the Westwood area, with rain** 308
watercolour

518 **Log Figure** 309
acrylic

519 **Jurassic Seascape - Westwood transformed** 309
oil on board

520 **Small pen sketches** 309
pen and ink

521 **Two sketches of man/fossil relationship** 310
pen and ink

522 **Colour sketch incorporating Fossils** 310
pen and watercolour

523 **Westwood Fossils** 311
oil on board

524 **Wood, Stone, Fossil, Earth – above Westwood** 311
acrylic

525 **Westwood Daydream** 312
oil on paper

526 **Westwood** 312
watercolour

527 **Sketch for 'Spring', 1st version** 313
pen and ink

528 **Sketch for 'Spring', 2nd version** 313
pen and ink

529 **Westwood Dancer** 313
oil on board

530 **Spring, 1st version** 314
oil on board

531 **Spring, 2nd version** 314
oil on board

4 The Stone Pit

532 **The Stone Figure** 315
pen and ink

533 **The Primitive Tribe** 316
pen and wash

534 **The Quarry Rockface** 317
pen, ink and watercolour

534A **A Limestone Outcrop** 317
pen and ink

535 **Hero in the Rock** 318
pen, ink and watercolour

536 **Giant Head** 319
pen and ink

537 **Three Giant Warriors** 319
pen and ink

538 **Fragmented Stone Man** 320
aquarelle pencil

539 **Moon with Fragmented Figure** 320
gouache

540 **The Stone Pit** 321
acrylic

541 **Rockface Warriors (based on fig. 537 sketch)** 321
gouache

542 **Untitled I (1980s)** 322
gouache

543 **Untitled II (1996)** 322
acrylic

544 **The Old Warrior** 323
mixed media

545 **Self-Portrait in the Stone Pit** 323
photo

546 **An Amazon with a Challenger** 324
pen, ink and wash

5 Postlip Warren

547 **Summer - Postlip Warren and Watery Bottom, Cleeve Common** 325
watercolour

548 **Autumn - Postlip Warren** 326
watercolour

549 **November - Rising Mist, Watery Bottom** 326
watercolour

550 **Postlip Maiden 1** 327
pen and wash

551 **Postlip Yellow, Watery Bottom** 327
pen and watercolour

552 **Postlip Valley** 328
gouache and watercolour

553 **Postlip Fragments** 328
gouache

554 **Postlip Maiden 2** 328
gouache

555 **Fiery Sky, Wanaka, New Zealand** 329
gouache

556 **Night and Day, Watery Bottom** 329
gouache

557 **Darkness at Noon, Postlip Warren, Watery Bottom** 330
oil on board

POSTSCRIPT   The Joker's Domain

558   **Freefall - Falling
(enlargement
of fig. 31)**   333
acrylic

559   **Regeneration**   334
gouache

560   **The Joker's Birthplace**   335
acrylic on board

561   **The High-railed Cot**   336
gouache

562   **Childhood of the Joker
(from frontispiece)**   337
gouache

563   **Dancing Tree Root**   337
acrylic

564   **Sketch for front cover**   338
brush and paint

565   **Neither Fish nor Fowl**   338
pen, brush and ink

566   **The Compere**   339
gouache

567   **Dancing Joker**   339
pen and pencil

568   **Woman and Joker**   339
pencil

569   **The Jester and
his Partner**   340
graphite powder,
pen, brush, chalk

570   **Tightrope Walker**   341
gouache

571   **The Old Clown**   341
gouache

572   **Clown with
a Bull's Horn**   341
finger paints, brush

573   **Quest of the Joker**   342
brush, pen and ink

574   **Backstage -
Some Aspects
of the Psyche**   343
acrylic

575   **Millennium Poster**   344
pastel

576   **Millennium Poster
(upside down)**   344
pastel

577   **Hello, Everybody!
(detail from fig. 178)**   345
oil on board

578   **Joker as Frog Prince**   345
ceramic

579   **Joker plays Enkidu
(detail from fig. 500)**   345
gouache

580   **The Maskmaker**   346
pen and ink

581   **The Maskmaker's
Choices**   346
pen and chalk

582   **Revised 'Spring' -
1st version (fig. 530),
amended**   347
oil on board

583   **Part of a Cork Tile**   347
photo

584   **Facial Features
in Cork Tile**   347
pen and ink

585   **Final Appearance**   348
pen, brush and ink

586   **Curtain Call**   348
pen, brush and ink

587   **A Backstage
Conversation**   349
pencil and graphite powder

588   **Strange Meeting
(The Cripple meets
the Joker)**   350-351
oil transfer with pen and ink

589   **Zany Prancing -
2nd version
(see fig. 574)**   352
gouache

PREFACE

We can all experience fear when we feel unable to cope with something in our lives. A certain measure of fear is basic to our lives and safety. This is a book about the effect of fear on my life, often combined with a sense of loss and abandonment. Though destructive, the fear has finally been helpful to me, offering many creative possibilities and renewed energies.

As young children, my brother Dave and I lived in the West of England and frequently spent time away from home at a farm or a Community in the Cotswolds. I felt that this showed Mum's displeasure with us and I tried to make a happy mask that would be acceptable to her. The cover smile became even more rigid when Dad died in 1933. His death caused a much greater sense of abandonment (I was now six) and one that made me cling more firmly to Mum.

Mum was now virtually penniless and she took us to live in her mother's house. There she started working even longer hours as a piano teacher. Her fees were so meagre that she barely met all our expenses. Dave and I found ourselves sent away again, but for much longer periods. Sometimes I was 'fostered out' for six to nine months at a time, mostly during my primary school years.

At the age of ten, I was hospitalised for three months with constipation; it was acute and quite possibly psychosomatic in origin. I spent many hours 'trapped' inside a high-railed cot with only one weekly visit from Mum. This prison-like existence cast many shadows later.

Dave and I were difficult to control and Gran complained of excessive noise. Mum sought help from a local church charity organisation that had connections with a non-fee-paying boarding school for children of single parents.

We found ourselves at Watford in what I felt must be an orphanage. One large bald-headed man there was known as 'The Bull'. He was someone we dreaded because he had such a reputation for caning boys. Evidence was to be seen in the communal showers: weals and welts on buttocks and upper legs. This member of staff soon became my first externalised monster, an ogre.

One thing relieved this dark episode: the art teacher saw I had some ability at drawing and offered encouragement, often putting my efforts up in the art room. When some of my pictures went missing, he explained that this should be thought of as a compliment, not a disaster.

Following the Munich Crisis in 1939, when war was imminent, children in the London area were sent away for safety. My brother and I were evacuated to our own home.

Dave and I were now placed in separate schools but, for me, settling in and concentrating proved impossible. My inattentiveness developed into a nervous tic, diagnosed by a psychiatrist as a 'nervous breakdown'. The remedy for this was that I lived in the country for a year with a farm labourer and his family in a small Cotswold village. Within days, I was splitting my time between schooling and farming, but only the farming proved satisfying. I mixed well with other boys of my age and was soon involved in the usual village activities of scrumping apples, being chased by the village Bobby, climbing trees for birds' nests and being surprised by a couple of girls who teased the lads by revealing their charms.

One day, one of the lads invited me and two others back to his garden shed. He lit a candle and lifted a newly hatched chick from his pocket; he held it over the flame and slowly roasted it to death. My feeble protest met with derision and much laughter. In moments, I became, in their view, an outsider from the gang. So I began to feel myself alone, an outsider. I had to put up defences against such harsh reality, as many children do when faced with cruelty to defenceless animals.

Isolated from former mates, I found solace in the countryside, just looking at plants and animals. It was then, sitting in a flower-filled meadow and viewing the lush landscape around me, that I knew what I wanted to do: I was going to be an artist.

Back at home - and much to my surprise - Mum fully approved of my plan and I was enrolled in the local art school immediately. The curriculum for a 13-year-old was simple, the three Rs for the first two hours, and the remainder of the day taken up with the sheer delights of drawing, modelling and learning basic techniques of perspective, colour theory, etc.

After two years' art training, I found an apprenticeship in a local aircraft component factory as a junior draughtsman for general engineering drawing. Because I had learnt to master perspective at the art school, I was taken on by the technical illustration department where I developed more skills and confidence. This period had to end abruptly when I reached eighteen, the age of conscription. What followed were three boring years as a storeman in the Royal Air Force. Without the consolation of drawing, I found a need to construct ever more effective masks to cover my vulnerability amidst crowds of strangers in close proximity. These masks became ever more rigid, like shields, and eventually like a total suit of armour so effective that I began to lose sight of my own identity. A profound negativity had established itself and I concentrated on survival until I was demobbed.

I enrolled for further studies at a college of art and later became a student at the Royal College of Art, London, supported by a government grant. Any true progress was inhibited by a number of emotional instabilities and depressions. I had a sense of failure which engendered a sudden desire to abandon creative work for some years.

During the next period of my life, I worked in a printing house as a designer, began to teach art part-time, got married and started a family. I gradually increased the amount of art teaching and reduced the hours of print work. New ventures in craft, theatre studies and book illustration carried me through to 1979 when I decided to retire early from teaching.

During the summer of 1980, I had an emotional breakdown which made the world a place of chaotic darkness for me that brought, paradoxically and for a brief moment, a sense of true freedom to express myself. In 1990, I had a further breakdown precipitated by a family crisis. This time I sought professional help from an art therapist. Gradually I began to understand that mask-making can have two sides to it. On the one hand, the mask is a protective device covering up our true nature; on the other, through art, the mask can be a means of self-revelation and discovery. Fear can be transmuted by our innate creativity.

The following pages show a long sequence of paintings and other art works developed over the period since 1980. For the first ten years, these emerged from my own need to understand myself, and over the next ten years from the professional input of a trained art therapist. Therapy helped unravel the personal history that had been long hidden away under a slowly disintegrating suit of armour.

PART ONE

Breakdown: The Pre-Therapy Years 1979 – 1990

CLOVER CLIFF 1979 – 1981 — 3
> Intimations of change, premonitions of emotional disturbance. Clover Cliff is a geographical location where significant change affects feelings of 'seeing' landscape

FREEFALL, AUTUMN 1980 — 15
> The breakdown day: an illustrated account of the day from the morning freefall through to noon, afternoon, evening and night

PERIPHERAL VISIONS 1981-1983 — 31
> Frequent morning depressions lead to 'reveries' or fantasies based on transformations of discarded clothing - things seen 'obliquely'

FIGURE ON A SWIVEL-CHAIR 1984-1986 — 37
> Search and discovery for a symbol which could represent ideas on transformations and spatial relationships

SKELETONS 1984-1986 — 47
> Skeletal forms found in the landscape - symbols of the victim, mortality and resurrection

DRAWING, PAINTING AND NURSING MOTHER 1986-1989 — 57
> On forming a closer relationship with mother through drawing, music and humour

MIRRORS AND REFLECTIONS 1988-1990 — 69
> Concerning fragmentation, dependency, changes in the relationship between friends

CLOVER CLIFF 1979-1981

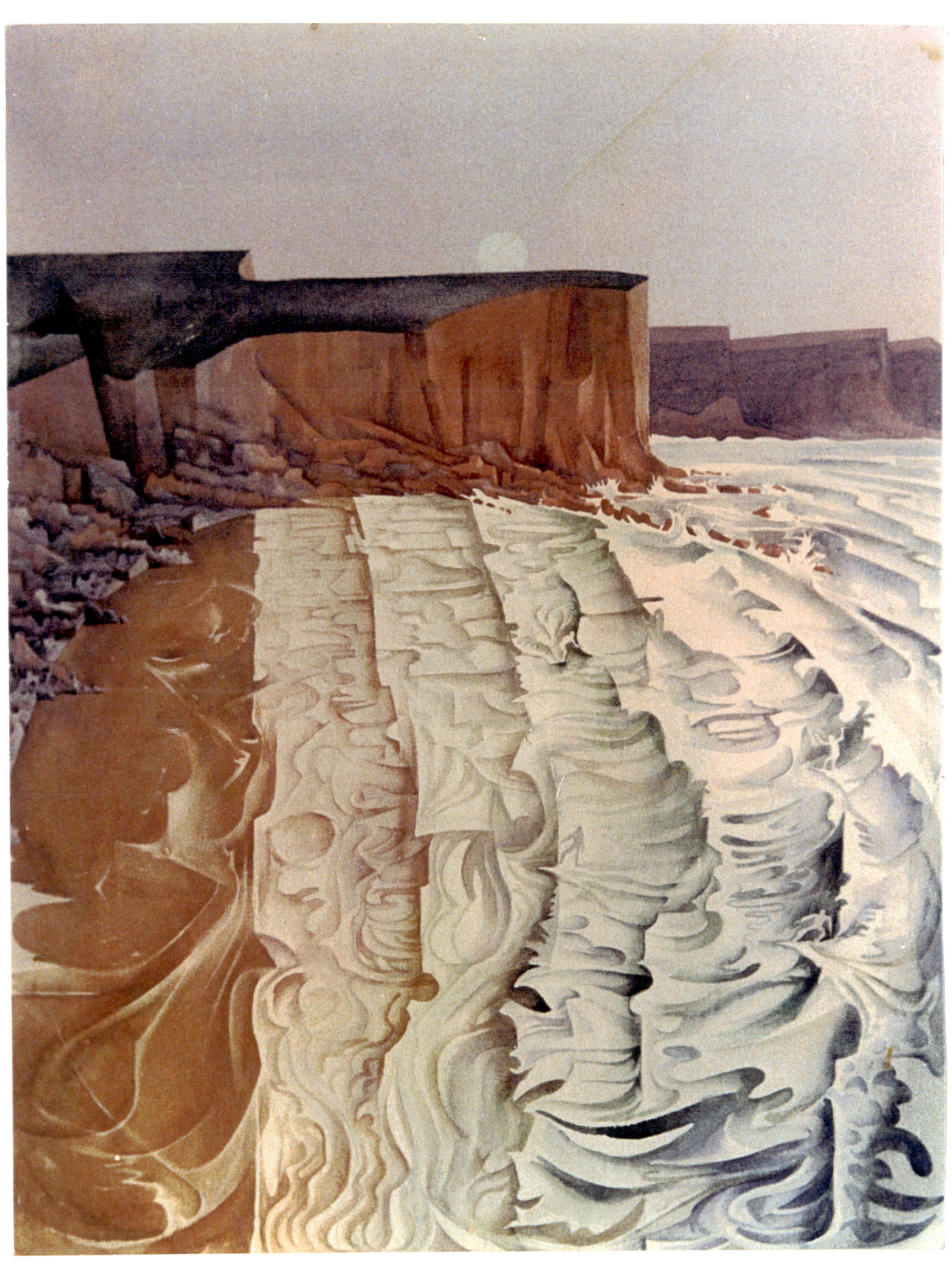

Fig.2 Surfers   Watercolour

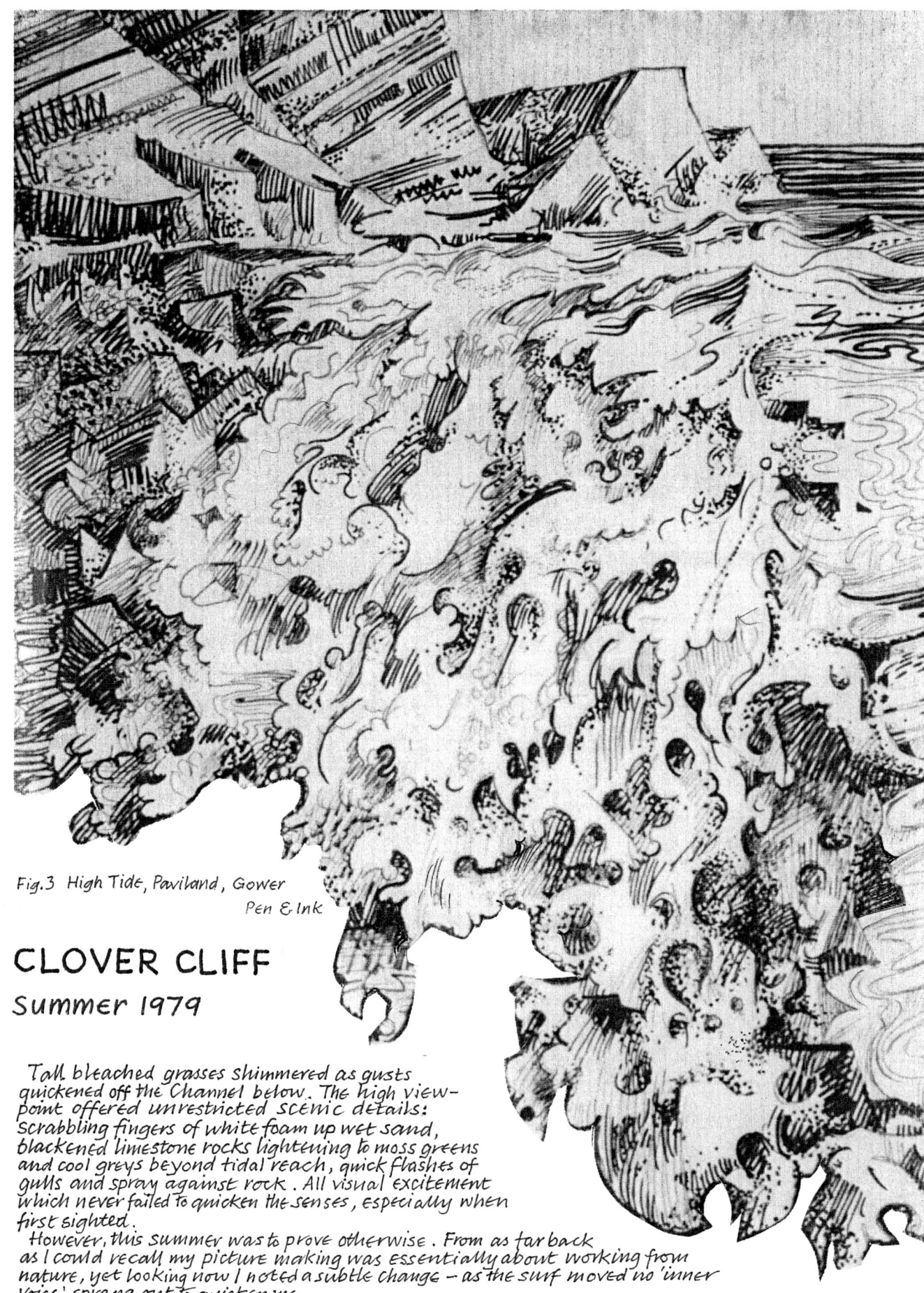

Fig.3 High Tide, Paviland, Gower
Pen & Ink

CLOVER CLIFF
Summer 1979

Tall bleached grasses shimmered as gusts quickened off the Channel below. The high viewpoint offered unrestricted scenic details: scrabbling fingers of white foam up wet sand, blackened limestone rocks lightening to moss greens and cool greys beyond tidal reach, quick flashes of gulls and spray against rock. All visual excitement which never failed to quicken the senses, especially when first sighted.

However, this summer was to prove otherwise. From as far back as I could recall my picture making was essentially about working from nature, yet looking now I noted a subtle change — as the surf moved no 'inner voice' sprang out to quicken me.

I knew this was a common experience in the creative process, that one worked through the dull bits and that the ebb and flow was an essential ingredient of painting, yet as I continued to stare at the beach below, it was as if, though standing on perfectly stable ground, a seismic shift had just that moment happened. There was a wave of acute anxiety as I realised that the tremor came from within, not from the surrounding landscape.

Ignorant of any therapeutic help or known methods which might help restore normality I nevertheless knew that some new and radical approach was necessary.

I took a week out from the usual pattern of painting and playing on the beach to spend the whole time with the kids, among rocks, pools and caves. Their shrill cries mingled with the gulls and the roaring surf to cast off the gloom of the moment, and restored a sense of hopeful optimism during this creative lull.

Then, quite suddenly, the lines of surf rushing the Gower beach offered something new. An awareness of certain shifts in the formation of surf movement hinted at a hidden imagery - one containing limbs, sinews, muscular forms and occasionally complete figures.

At the same time on a wet indoor-games morning I glanced into an old cracked mirror in the cottage and saw a misalignment of my features corresponding to the surf lines.

The surf and mirror images became the precursors of something completely new.

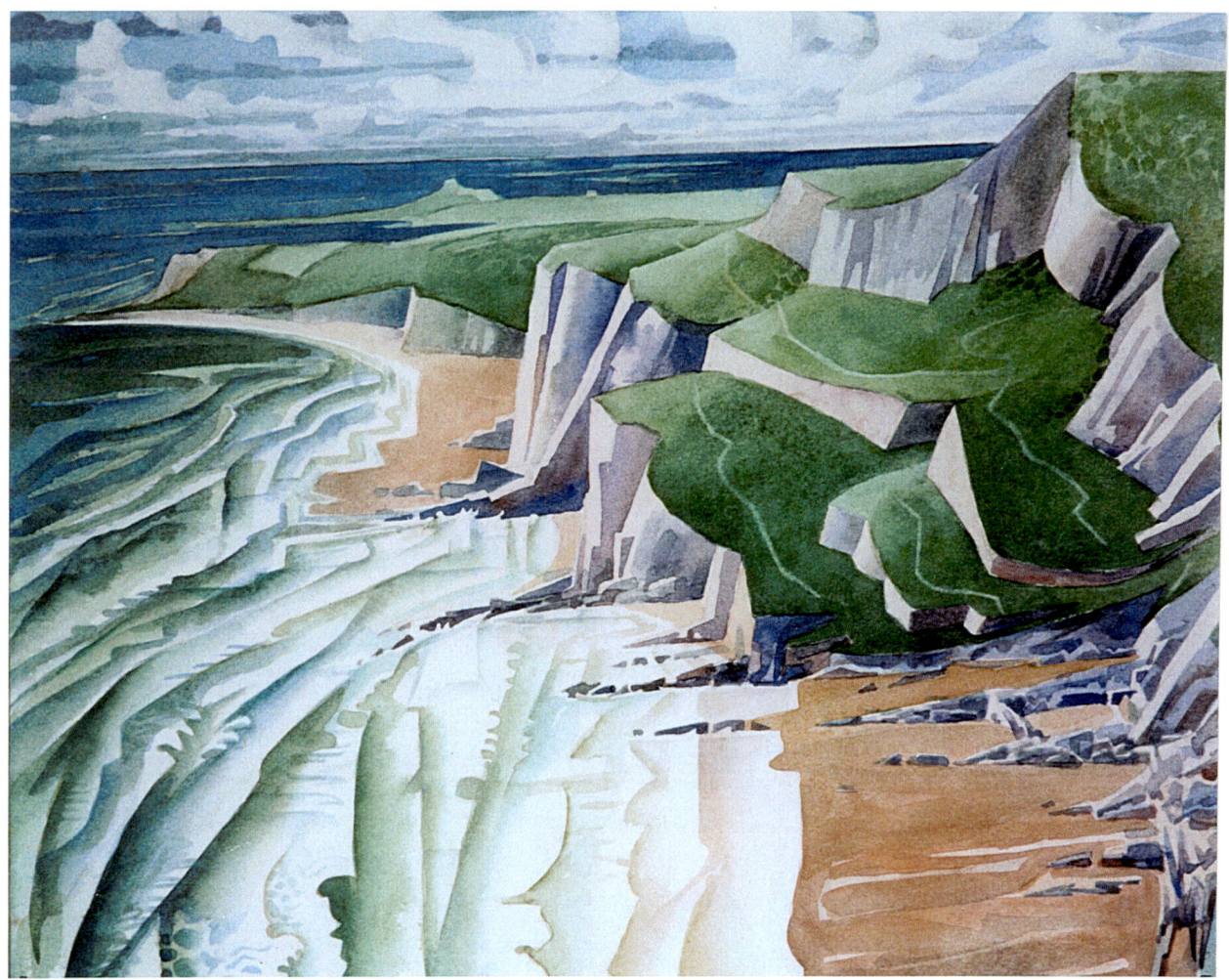

Fig.4 Surf Lines - Towards Worms Head   Watercolour

THE SURF PAINTINGS - FRAGMENTATION

Following the mental blockage and intimations of change in the summer of '79, a series of drawings and paintings evolved in the studio.

Over the next year or so many pictures with a large number of studies developed, trying to recapture this new awareness of figures in the surf movement. Various images suggesting parts of men and monsters, fish and birds, reflected inner feelings of change.

In retrospect a form of self-therapy was perhaps operating, making inroads into my earlier traditional work.

The surf pictures became highly stylised, even obsessively so, and developed into very formal compositions (fig 4). Many had a decorative, Art Nouveau feel (figs 5-7). Then, following the first cracked mirror sketch (fig 8), ideas combining this with surf lines followed (figs 9-13).

Later, the surf pictures ceased and a group of sea portraits became a new obsession (figs 14-16).

Closely related to the surf pictures was a portrait worked on at the same time (fig 17), a torn paper image, echoing the surf lines. And then, in another portrait, I repeated the idea, but by cutting instead of tearing. (fig 18).

Alongside this interest in the sea I had also looked at the cliffs, made studies of other hidden forms and developed one painting into figures enclosed by the rock (fig 19).

Finally, during this work in coastal scenes, some experiments with mixed media, making reliefs and also broader ranges of figurative work were developed (figs 20-22).

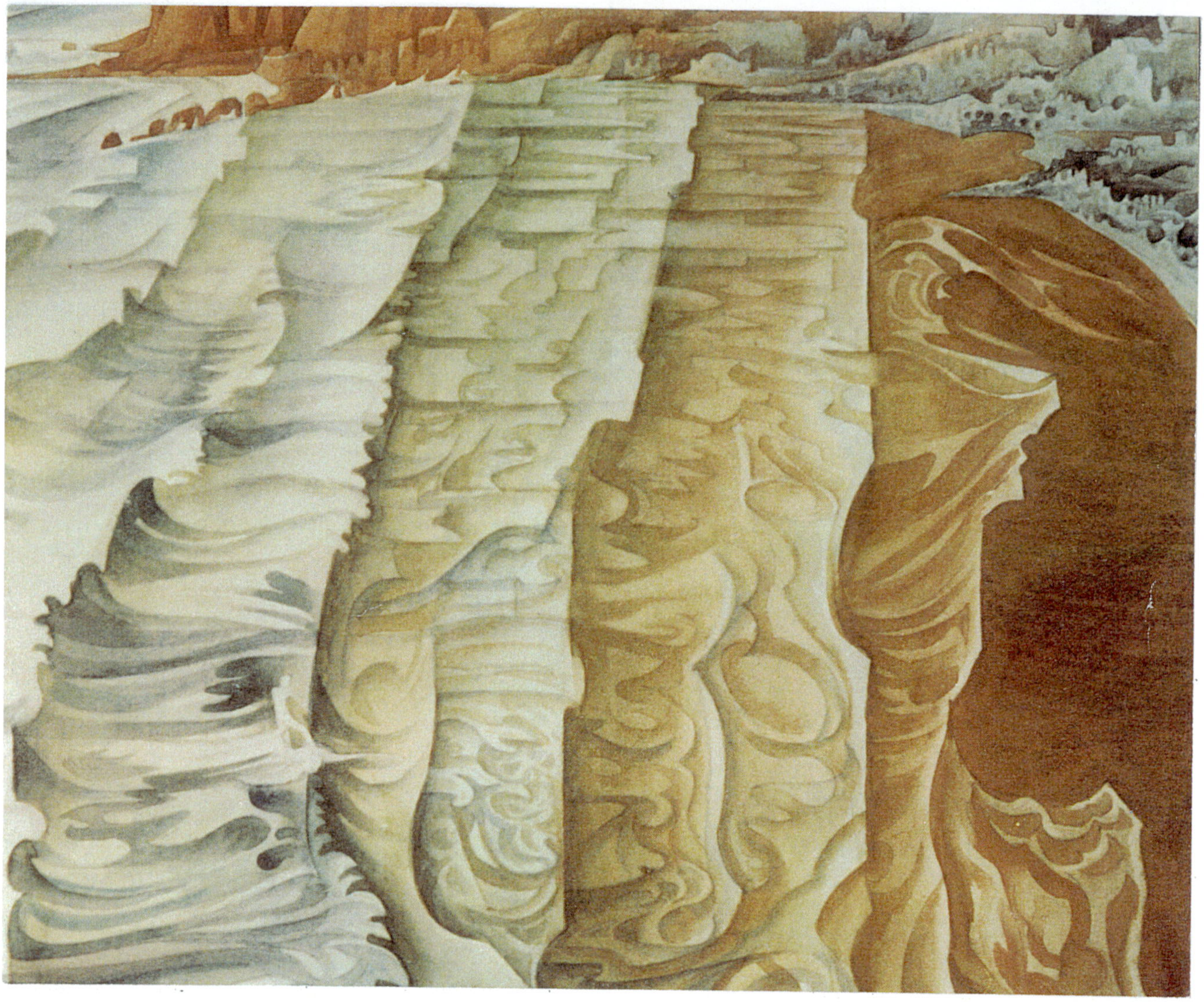

Fig.5 Mewslade Surf   Watercolour

Above, Fig 5: A standing figure heads in the surf, a fish stands on its tail - also some Art Nouveau effects.

Right Fig 7: Gower Surf - Night. Another stylised arrangement of cliffs and surf.

Below Fig 6: Leaping over the rocks a menacing wave threatens to overwhelm the onlooker, a reflection of the feelings of anxiety at this time.

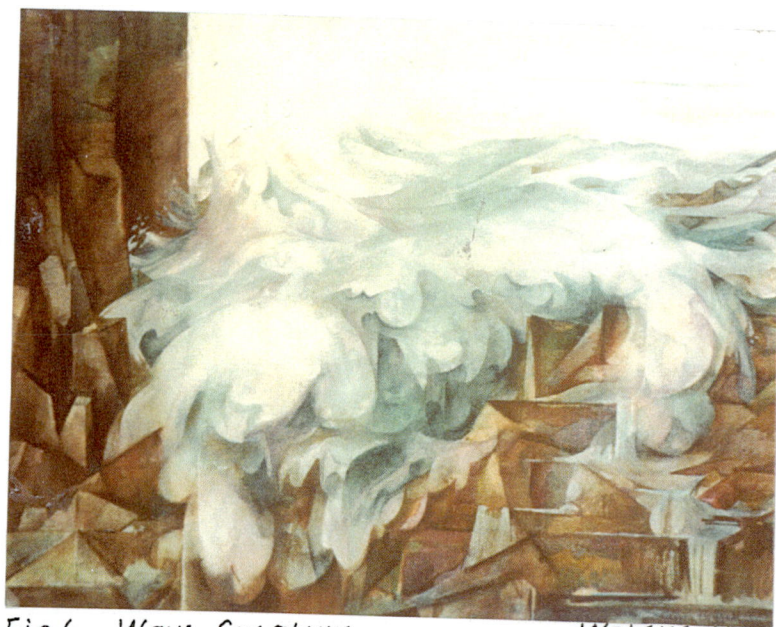

Fig.6 Wave Creature   Watercolour

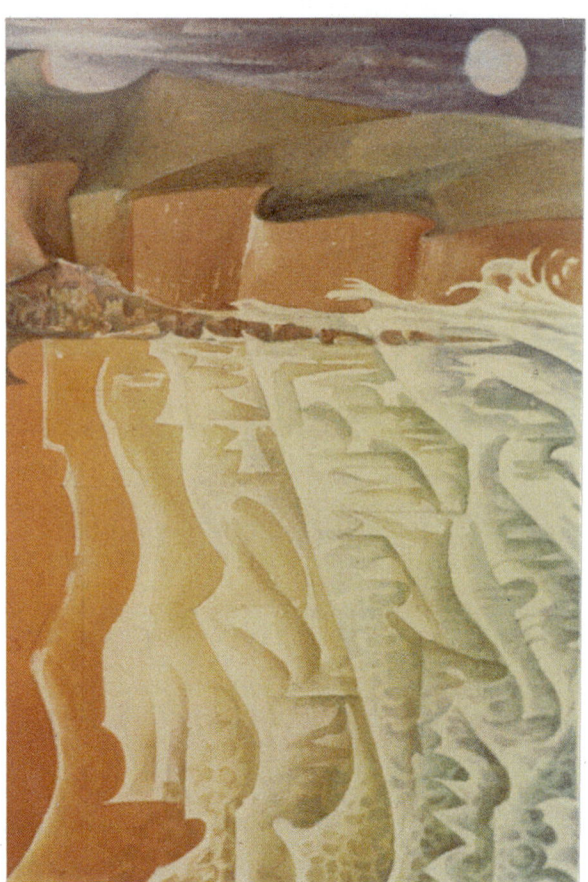

Fig.7 Gower Surf-Night   Watercolour

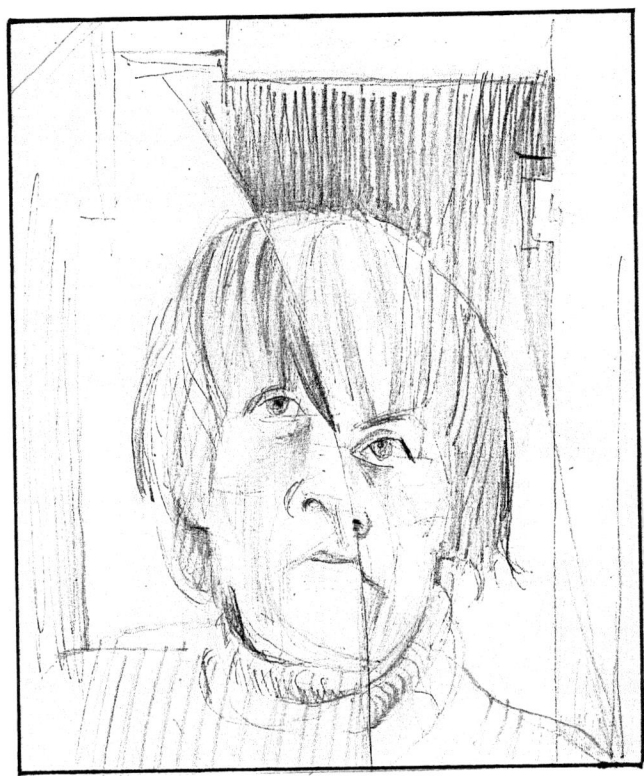

Fig 8: The Cracked Mirror. The first of many self-portraits to combine watery elements with portraiture

Fig 9: One of many sketches which introduced the face into surf-lines.

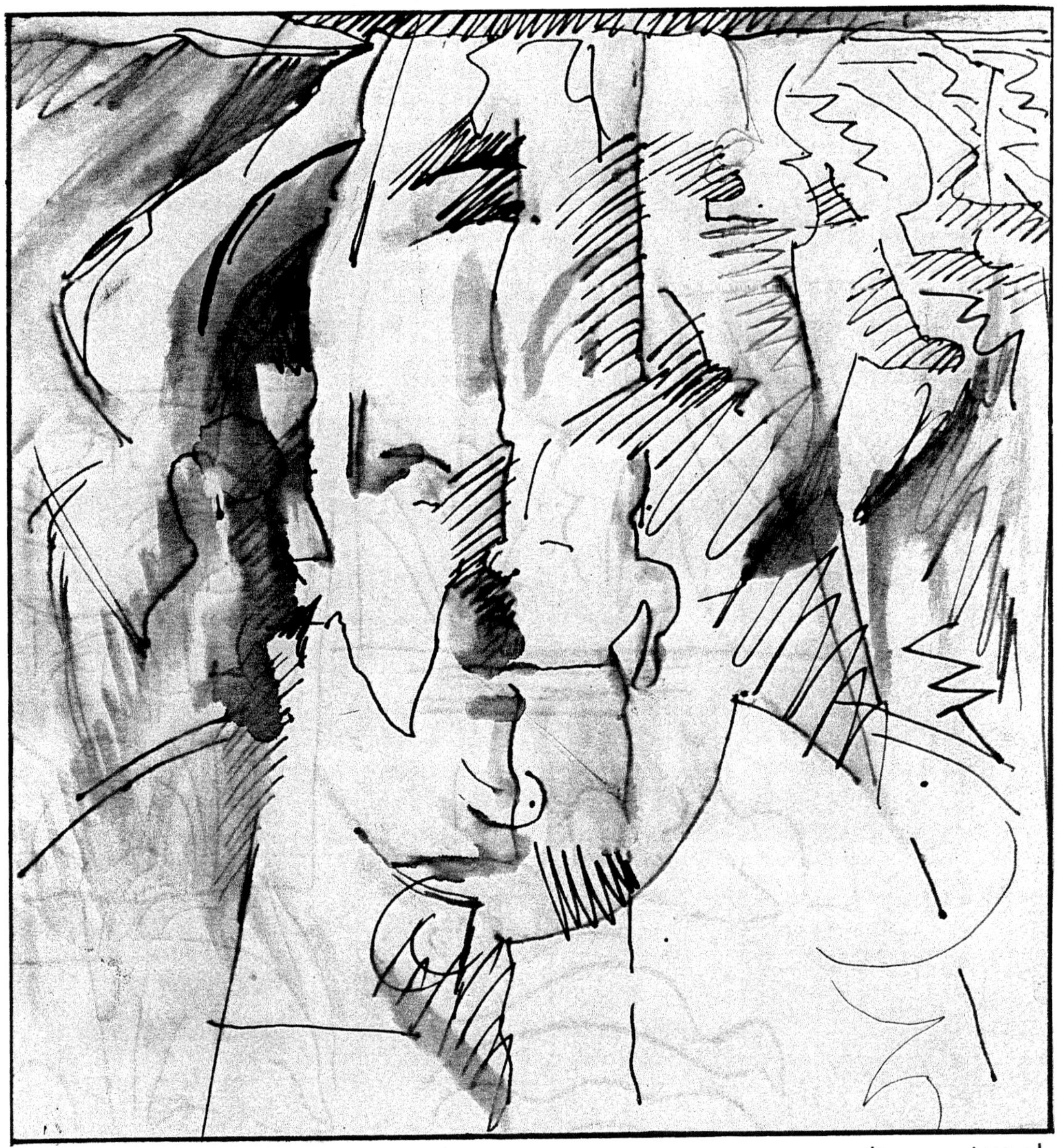

Fig.8 Reflection in a Cracked Mirror   Pencil

Fig.9   A Face in the Water   Pen and Wash

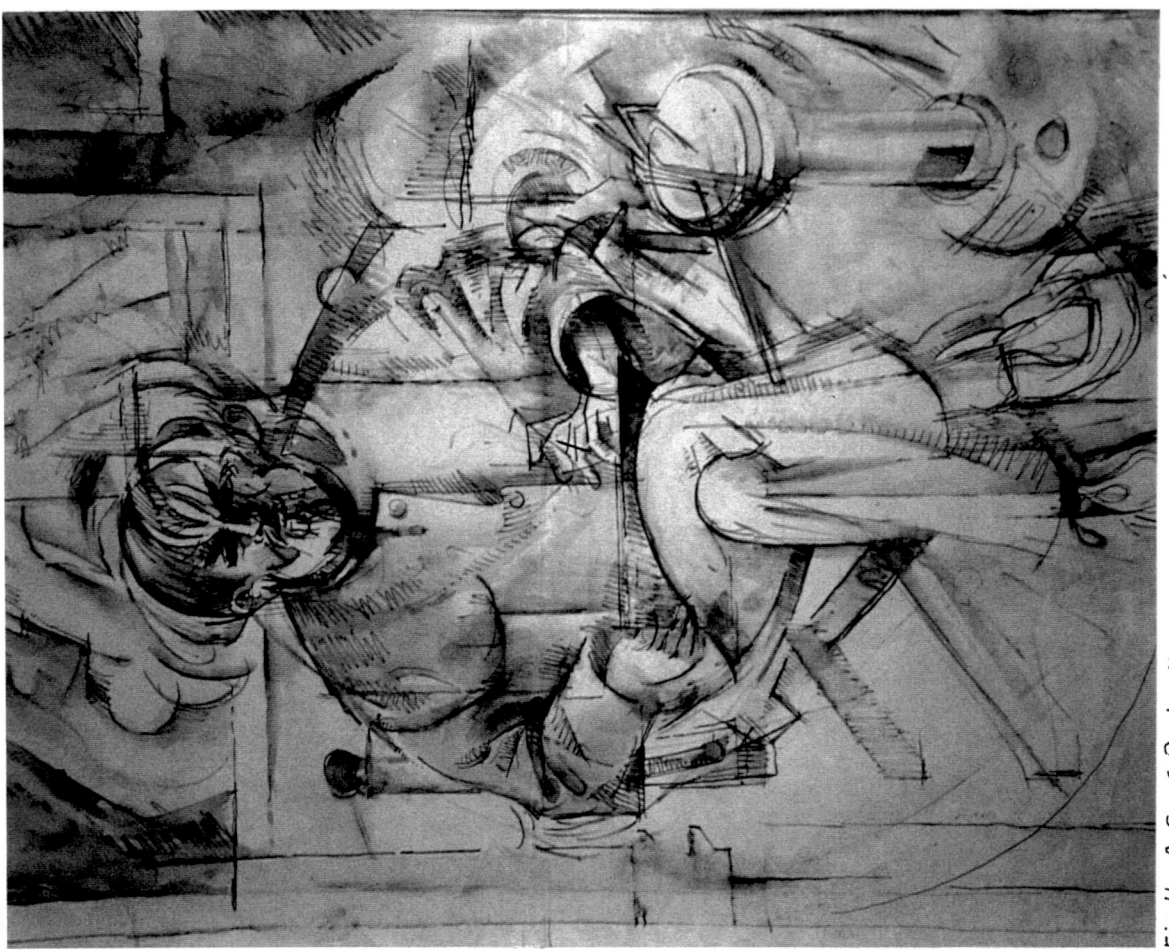

Pen & Wash

Fig.11: A Surf Portrait

Fig.11: The surf cascades down over the head, then into the arm and hand holding the pencil.

Fig.10: A further development on the theme of face in the surf.

Fig.10. Face in the Surf

Pen & Ink

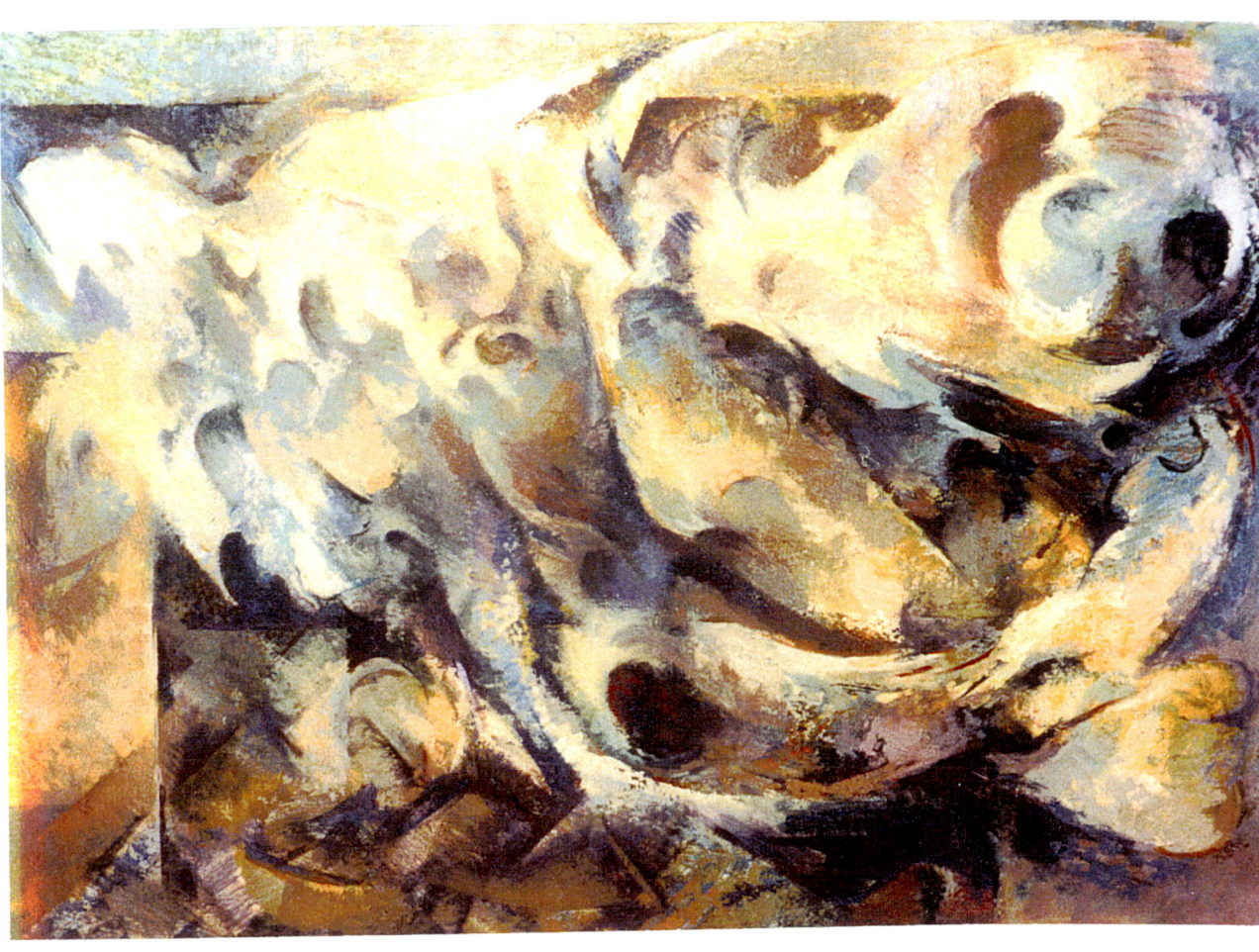

Fig.13 Wave Figure   Oil on Board

Fig.12 . Surf Man – Earth Woman   Watercolour

Above: Further development – the Surf Man gains company of an Earth Mother.

Right: The reclining figure, contemplating the sea, is transformed.

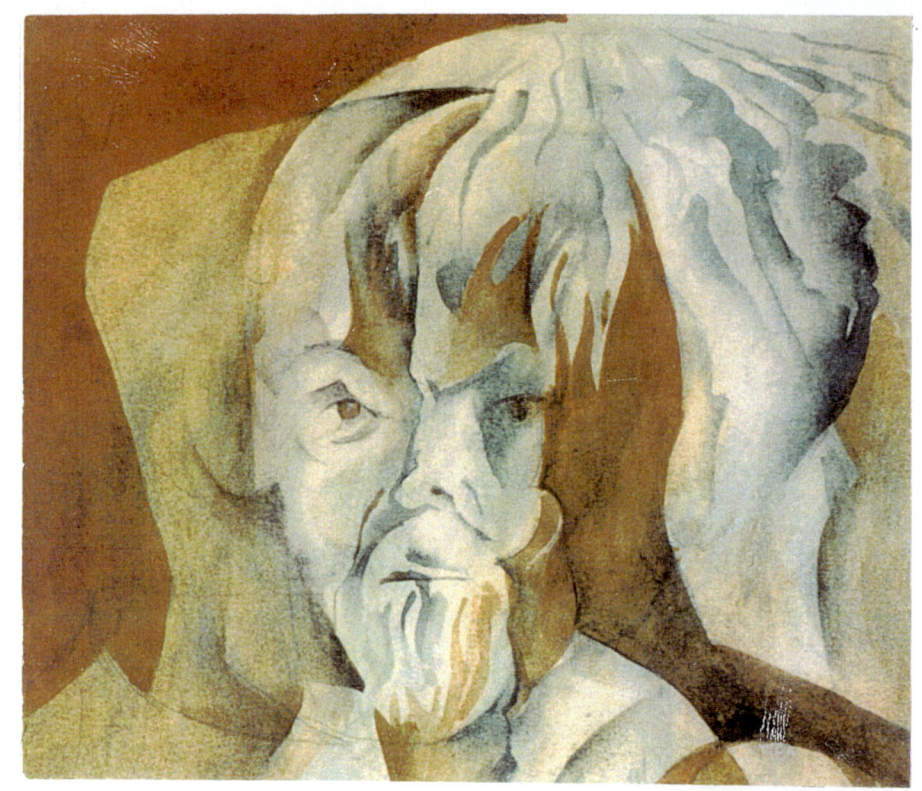

Left: First of six watercolour paintings following the series of pen sketches.
(See figs. 9, 10 and 11)

Fig.14 Surf Portrait   Watercolour

Below: A Sea Portrait, evolved from the watercolour series above. Worked in relief with mixed media: sand, acrylic paste, string, card and acrylic paint.

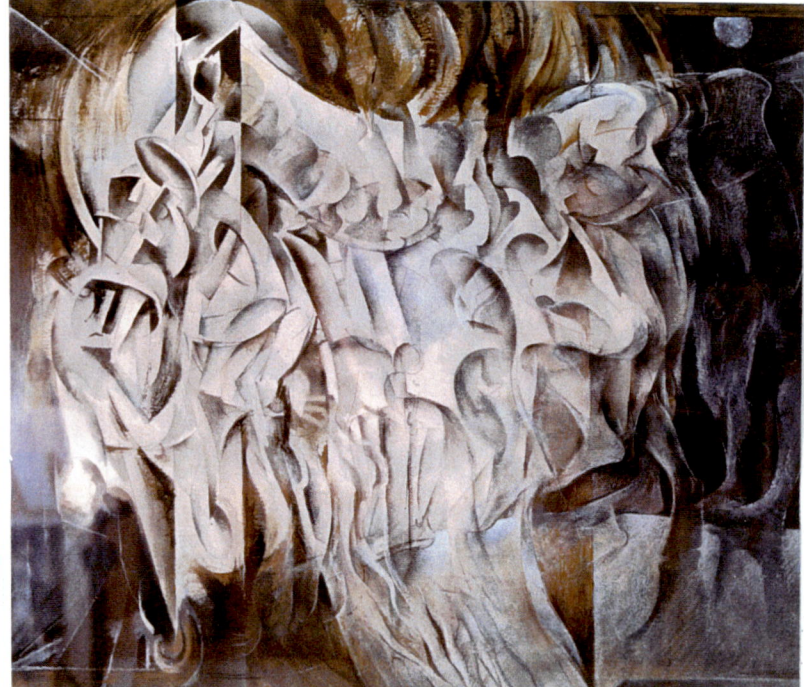

Fig.15 Sacrificial Head   Watercolour

Above: This painting sinks like a lead balloon through sheer overloading of equal 'wavelets' across its surface. It cancels itself out by lack of variety and tries to say too much — a sequence of lines for the walking figure; a large head and hints of other ideas — all overdone, obsessive and morbid.

Failures like this can sometimes help to clarify what needs to be said.

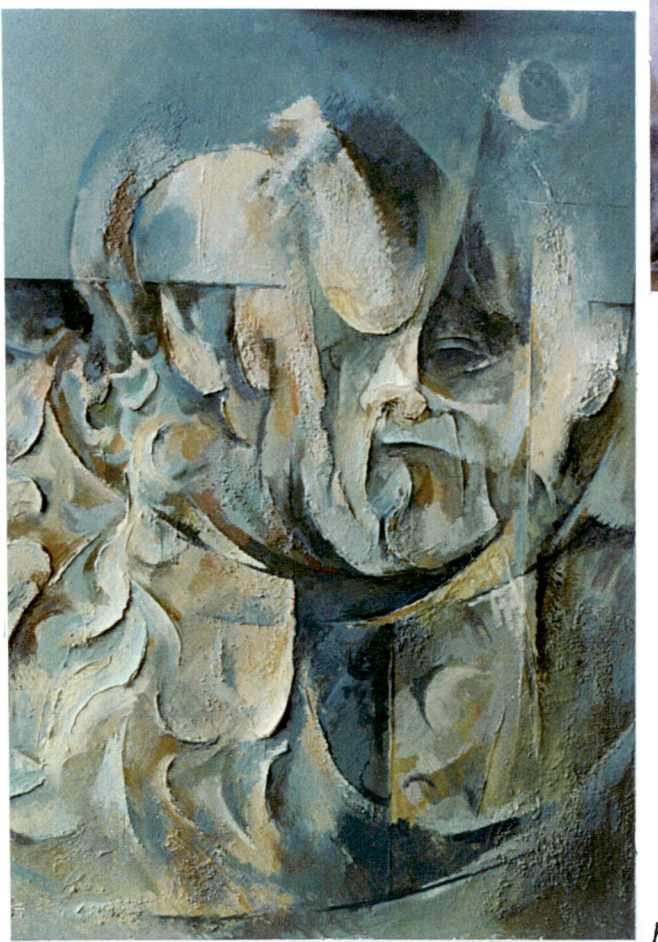

Fig.16 A Sea Portrait   — Acrylic on Board

TWO 'REASSEMBLED' SELF PORTRAITS

Below: Crayon drawing, torn and glued to a backing sheet to create a new image, fragmented and floating

Right: Painted then cut into strips, slightly shifted about, reflecting a state of indecision.

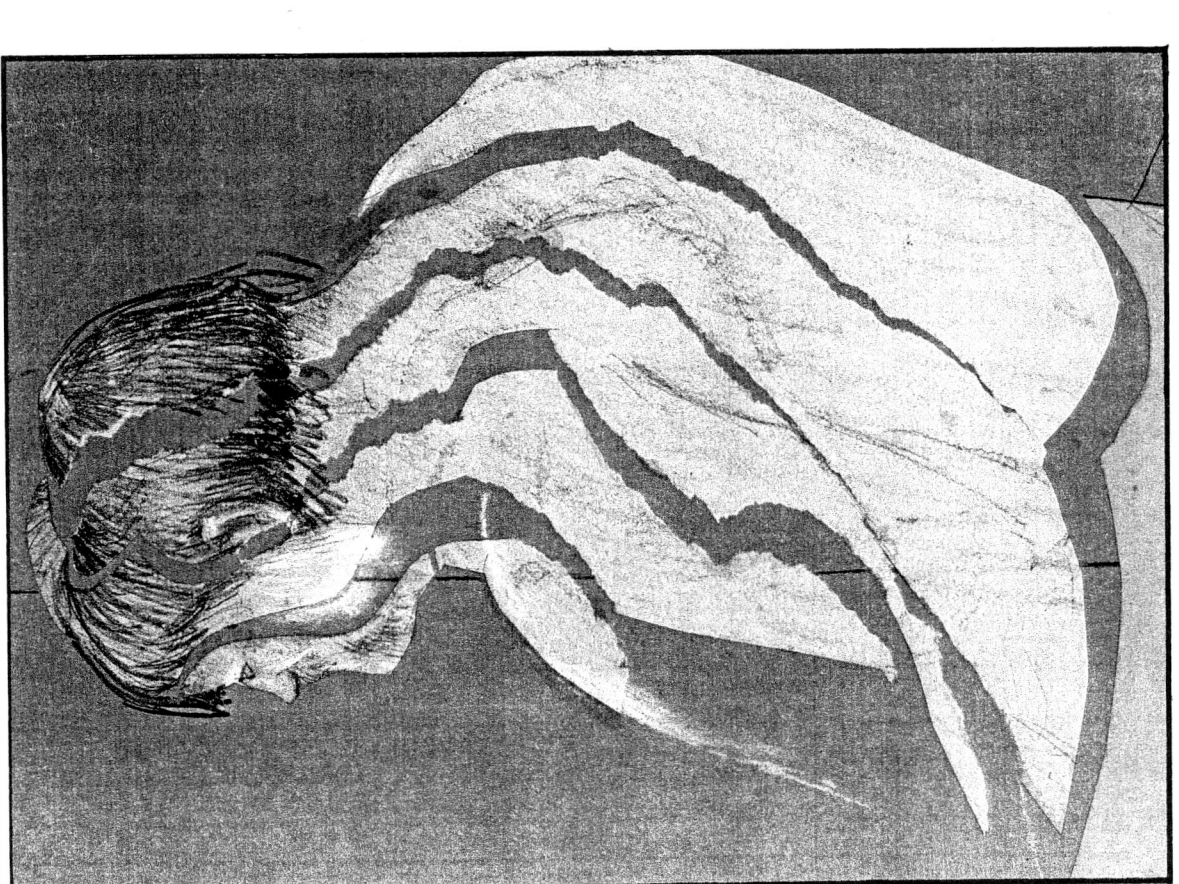

Fig.17 Fragmented Portrait — Torn & glued drawing

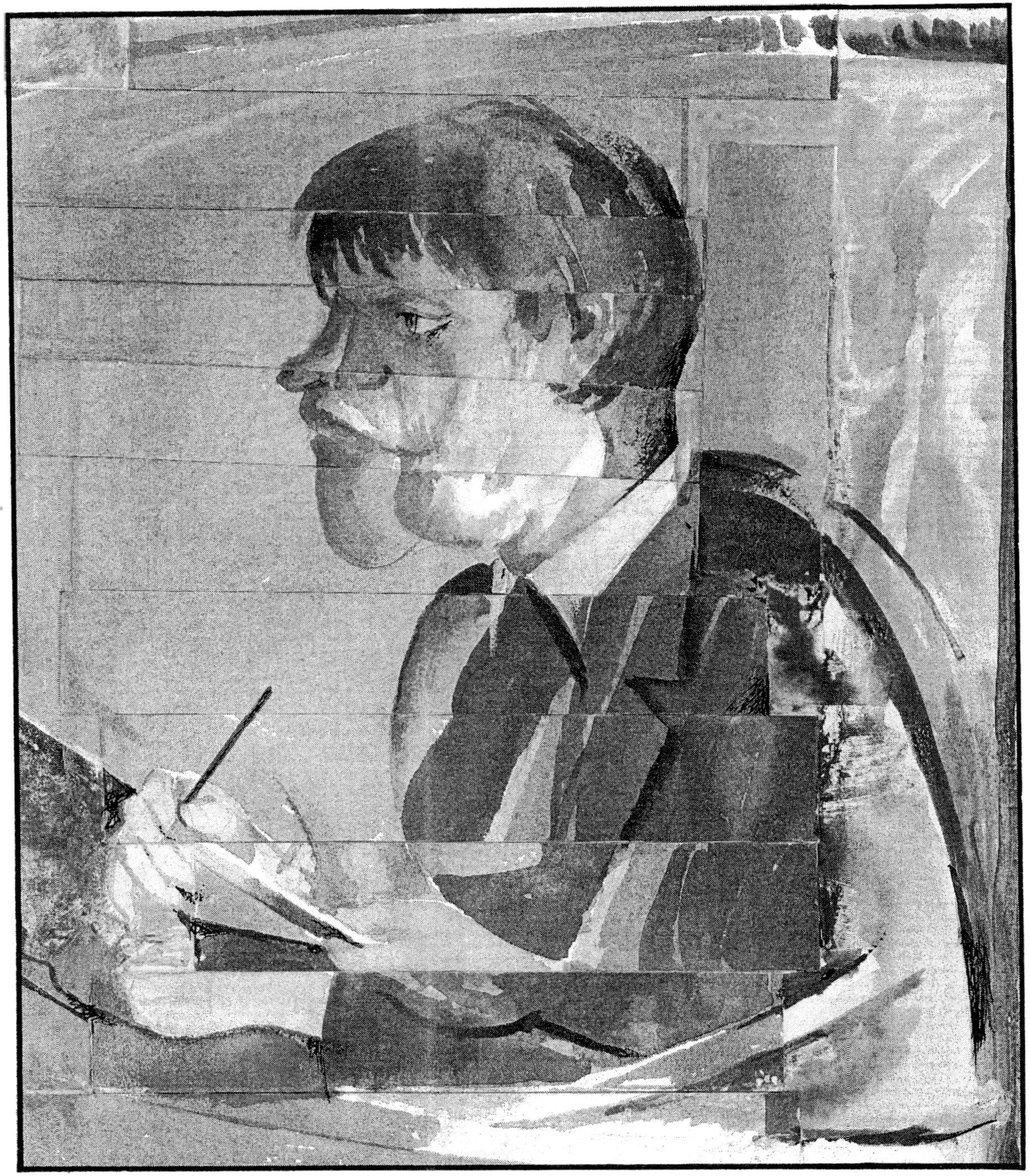

Fig.18 Artist and his Double — Watercolour, cut and reassembled

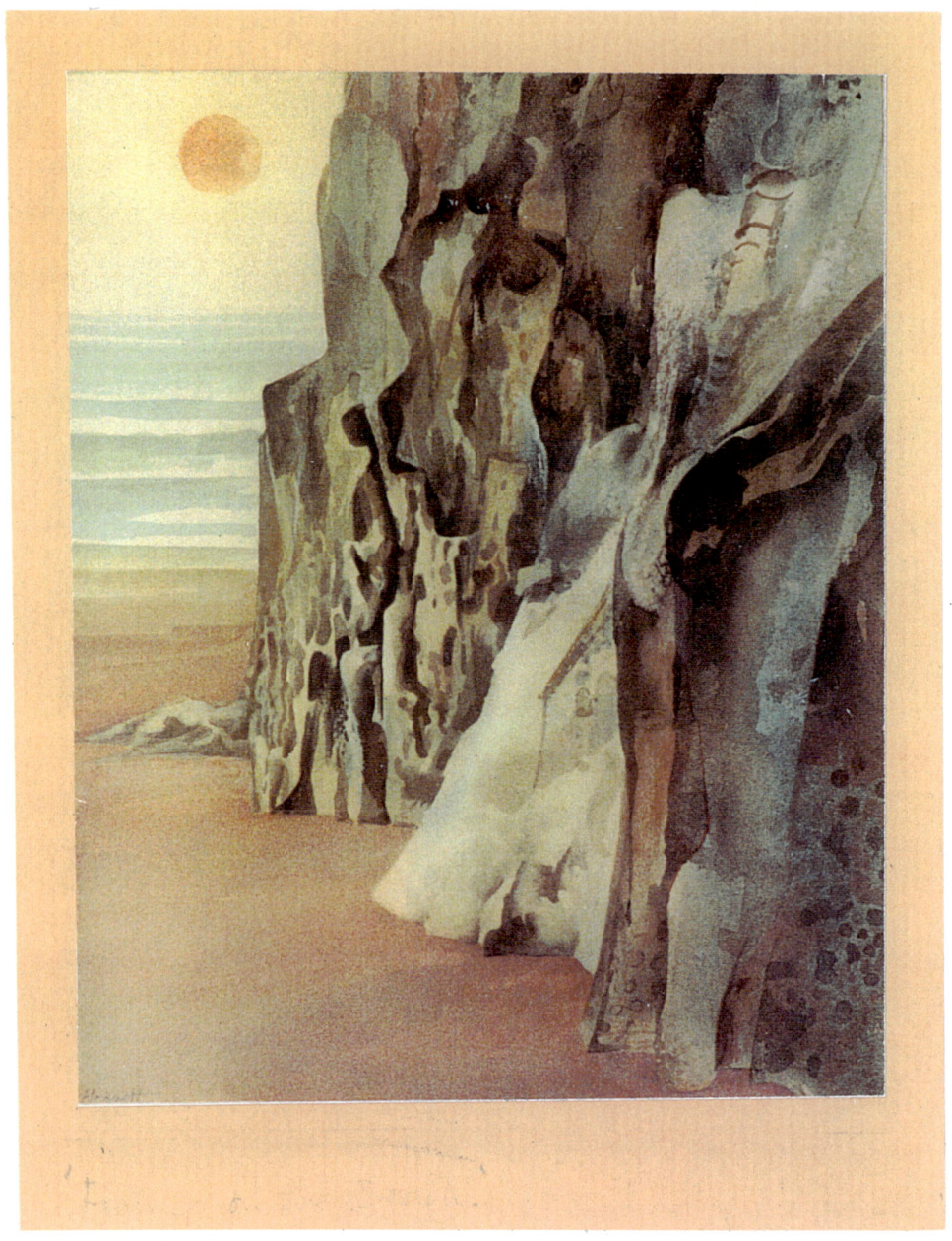

Fig.19   Figures on the Beach   Watercolour

Above: These anthropomorphic forms stand, lean or sit filling the cliff-face on the silent beach. Reflecting the inertia of a depressive state of mind they wait, ossified, to be slowly worn away by time. Their features steadily erode into the sands.....

Opposite page: Fig.20 - Influenced by lines of surf and mirror, reflections move as if affected by the wind, floating backwards, its shadow waits patiently.
  Fig.21 : The figure stands poised, trying to decide into which mirrored space it might enter......

  Fig.22 : A fanciful version of Aphrodite rising from the sea. Made up of wave and cloud forms, about to walk onto land.....

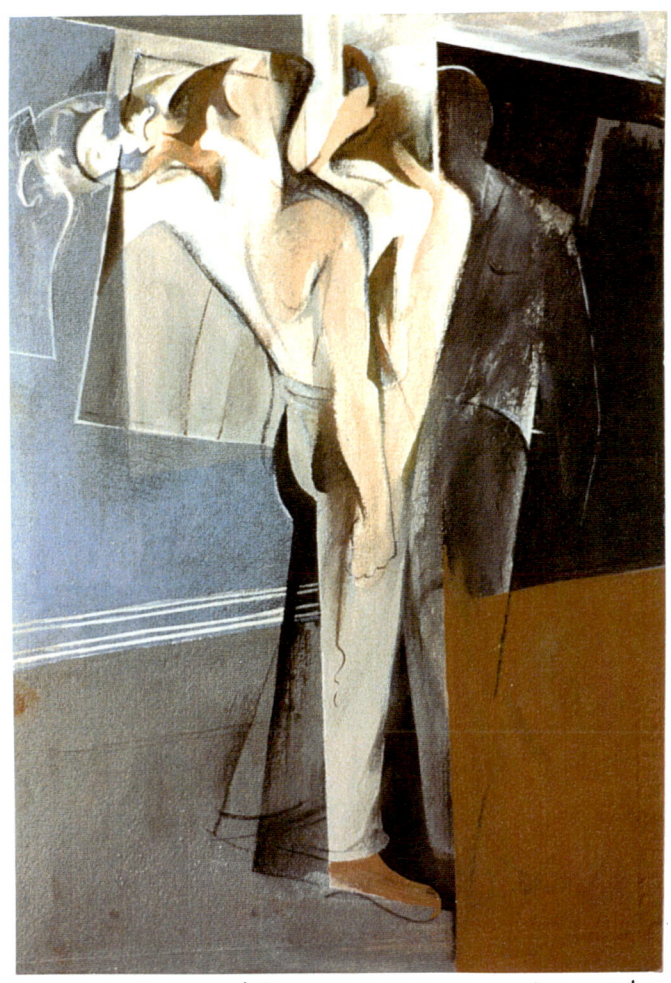
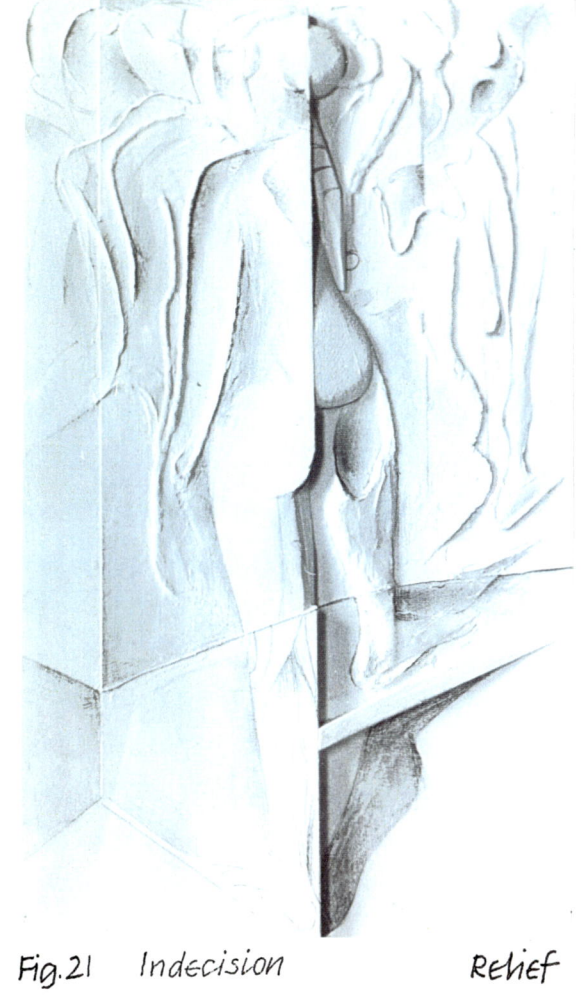

Fig.20 Mirrored Image   Gouache   Fig.21 Indecision   Relief

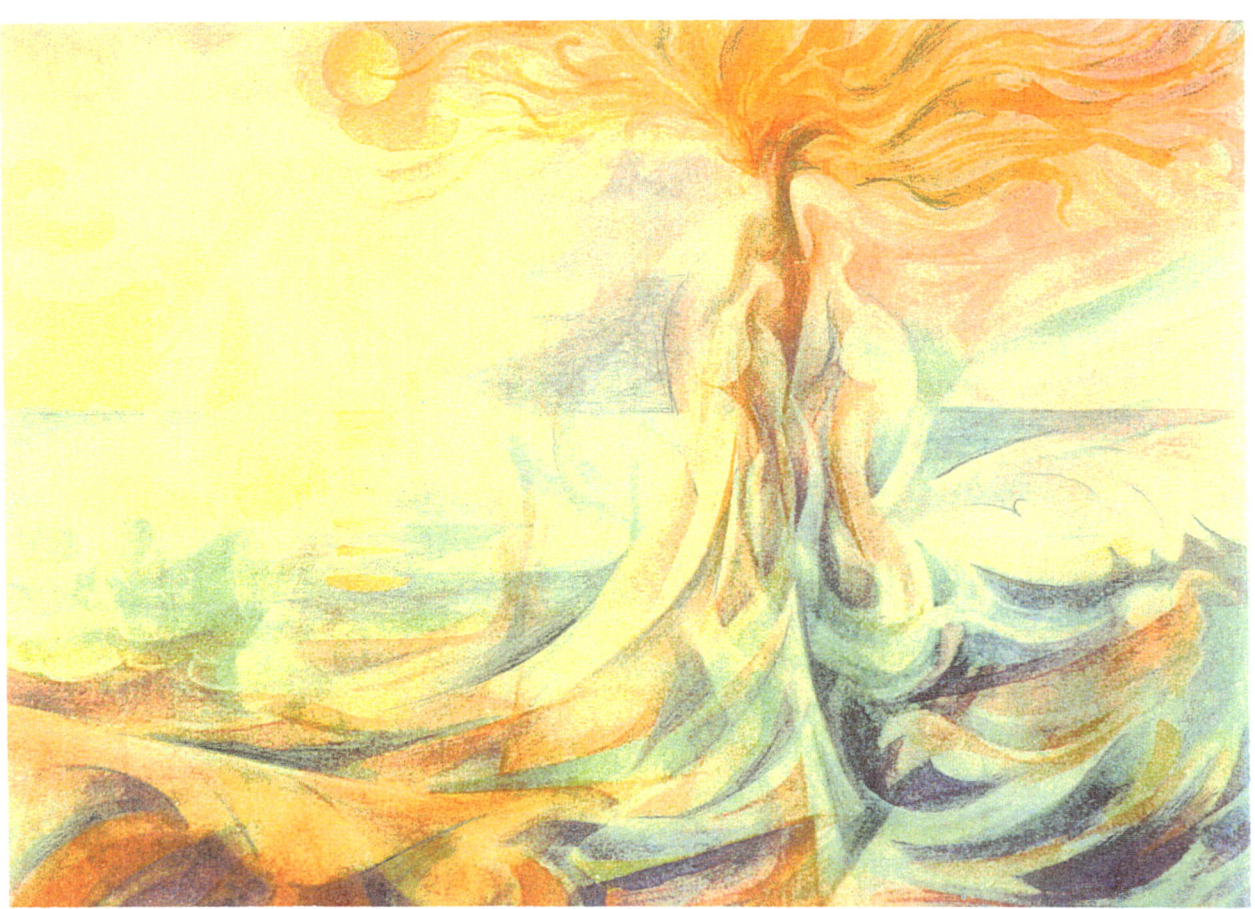

Fig.22 Aphrodite   Watercolour

A Serpentine Premonition

Following the many watery images in these pages, I felt a need to redress the balance with another stone form above the the beach.

Whereas 'Figures on the Beach' (fig 19) had elements of pure fantasy (the human shapes) within the rockface, the 'Stone Serpent' (fig 23) was already visible to a certain way of looking — projecting, as I was, the image 'serpent' into this particular lump of limestone, because it contained certain attributes associated with a snake-like creature. It reared up at the front, hugged the ground behind, had a narrow slit mouth which could conceal a forked tongue,.. etc.. ...

It was possible that I was ready to receive just such an image as an harbinger of the emotional 'fall' which was to occur during the following year.

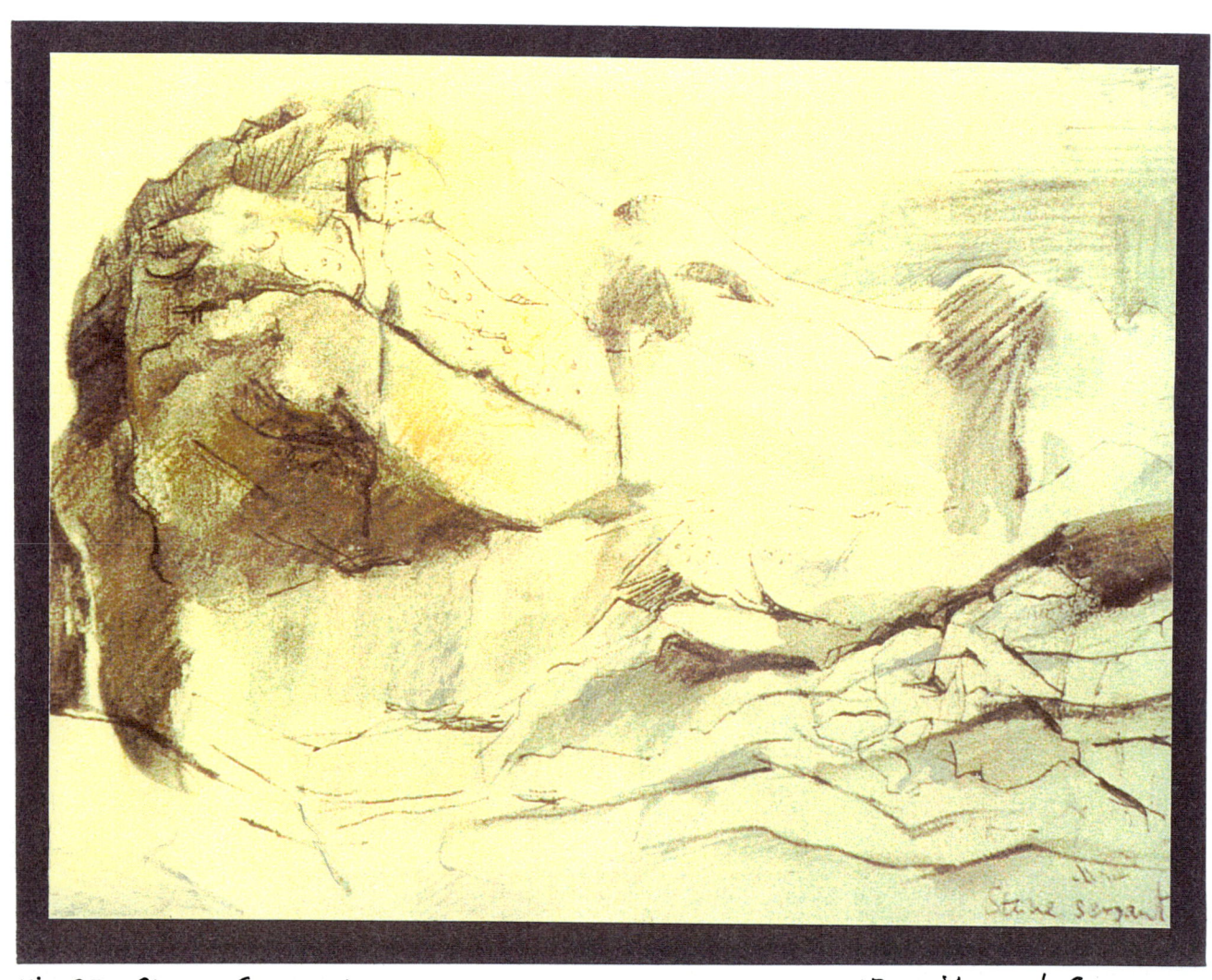

Fig.23 Stone Serpent   Pencil and Crayon

FREEFALL, AUTUMN 1980

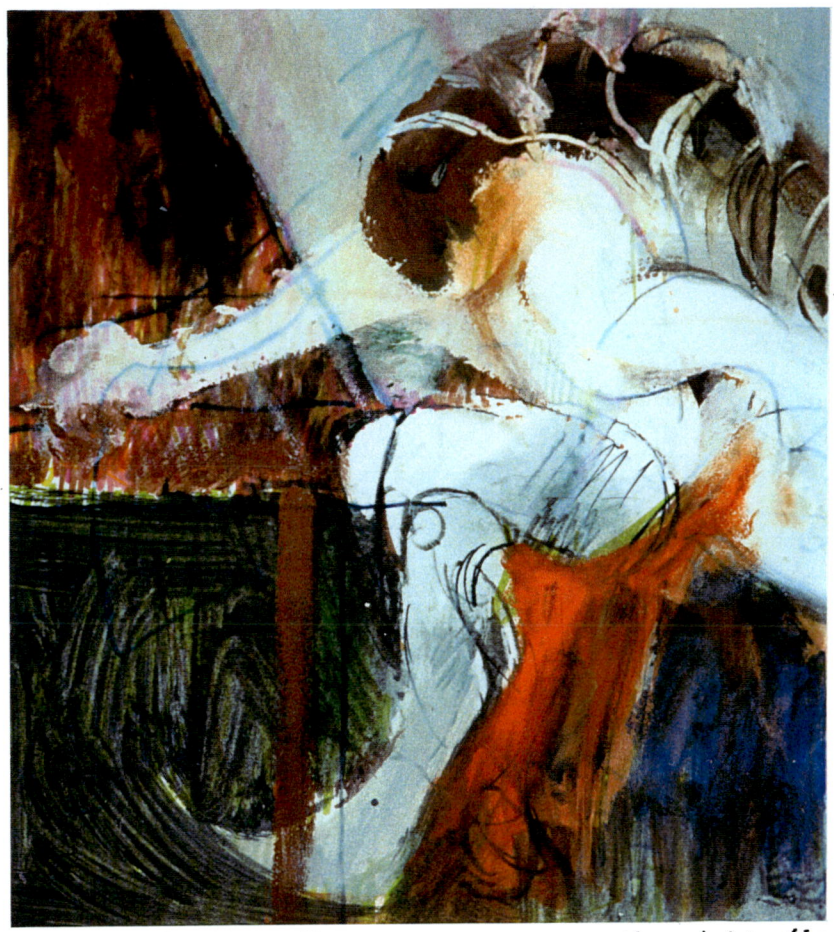

Fig. 24   Dizzy Spell   Mixed Media

The memory is as vivid now as twenty years ago when the world I'd known collapsed about me. One minute reading at the table, the next, staring into a black hole - the intervening moments an affront to logic and sensibility. As a cardsharp might flick his pack from hand to hand I gradually separated out into pieces from the chair, cascading to the floor, slithering deep into shades of darkness.

Was it an hour or just a few moments before I crawled across the floor and opened the door? A brilliant light flooded the hallway from the right, to the left a deep space opened up, completely black. Why the pause, the hesitation, before choosing a move towards light rather than dark? Did the world outside still exist? Finally I moved slowly, step by step, out into the blaze of sunlight in the garden, walking the length of the path and finding, leaning against the garden wall, an old chair.

I sat down quietly and waited for a sense of calm. A feeling of normality returned and eased my acute anxiety — but only briefly.

I found myself reaching out for a large, rusty nail (the details seemed highly significant). Gripping it tightly so that the knuckles shone white on my hand, an image of Christ crucified appeared — I felt as if nailed to the wall.

Later I found myself walking along a pavement, petrified that the flagstones would open up into unknown spaces. Also I had the impression that I looked odd, that trauma was transforming my features, so I kept glancing downwards to avoid contact with the eyes of strangers.

I had intended to walk back home but instead found myself walking in the opposite direction to a friend's house where I was received with much generosity. Given a comfortable sofa for the night, I nevertheless slept badly. My manic state would not allow me to sleep although I was totally exhausted.

Days, then weeks passed, until some psychic energy restored my ability to recapture the various experiences onto paper: a long sequence of sketches, drawings, paintings and relief modelling, reliving this extraordinary day. This section is a visual record of this day.

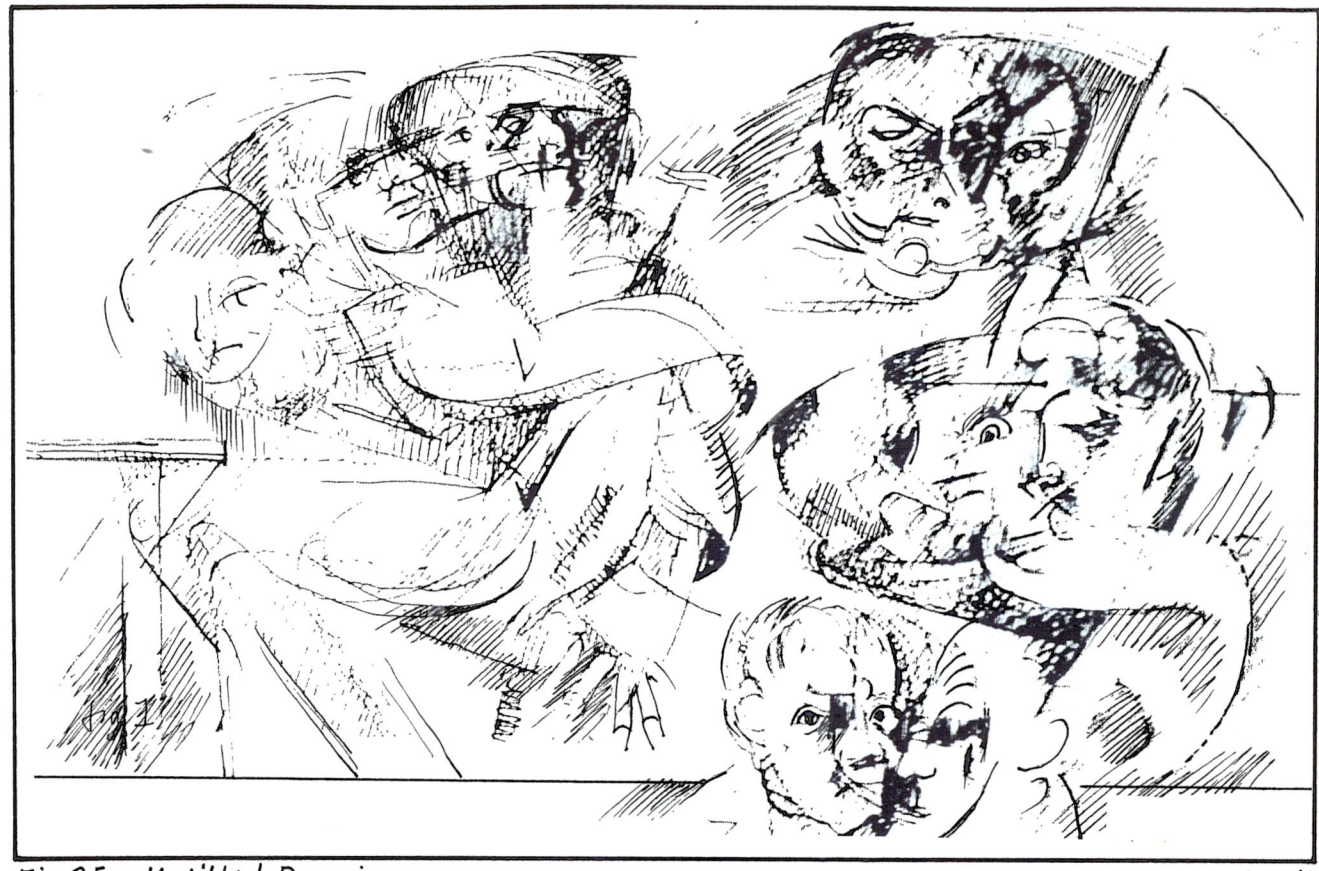

Fig.25   Untitled Drawing   Pencil

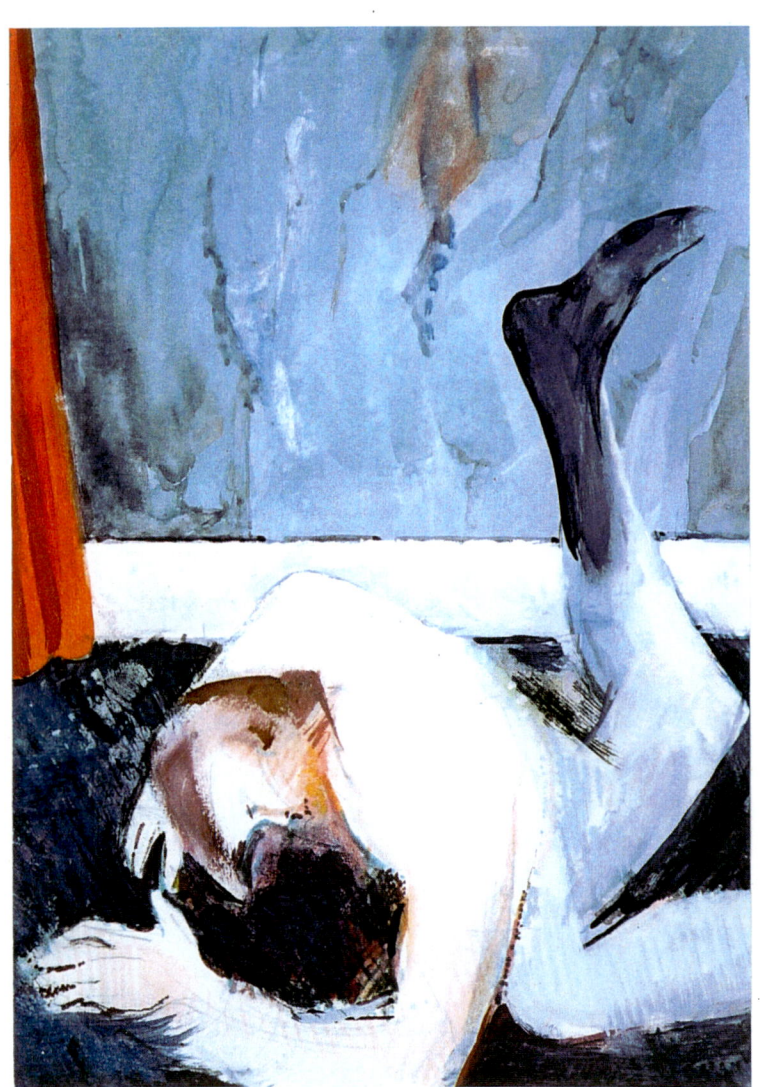

EARLY MORNING

First attempts trying to recapture the feelings of 'the fall'- the first moments/movements of the day:

Fig.25. Pen sketches of the moment of turning, twisting on the chair.

Fig.26. Looking into the black hole. Limbs akimbo, everything in flux, the wall melting down, the figure falling into the abyss. The main trunk of the body superfluous, only the limbs flailing about.

Figs.27 & 28. The head turning before the fall.

Fig.29 One of many drawings that attempted to show the complete movement from sitting in chair to the fall to the floor, designed like an open fan.

Fig.26 - Freefall. Original Colour Sketch.   Mixed Media

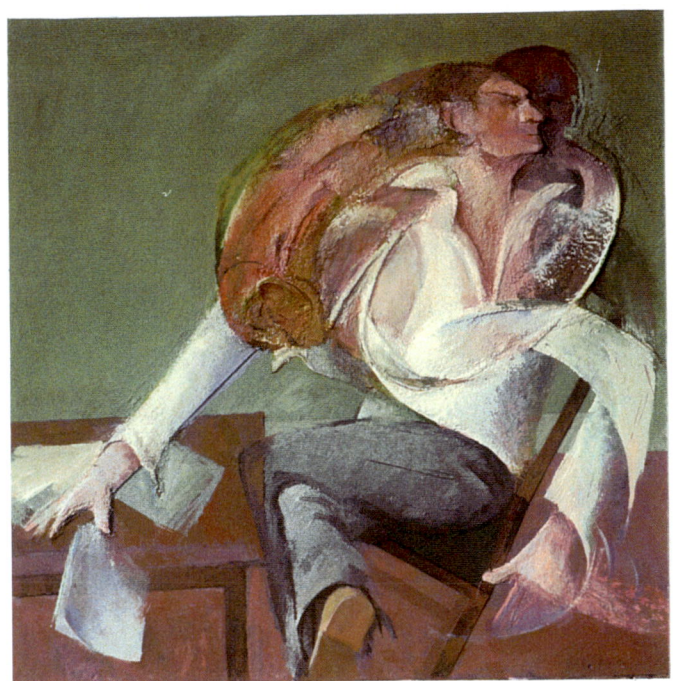

Fig. 27 Untitled   Mixed Media

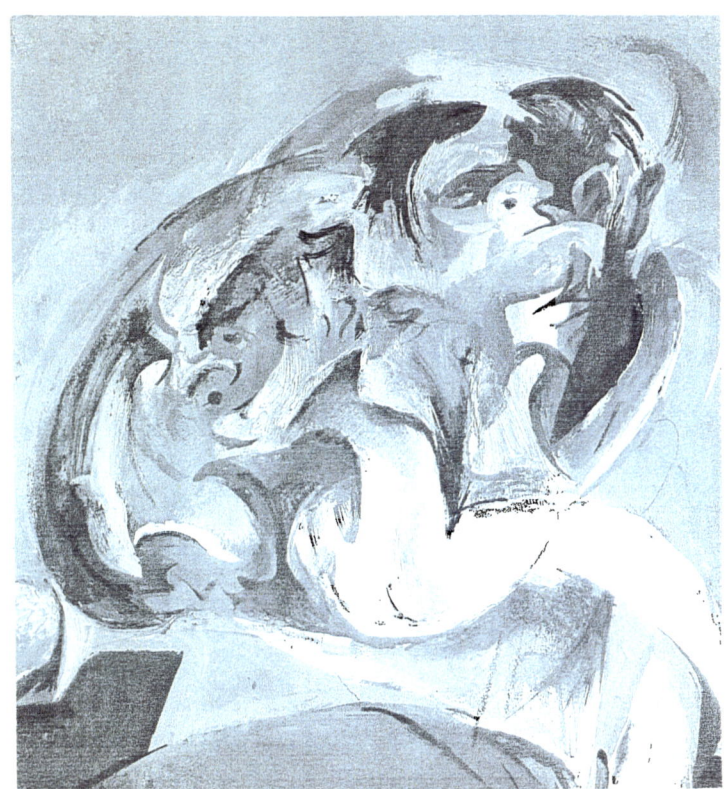

Fig. 28 Untitled. (Original Sketch)   Gouache

Above and Right: A white bird kept re-appearing in sketches and paintings of this turning movement. I came to see it as a symbol of the change caused by this precipitous fall.

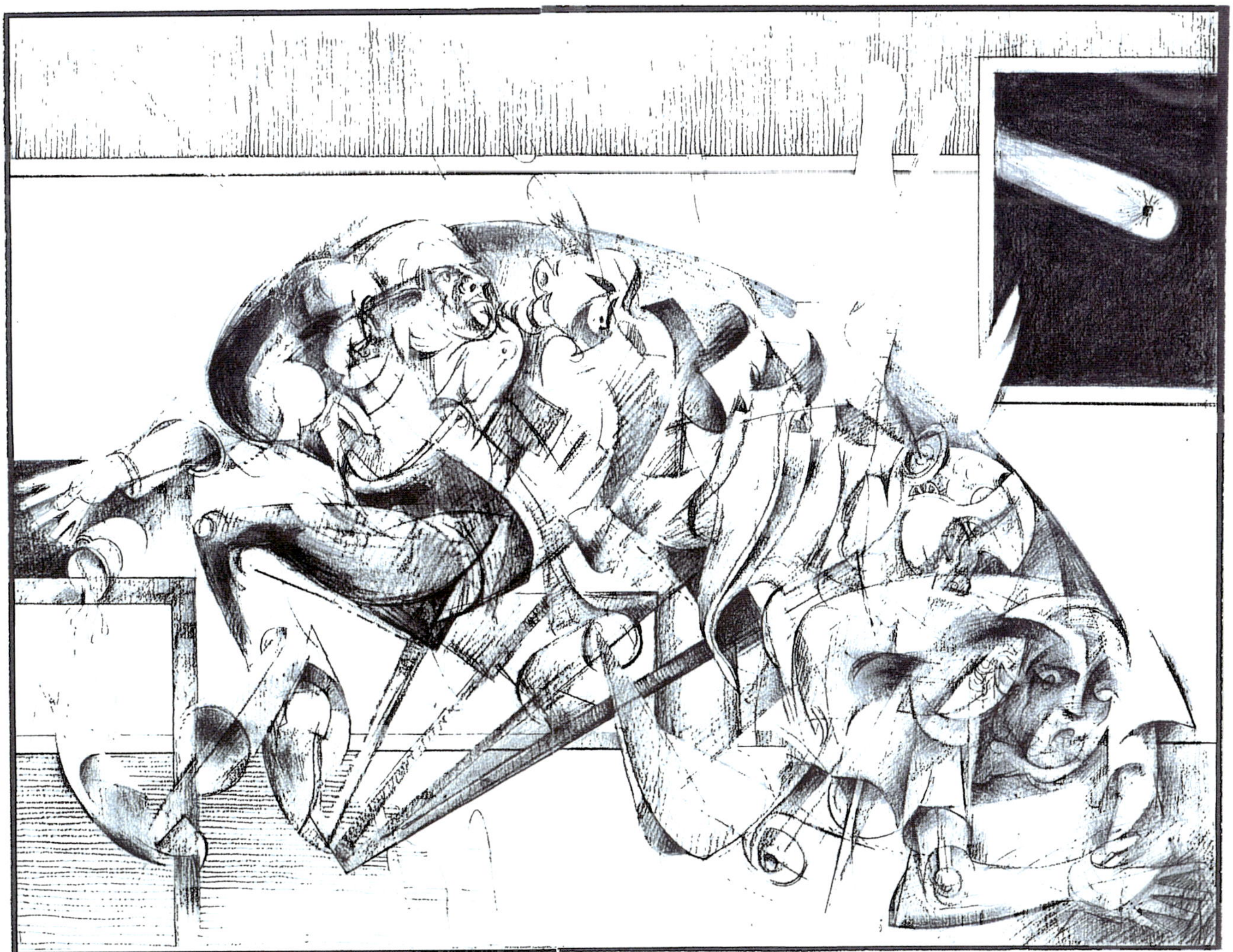

Fig. 29 Spillage (of cup of coffee; of self; of Halley's Comet).   Pencil

17

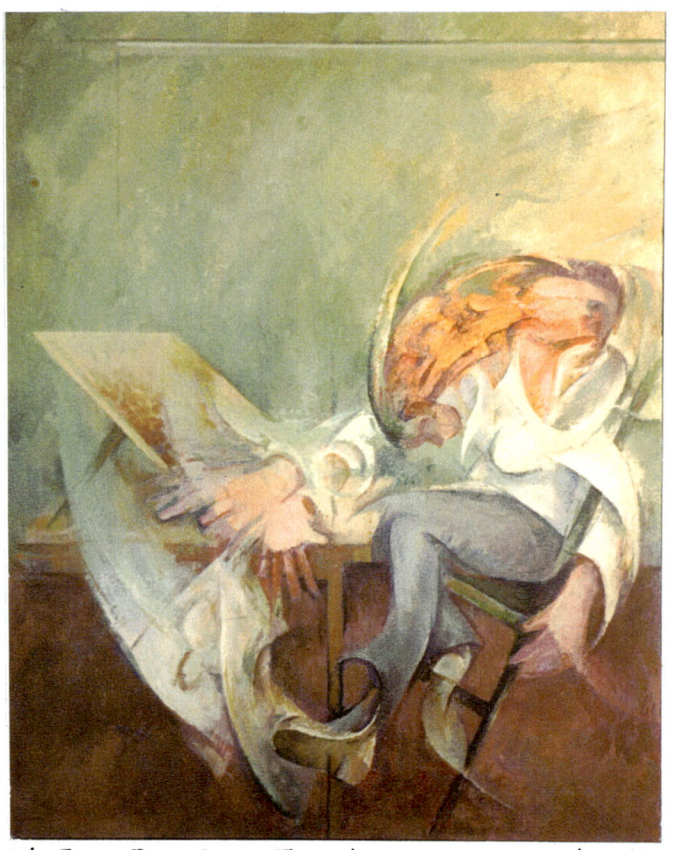
Fig.30 Freefall - Turning   Acrylic

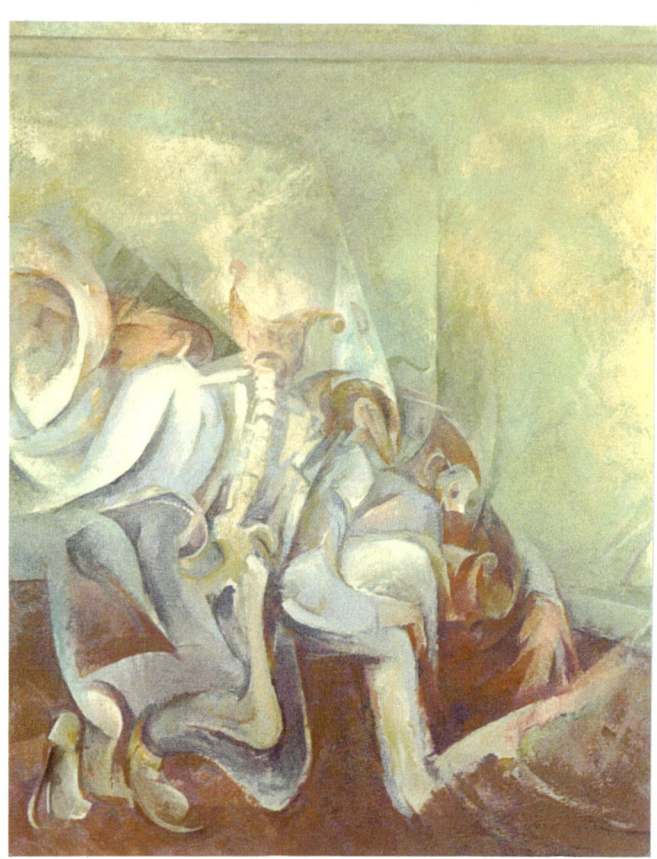
Fig.31 Freefall - Falling   Acrylic

These four paintings attempted to convey the feelings of the first part of the day. It came to be entitled 'Freefall' after the novel of that name by William Golding. I'd felt certain resonances to my own situation. I had developed a habit of photographing 'work in progress' as a method of retaining images I'd all too often destroyed and later wished I'd kept. My indecision at the time led to constant modification and obliteration of work. Of the four paintings only one remained unscathed —

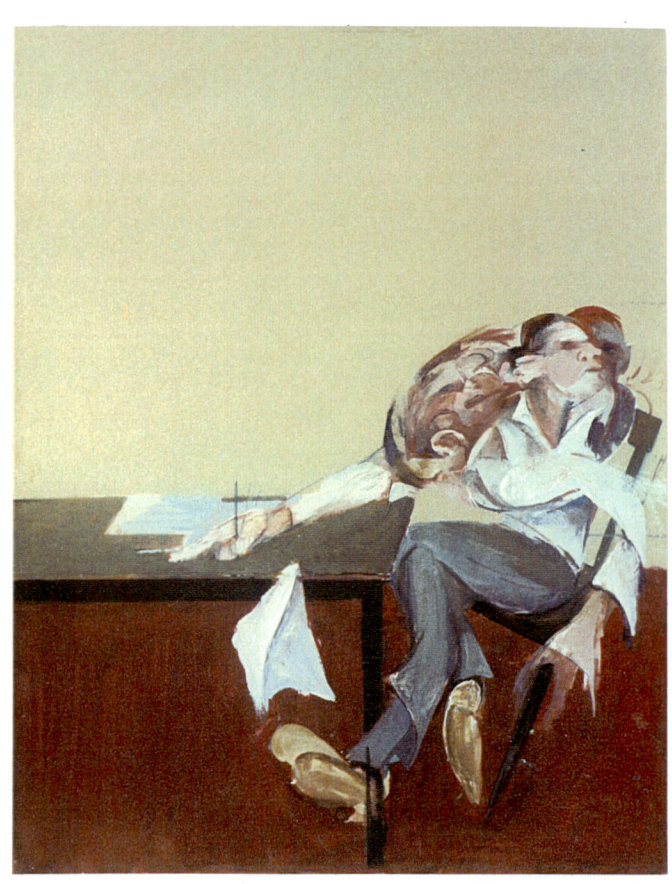
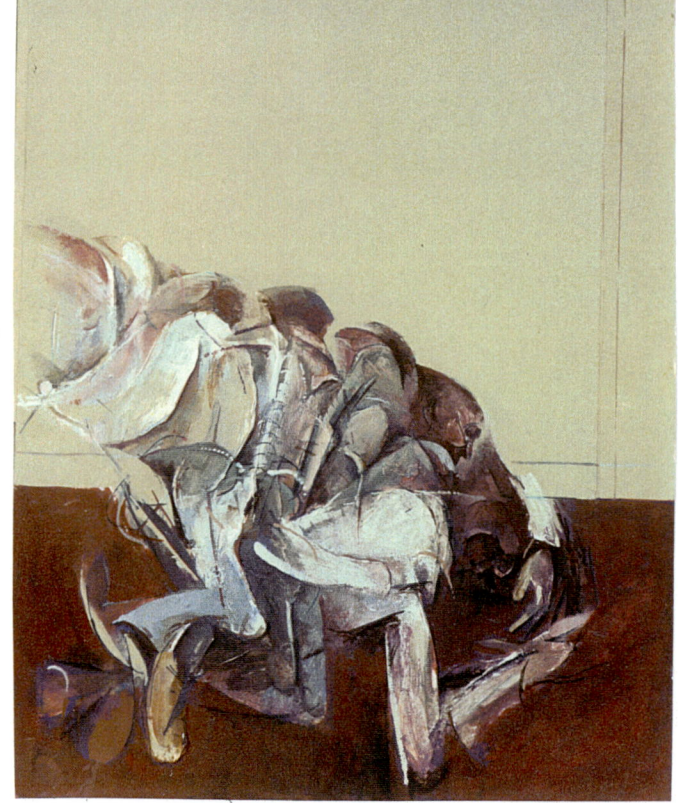
Fig.34 Freefall; a Diptych (final version of Figs. 30 and 31)   Gouache & Acrylic Paste

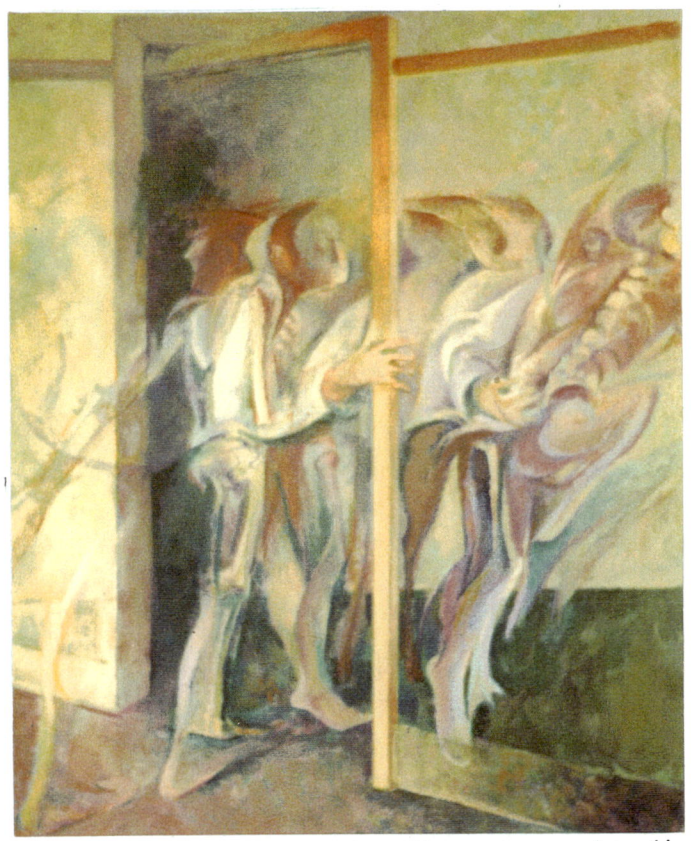 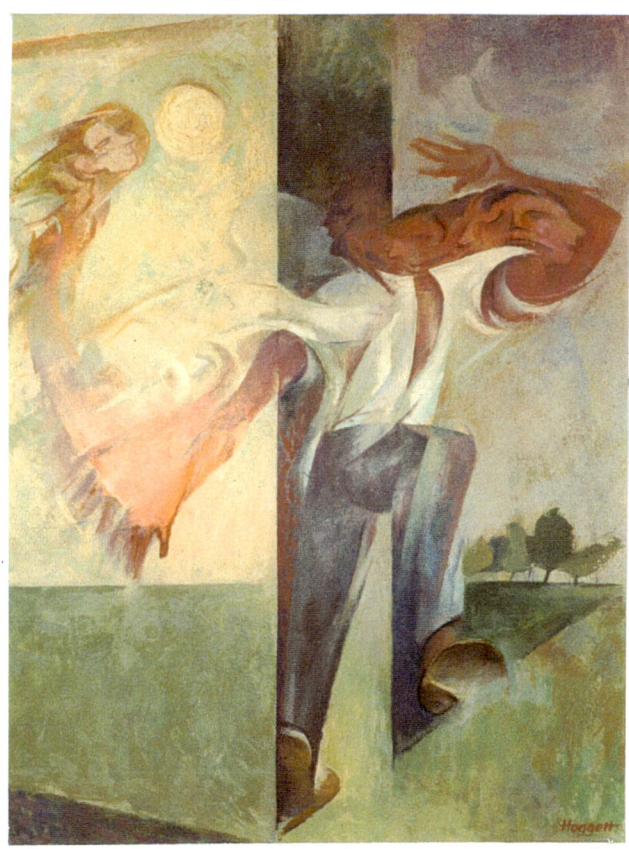

Fig.32 Freefall – Passing Through   Acrylic   Fig.33   Freefall – Breakout   Acrylic

Fig.30 'Turning'. The 'Falling' episode was changed beyond recognition and is now a more abstract 'slithering' interpretation (now Fig.54). The 'Passing Through' was developed, the part beyond the doorframe painted out and replaced with a picture on the wall. (Fig 32 became Fig 41). Fig 33 'Breakout' was destroyed altogether. I didn't want to show a romantic and sentimental side which I obviously knew I had. Hiding myself still played a large part in my work.

BREAKDOWN MORNING
Variations on a Theme

Right: A late development on 'Falling'. Using a plaster bandage over a prepared card structure mounted on board. In high relief it relies on oblique lighting to show form.

Below: Another part of the sequence — crawling away from the 'black hole'.

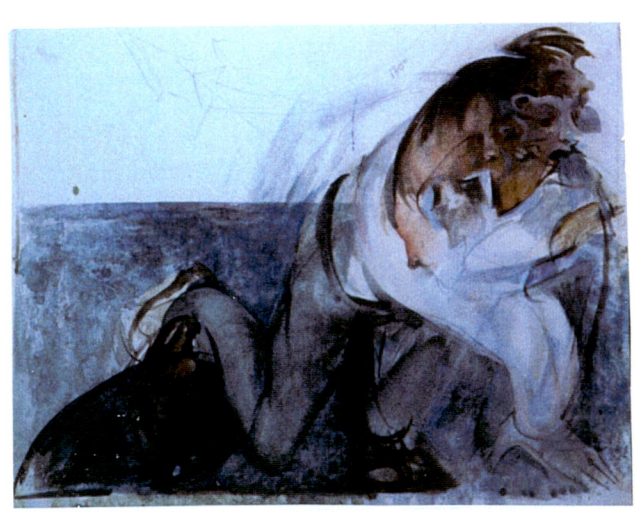 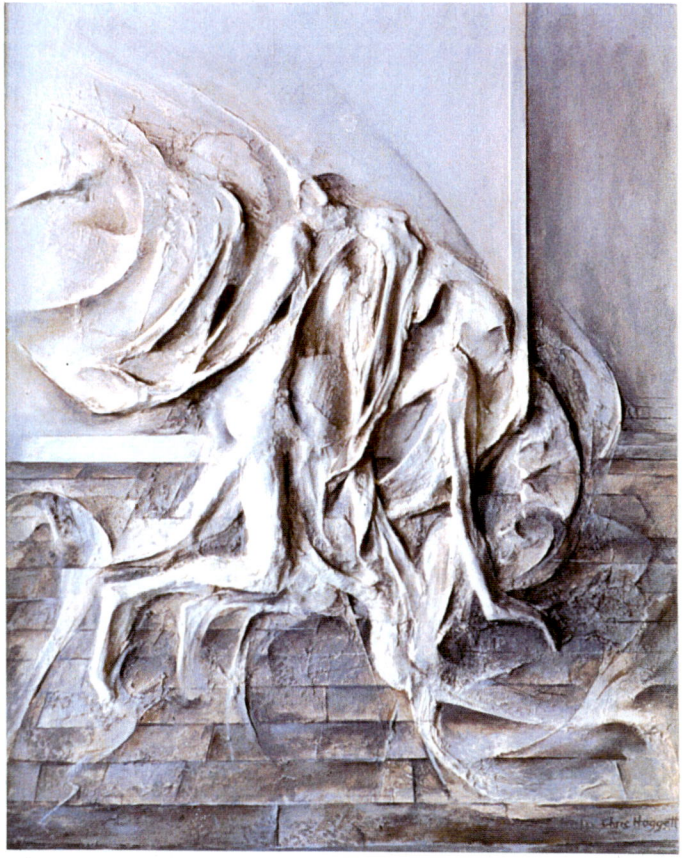

Fig.35 Out of the Black Hole   Watercolour   Fig.36   Freefall (The final statement)   Relief

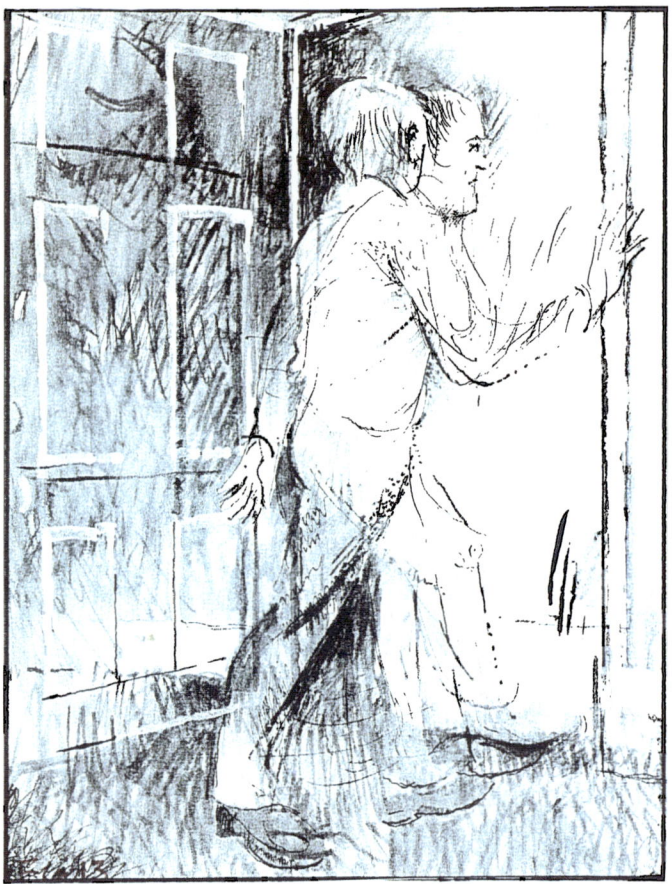

Fig.37. Passing Through - Original Sketch   Crayon

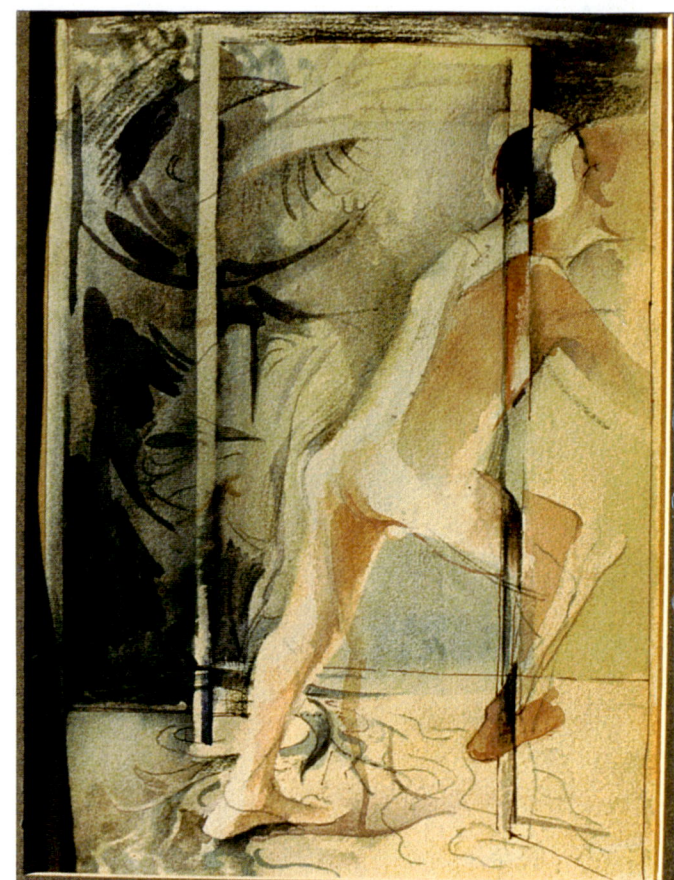

Fig.38 Passing Through - Nude Version. Watercolour

Variations on a Theme – Pausing, then Passing through the Doorway

Top Left: First sketch – looking both ways then exiting right.

Bottom Left: Falling through. Collapse of figure and doorframe.

Top Right: Nude version with heightened drama of threatening shadow.

Bottom Right: Strong emphasis of figure's movement towards the sunlight.

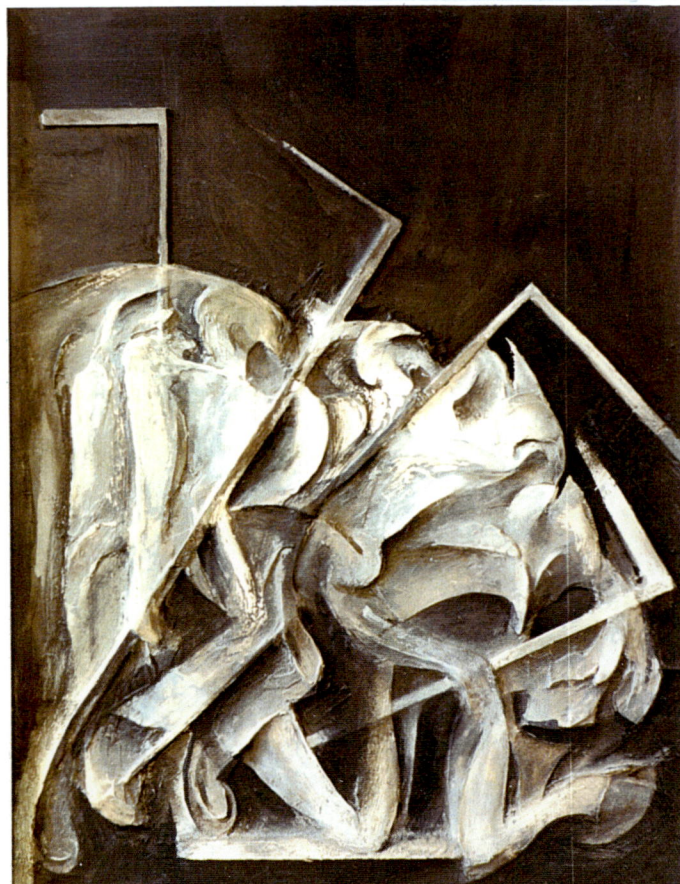

Fig.39. Figure Falling through Doorframe   Relief

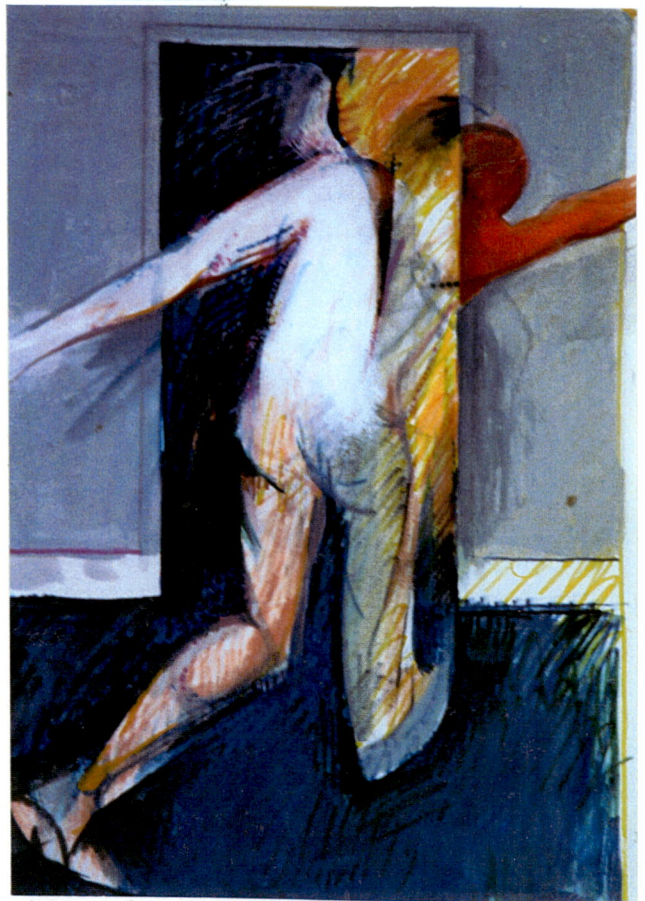

Fig.40. Passing Through.   Mixed Media

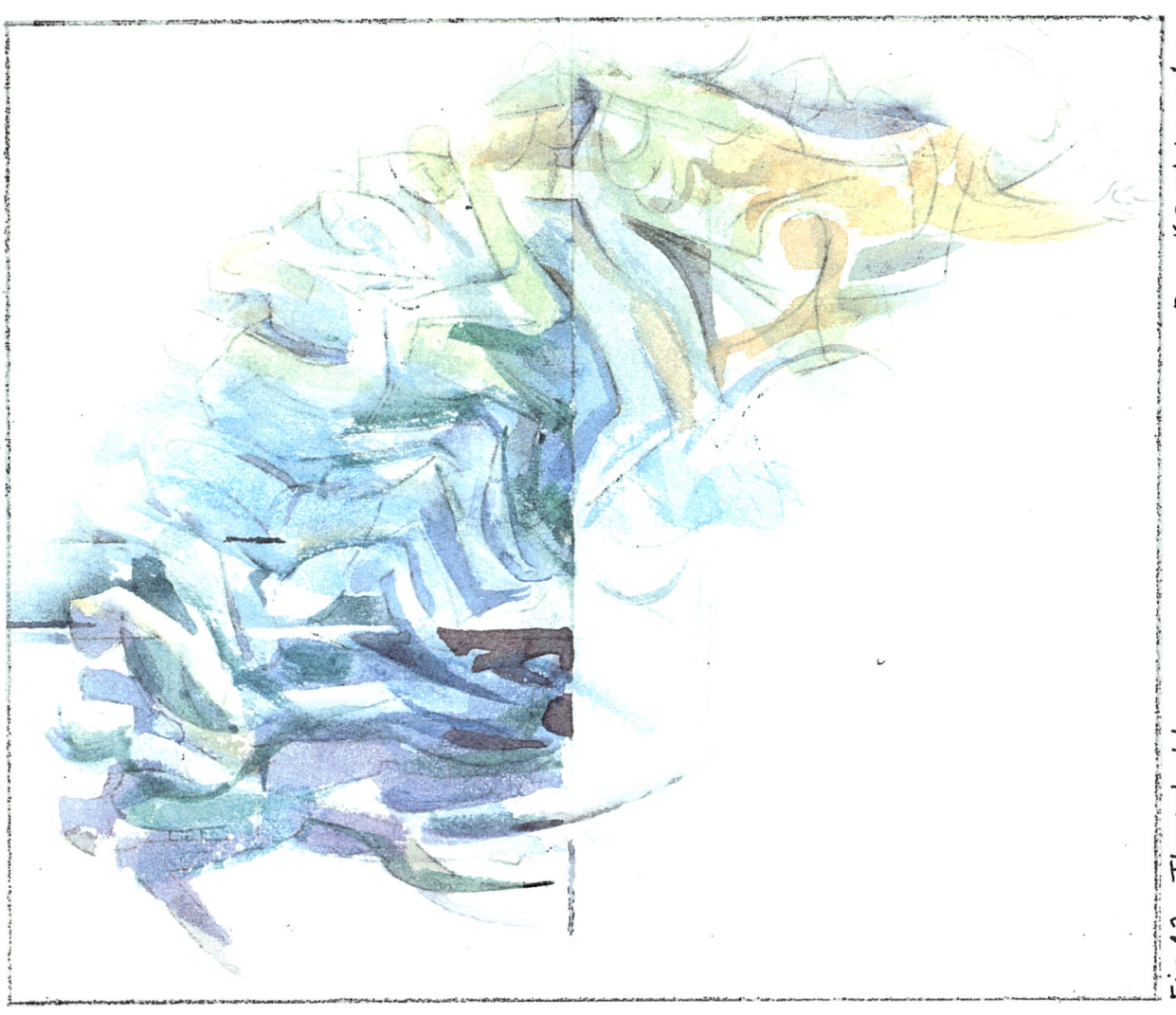

Fig.41 Passing Through - final version Acrylic Relief

Above: The reworking of Fig.32 on page 19. (The figure persists nevertheless in 'passing' in the framed picture).

Fig.42 Threshold Pencil & Watercolour

Above: One of the first sketches exploring the idea of passing into a new environment — including a vertical fall.

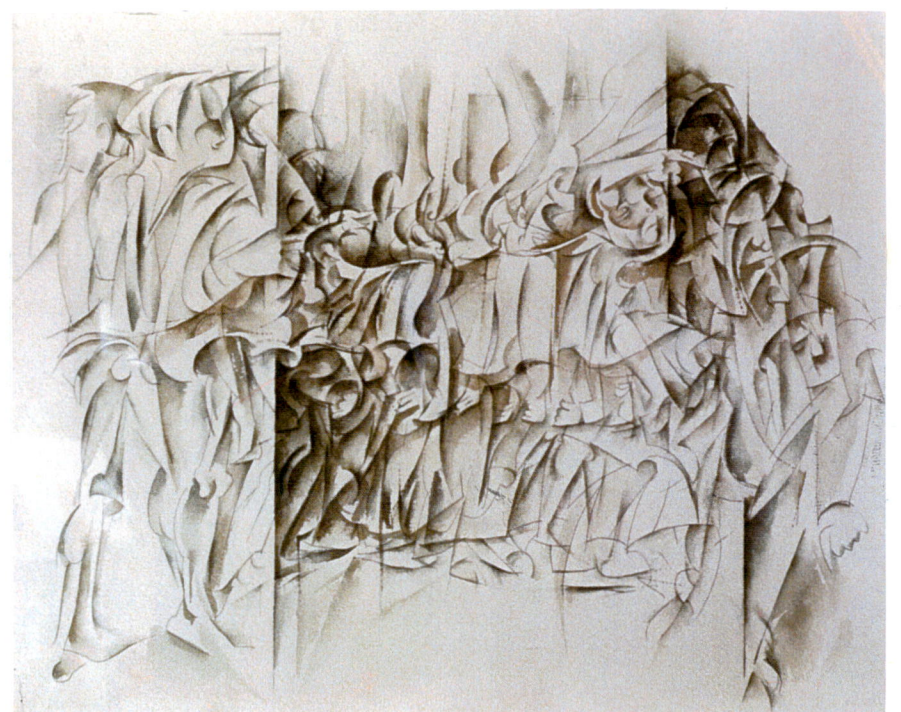

LATE MORNING – RUSHING ON

The 'Crossing the Threshold' sketches (Fig.42) led to the idea of passing through environments and a group of coloured sketches evolved into a few finished works. A lot of restlessness is evident in these later works.

I was all for 'moving on', anxious to reach the next, then the next, etc. – ever searching.... Yet the work itself indicated the effort to understand the situation, trying to recreate the moods of that day in visual terms....

Fig.43 (left) shows vertical planes: kinds of thin partitions or gauzes, where there are moments of hesitation before rushing through towards the next place.

Fig.43 Figure passing through Three Environments   Pencil and Watercolour.

Below: A combination of 'Figure passing through three Environments' with the seated figure in Fig.45. The idea was to stress the anxiety felt by the seated figure as he holds open the door for his subsequent journey into the unknown. – only to find himself back in a chair equally anxious. As he passes through the central 'room' he experiences a brain storm or emotional high as some atmospheric activity surrounds his head. I felt at the time that this was an attempt to convey the emotional swings of mood prevalent at the time. This painting was later destroyed – as a failure.

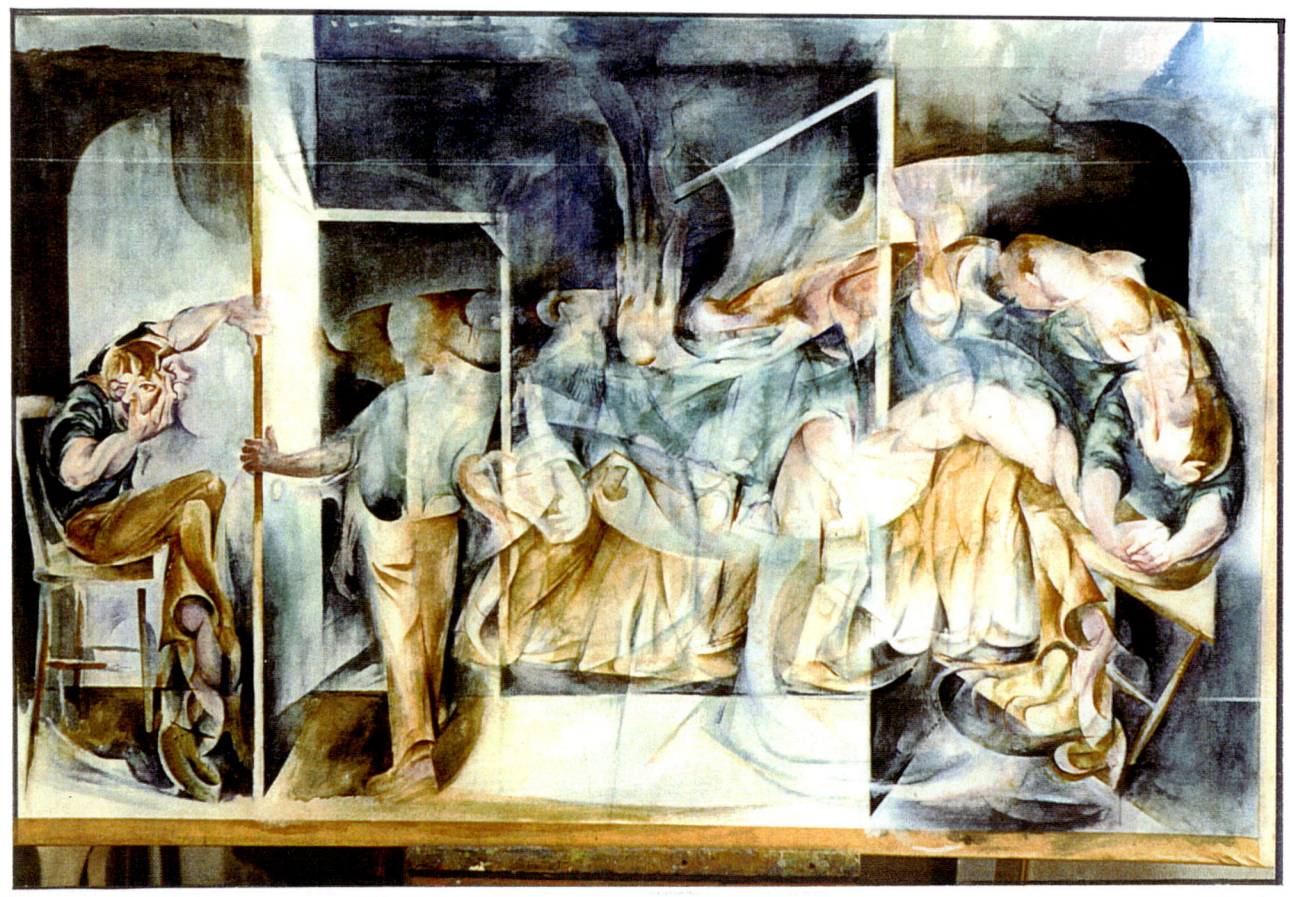

Fig.44   A Psychic Journey   Watercolour

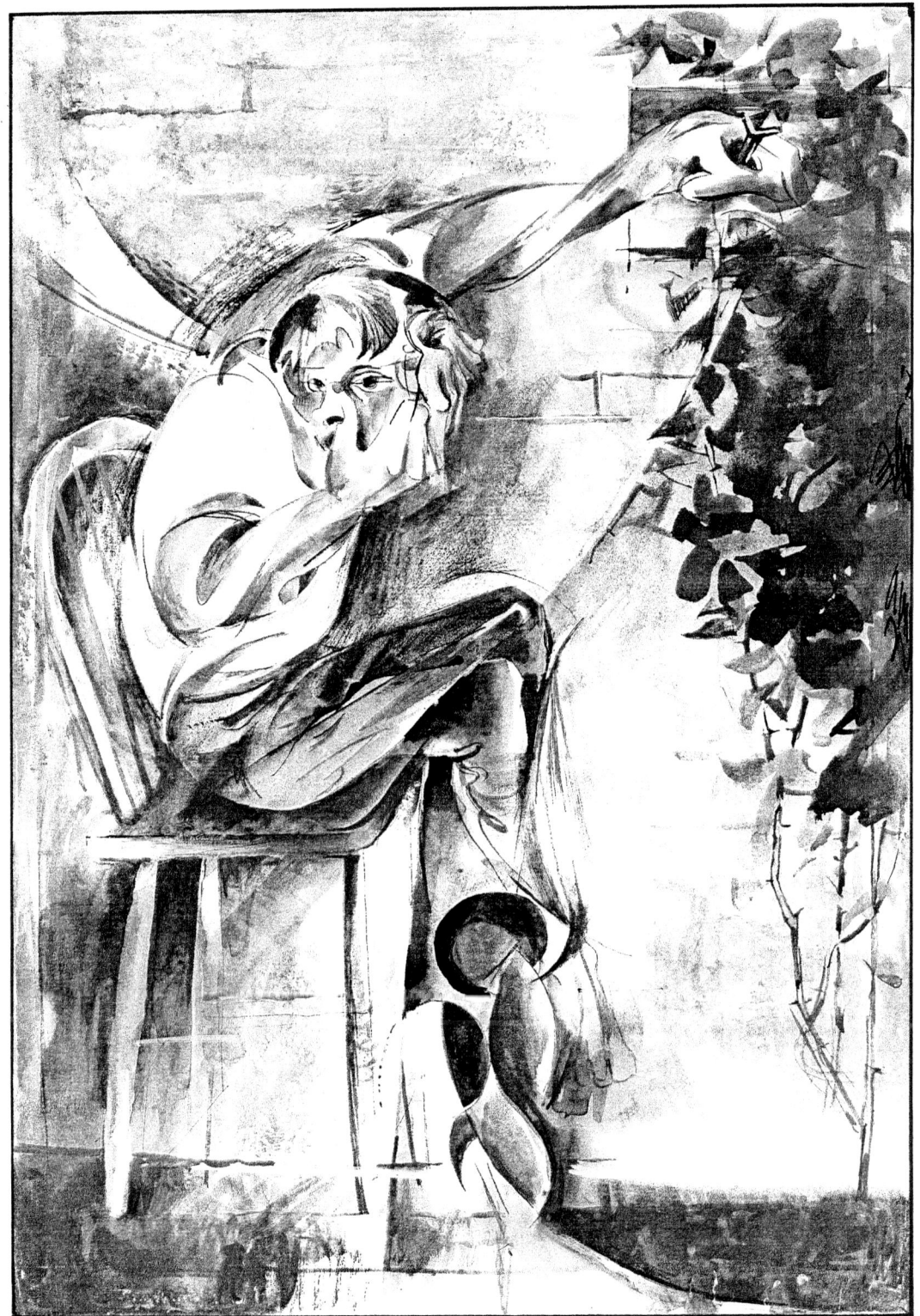

Fig. 45 Figure in a Garden   Watercolour

MIDDAY-IN THE GARDEN

Seated now on the chair at the bottom of the garden, I rest for some moments, anxious and tired. Seeing a wall nail I clutch at it and feel as if involved in a crucifixion - I am crucified. I relax then, until the anxiety returns. The whole figure expresses for me the fear and retention of fear through the distortion of the limbs. The entwining of my legs symbolises the 'screwed-up' tension within - in fact I'm inclined to screw down into the earth, hiding from unknown implications relating to the breakdown.

The hand gripping the side of the face hints at the pulling away of one of the many masks I'd created over many years, protecting my vulnerabilities and feelings of inadequacy.   A sense of change is imminent.

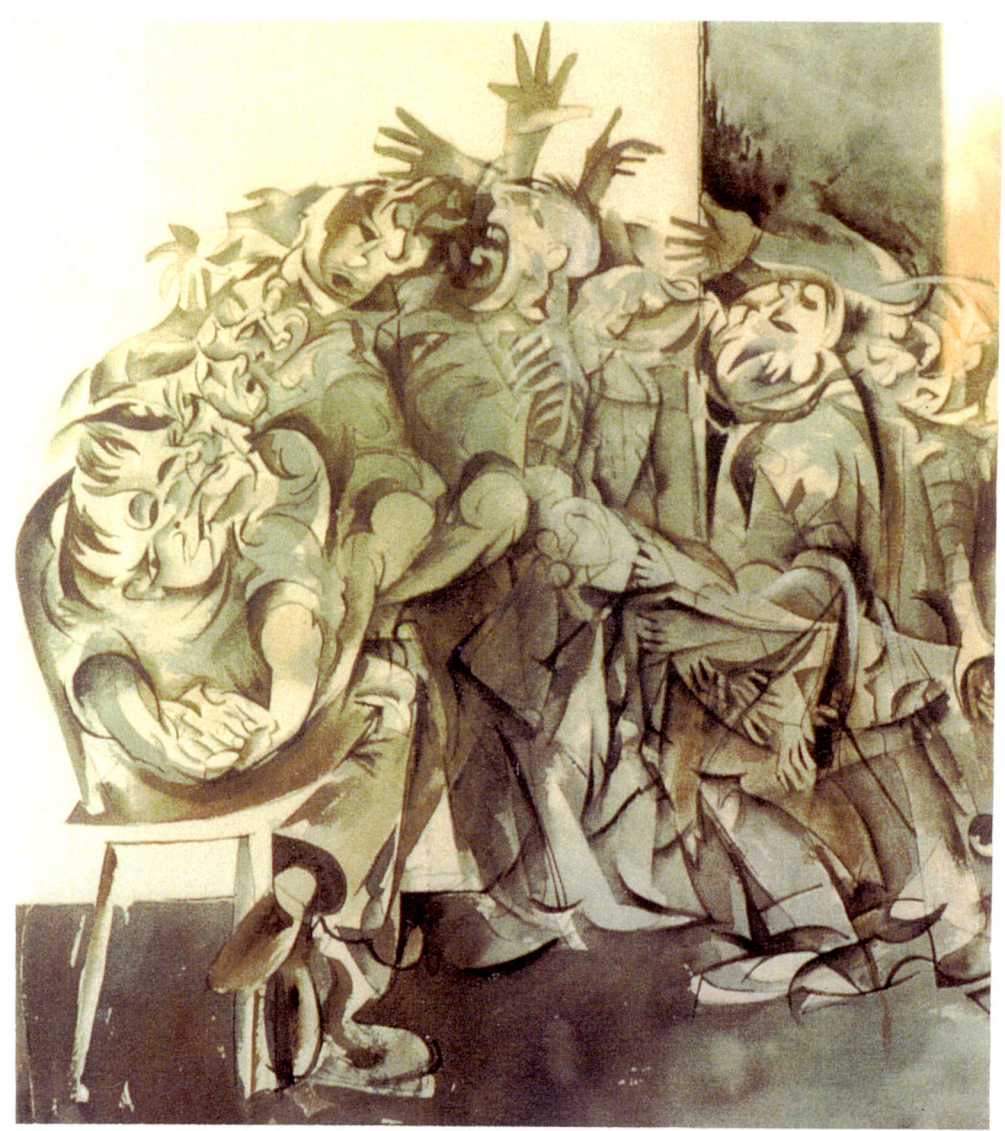

Fig.46 Figure falling into a Chair Pencil & Watercolour

FIGURE FALLING INTO A CHAIR

The chair position and direction of the figures contradict the other paintings on this theme of collapsing into a chair. Now moving from right to left it feels 'odd' as if deliberately going against the grain - or was this the point......

The movements, gestures are theatrical: faces scream, look anguished, heads turn upside down (echo of Chagall); hands take flight, flutter or are wrung in distress. I think this was the final expression of the garden experience, or ideas and images arising from it. Painted many months, possibly a year later.

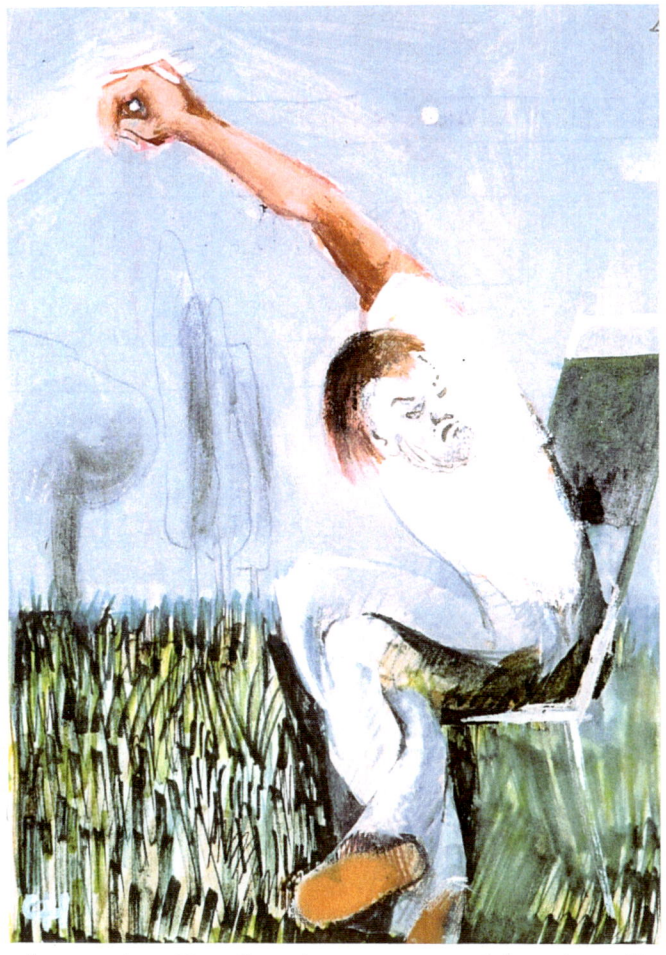

Fig.47. A walk along a Pavement.   Acrylic Paste

AFTERNOON - MOVING ONWARDS

Fig.47. Departure from the garden into the street. Walking along the pavement I sense that the surface is unstable, that the flagstones move as a wave, rising slightly, tilting downwards then rising again. I must be careful not to trip up and fall in.

Fig.48. Further thoughts on the garden scene. The wall has vanished - now aware only of the large nail, suspended in space by psychic determination.....

Fig.49. Crossing the road as swiftly as possible before the Macadam melts and I'm swallowed into its black depths.
There is a feelings of persecution, that perhaps I'm an alien creature.....

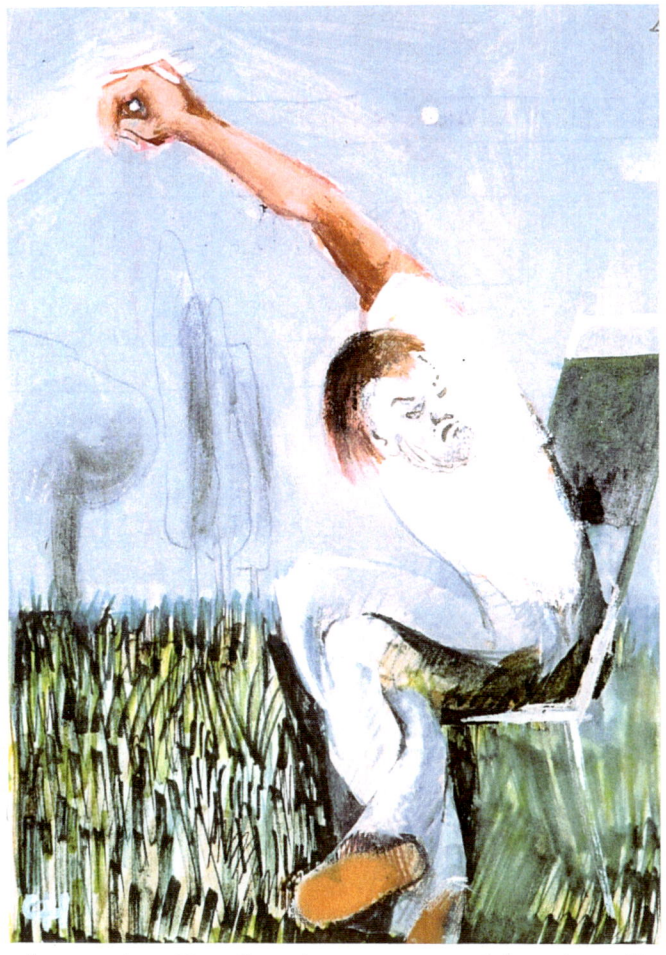

Fig.48. In the Garden   Mixed Media

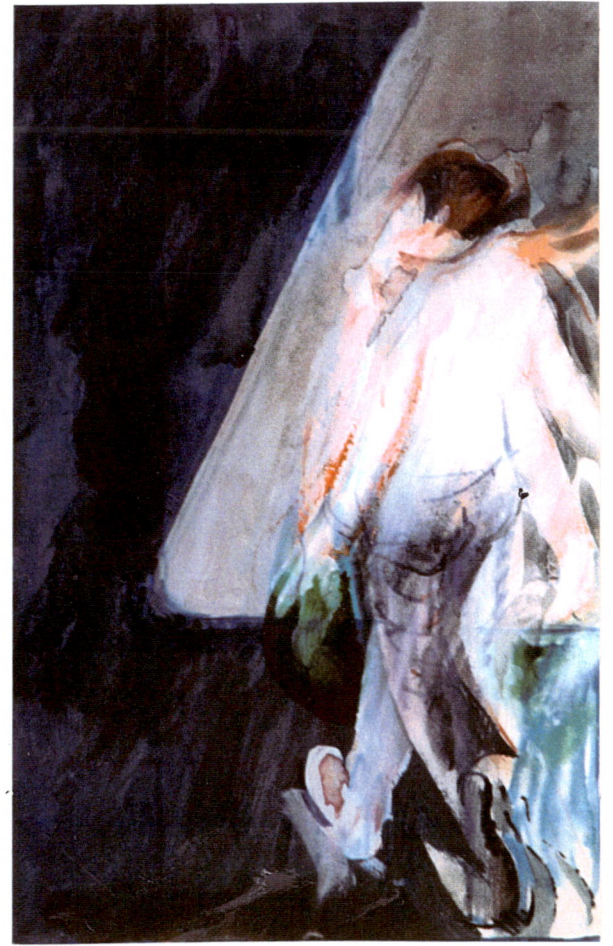

Fig.49. A walk across the Road. Mixed Media

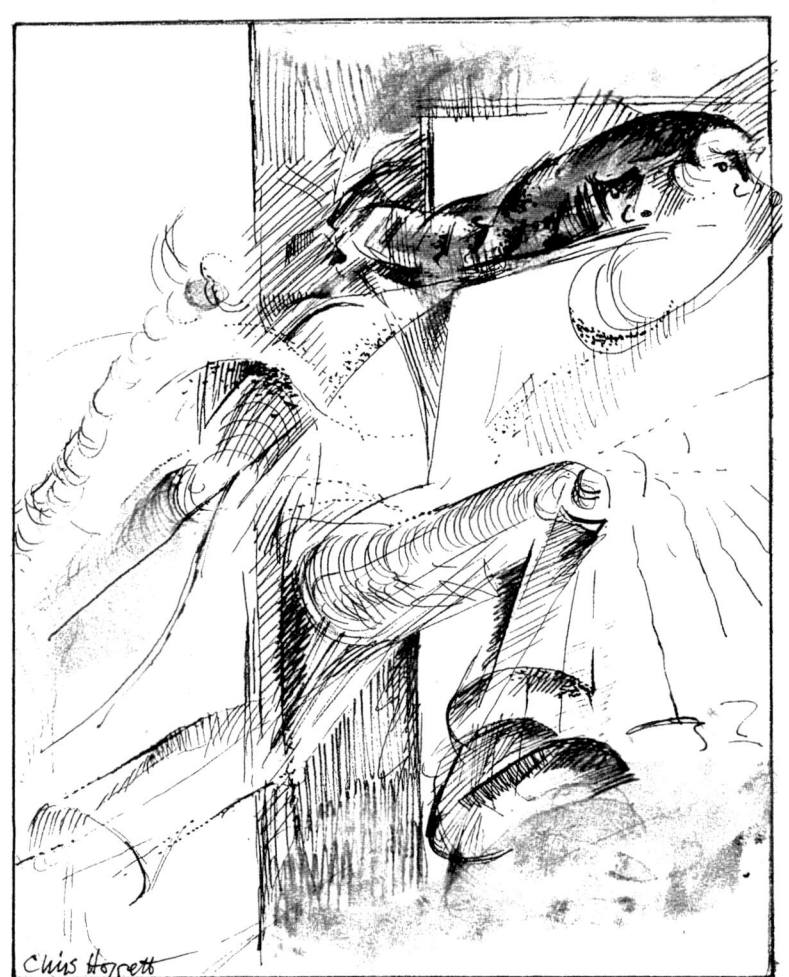

Fig.50 Escaping the Wall. Pen & Ink

EVENING

Having settled quietly for the evening in a friend's house I hoped for a quiet evening but the internalised activities continued. Escaping from a hitherto unknown darkness, my mind seemed to act like a film projector, showing repeated images of flight and escape - but hopefully into a more restful environment.

Frequently a narrow space between two walls, through which I have to pass seems to close. Perhaps I will be squashed between them?

A feeling of claustrophobia seems closely linked to this narrow space, (see dream 2 and illustrations on pages 83 and 84).

Fig.51 : Hints of an additional fear begin to take hold - of my hand!
A coat I keep dragging behind me transforms itself into a wolf-like head holding on to my fingers.

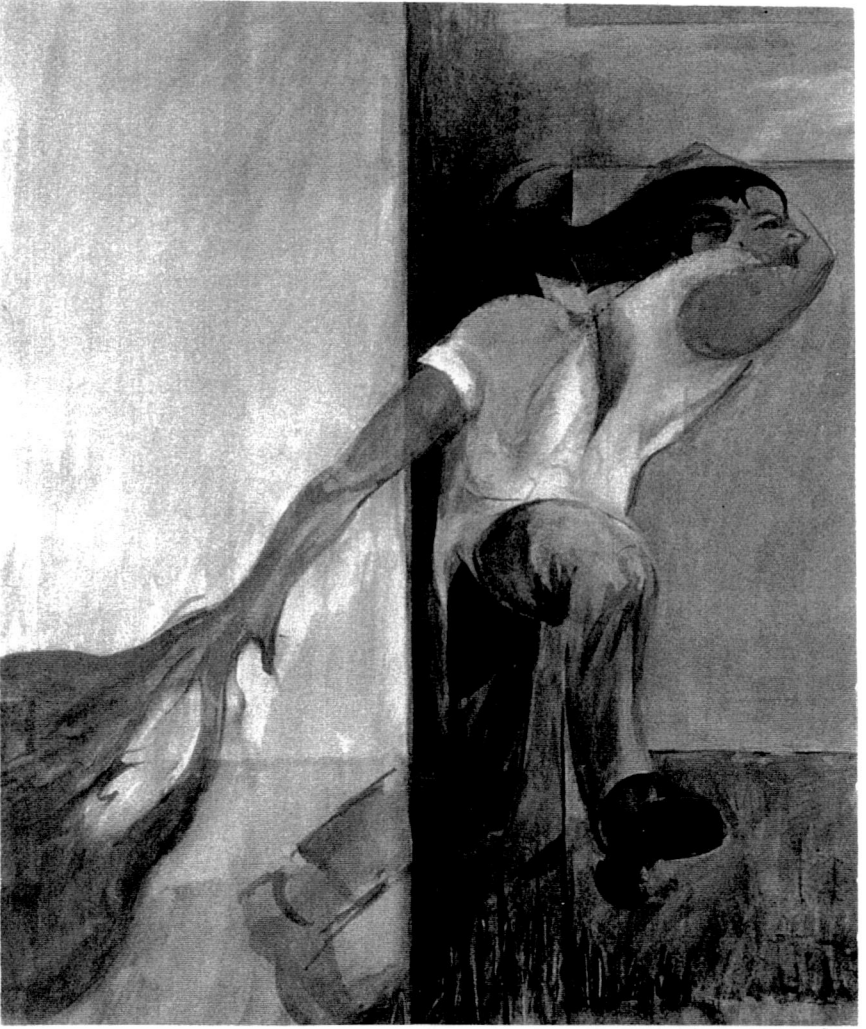

Fig.51 The Trailing Jacket. Watercolour

NIGHT AND BEDTIME
(end of a Breakdown day)

These sketches sum up the mood at the end of the day - the night hours of sleeplessness.
The foetal curved position expresses the infantile vulnerability, hugging the self.

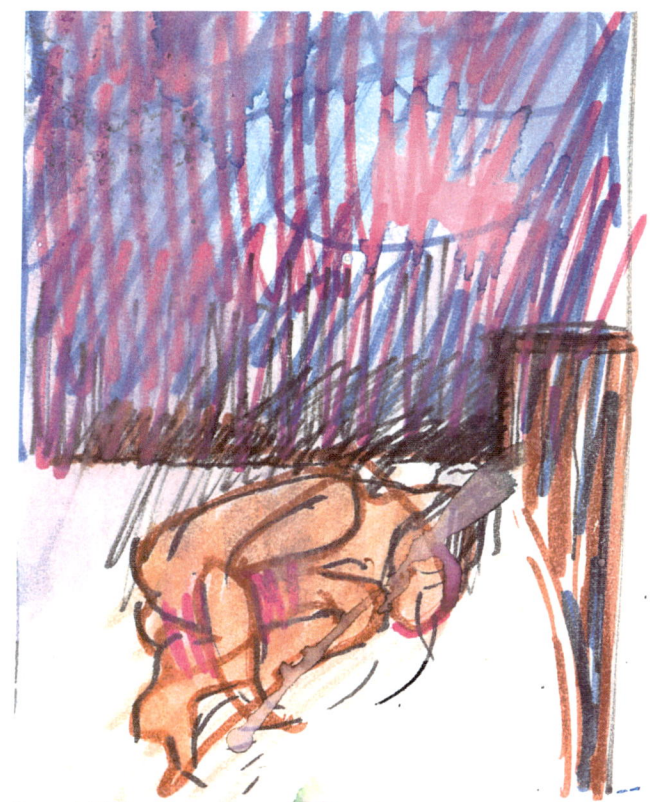

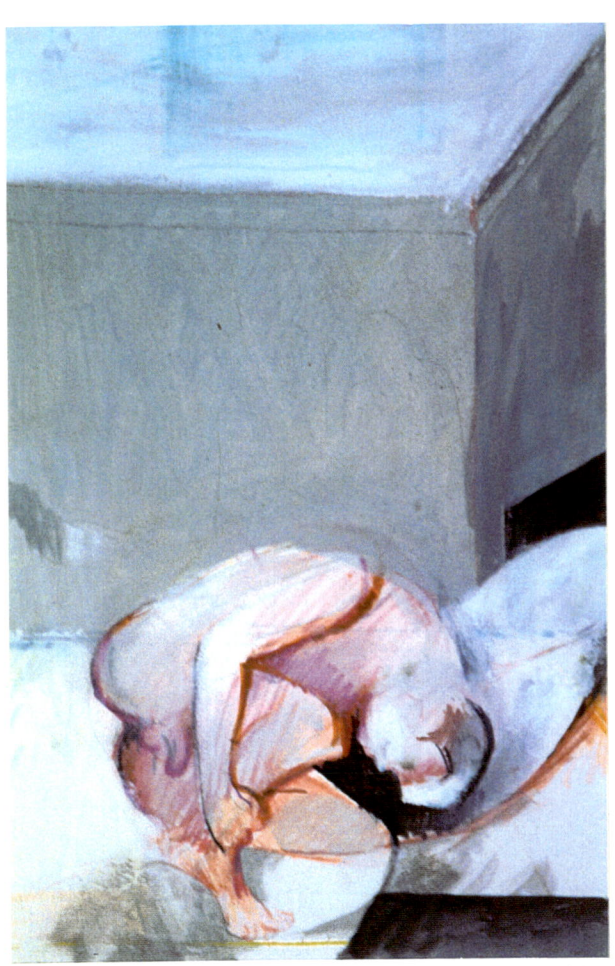

Fig.52. Foetal Curved   Mixed Media

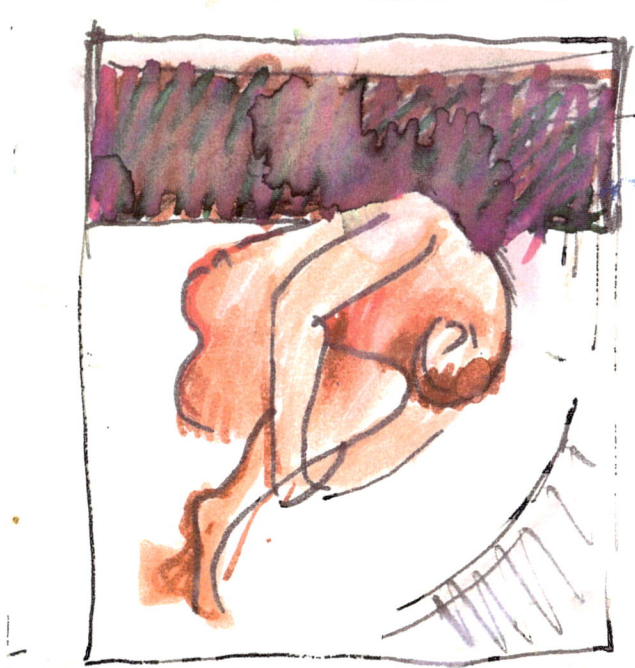

Fig.53 Two Sketches   Coloured Inks

Lack of sleep continued for some time, certainly for many weeks until I was advised to seek help, have controlled medication, sleep properly and slow down to awaken like Rip van Winkle, refreshed. However I rejected all this, chose a more laboured way out of the problem, sketching occasionally, walking a lot until I found a pattern of normal sleep again.
The sections which follow are more or less in chronological order but having never kept a diary and only occasionally dated my work, there is an element of guesswork involved. What is certain is that all the events occurred approximately at this time in the eighties and many of the moods and feelings recorded in visual terms, some obsessively repeated, usually because the 'happenings' seemed significant at that time.

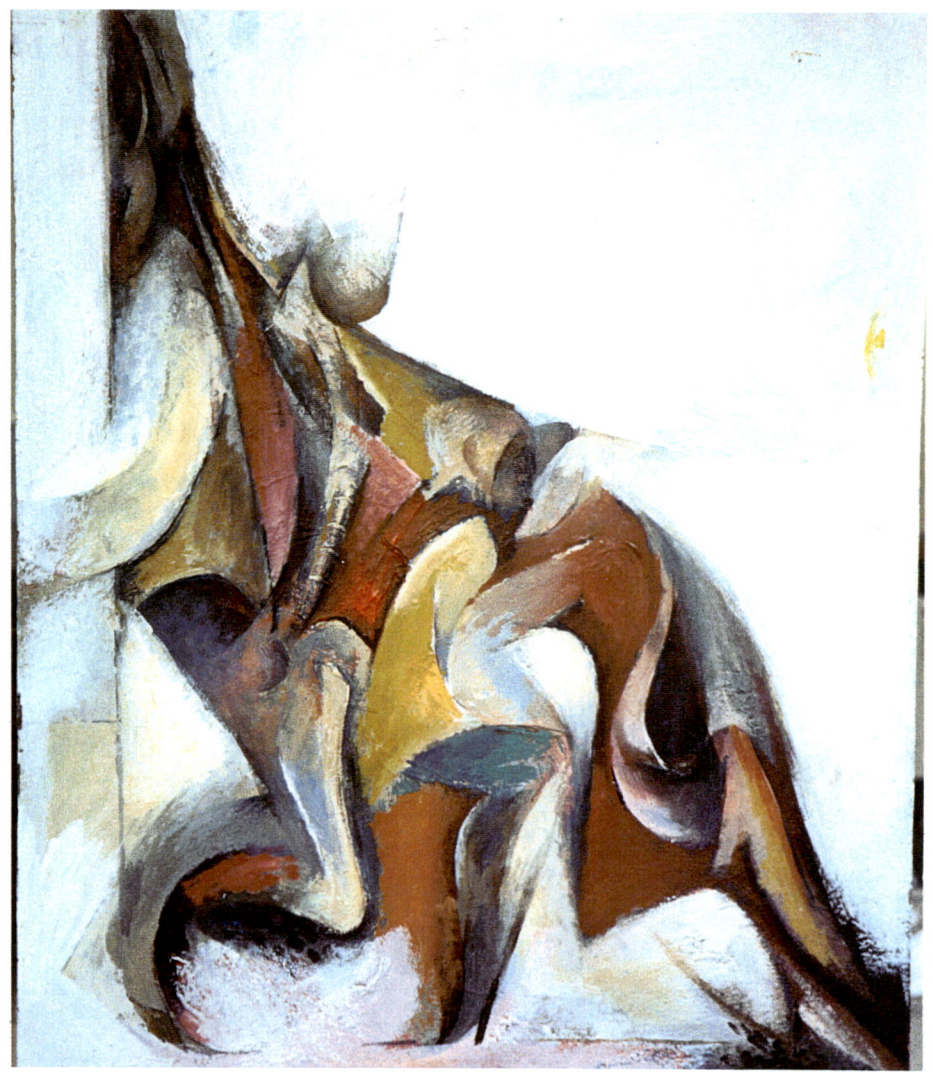

Fig.54   Re-working of Fig 31. (Unfinished)   Oil on Board

An almost total obliteration of the original painting (Fig 31) except for the spinal column and femur of the central left figure. At the time of re-painting the early version seemed to convey something of the flickering mood swings of that morning (a jester's headpiece, a mask and the skeletal parts of mortality). Two years later this more abstract version corrected what I thought had been too complicated and 'fussy'. A mistake. It's usually better to work from the original idea in order to make comparisons — it may then lead to a third version with further interesting developments. No matter, this possible error of judgement helped to remind me not to rush into unnecessary re-workings on top of old pictures.

VARIATION ON A THEME - 1

Right: 'Celestial Freefall'. A nebulous skyscape with a falling figure — seen as either man or bird. Stars, planets and raging winds surround the figure.

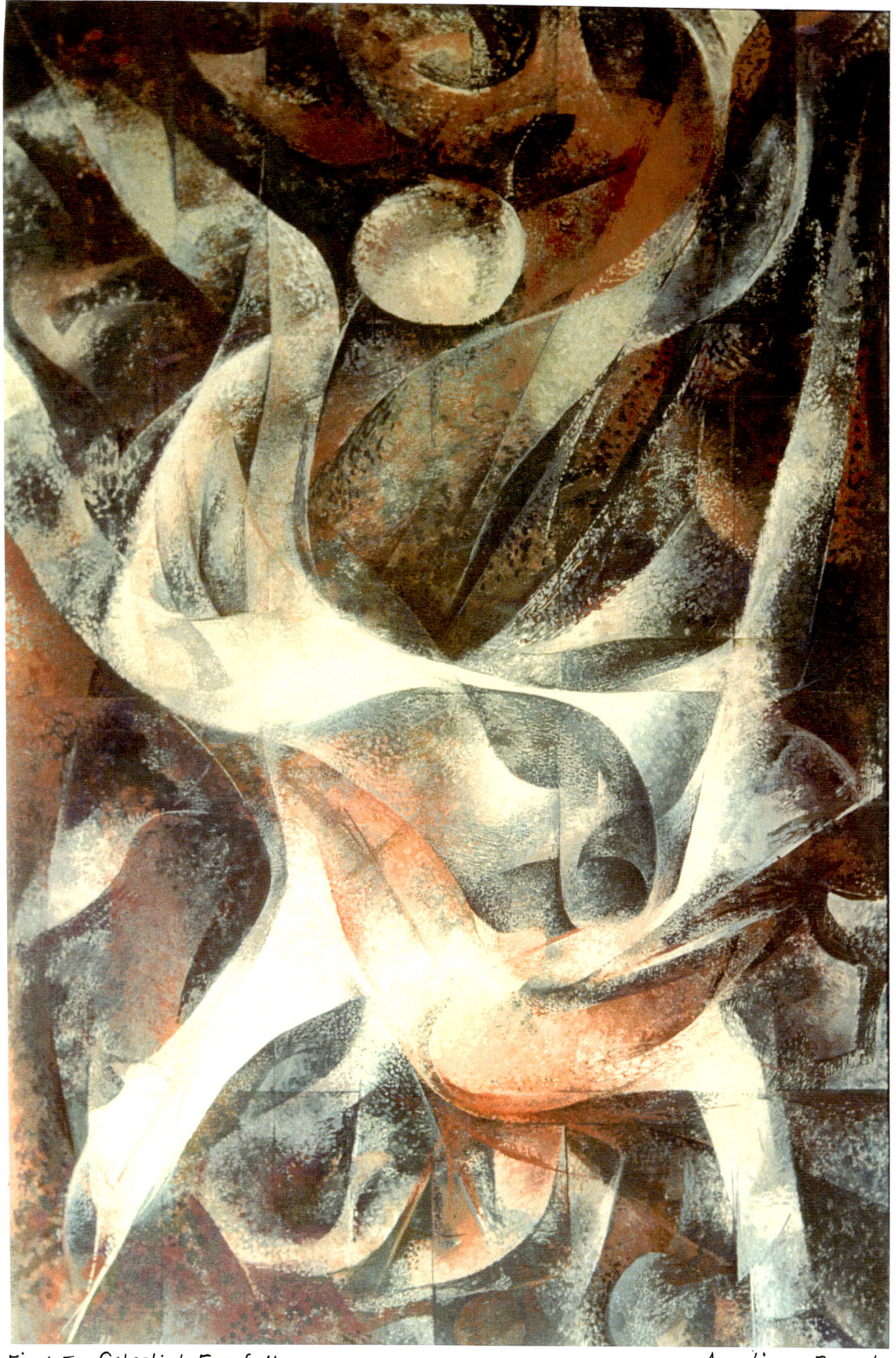

Fig 55 Celestial Freefall   Acrylic on Board

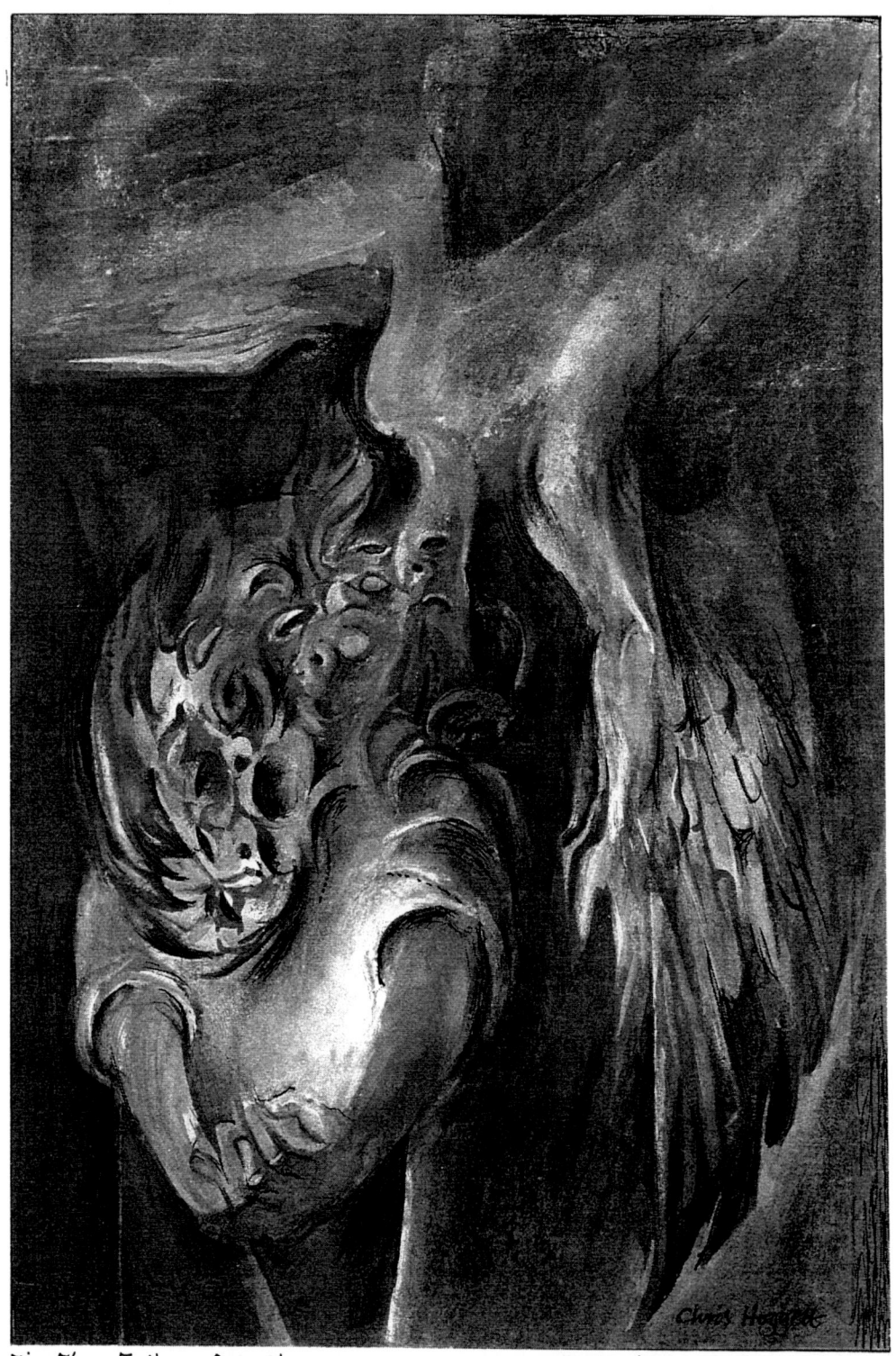

Fig 56 Fallen Angel   Watercolour & Gouache

VARIATION ON A THEME – 2

'Fallen Angel'. No particular crime or misdemeanour came to mind when this was painted, unless despair could be seen as an aspect of guilt. This seems to be expressed through the angel's contorted features empathising with that of the anguished self.

PERIPHERAL VISIONS 1981-1983

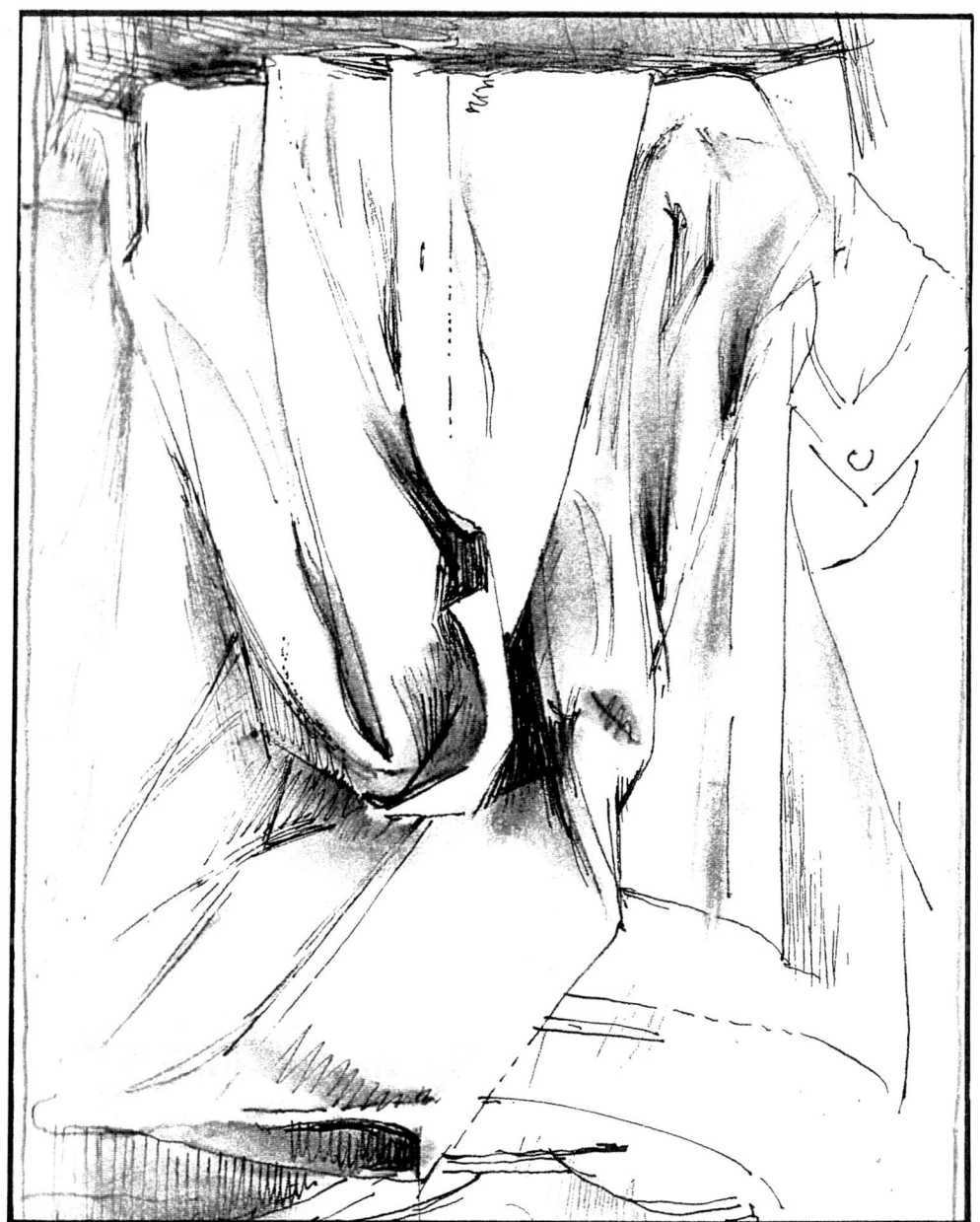

Fig. 57   The Basic Stuff (discarded clothing)   Pen & Wash

Morning depressions frequently led to periods of lassitude, diminishing drive and energy and consequently longer moments of staying in bed. With a reluctance to read, or listen to the radio, I'd gaze abstractly at nothing in particular, allowing an unfocused vision to meander about the room. One morning with this peripheral way of looking I was surprised to find a figure slumped in the chair at the end of the bed and instantly re-focused onto a heap of casually discarded clothing from the evening before.
 I now deliberately repeated the experience, unfocused and then focused — I found the apparition again.
 This experience recalled many 'day dreams' from the past, like Leonardo's images from old walls, seeing creatures in clouds and similar transformations. All common enough and therefore not of much importance — except these clothing images occurred so often as to signal a need to record each 'transformation' which echoed a sub-conscious mood so accurately. The 'slumped' cloth reflected the 'slumpiness' within my inner lassitude......
 After the first few 'visions', I kept the chair in the same position and sketched other 'cast-offs'. This continued for many months until the interest flagged and the transformations ceased......

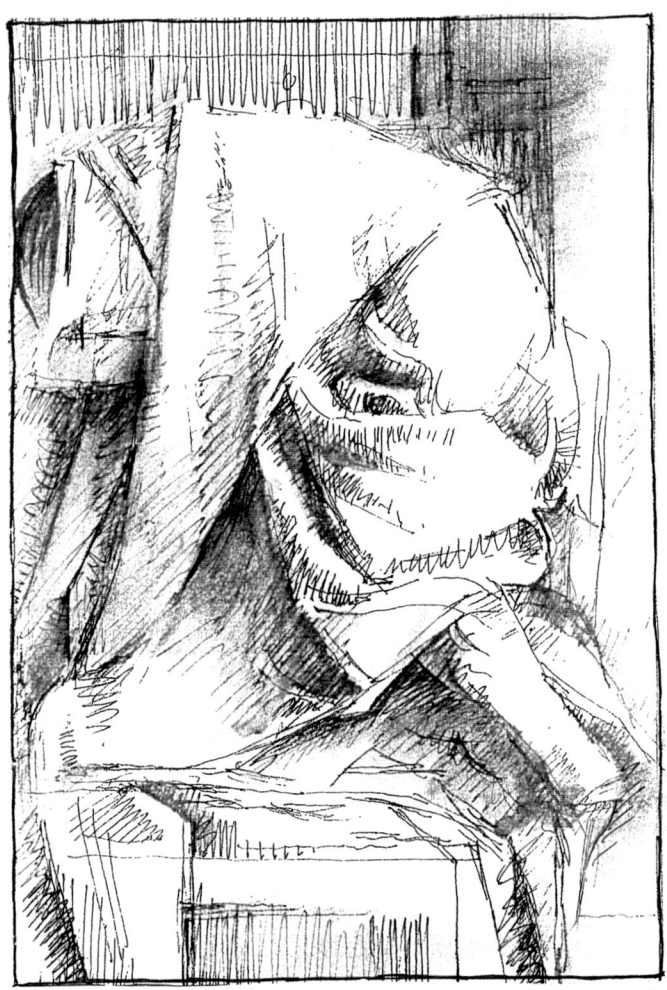

Fig. 58 Slumped - N° 1   Pen & Wash

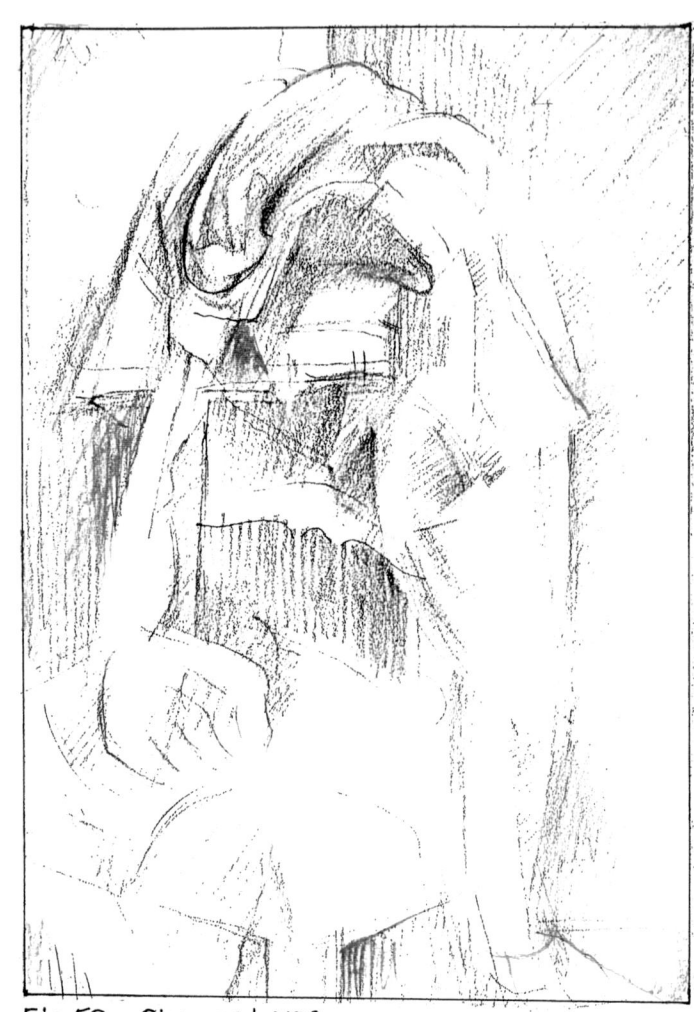

Fig. 59 - Slumped - N° 2   Chalk

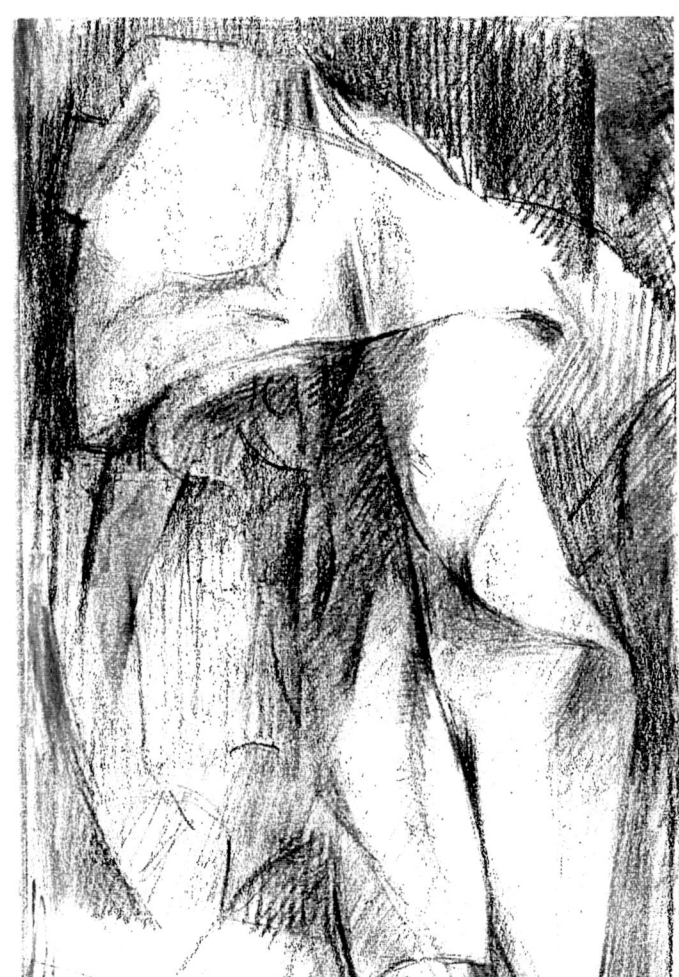

Fig. 60 - Slumped - N° 3   Chalk

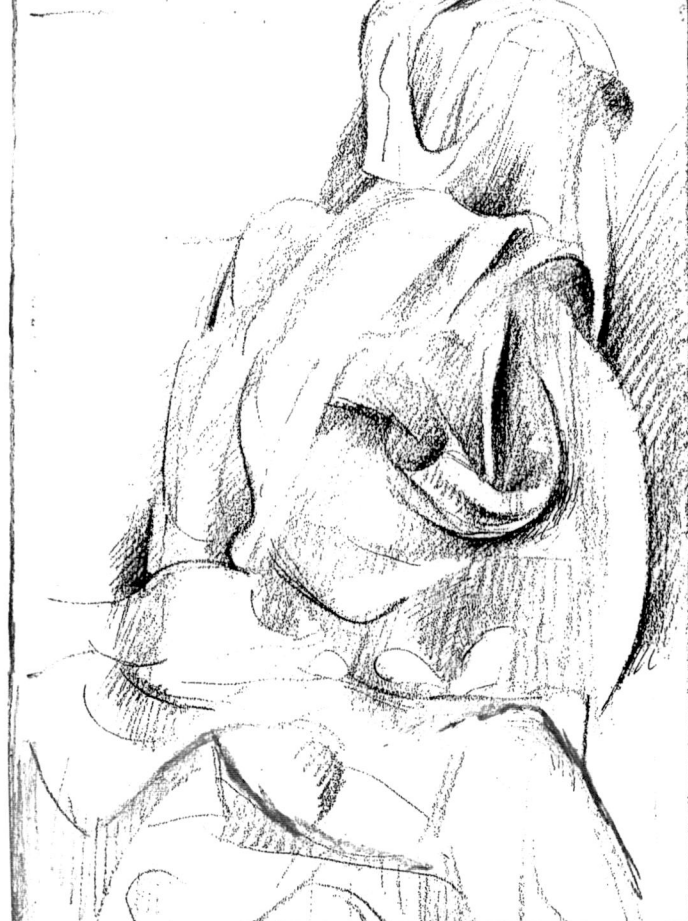

Fig. 60A Untitled   Chalk

All the sketches of clothing fell into two categories: 1 - anthropomorphic heads and figures, or 2 - animal and bird forms. Sheets rumpled on the bed assumed the forms of landscape: fields, hills or lakes.

All seemed to reflect some inner need — perhaps a search for the sources of this deep confusion and ambiguity. Whatever, the whole group of drawings of which this selection represents about half, came to be a great therapeutic help at this time....

Fig.57 (page 31) 'The Basic Stuff' - shirt, trousers over back of chair - no obvious 'inner' vision.

Figs 58-60. Variations on 'slumped over' figure reflecting the inner feelings.

Fig.60A. Figure more erect, head lifted up.

Fig.61. 'Melancholic Face', reminding me of a former tutor - John Milton.

Fig.62. A head with a pensive, questioning look - a touch more optimistic.

Fig.63. A curious bundle, until I 'recognise' a clown's face appearing from behind - felt a more hopeful time ahead when I saw this.

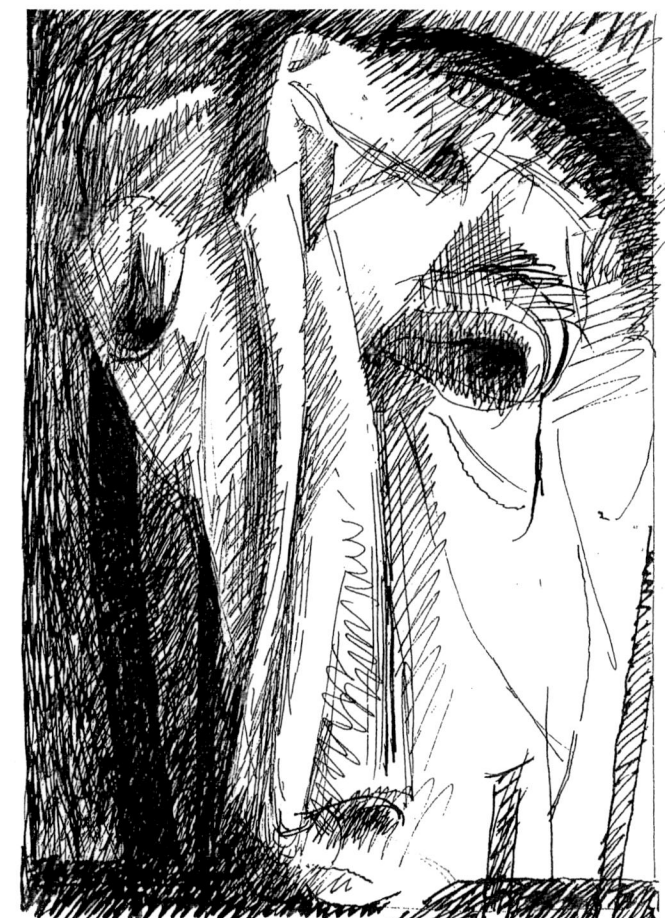

Fig.61 Melancholic Face — Pen & Ink

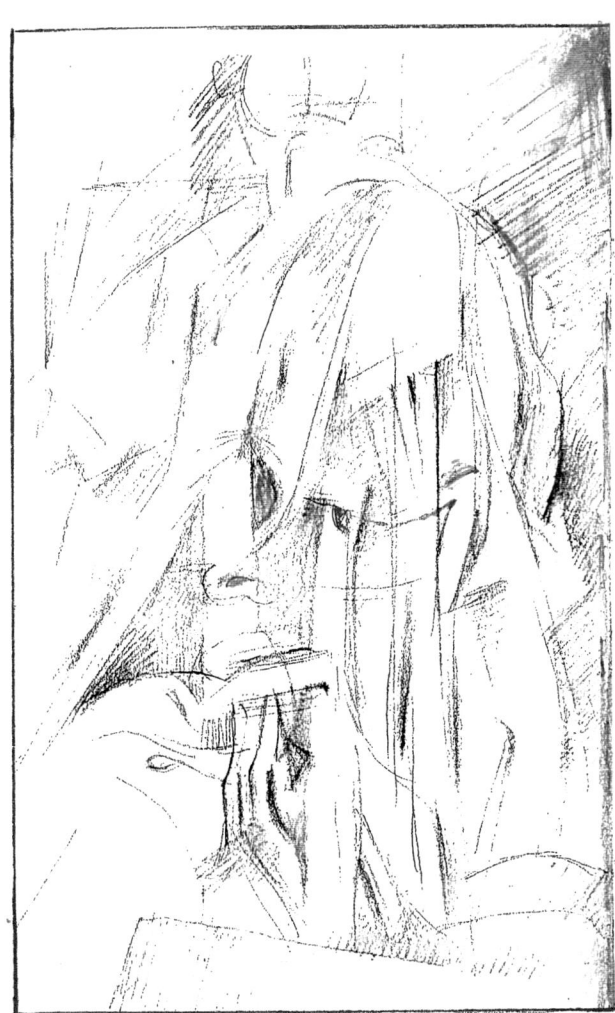

Fig.62 Pensive Head — Pencil

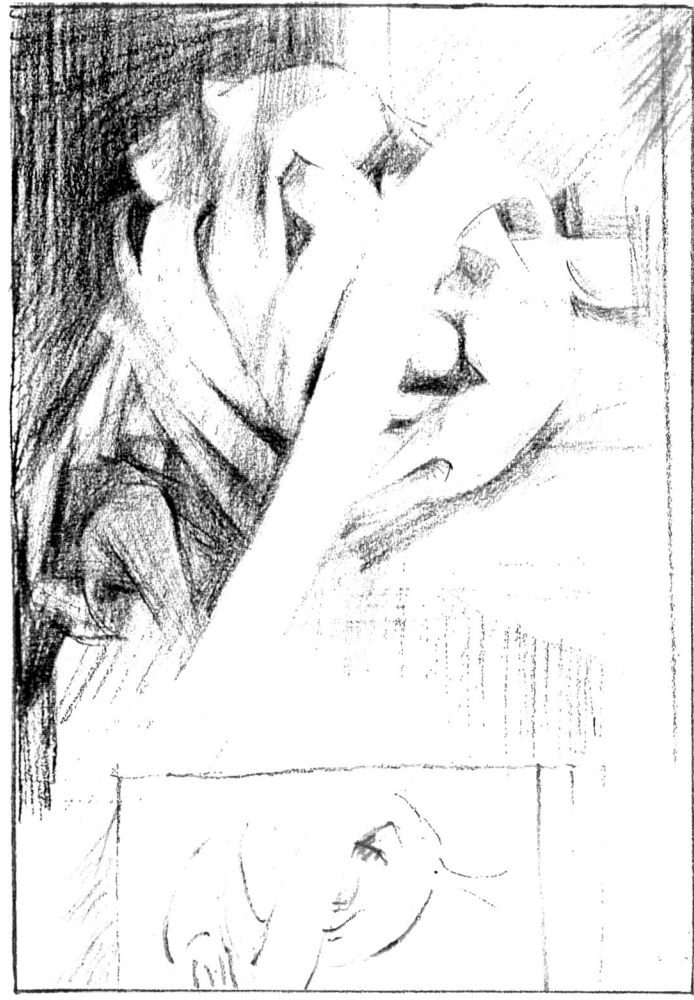

Fig.63 Bandaged Clown Face — Chalk

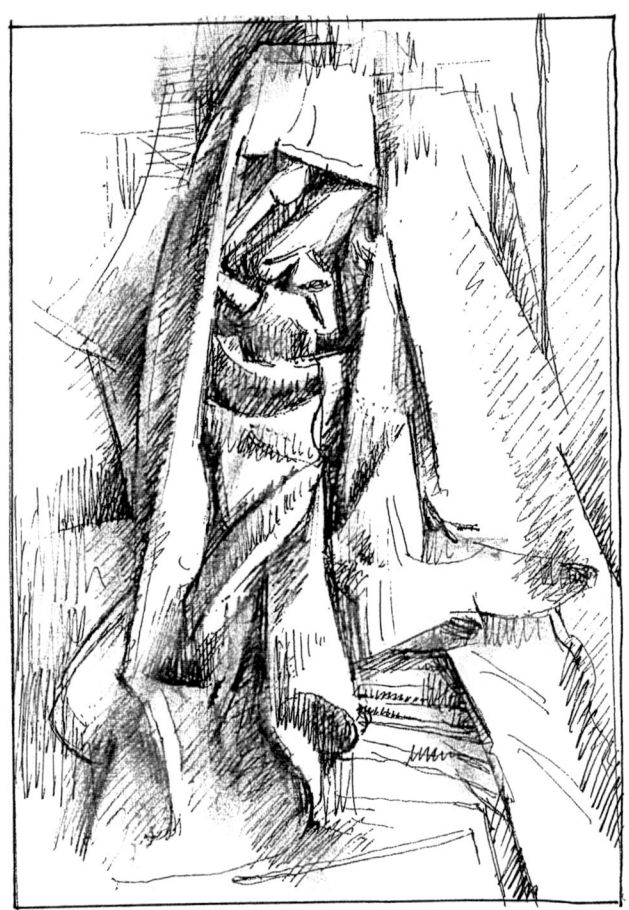

Fig. 64 Water Turbulence   Pen & Ink

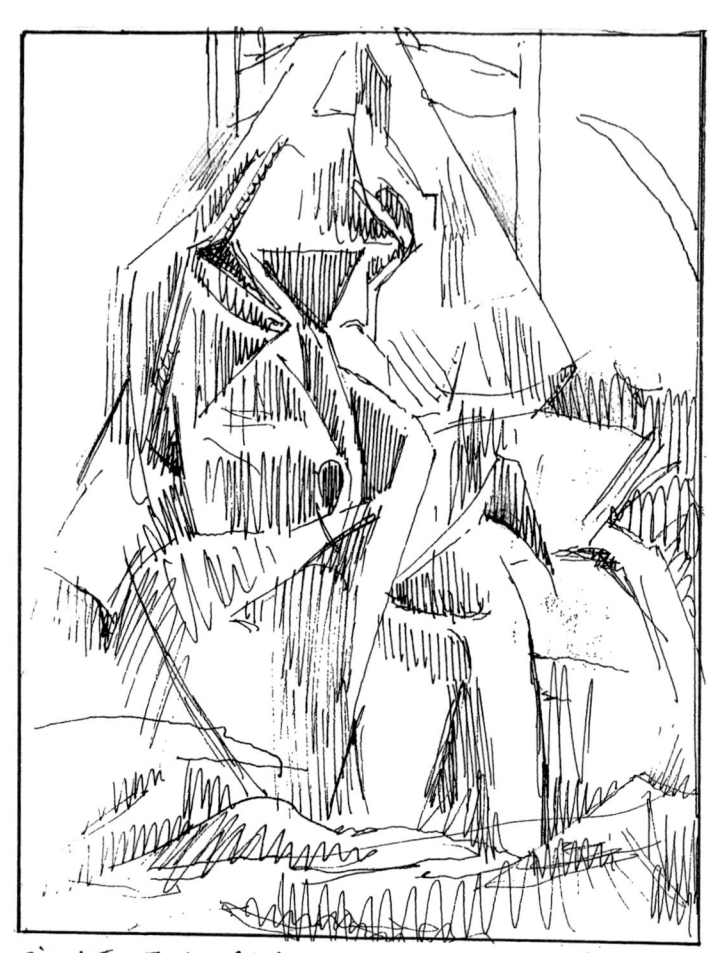

Fig. 65 Fall of Water   Pen & Ink

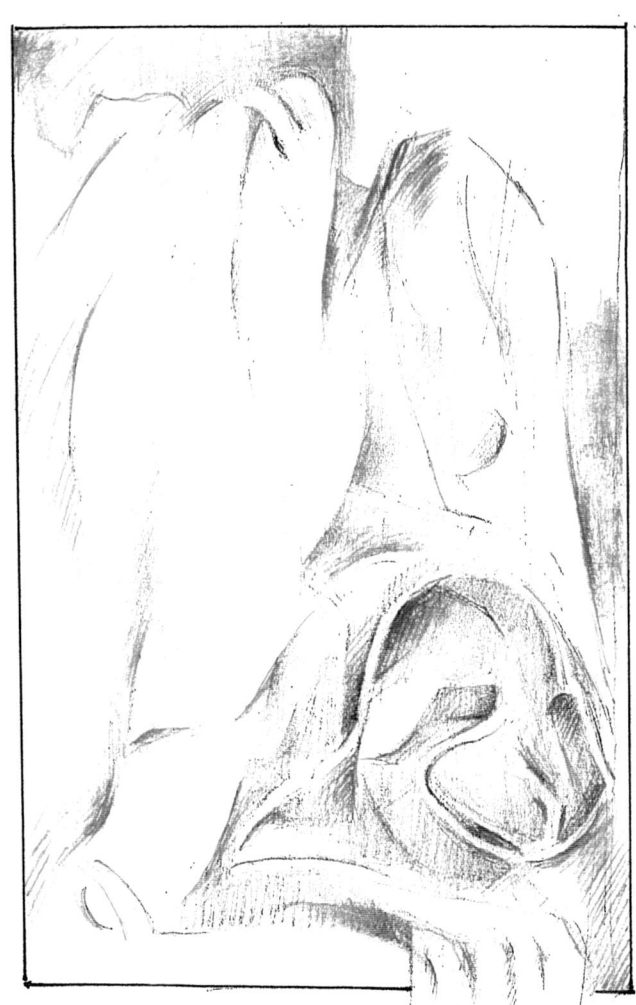

Fig. 66 Canine - or Vampire   Chalk

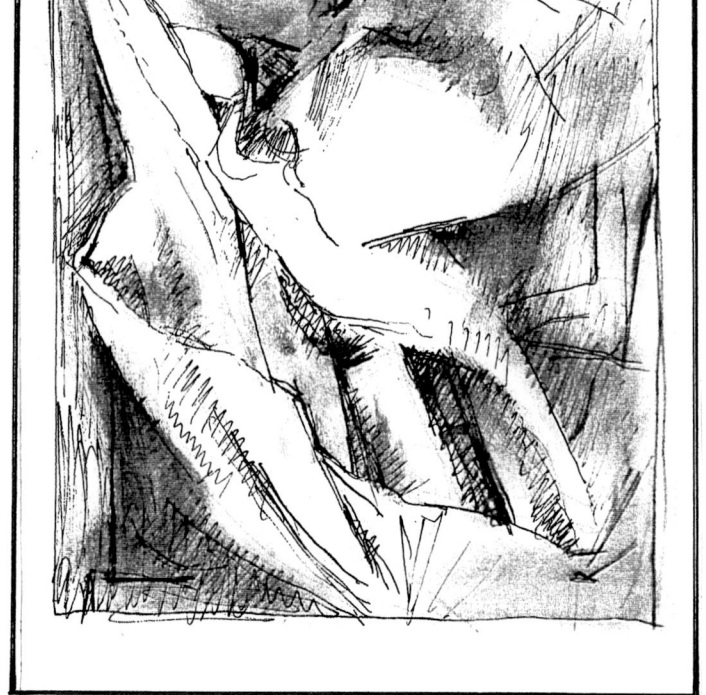

Fig. 67 A Mystery Figure   Ink & Chalk

WATER · FIGURES · ANIMALS · BIRDS

An assortment of 'findings' - I feel each of them as an 'entertainment' when completed - they all seem to express internalised moods and anxieties.

Figs 64-65. Forces of nature, cascading between banks, a swift river. Also, a waterfall spreading out down rocks.

Fig. 66. A canine form - or a vampire with towering wings.

Fig. 67. Sinister fragments of what.....? It's the unknown which disturbs.......

Fig. 68. Another slumping figure, yet bovine (because of horns?).

Fig. 69. A powerful image: the open end of a sleeve forms the head of a bird of prey.

Fig. 70. A large owl form.

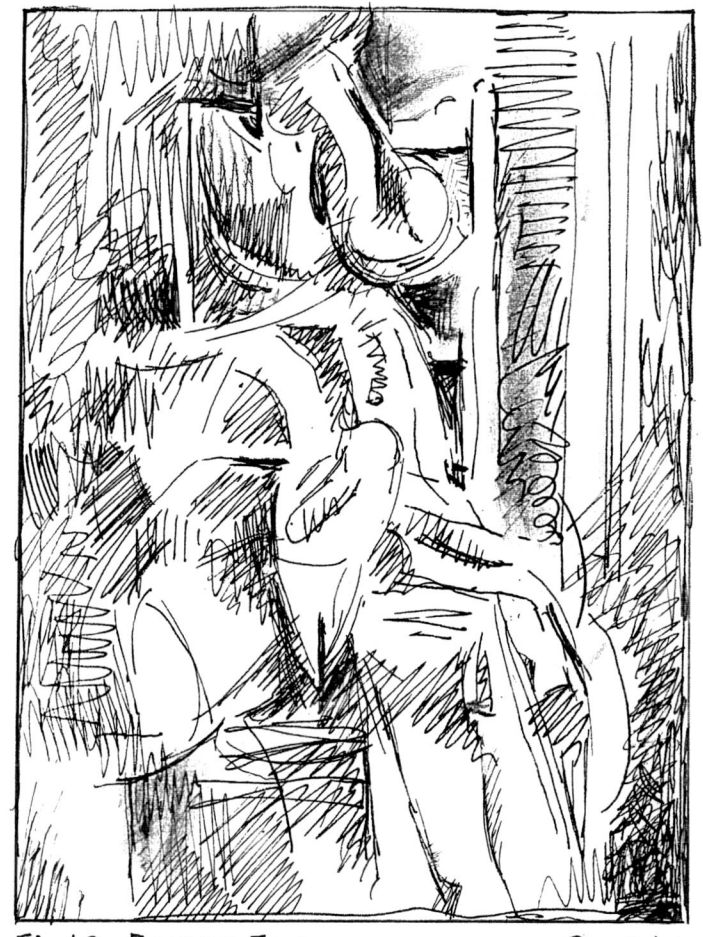

Fig. 68 Bovine Form — Pen & Ink

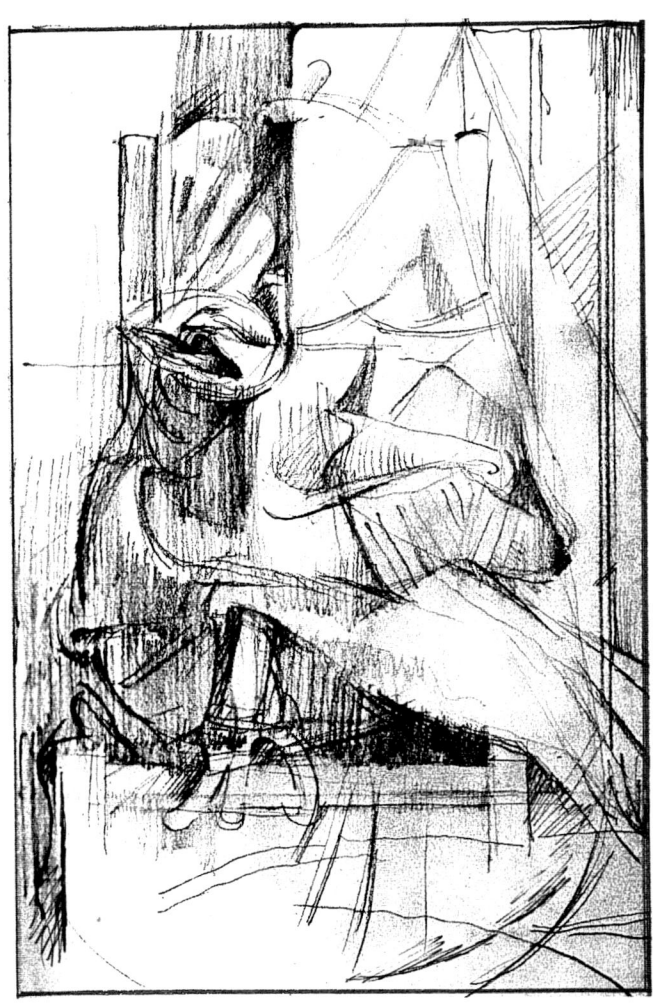

Fig. 69 Bird of Prey — Pencil

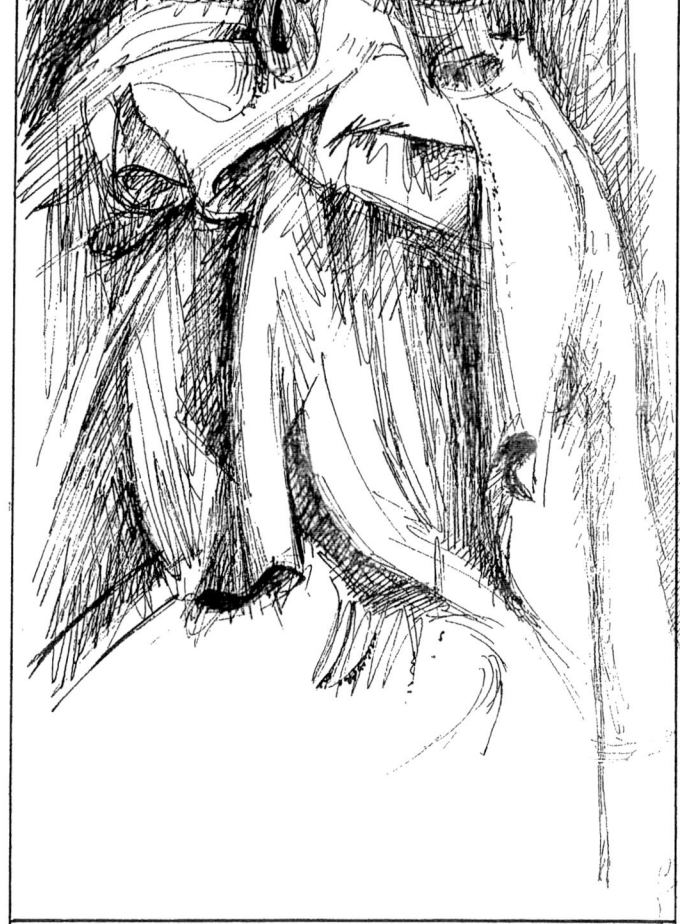

Fig. 70 Owl — Pen & Pencil

BED COVERINGS: Quilts·Duvets·Sheets

Large pieces of fabric offer correspondingly bigger imagery, usually landscapes

Fig. 71. Figure 'found' in a duvet.

Fig. 72. Fields, hedgerows and hills - in a patchwork quilt.

Fig. 73. Mountainous landscape with a lake or reservoir - Blue hot-water bottle lying partially hidden by folds on a light brown Duvet cover.

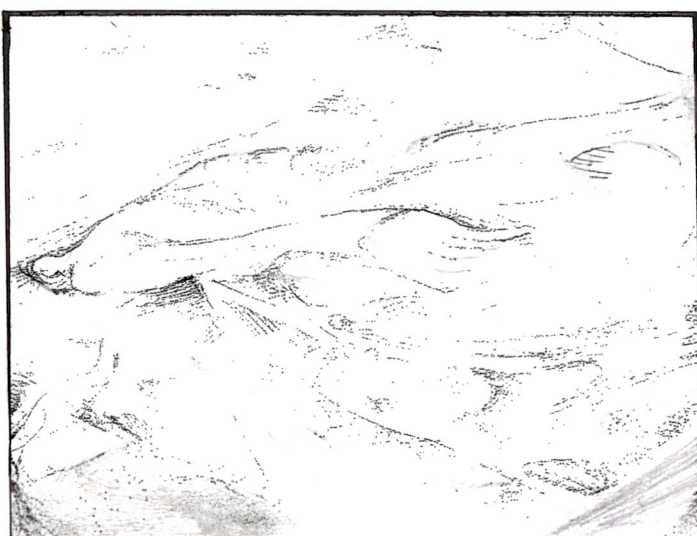

Fig. 71 Figure in a duvet   Pencil

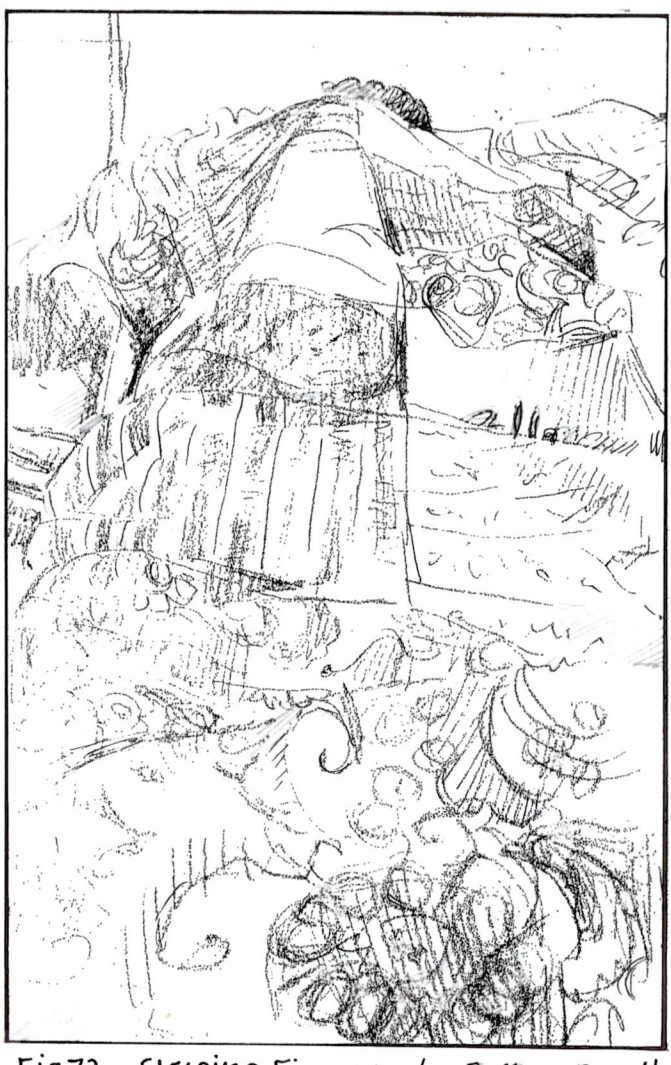

Fig. 72 Sleeping Figure under Quilt   Pencil

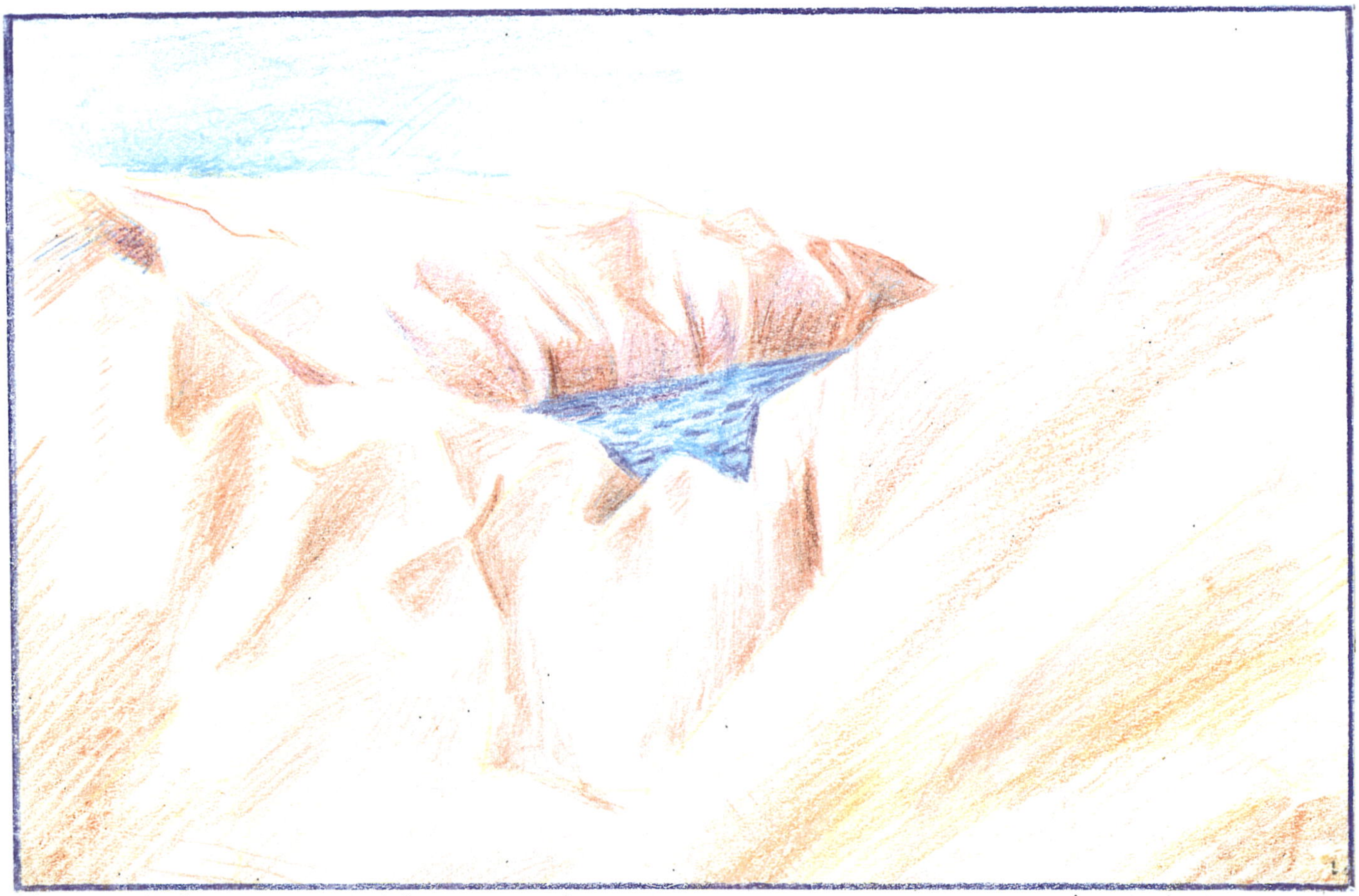

Fig. 73 Lake surrounded by mountains.   Coloured Crayons.

FIGURE ON A SWIVEL-CHAIR 1984-1986

The paintings and drawings relating to the breakdown had, with hindsight, eased some of the negativity and collapse of self-worth experienced at the time.

Although I'd little knowledge of the nature and causes of the breakdown, or of the overwhelming fear it engendered, I did recognise a desire to search for a meaning behind this fear.

Unable to look directly into this 'dark hole', it was nevertheless possible to find an oblique way via the visual 'record' of the event — the continuing series of works about the experience.

No longer felt purely as a negative experience, the very word 'breakdown' began to take on a new face — perhaps it was a harbinger for change and new growth. A sign of a more optimistic approach occurred the moment I termed it 'breakout'. 'Out' had spatial connotations which implied a horizontal forward movement whereas 'down' implied a vertical inertia. This new optimistic emphasis brought forth its own problems however. The idea of a breakout created a kind of tidal wave with uprooted emotional flotsam suddenly apparent on the surface. Now aware of manic phases when extravagant spending sprees occurred — and of the constant aggravation forced onto others. This together with countless sleepless nights. Then the physical inertia, the 'cotton-wool' white-out of ideas, action and decision making during the depressive periods. Between these swings of mood were occasional frenetic searches for dogmatic certainties to prop up the fragile self image.

All these swings of mood were masked by a calm public image — a 'Business as Usual' persona.

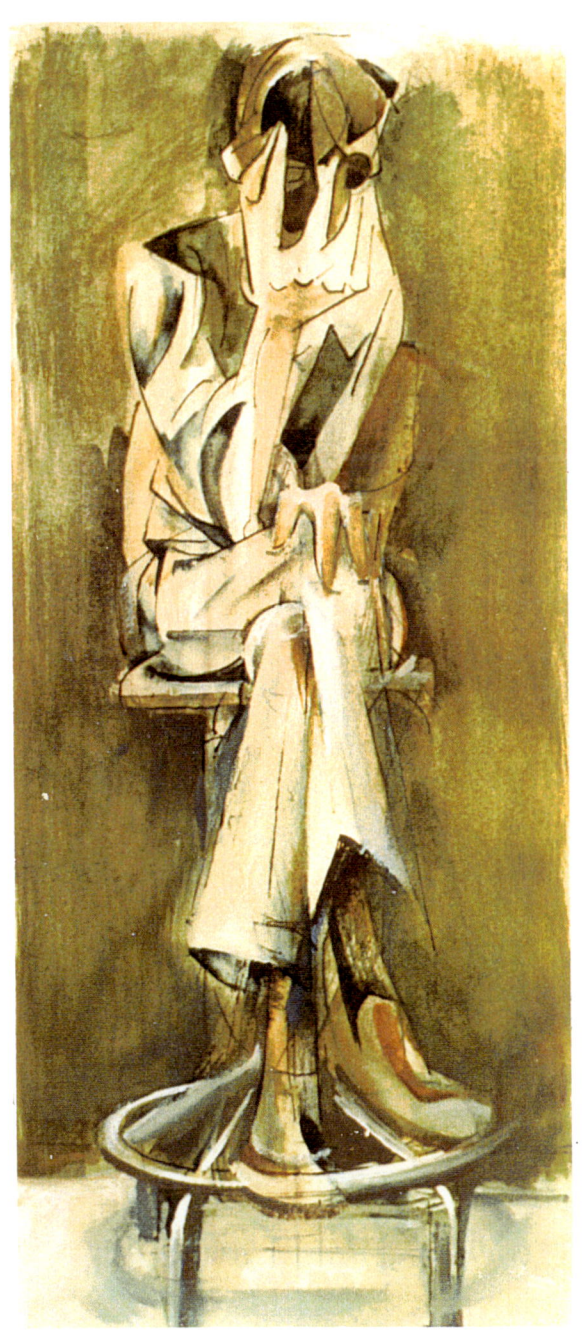

Looking now for some visual image which might help clarify the duality between stormy depths and a calm surface I found an idea had then established itself firmly in the mind. For some time I had been perplexed as to how I might find this image when I realised my swivel-chair, which I had often used when at the drawing board, could stand perfectly still at its base while also turning about at a higher level. Could there be possibly an analogy here?

Immediately taking on a new life, a little like Dr. Who's phone box, the swivel-chair could (like the Tardis) transport me through 360 degrees, if not yet through a time warp.

Curiously enough, after many months of working on some thirty or so variations on this theme it did begin to feel that elements of spatial 'travel' were indeed beginning to happen.

A small pencil drawing version showed movement towards dance, the foot rail spiralling up to meet the dancer-cum-sitter's hand — he is no longer a 'Figure on a Swivel-chair' (see Fig 89).

Following this, another altogether darker pen and wash drawing seemed to show a perambulating figure, no longer confined to his fixed position but now a 'cyclist' pedalling off somewhere. Perhaps the swivel-chair had been transformed, had become my own time machine. (Fig 91)

It was at this point that the 'machine' vanished completely for I found a figure dancing in a twirling fashion with his own shadow. Months later I painted a tightrope walker attempting a balancing act on the highwire. The shadow was still there — the picture seemed to be an extension of the dancers. Much later I looked back on this series as a therapeutic self-help programme......

Left: Fig. 74. Stationary figure on swivel-chair (early sketch has figure immobile). Pen & Watercolour.

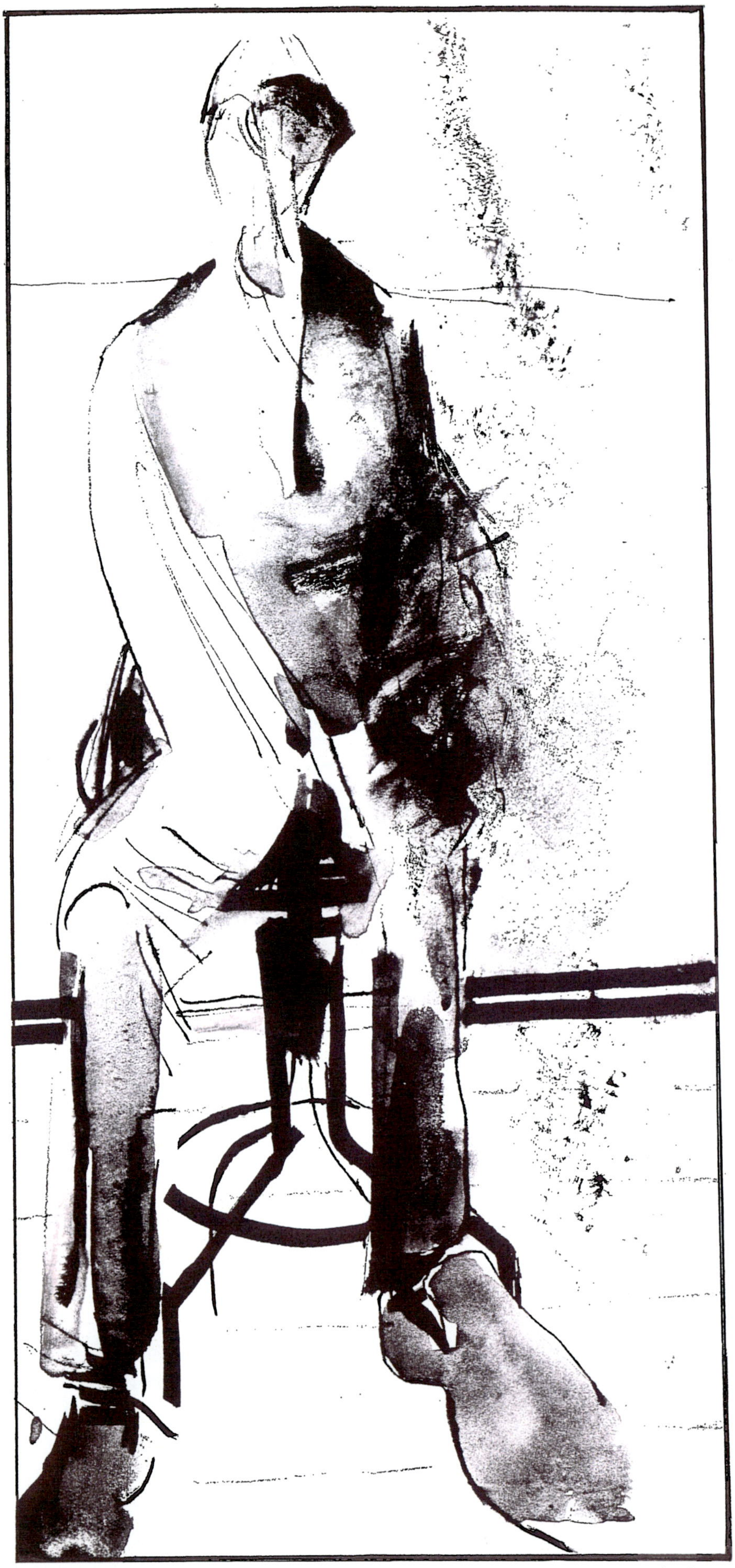

Fig. 75 Untitled.   Pen & Wash

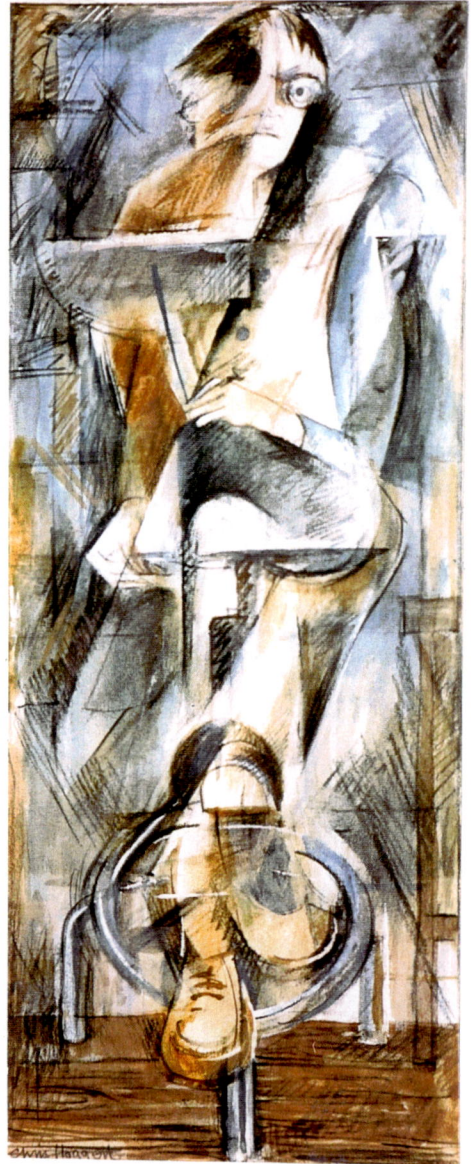

Fig. 76 Seated Figure 1 Watercolour

Above: As the figure turns through 360°, momentary glimpses of a hand, knee or a chair-back catch the eye then slip back into space – moments of clarity, moments of obscurity.

Left: A compulsion to seek a leaner, narrowed appearance. This is pursued further in figs. 79 and 80.

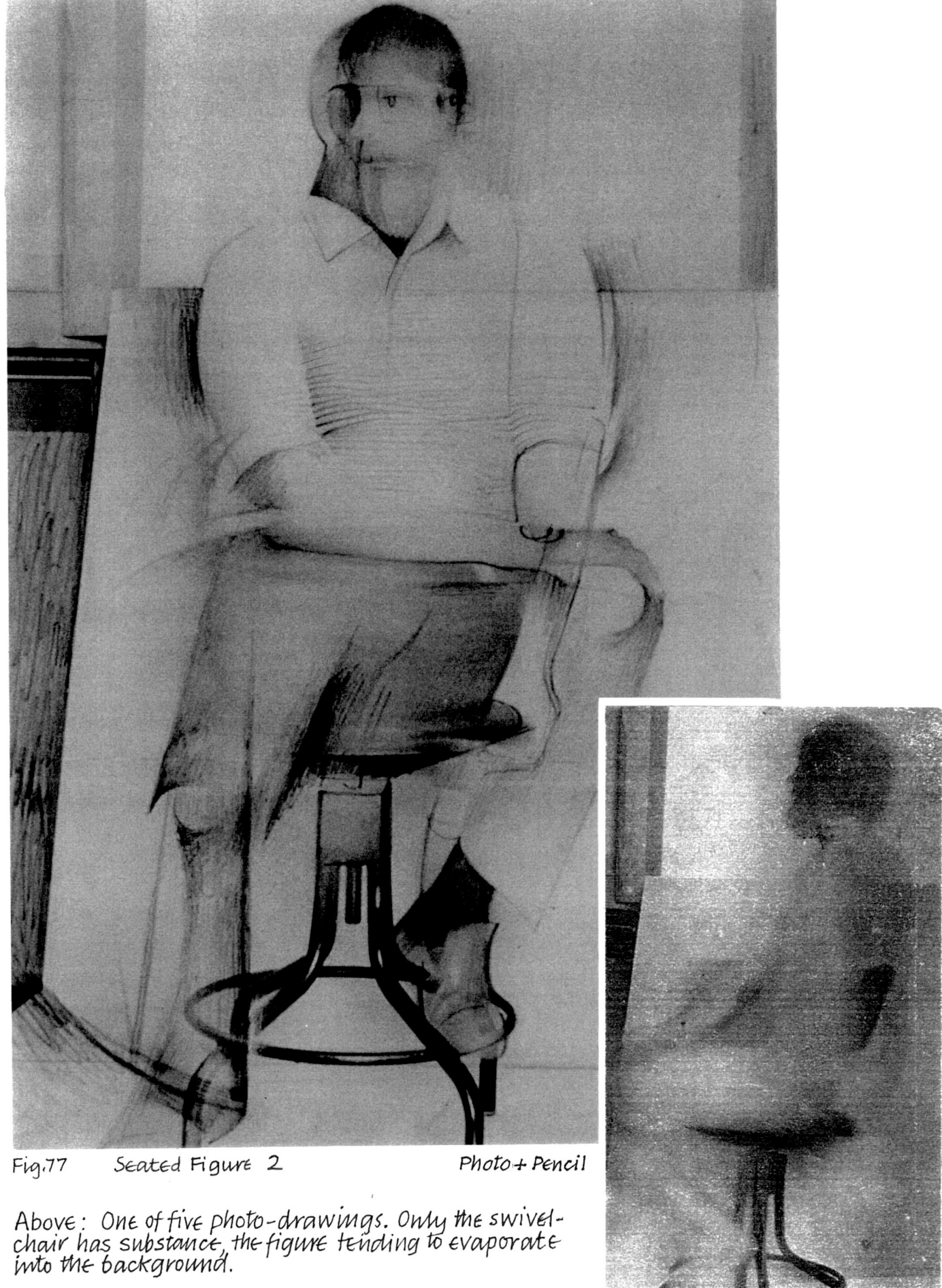

Fig.77   Seated Figure 2   Photo + Pencil

Above: One of five photo-drawings. Only the swivel-chair has substance, the figure tending to evaporate into the background.

Right: One of many small photo-prints untouched by the pencil — a twirling ghost image.

Fig.78 Seated Figure 3.   Photo

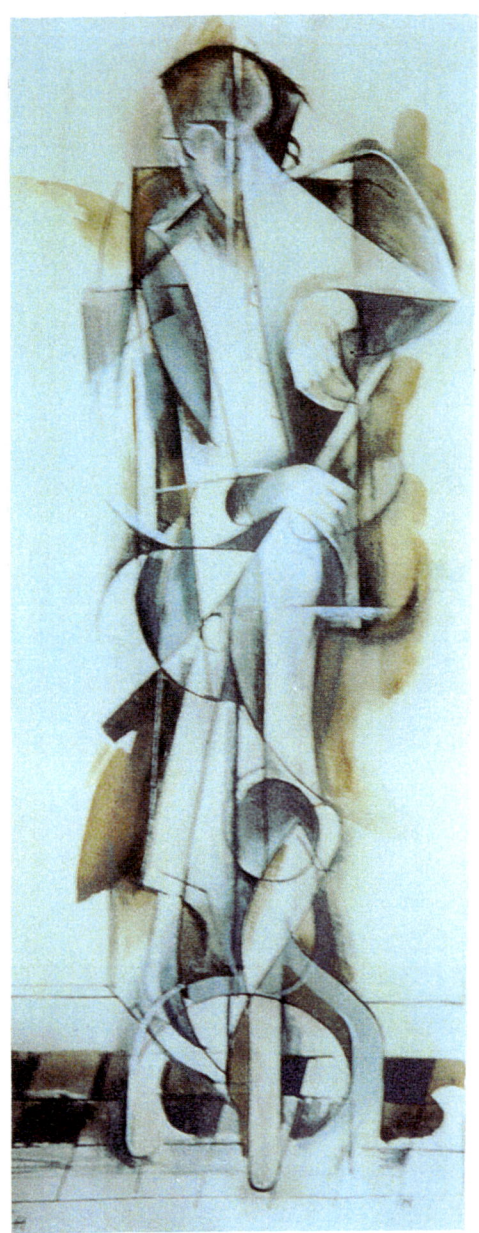

Fig.79 Seated Figure 4. Watercolour

Above: The figure becomes more scant, thinned down - here with the aid of geometrical shapes slicing through figure into space

Right: Perhaps to condense the subject even further it would be possible to arrive at its essence?

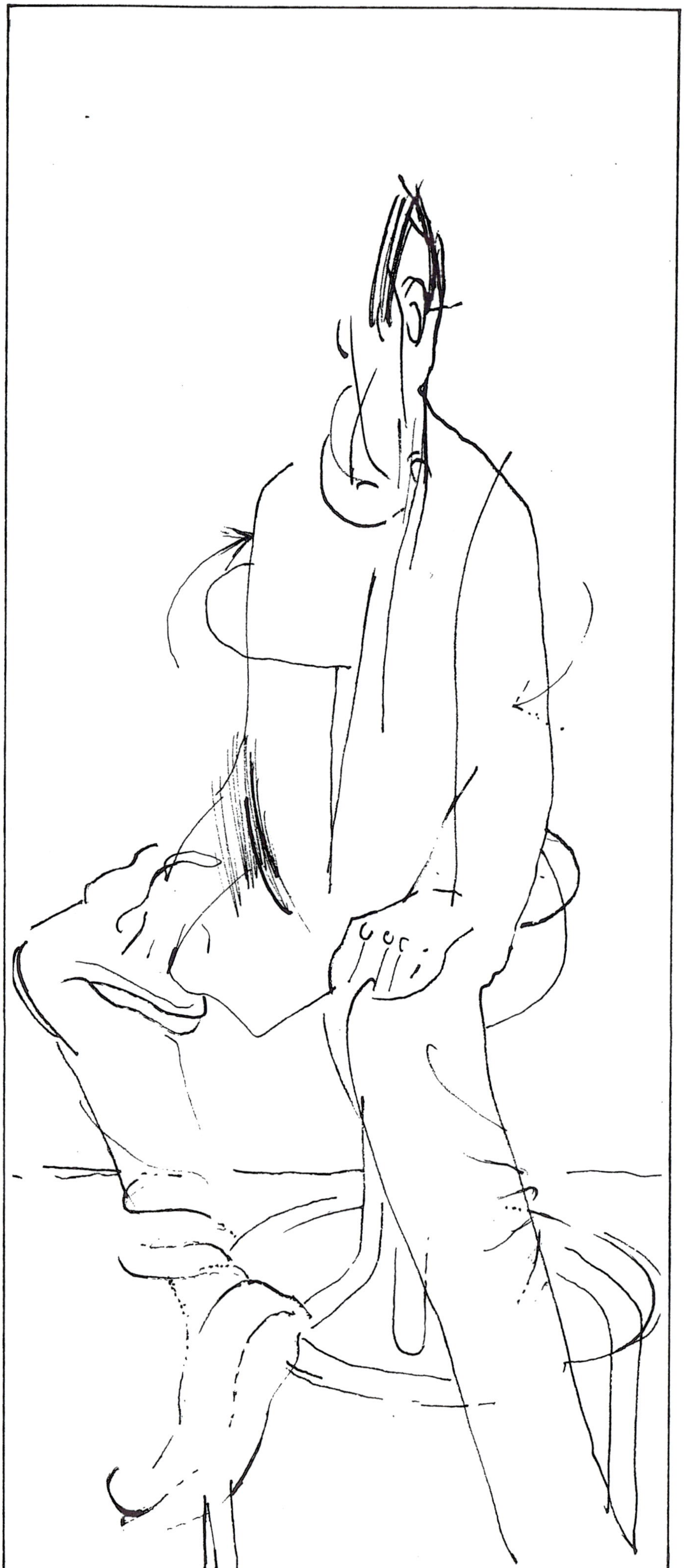

Fig.80. Seated Figure 5 Pen & Ink

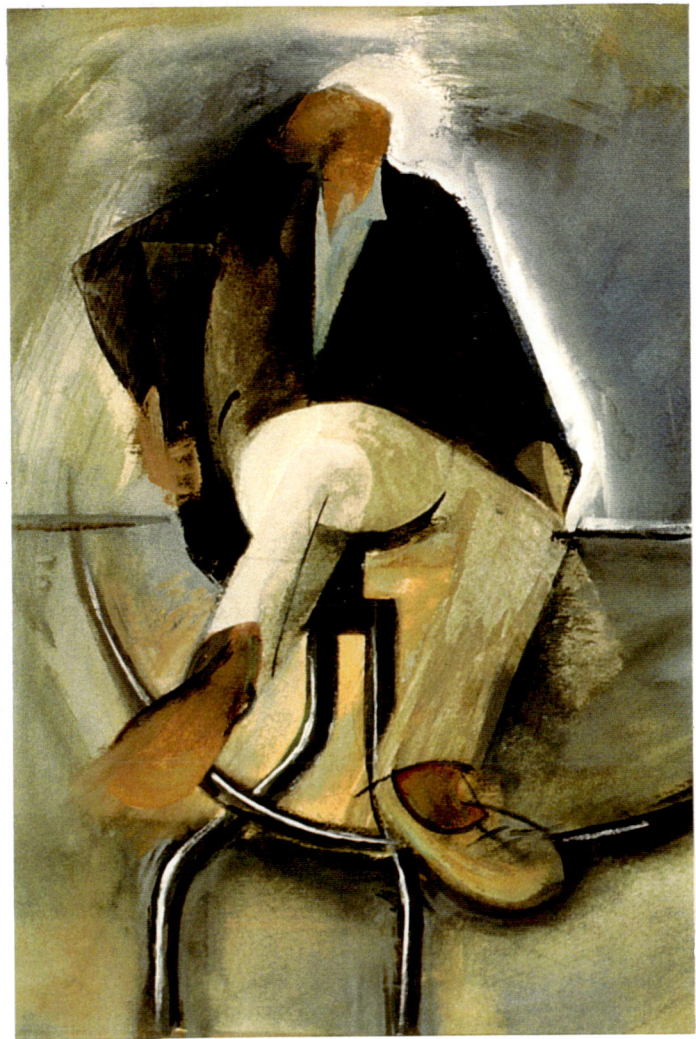

Fig. 81   Seated Figure 6   Gouache

Left: The subject of the figure with chair had been the only consideration (as here), but now a need for a setting or background rather than just an empty space took hold. Floors, walls, furniture, etc., became equally important. See the painted reliefs in figs 84-87.

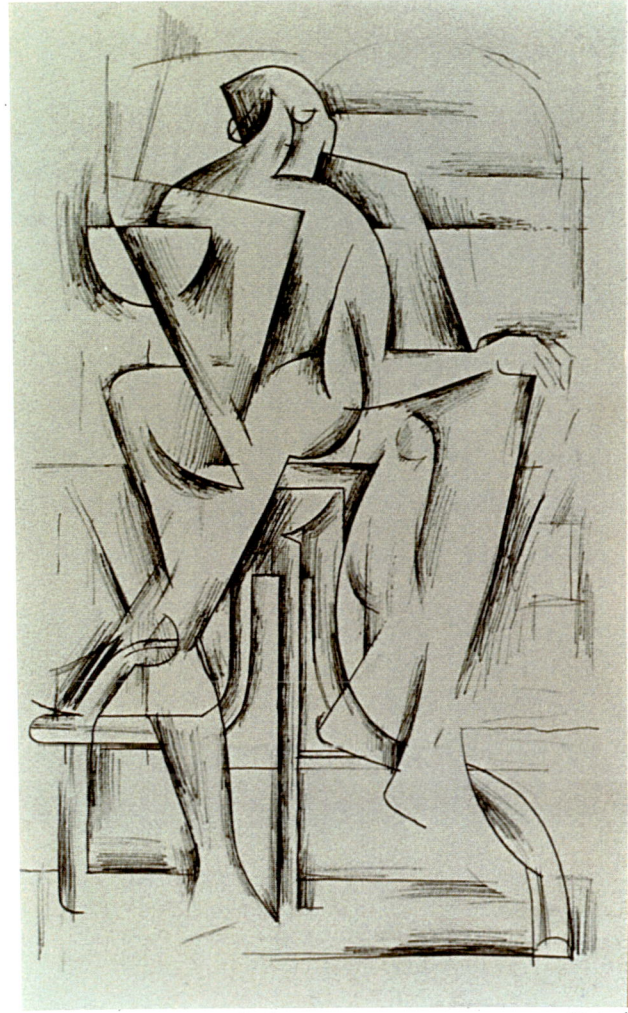

Fig. 83   Seated Figure 8   pen & Ink

Above: A hint of building structures lies behind this figure and chair. The figure also takes on a more animated dance-like movement. See painted development in figs. 88 and 92.

Left: Figure on a bar-stool in an isolated corner of a room. The figure ready to move away perhaps from the precipitous floor

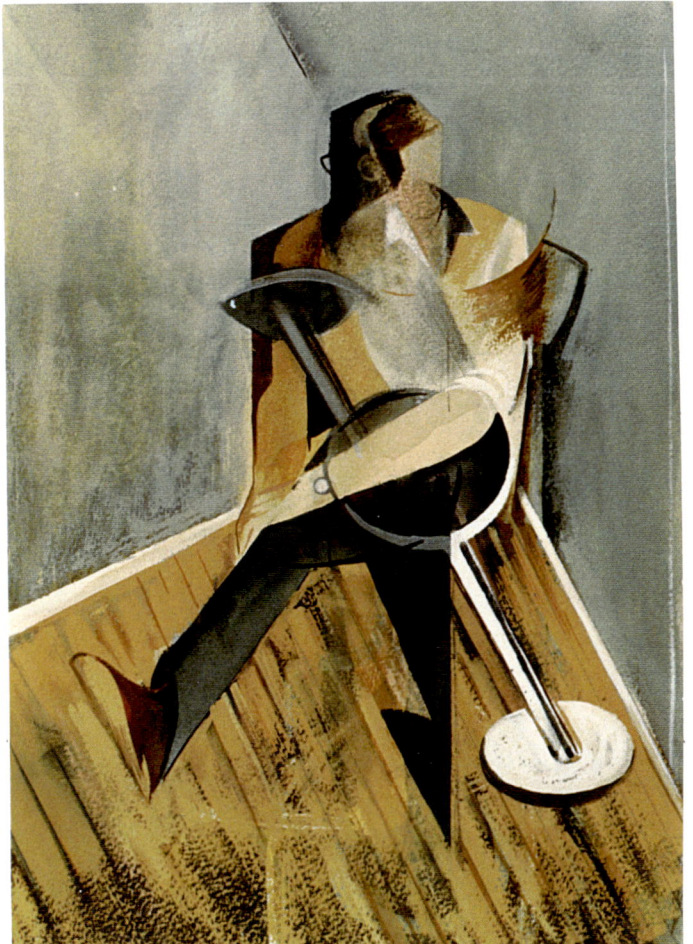

Fig. 82   Seated Figure 7   Gouache

41

Fig. 84 Seated Figure 9.   Mixed Media-Acrylic

RELIEF COLLAGES

Left: Many different materials (vermiculite, sand, other granular things) were glued to a base board to give deep relief to parts of the work. This helped to achieve textural qualities before painting.

I felt the purpose was to produce something more tangible — a contradiction to the very purpose of this theme of ambiguity and amorphous qualities of a turning figure.

Yet this paradox did seem to be the purpose of these three reliefs........

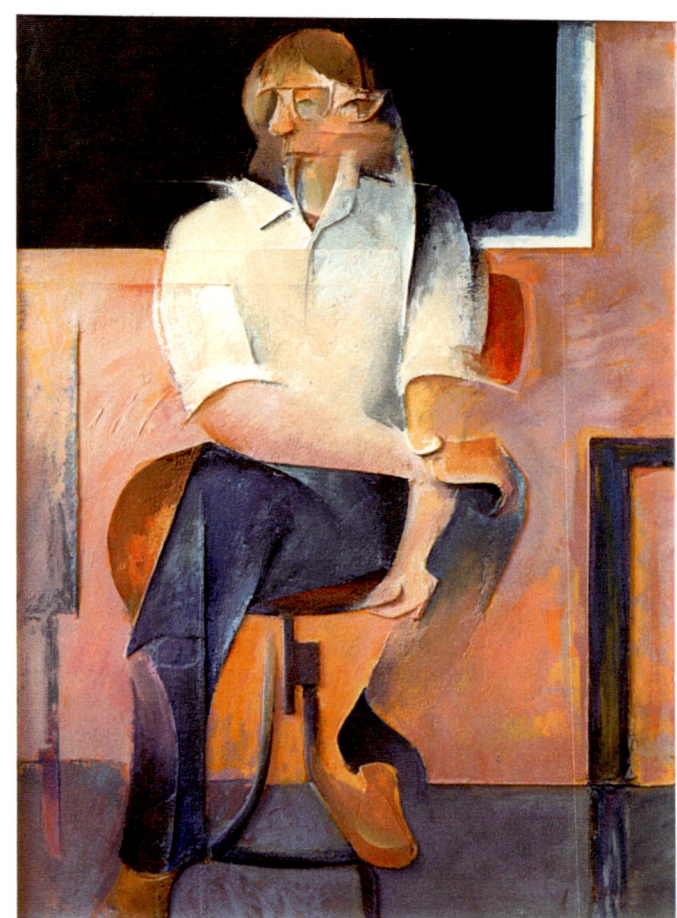

Fig. 85 Seated Figure 10   Acrylic Paste & Paint

Above: Textural elements through brushwork. More use of graduated tone and colour to aid the movement of the turning figure.

Left: A decisive cut through a side profile as the front face looks into the mirror, working on a self portrait. The final result was too complex and confusing and needed reworking........

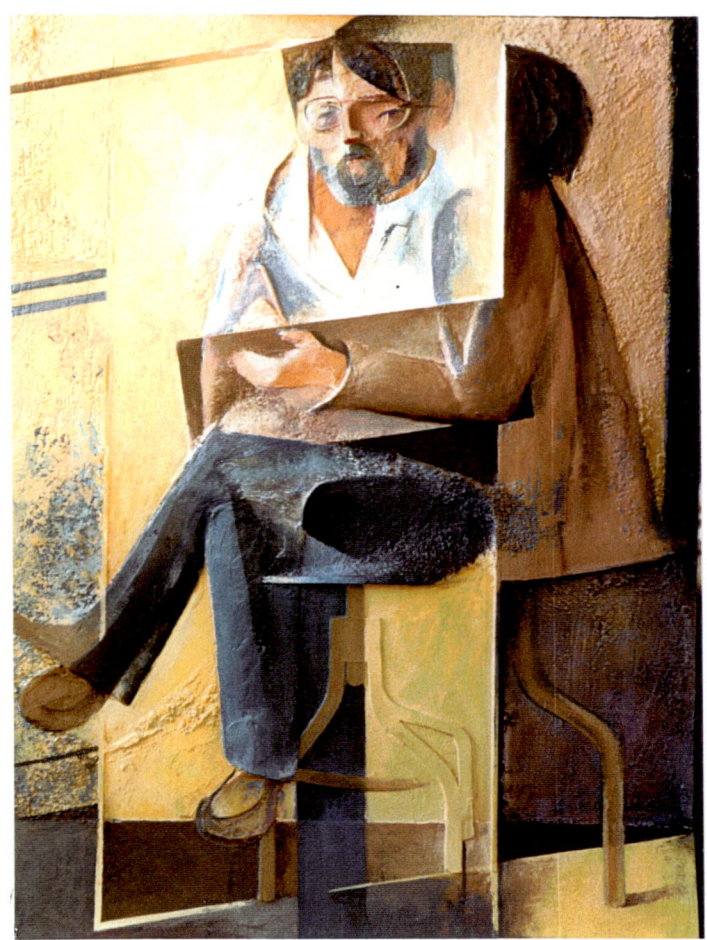

Fig. 86 Seated Figure 11   Mixed Media-Acrylic

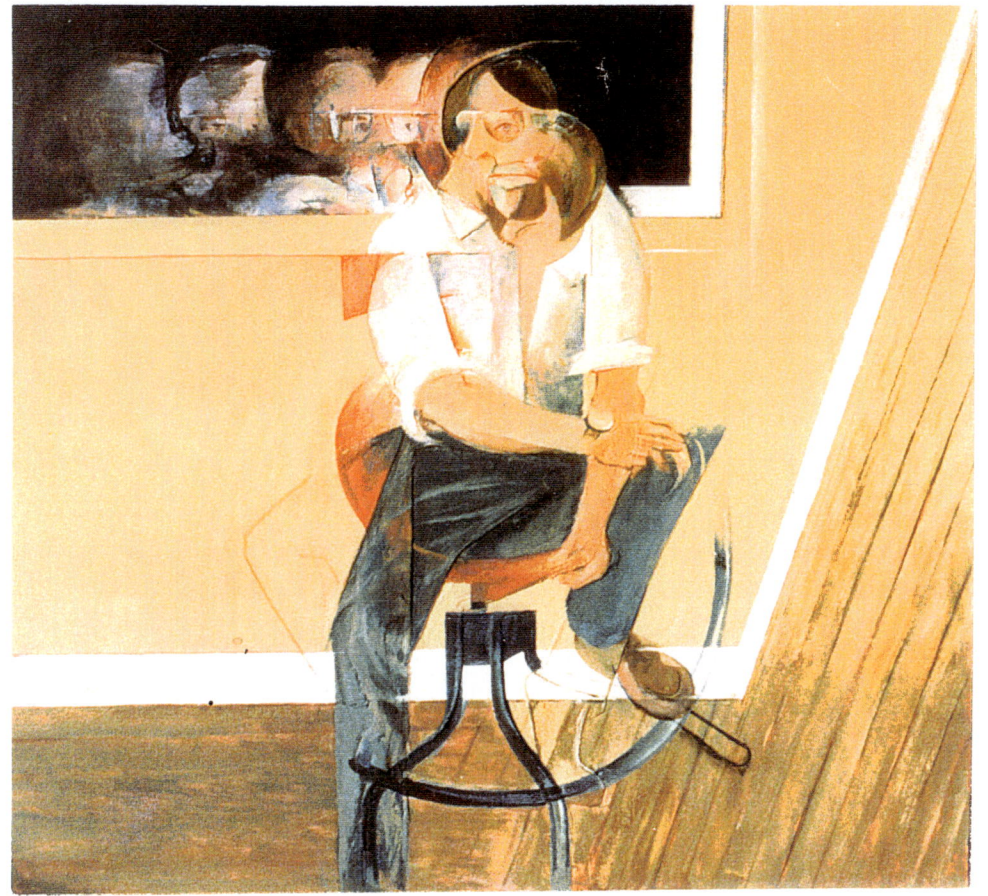

Fig. 87 Seated Figure 12   Mixed Media - Acrylic

Above: Painted at the same time as reliefs (opposite) this painting was reworked because of a new interest in horizontal against vertical movement - the head is the fulcrum or turning point - the eyes/glasses stretch across a black window, the head takes a downward shift.
  Interest in the plate-tech tonics of volcanic zones probably influenced the painting. (see page 243).

Right: As the chair begins to lose its structure, so the sitter's doubts increase - a look of apprehension flits across his features......

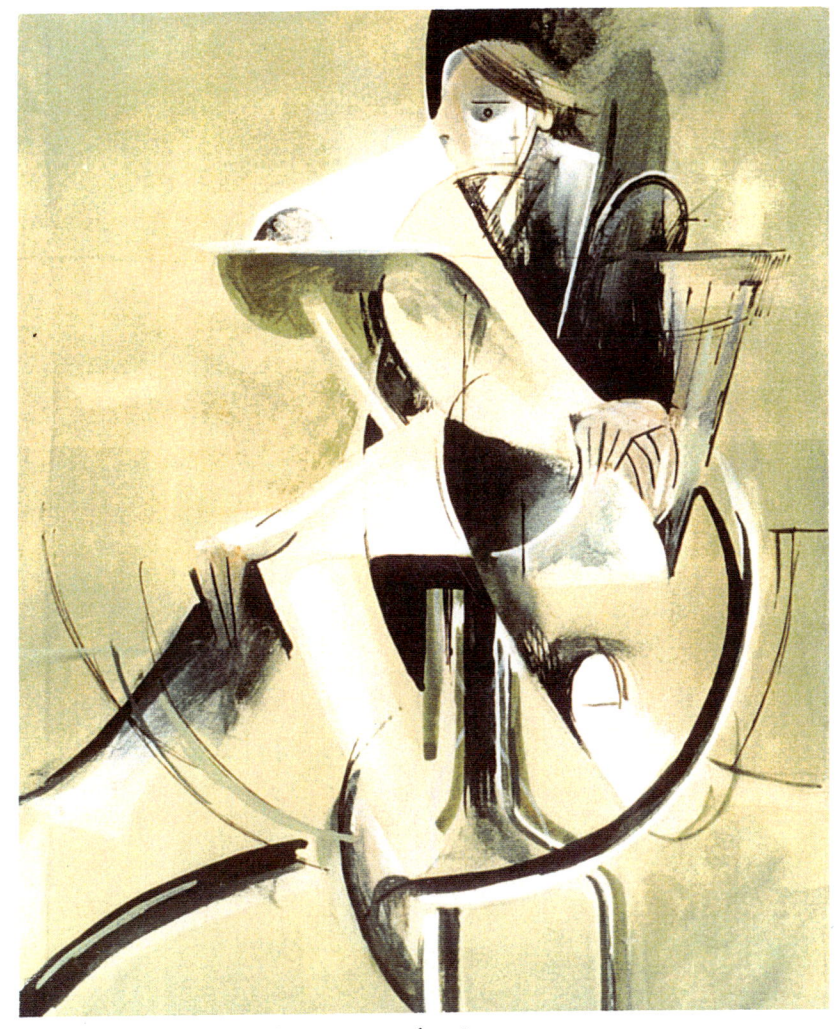

Fig. 88 Seated Figure - Spinning.   Ink & Gouache

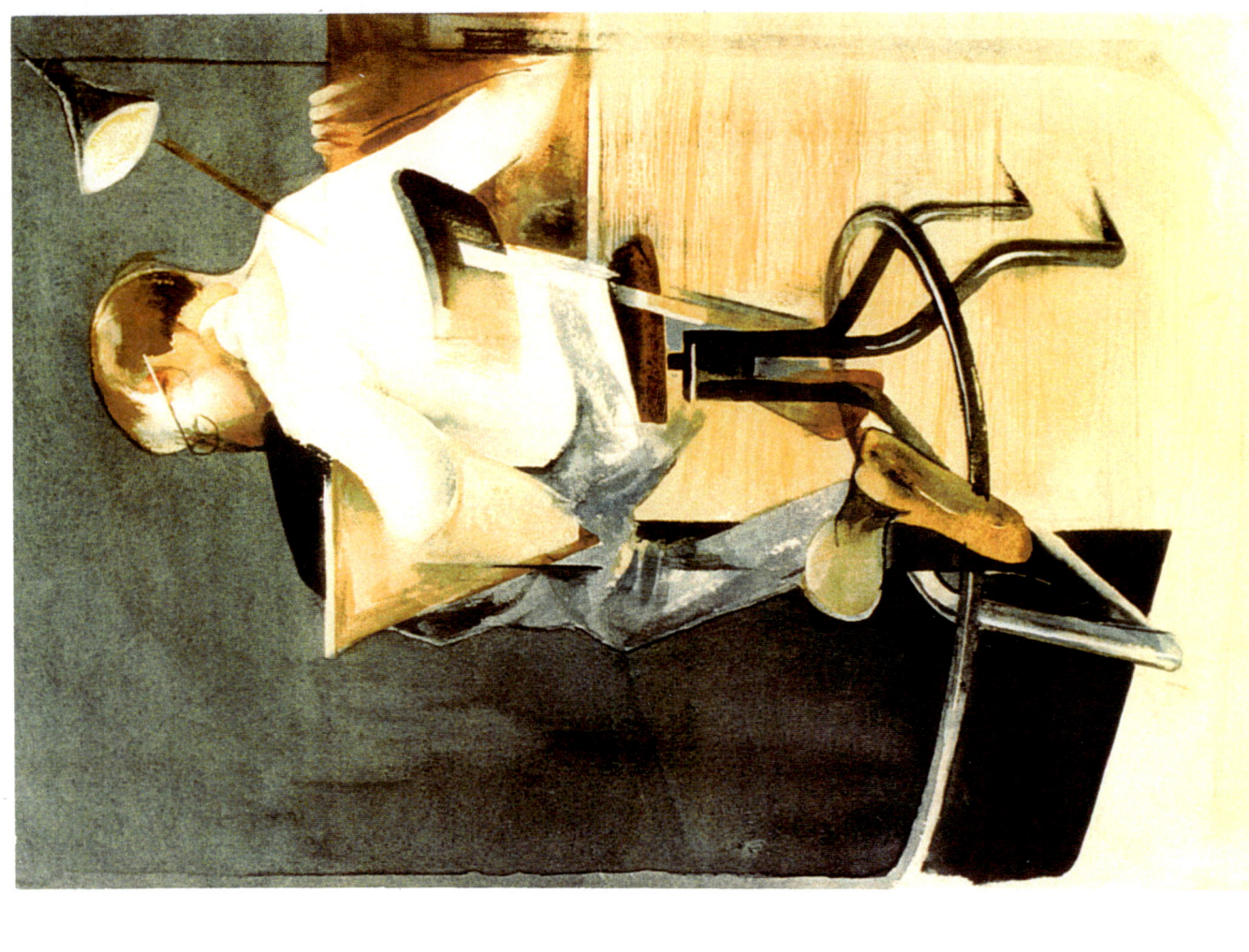

Fig. 89 The Dancer   Pencil

Fig. 90 The Draughtsman   Watercolour.

Above: The foot-rail begins to unravel, rises up to meet the sitter-cum-dancer's hand. It's time to leave the 'time machine' and move into new territory.

Right: An ambiguity resides in the figure at his drawing-board. The board can be seen to advance or retreat as the draughtsman contemplates his shadow 'behind' the board. The foot-rail is capable of spinning one or other into action.

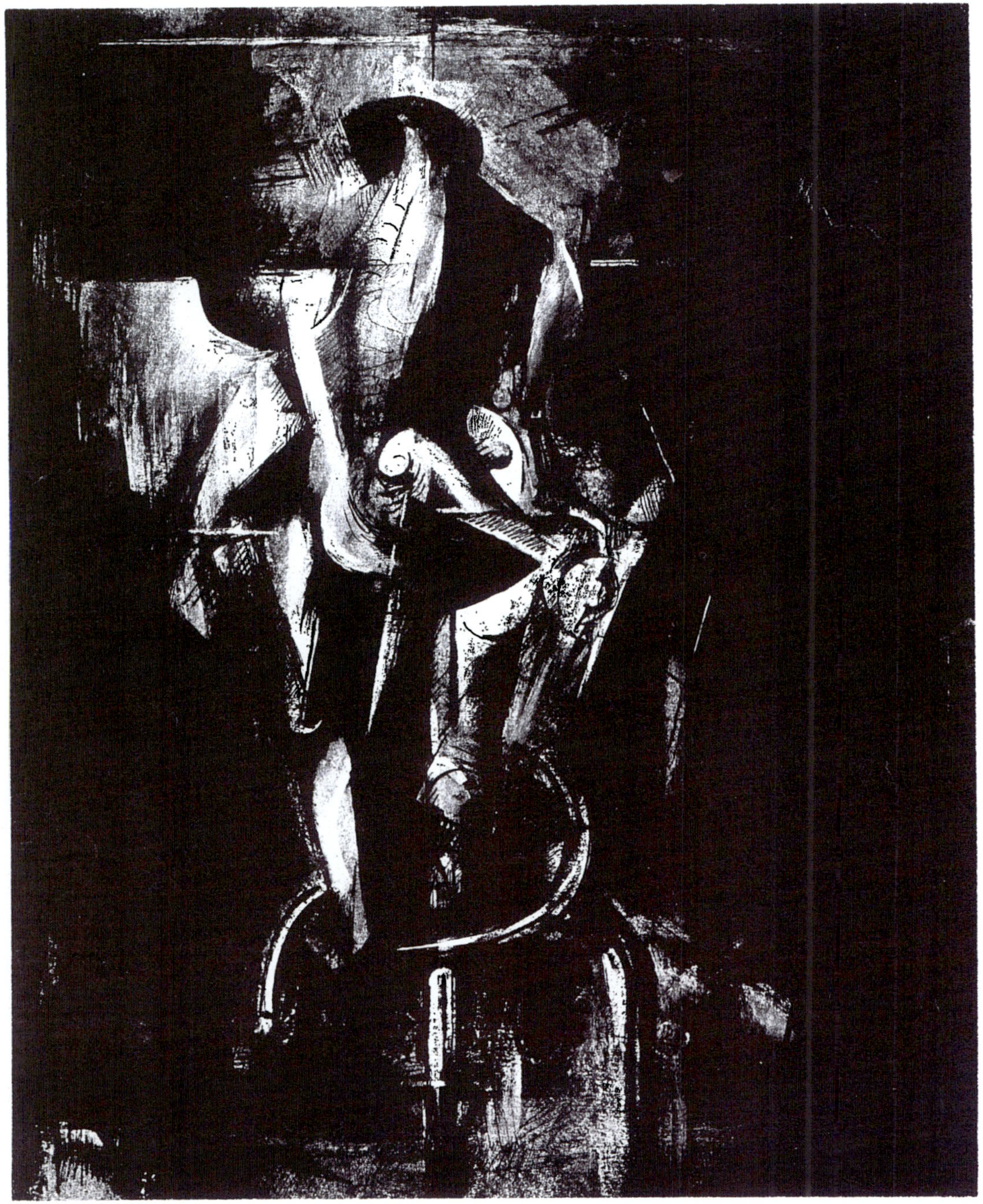

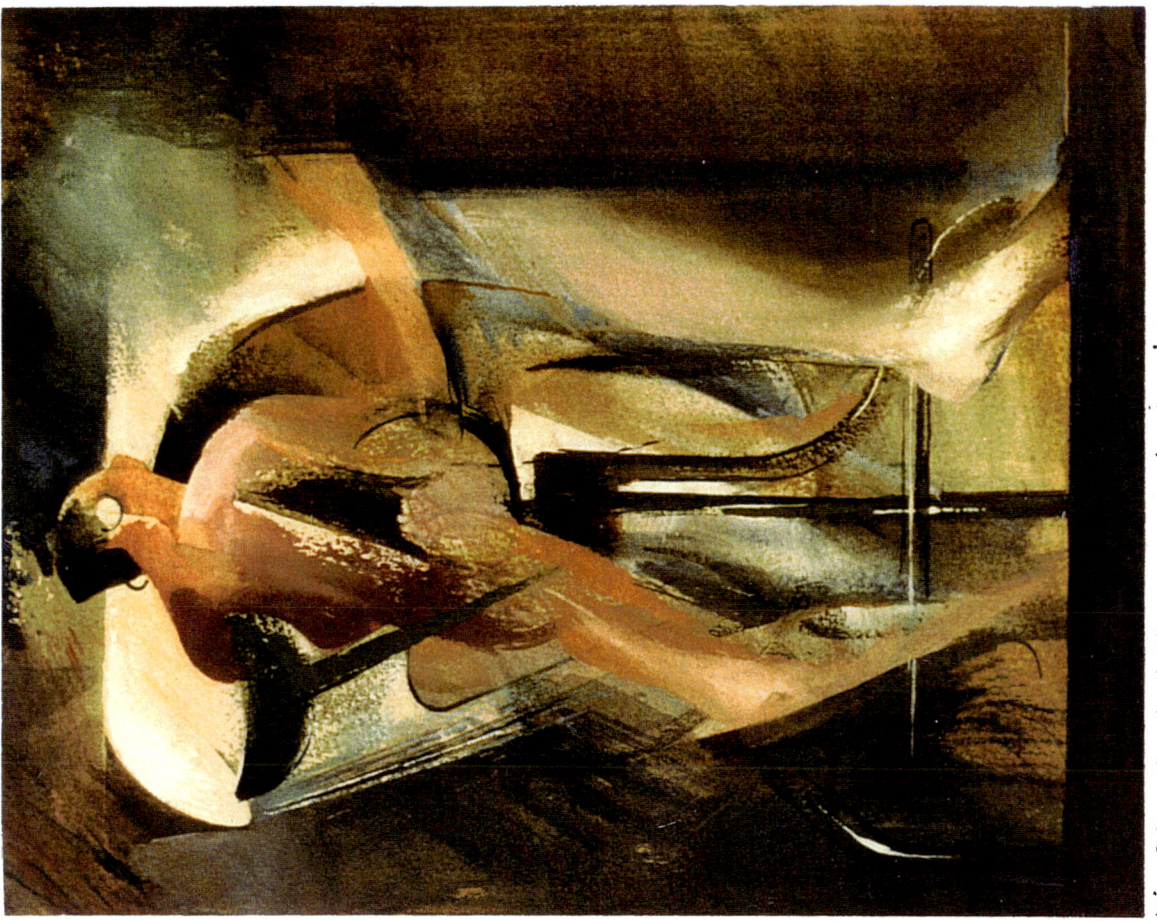

Fig. 92 Seated Figure – Nude Version   Gouache.

Above: Developed from pen sketch (fig 83), this nude version is unwinding or loosening-up, stepping out from the chair.

Left: The chair becomes a bicycle – or possibly a tricycle as the rider/sitter decides it is time to move on – yet the way ahead is dark and ominous.

Pen & Wash

Fig. 91 The Cyclist

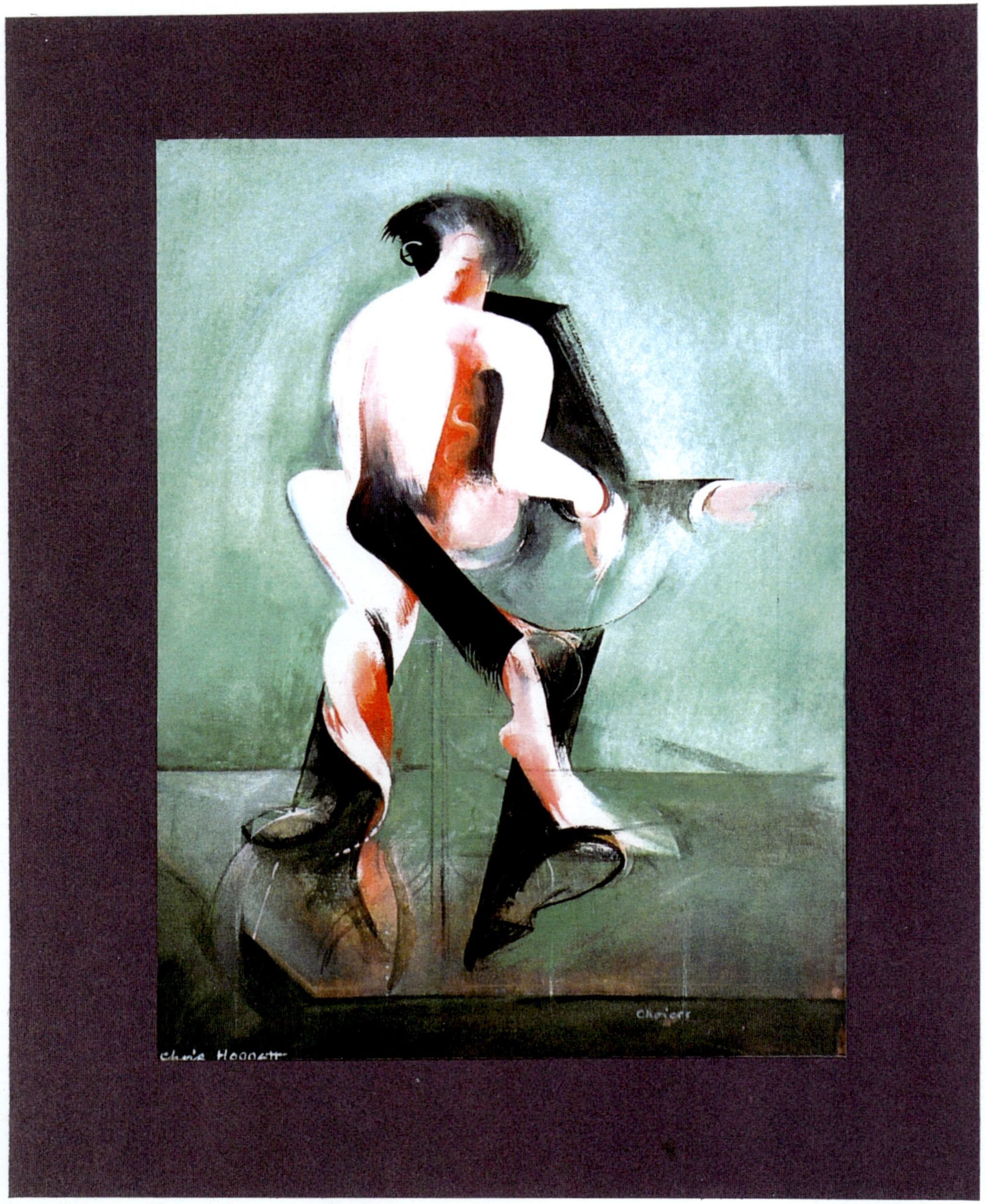

As the chair transformed itself into a vehicle (fig.91) and the figure pedalled away, it followed that the chair could be removed entirely. So what would happen to the figure? The two final pictures in the series attempted to answer the question:

Left: The figure is now dancing with his own shadow (fig 92 is a possible precursor)

Below: The figure is above the circus ring — one couldn't ask for more space than this — it's now become a balancing act.

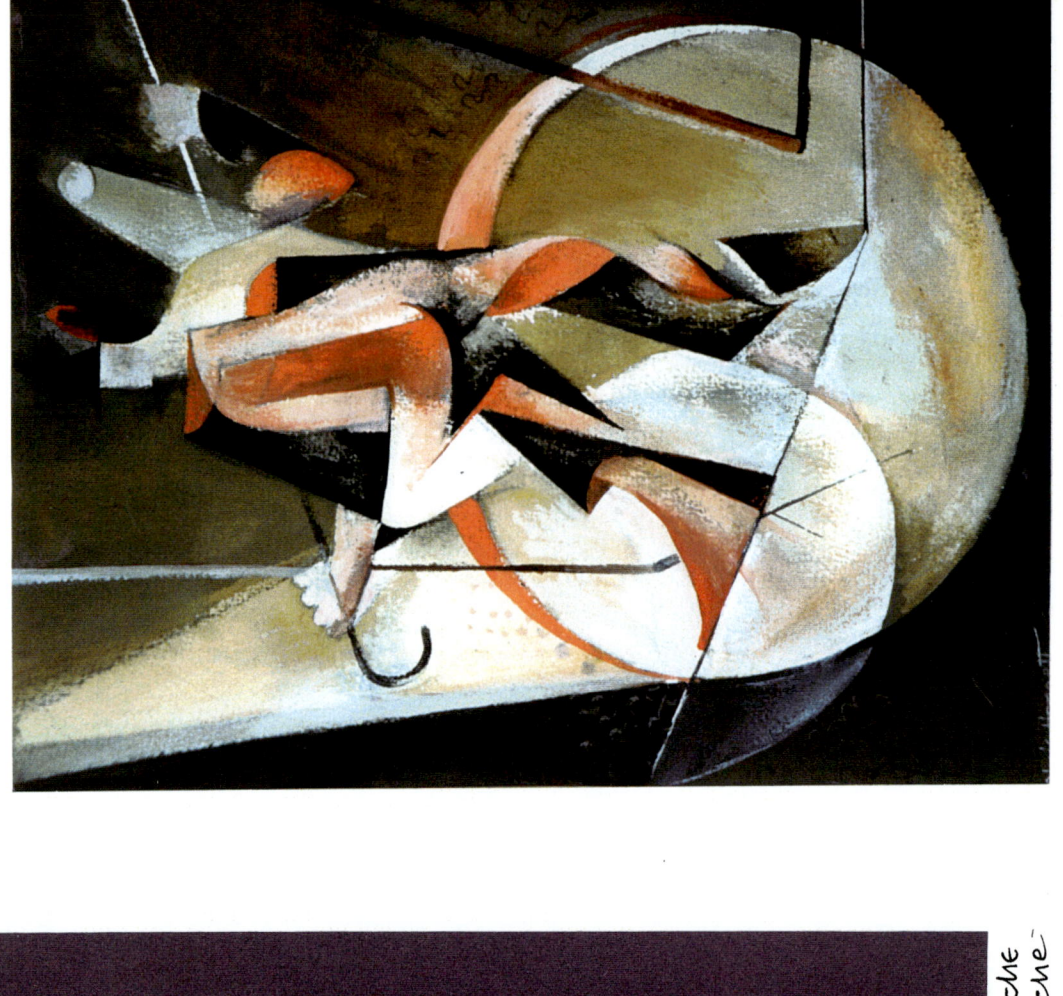

Fig.93 Dancing with one's shadow.   Gouache
Right: Fig.94. Tightrope Walker   Gouache

46

SKELETONS 1984-1986

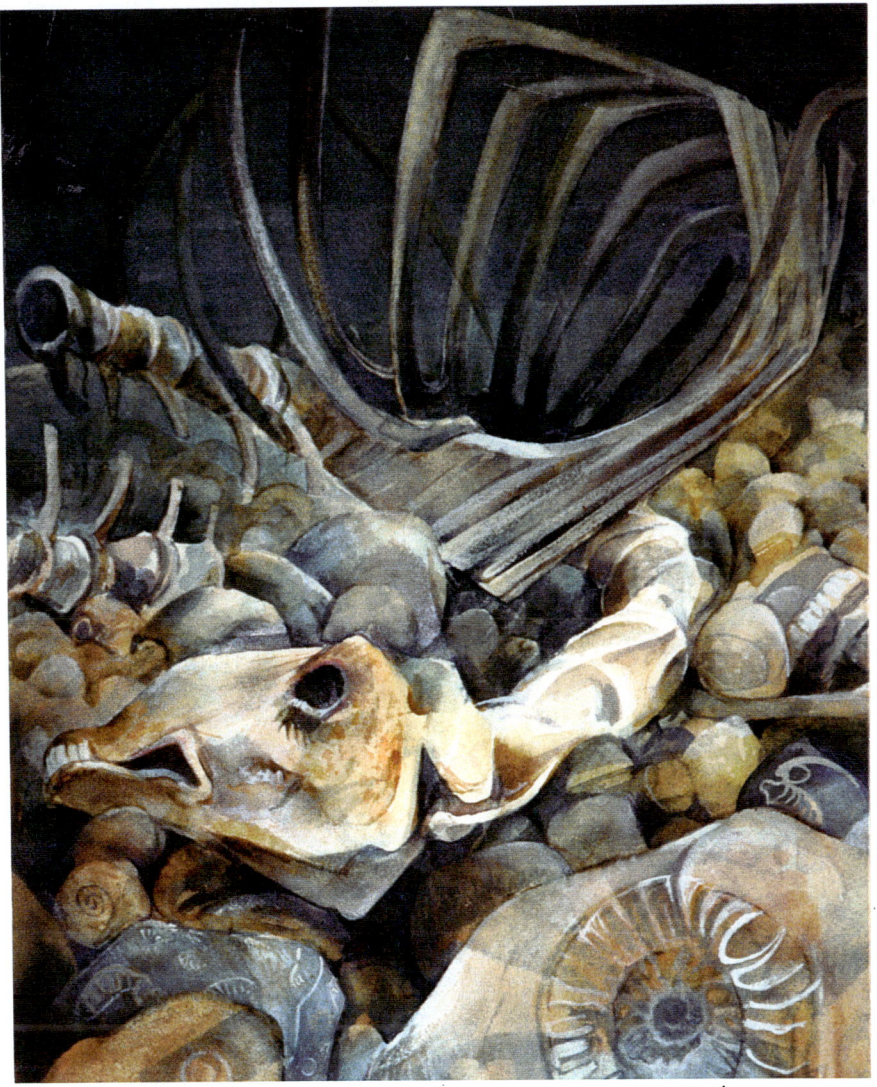

Fig. 95   On the Beach   Watercolour

The skull collection started in the 1960s. First I acquired an ancient human medical specimen with a finely textured patina, then a deer with an elegant pair of antlers. These were soon followed by three sheep and a small dog skull. The collection gained momentum when I visited a local butcher who soon found me a large horse, a cow and a pig. Then I picked two delicately boned herring gulls off a beach and was given a sea turtle. Together with assorted rocks, pebbles and shells these formed a useful group of natural objects for drawing classes.

During the early 1980s I was intrigued by a discovery near Clover Cliff headland. An almost complete skeleton of a sheep was lying in a slight hollow, the head detached and two front legs scattered. Compelled by a need to record the impression and the effect it had on me, I made two pen & wash studies - and then wondered why I did this. I could not find morbid or romantic connotations, although I could recognise some aesthetic content - a subtle turn along a scapular edge, tonal and colour contrast of sharp white ribs with brown tufts of wool on cheek and ankles.

Yet I felt something more than this, something disturbing, a symbol I couldn't relate to at the time.

Beachcombing in the Gower a year later I made a gruesome find which offered a possible answer to the skeleton discovery and its consequential emotional reaction. A dead sheep, its front and rear pairs of legs separately trussed and its belly slashed along its length lay on the upper beach. It looked a sacrificial victim, probably thrown from the cliff above. I began making connections with the earlier find and soon found myself involved with a small group of watercolours on the theme of a 'Bone Chalice'. They seemed to echo and reflect on an inner anxiety I'd not encountered since childhood - that of feeling a 'victim'. An acute trauma had been reawakened.

The obsession to search and paint continued as I found further sheep skeletons, some being re-invented into a more fantastical nature which continued until some inner tension seemed to lessen, bringing this series to a natural conclusion.

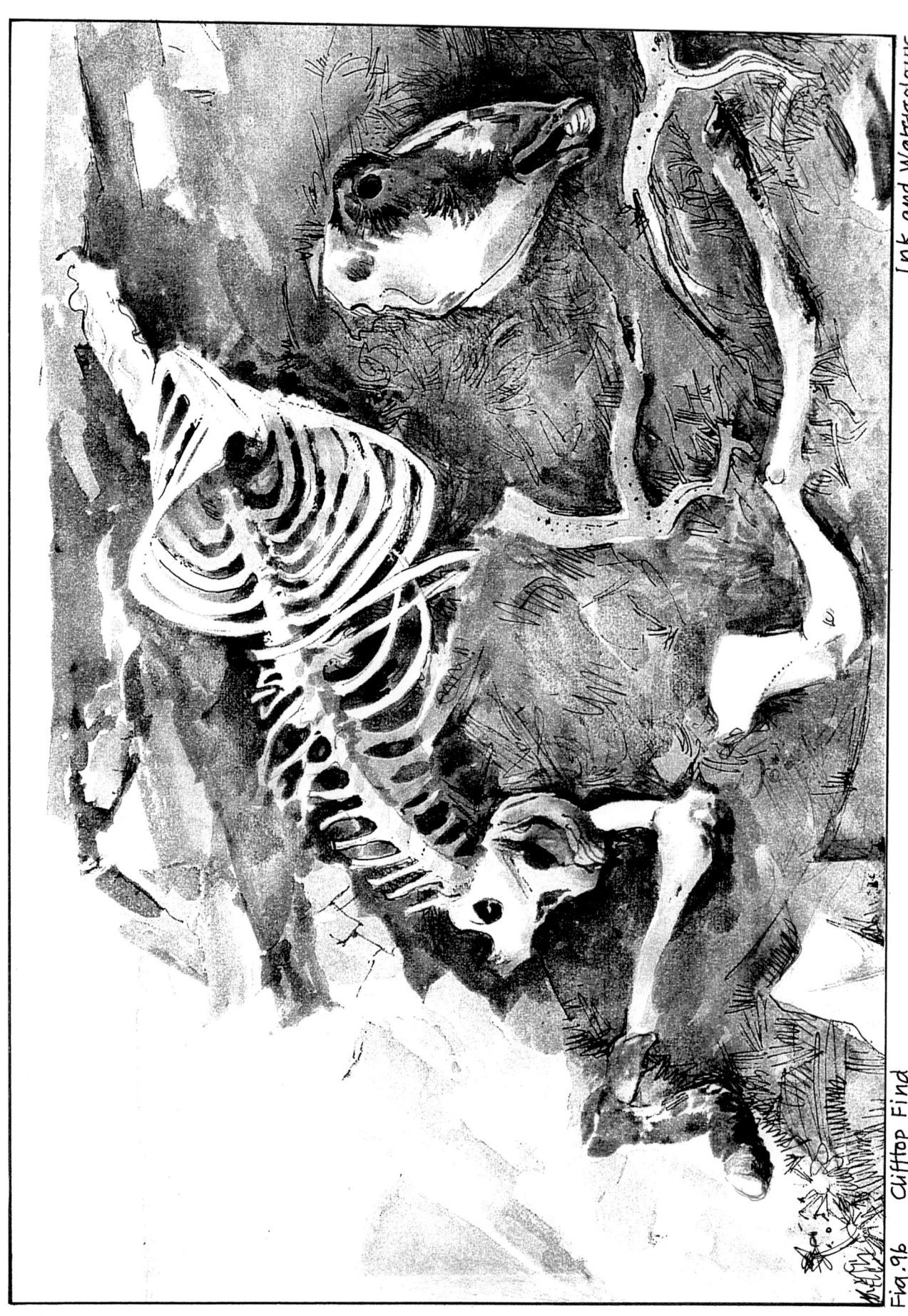

Fig. 96 Clifftop Find Ink and Watercolour

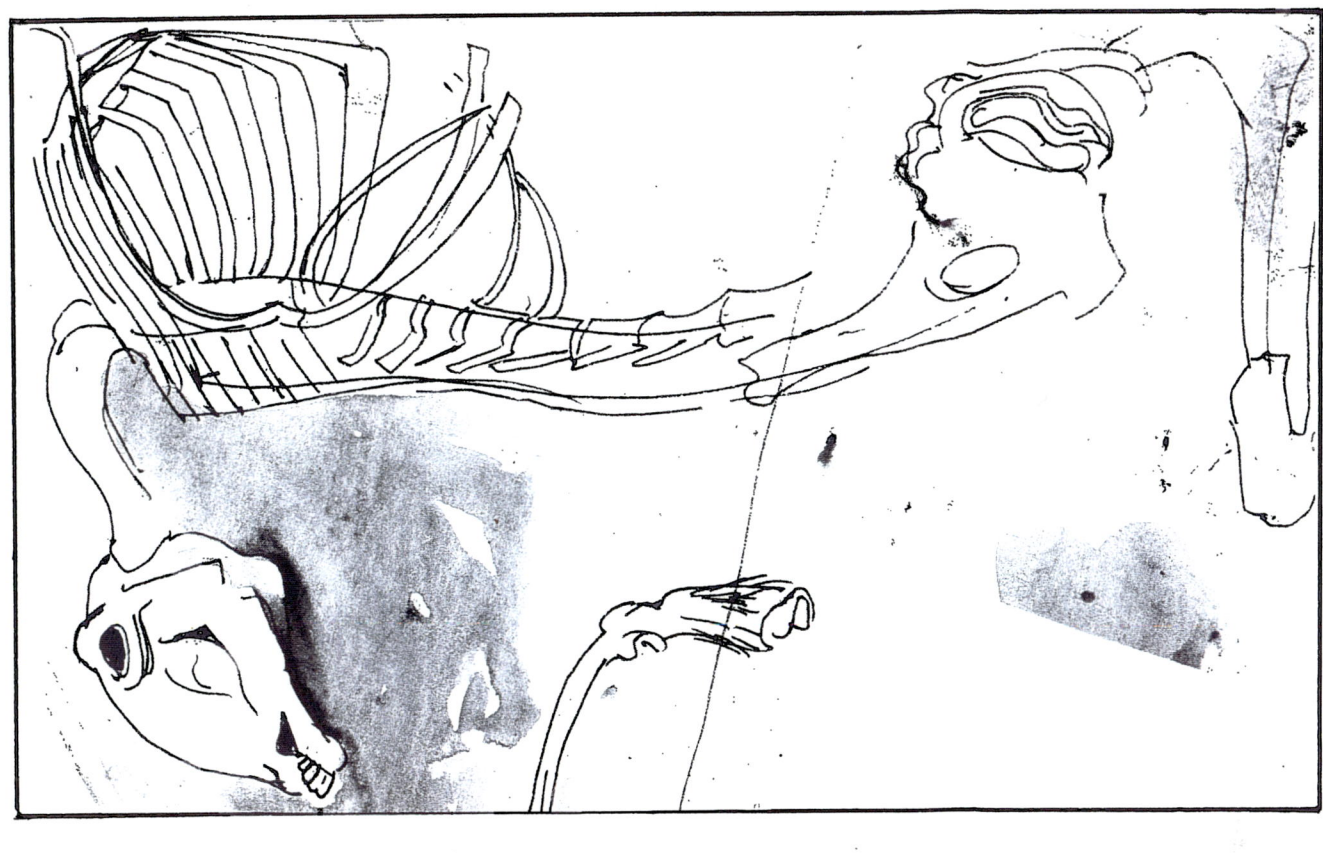

Fig. 98   Skeletal Sketch   Pen & Wash

SHEEP'S SKELETON ON A GOWER CLIFFTOP

An almost complete sheep's skeleton discovered on a clifftop above Mewslade Bay in 1984 engendered a sequence of pictures.
Above: Skeletal arrangement as found and immediately sketched.
Right: From another viewpoint with the head 'replaced' to the top of the spine.
Previous page 47: Skull and ribcage rearranged for a beach scene.
Below: A painting based on the drawings, arranged on a linear grid structure not-unlike a map; the skeleton suspended and incorporated into a background of clifftop and face, with stones, pebbles, gorse, backed by the shore, sea and a full moon.

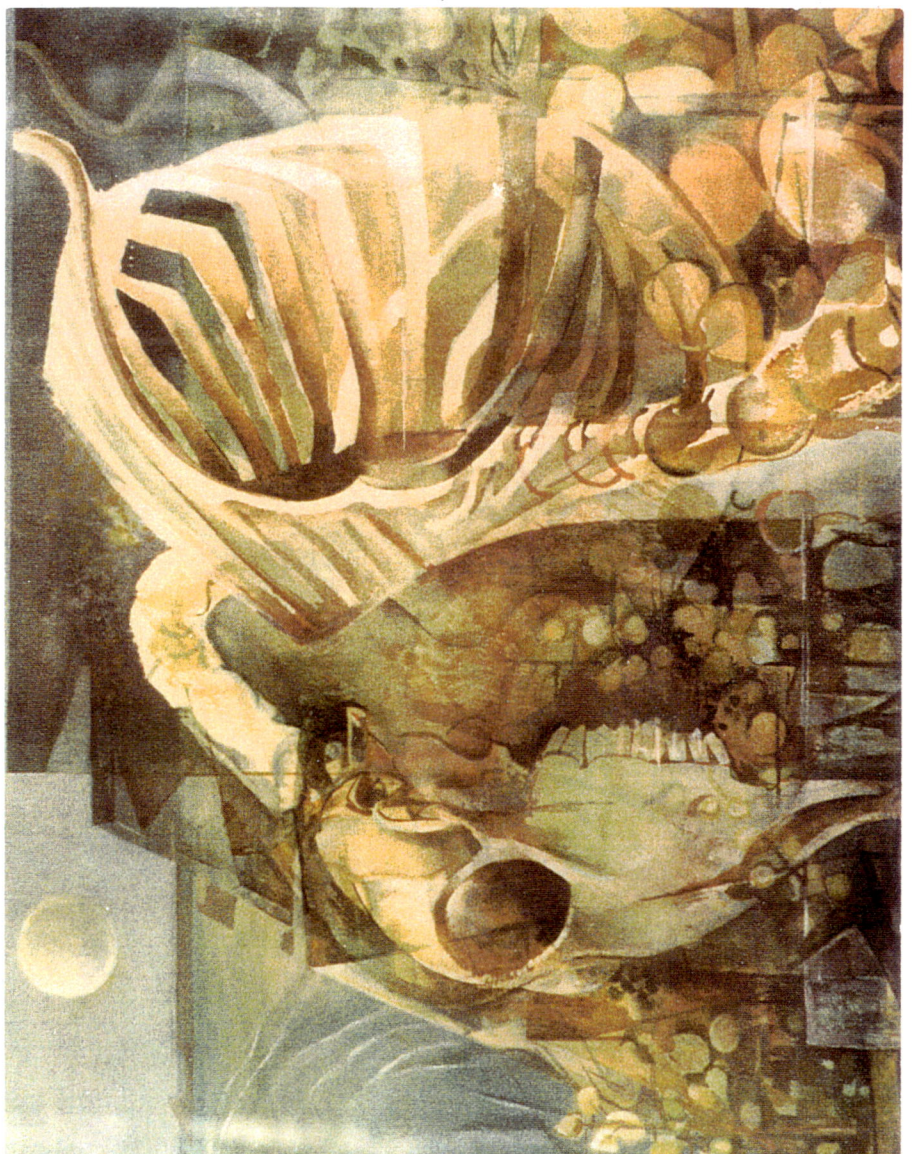

Fig. 97   Skeletal Form – Gower   Watercolour

49

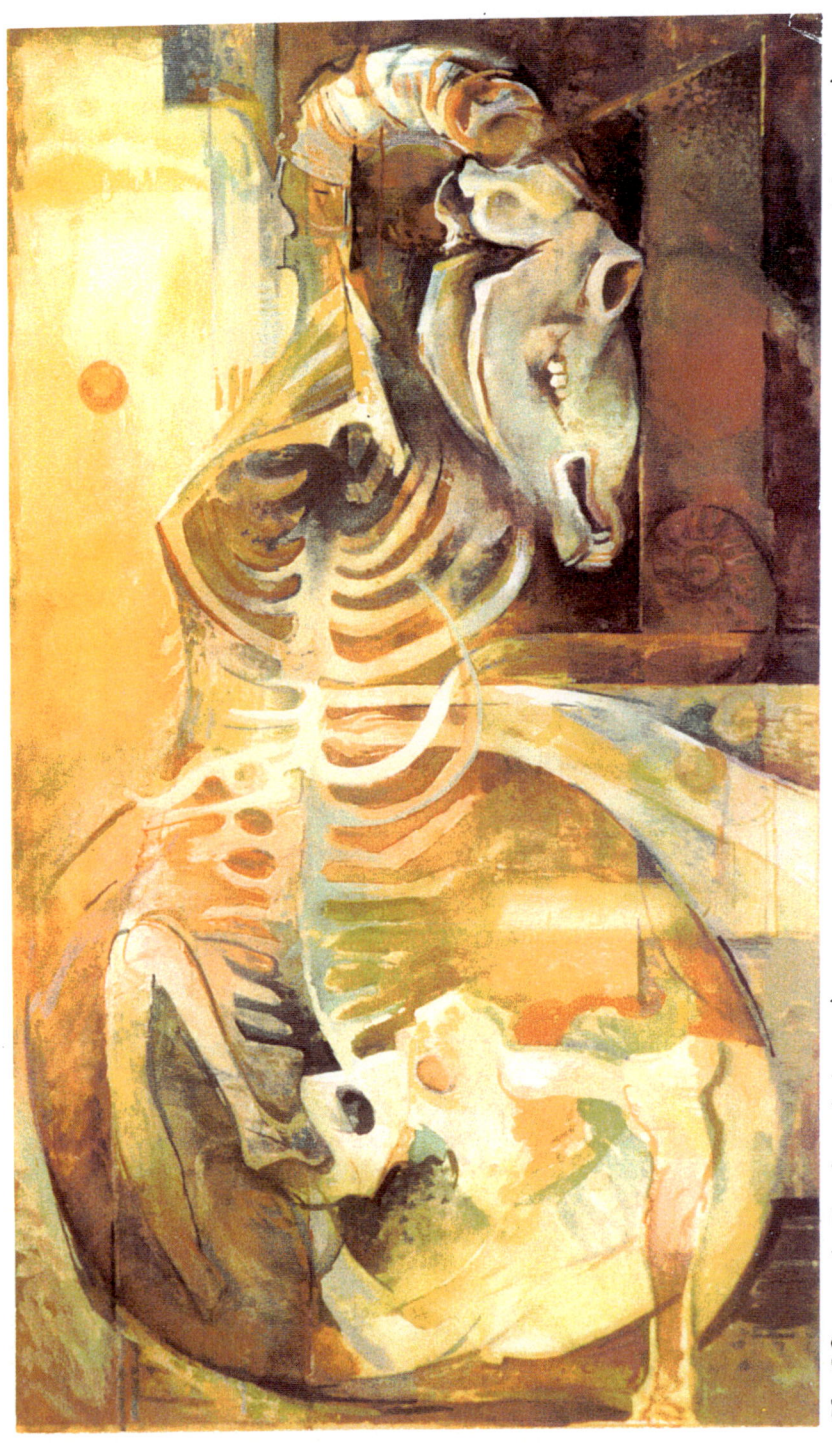

Fig.99   A Skeletal Landscape   Watercolour

A SKELETAL LANDSCAPE

The original skeleton study (fig 96) was reworked many times (with hindsight, obsessionally so, for I found many pictorial ideas from such a small source). In this re-interpretation the skeleton now extends over the full width and height of the picture — a cavernous underworld with peripheral hills and coastline.

Reading a Gower pamphlet on an important archaeological site close-by our holiday home - probably influenced the basic structure of the painting. (The discovery of the Paviland cave unearthed a ceremonial burial of a young male, dated to 26,000 years ago. Grave-goods included artefacts of mammoth ivory and some 4,500 finds of bone and stone-tools.) A more psychological search for my own 'underground' areas could be surmised from the depths around the skull.

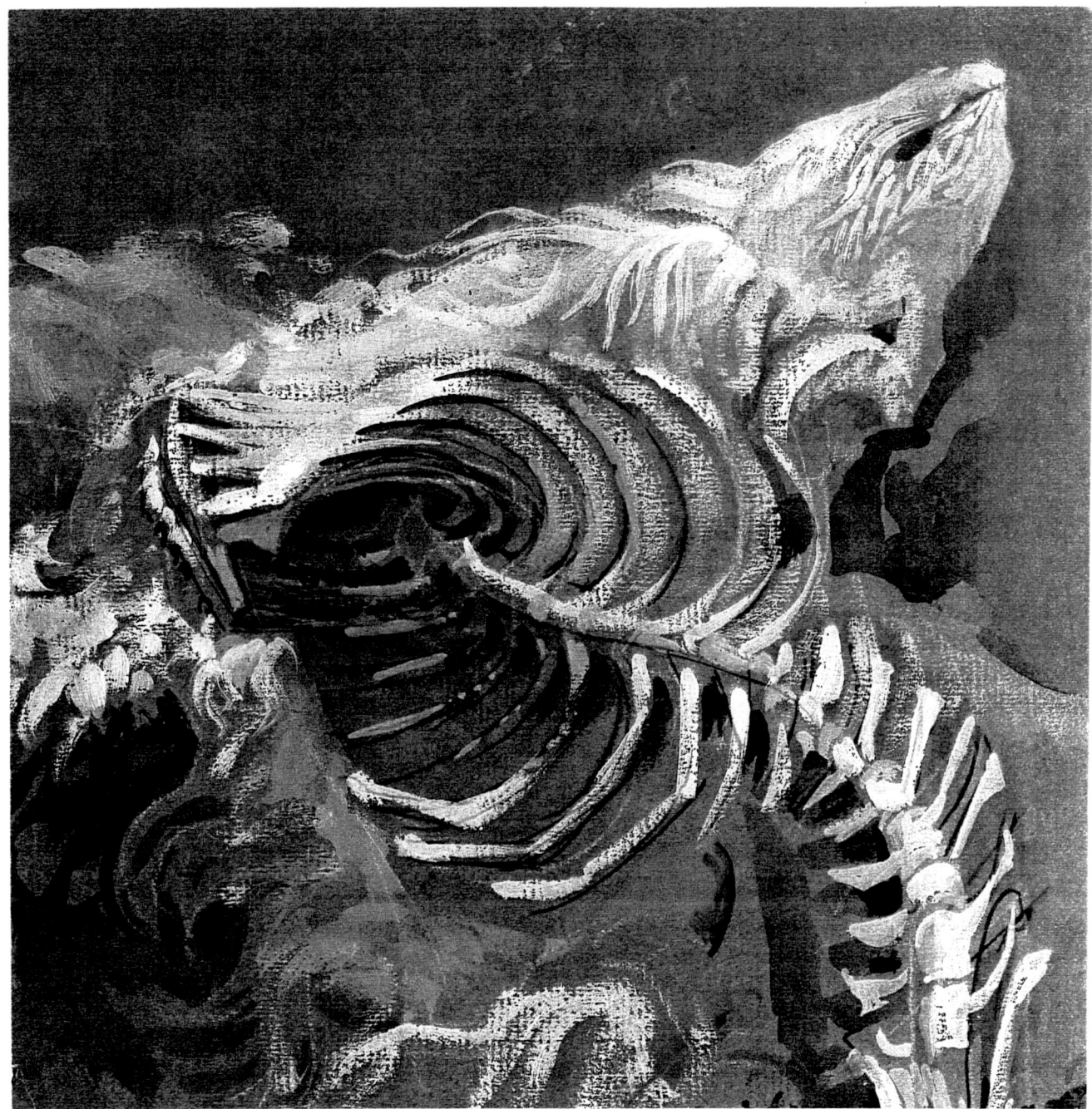

Fig.100 A Sheep's Carcass   Pen and Gouache on toned paper

A LAKE DISTRICT FIND

Stimulated further by this discovery on a mountain in the 'Lakes' I made sketches and took photographs of this more 'complete' sheep's carcass. After the birds and weather had cleaned out the interior, the superb form of the skeleton could be observed – the pattern of ribs centred and structured around the S shape of the spinal column.

Often disintegration and destruction can reveal their own hidden beauty – this can especially apply to old tree forms (see Paul Nash and Graham Sutherland).

This gouache study was painted from an earlier drawing.

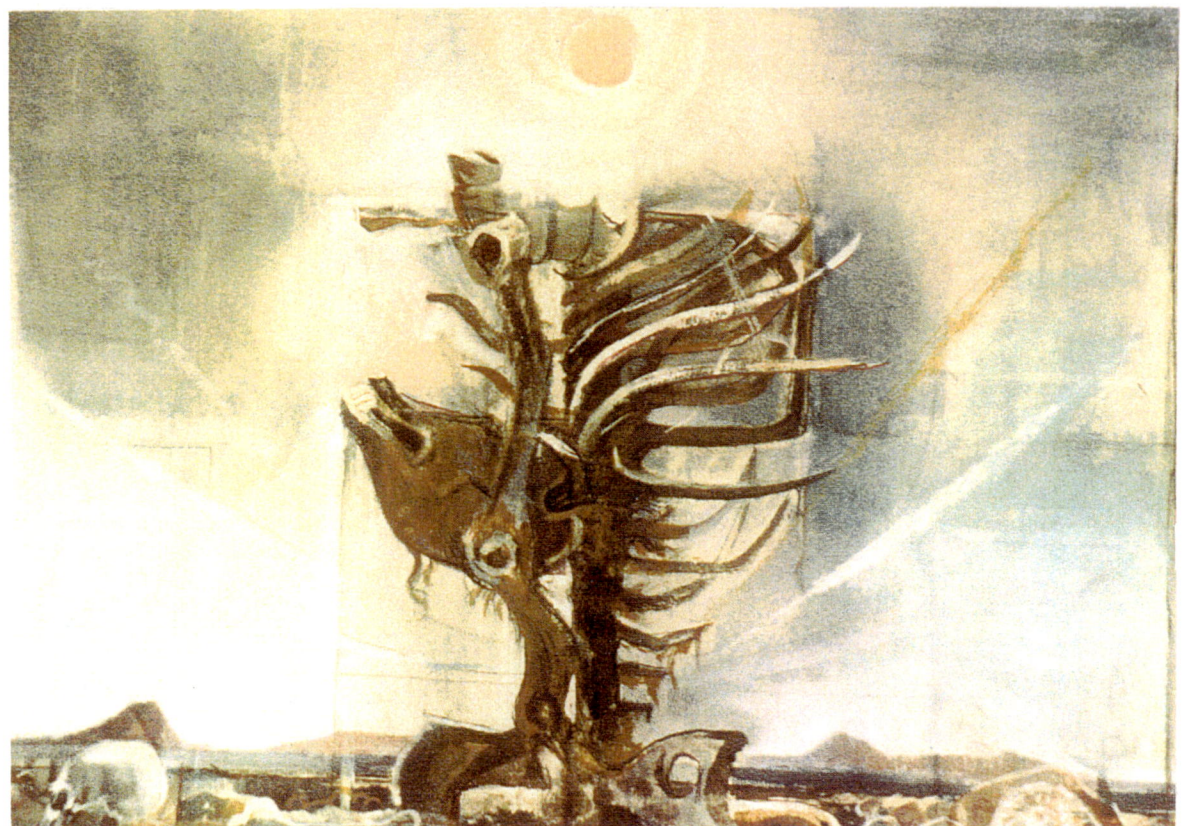

Fig. 101   Chalice in a barren landscape   Watercolour

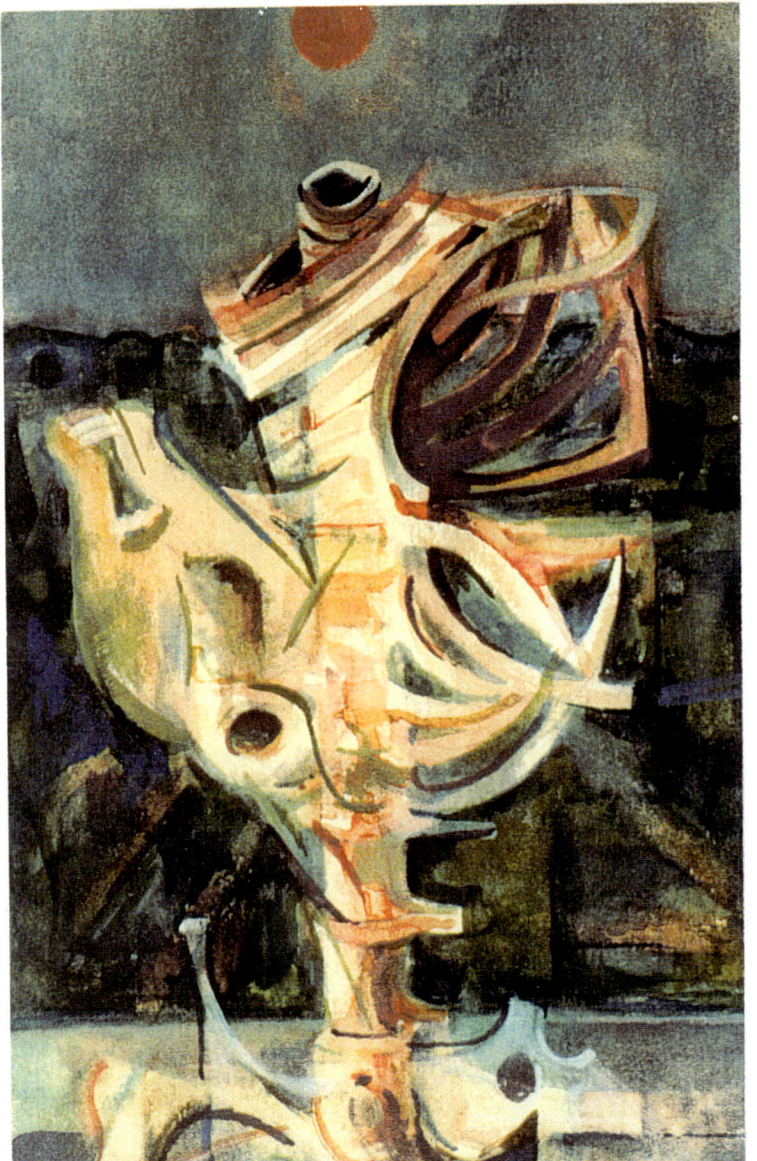

THE CHALICE

This group of five chalices shows the change of content and subject matter after the discovery of the 'killed' sheep.

A religious, spiritual presence is hinted at by these transformed skeletons. These are now symbols of sacrifice, of offerings to a God or gods.

Also the sheep becomes the 'Lamb of God' — the sacrificial victim.

Above: The bone chalice stands on a great plain littered with skulls, stones and fossils set against a distant range of mountains.

Left: A complete rearrangement of the bone parts to form the chalice which stands on a slab or altar. The chalice is to be offered up to the red sun-god, suggesting some ancient rite.

There is an ambiguity about all of these symbols of sacrifice — whether they are pagan, Christian or whatever — but each emphasises the idea of the victim which is to be 'offered up'.

Fig. 102   Bone Chalice - 1   Watercolour.

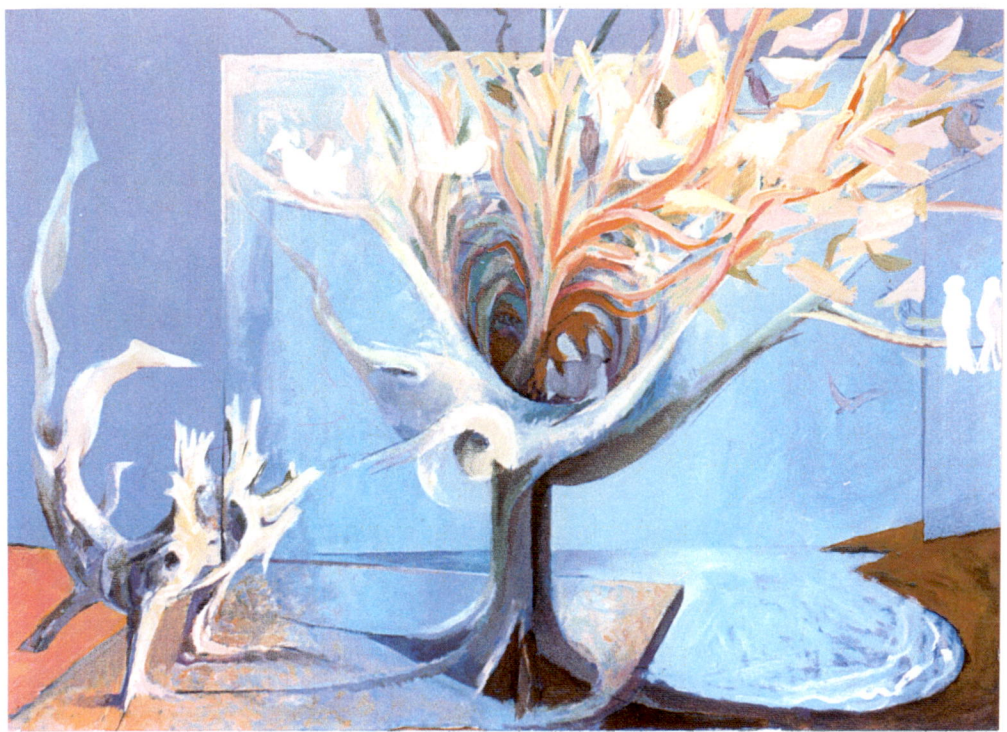

Fig.103   Tree and Tree-root Chalices   Acrylic

I feel that each chalice was a reinvention of the original carcass, the skull and ribcage making the cup and the spine and legs serving as supporting stem and base. The version above is lighter in mood, the carcass transformed into a tree with doves resting in its branches, as a tree root dances in attendance.

Below left: Another variation on the tree form, turning and swirling.
Below right: A more contrived reworking, with a lush landscape filling the cup to overflowing. The individual parts are more clearly defined.

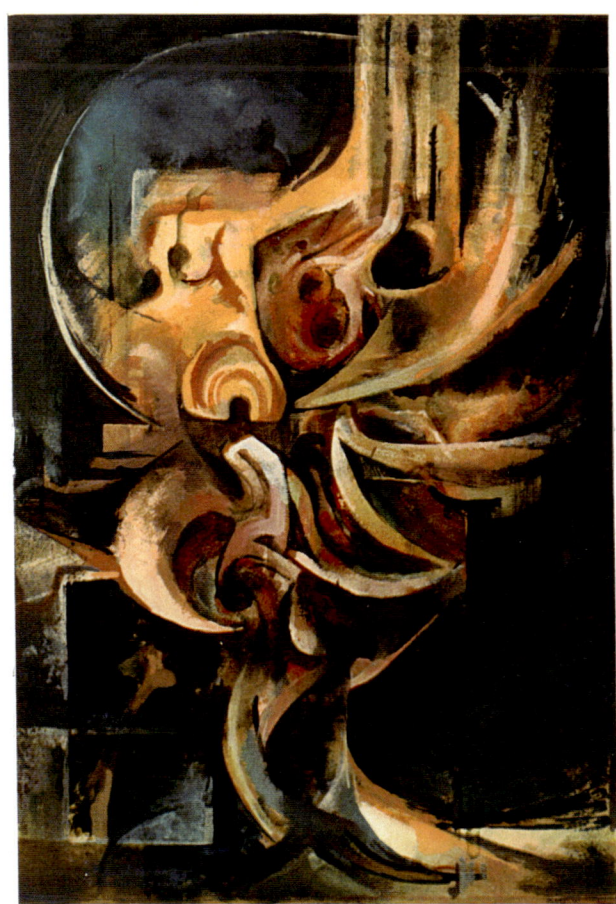

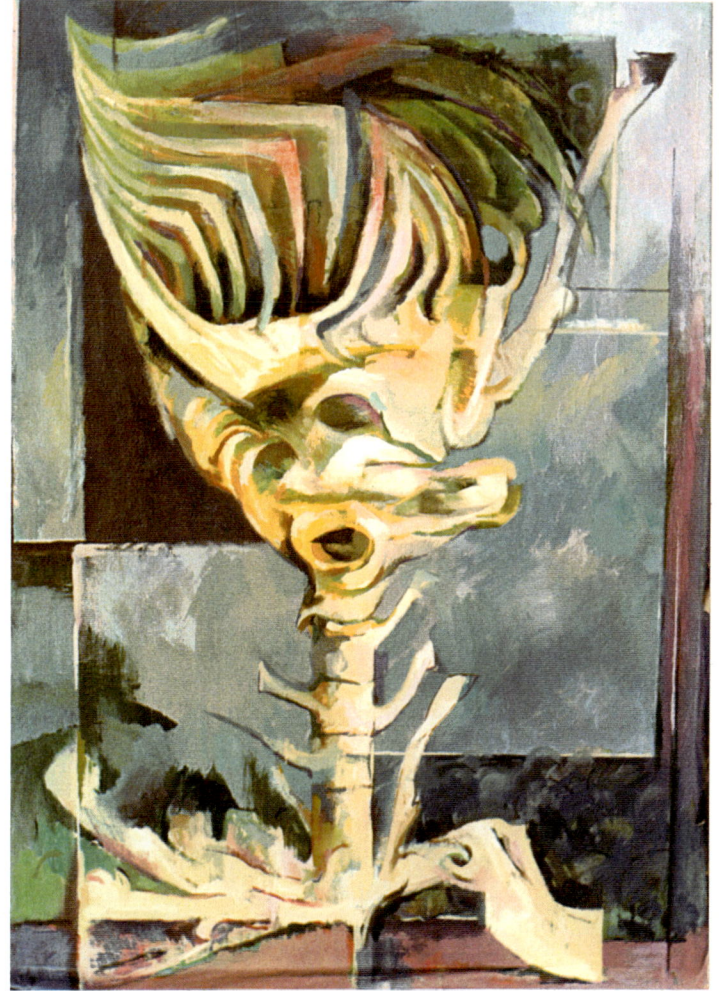

Fig.104 Tree Root Chalice   Gouache   Fig.105 Bone Chalice - 2   Gouache

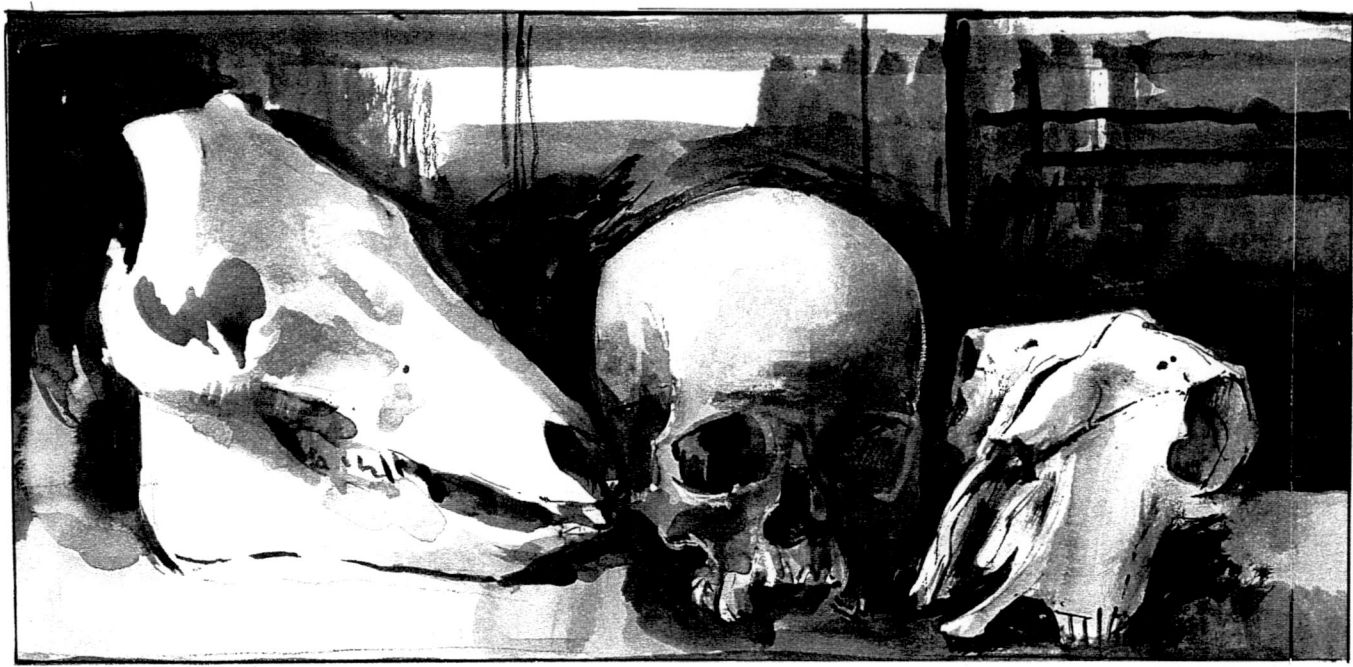

Fig.106   Three Skulls   Watercolour

Encouraged by a release of creative energy from the series of skeletal paintings, I started redrawing the skulls from my collection. From the studies I returned to the landscape subject again with more interest in my local area of the Cotswolds.

Above: A pig, a human and a sheep's skull from my collection.
Below: A large sheep's skull underlies the structure of these local landscape scenes.

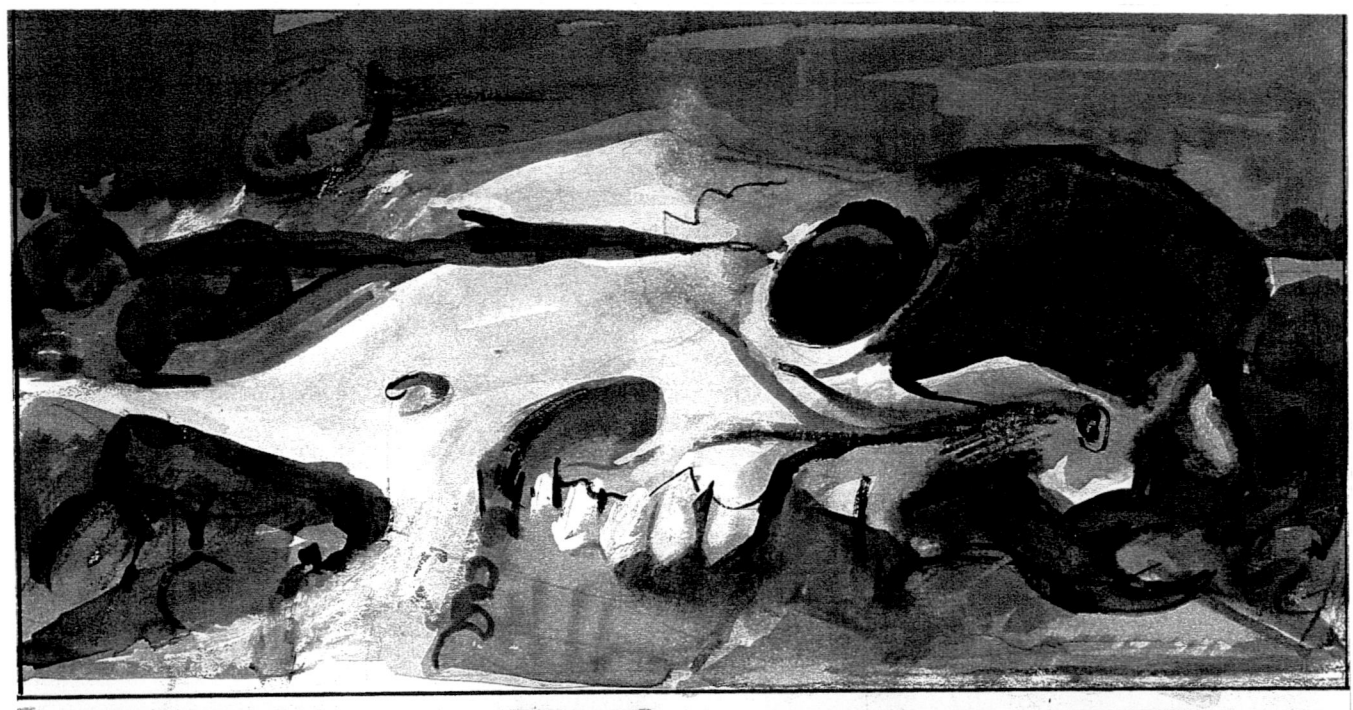

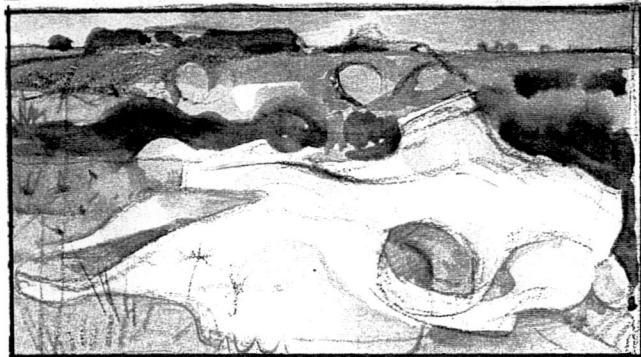
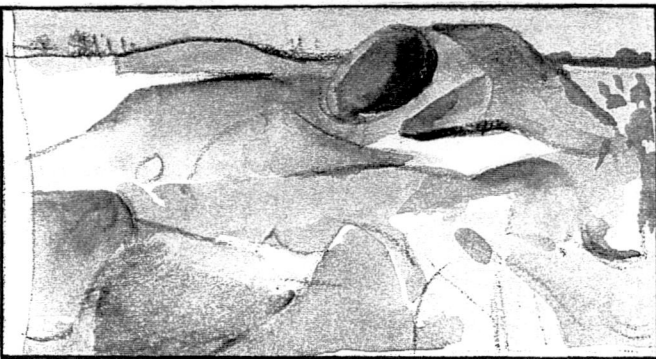

Fig.107   Three Skull Landscapes   Watercolour

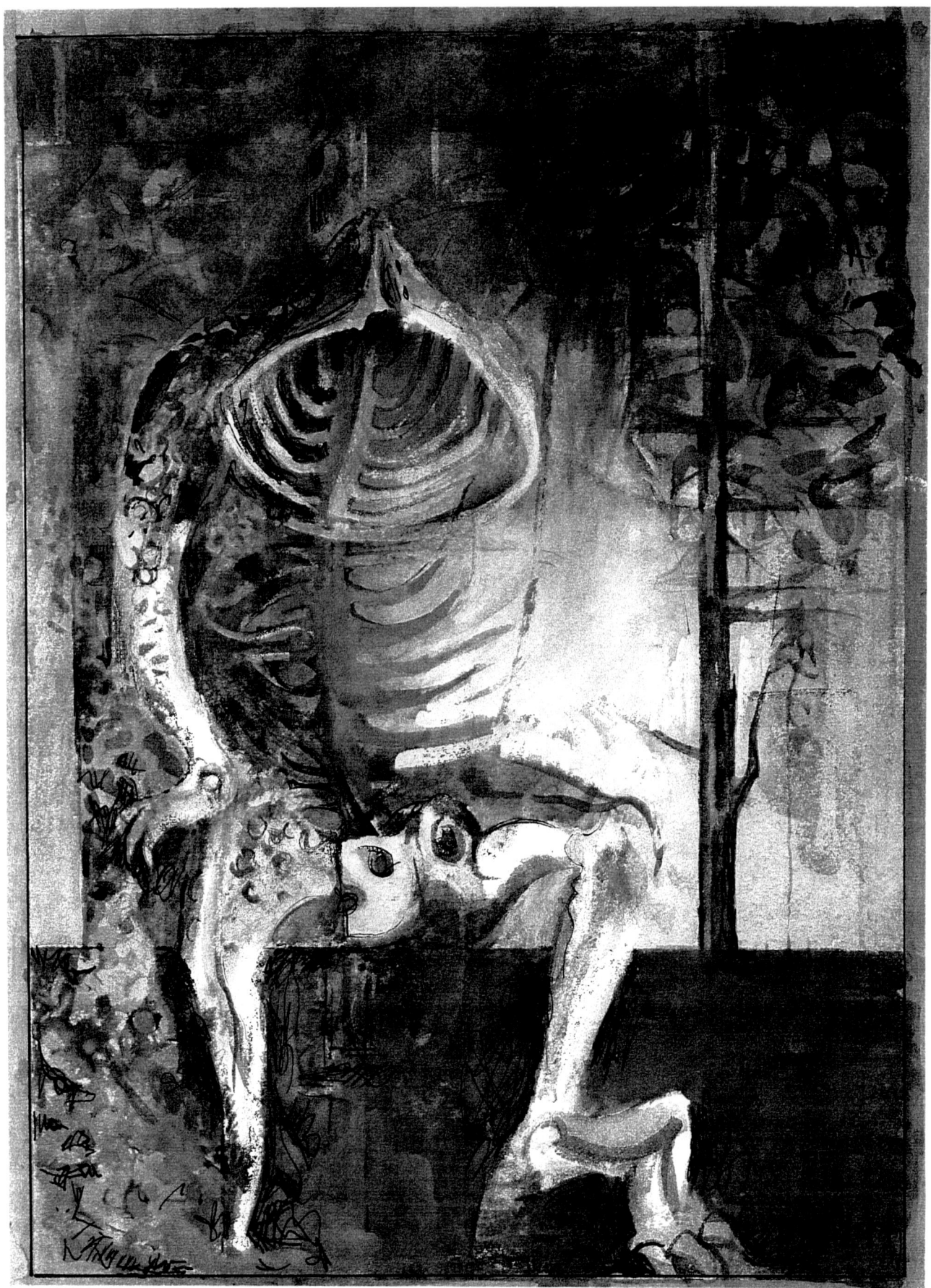

Fig.108 Bone Spectre	Ink & Watercolour

A SPECTRE

Using the rib cage from the original drawing (fig.96), it now becomes an alien's mouth whilst the pelvis and leg bones are rearranged and partly covered with a mottled skin to the left side of this sinister spectral figure — one of three fantasies worked on during a somewhat Gothic (romantic?) frame of mind.

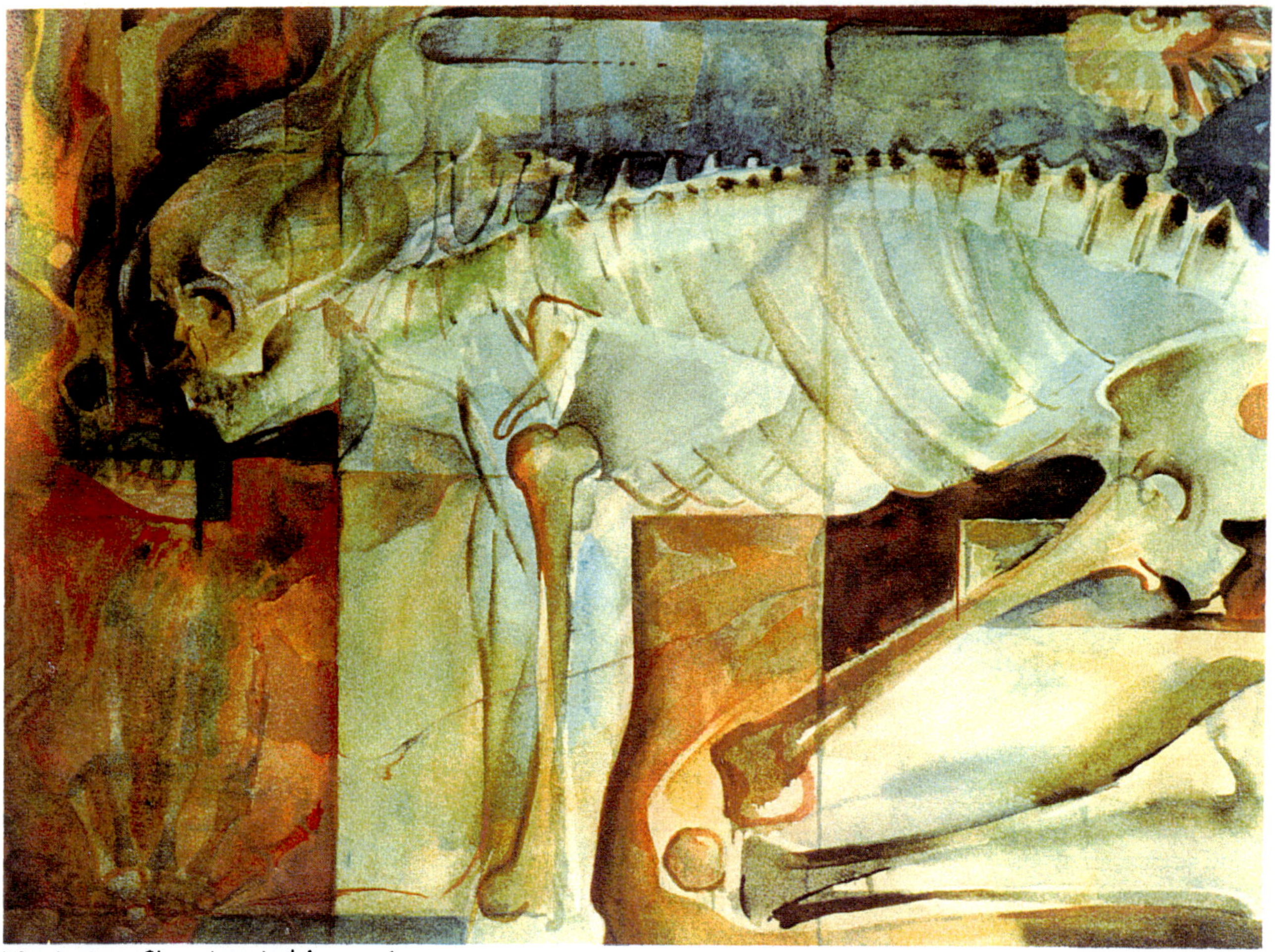

Fig.109 Claustrophobic Burial   Watercolour

Subconscious fears rise to the surface. Claustrophobia, of being enclosed, buried, entrapped in a vacuum, cave or grave. All these are implied in the painting above. Below, the fear is more of drowning, or suffocation below the soil or in liquids. The humanoid figure has retained a sheep's head.

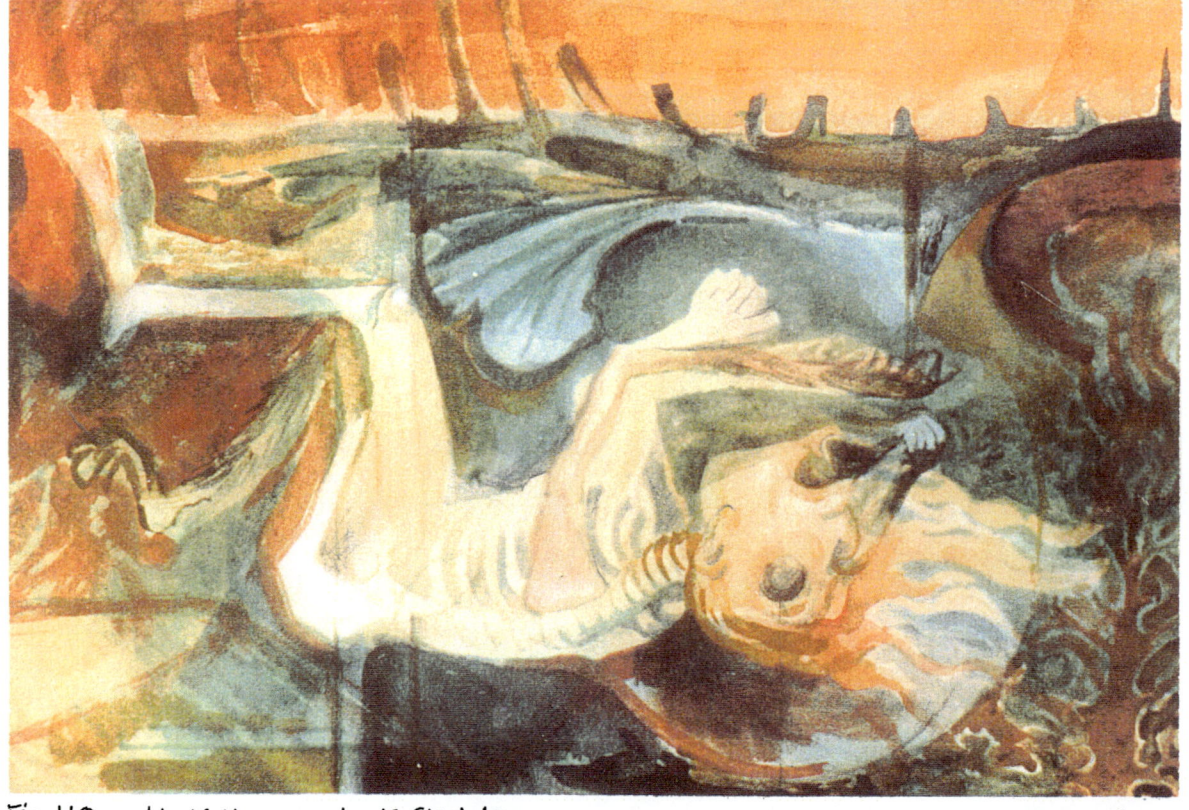

Fig.110 Half Human, half Skeleton   Watercolour

DRAWING, PAINTING & NURSING MOTHER 1986-1989

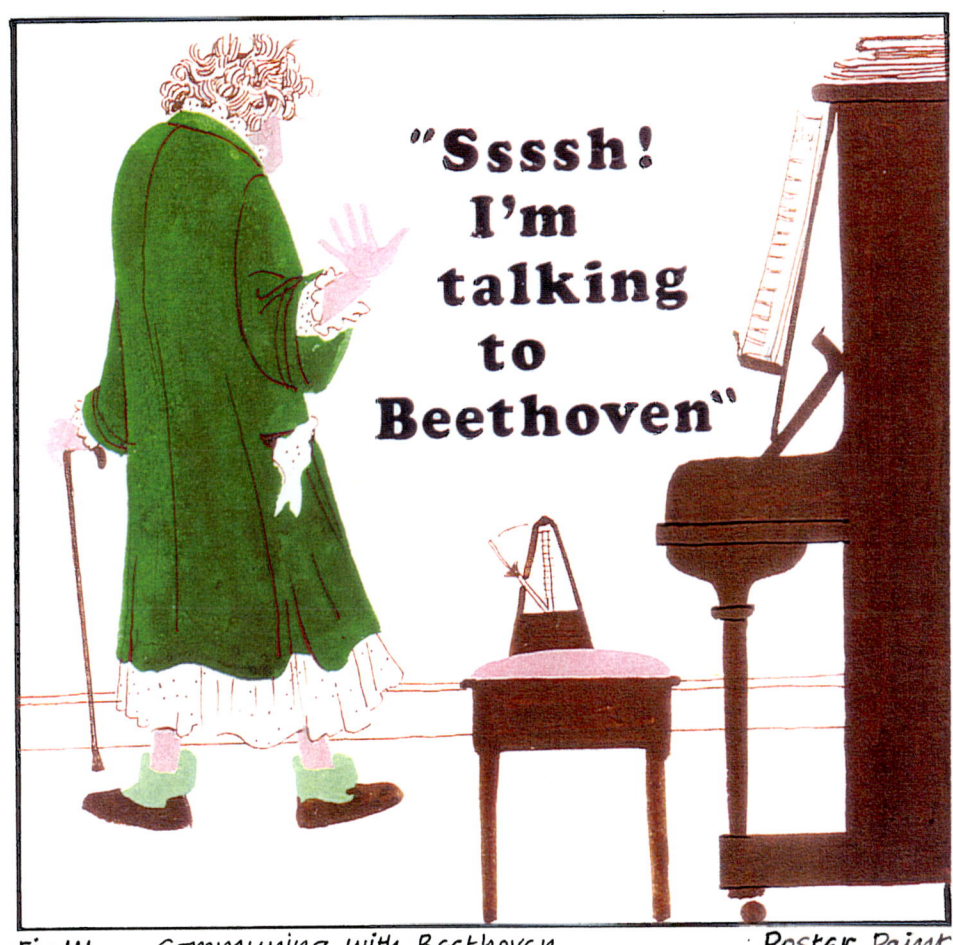

Fig. III   Communing with Beethoven   Poster Paint

Foetal curved, holding my hand and gently smiling, I knew she'd died. Mum at ninety-four had had a tenacious hold on life, but following a third hip operation she never countered the infection and died in hospital in February 1989.

Four years earlier, Alfred, who had cared for and nursed my paraplegic brother in the past, contacted me again on hearing of Mum's increasing fragility, and offered to return and assist with nursing and care. Alf was one of those precious finds – a dedicated carer and trained nurse who chose freelance voluntary work in exchange for free board and a minimum wage.

With this generous offer we decided to share the nursing, Alf taking on evening and night duties and I the day-time help. An ulterior motive also contributed to my decision to help Mum – I felt a need to reconcile myself with someone with whom, throughout childhood and beyond, I'd not formed a close relationship. A large amount of shared time would now become available to us and something creative might develop. It did, although not quite in the way I'd expected.

Each morning, on arrival, mum and I would deal with any problems of the moment. If she was sleepy, I'd go upstairs to a temporary studio and work, returning only when I heard her buzzer – which sounded fairly frequently. Over a period of time I found myself often working in her room finding much material for drawing her in her various mood swings.

This usually led to interesting results on paper, whether as drawings in pen and ink, crayon sketches, pencil or small watercolours.

Many 'reveries' arose during our days together but four in particular began to dominate: Music, the piano and the 'Great Masters', Visits from the Queen, the 'Cat Plague', and matters relating to the 'Missing Handbag'. The constant anxieties Mum attached to these matters could at times become very tedious and irritating, but I discovered that the artwork relating to them was also therapeutic and, fortunately, also a source of entertainment for us both. Mum enjoyed the drawings and frequently laughed at her own foibles expressed in the work – especially when she was lucid.

Music had always been central to her life. A piano teacher for over fifty years, she continued into her mid-eighties, then played for herself until deafness distorted the quality of sound in her performance which made her retire. An attempt to fit her with a hearing-aid proved futile. One day, after about three days of use, with an oath, she threw it away in disgust, never to use it again. From then on, for the remaining three years of her life, she wanted me to play her favourite pieces on the piano from her three Bs (Bach, Beethoven and Brahms) and also a few works by Ravel, Debussy and Poulenc. A strong German-French tradition held sway. The Russians didn't get a look in - Rachmaninoff was out (too sentimental). Others like, say, Bartok were also out (too modern). This was fortunate for me as the last two required a far better technique than I possessed. Some of Mum's most entertaining remarks sprang from musical associations which, in turn, led to many quick sketches with her quotes included. I also wrote a poem relating to this time (page 66).

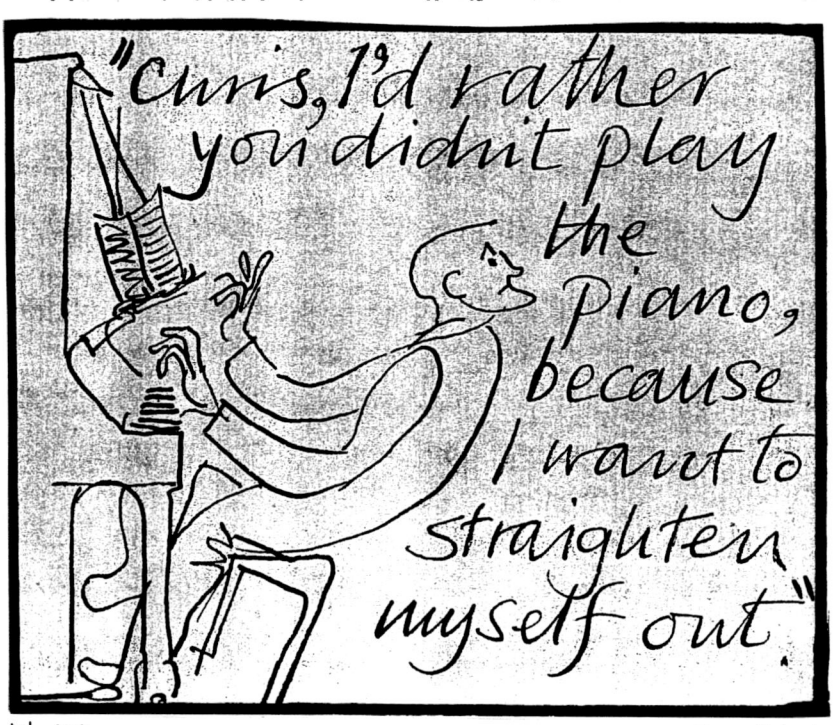

Fig.112   Pen & Ink

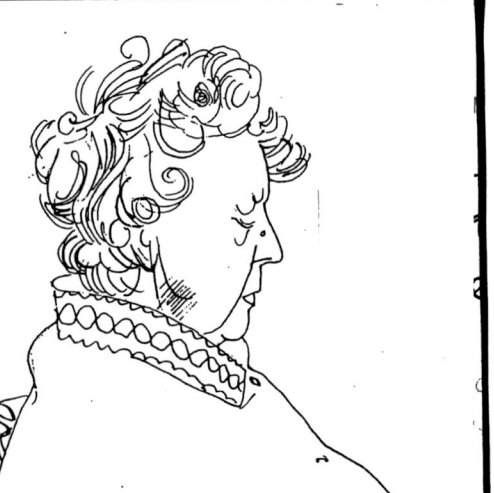

Fig.113   Pen & Ink

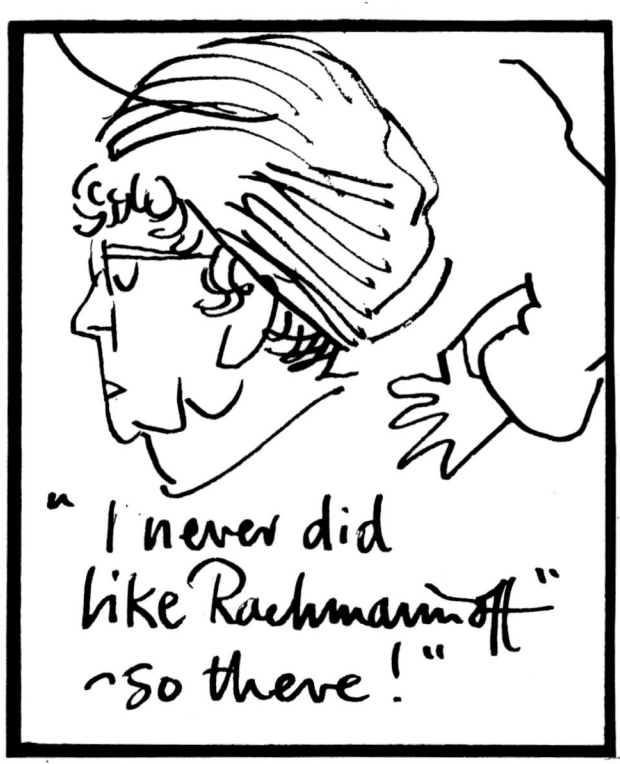

Fig.114   Pen & Ink

MUSICAL VARIATIONS

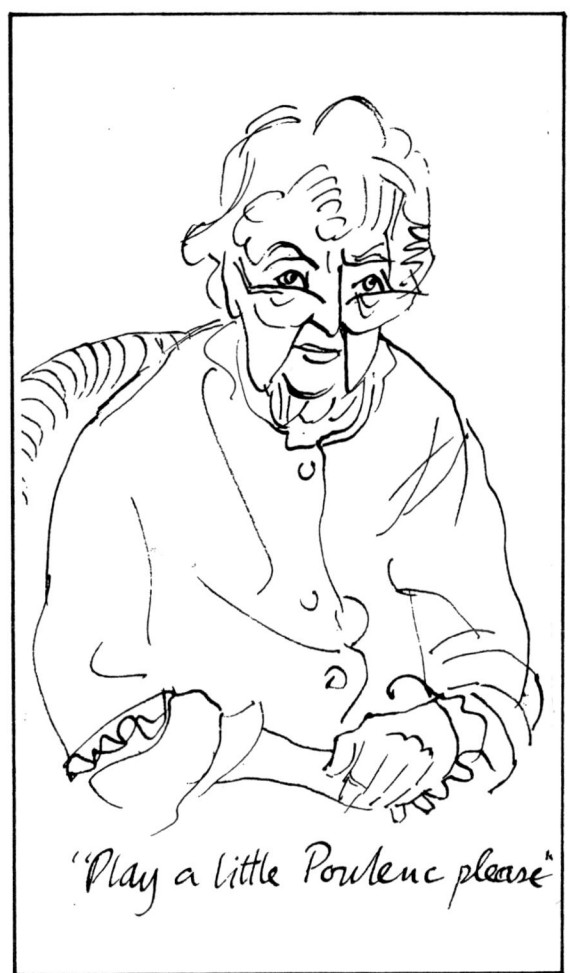

Fig. 115   Pen & Ink

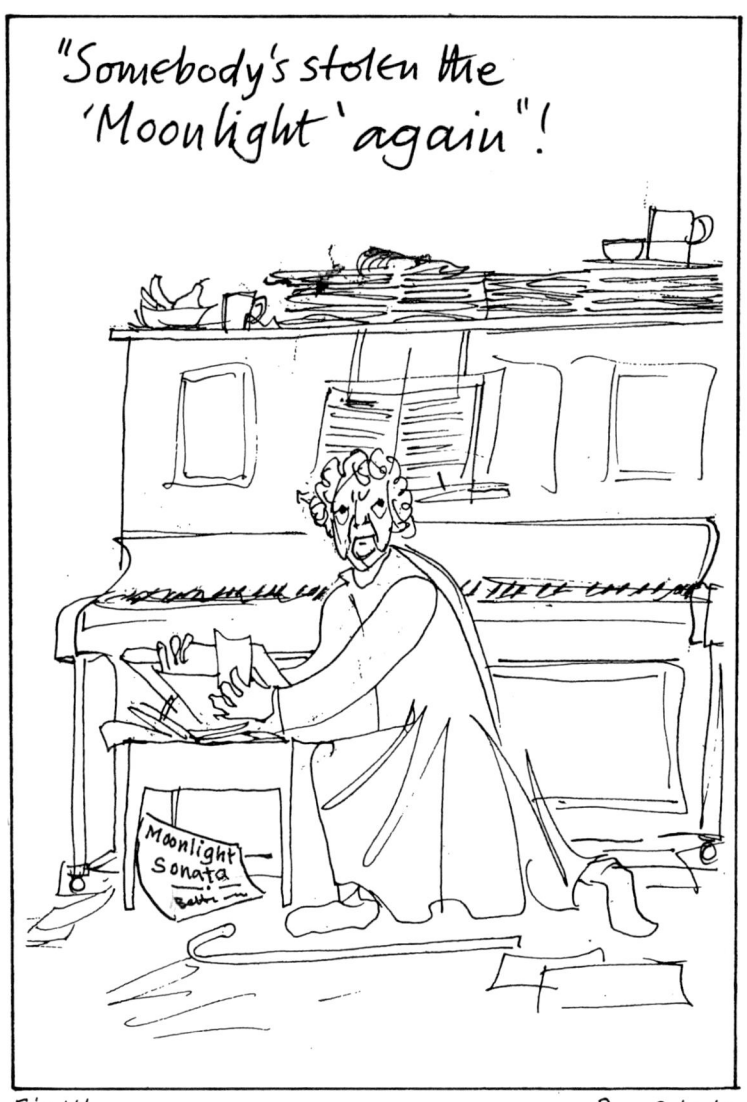

Fig. 116   Pen & Ink

THE QUEEN'S VISIT

The journey from home to Mum's house often held for me a certain anticipation, as the greetings I received were invariably unexpected. Usually some surprising remark would greet me on opening her door. 'Why dear, you've just missed the Queen, perhaps you could arrive earlier next time' or, 'Would you open the front door to welcome Her Majesty', or again, 'Hoover the carpet Chris, before She arrives'.

Once, arriving late, I found her kneeling, begging that older people might be excused this difficult task of curtsying. On other occasions roles would be reversed and I was expected to treat her with a little more deference, she taking on the role of Queenship — 'You may leave us now' etc... These 'Queen and I' conversations rarely lasted more than a few minutes but their impact as visual material was considerable with many sketches illustrating these moments (figs 117-123).

Often our talks became surreal when another 'guest' entered the conversation — only gleaned as I heard queries or answers addressed to other parts of the room, totally unrelated to our earlier talk.

One day Mum asked for a permanent wave 'before the Royal presence arrived for tea', and a hairdresser was brought in, a rare extravagance indeed, indicating the importance of the coming honour. Looking at the crayon drawing done at the time recalls the mood of the day — the fixation on Royalty, the hair rising up, embracing the space in the room, a 'permanent wave' enclosing Mum's internalised Queen (fig 123).

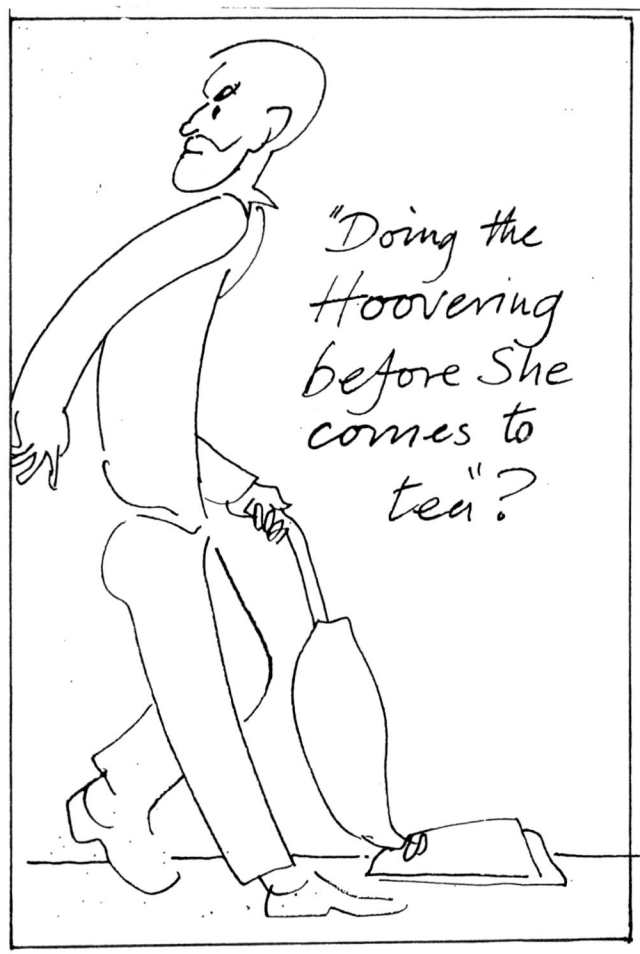

Fig.117 Pen & Ink

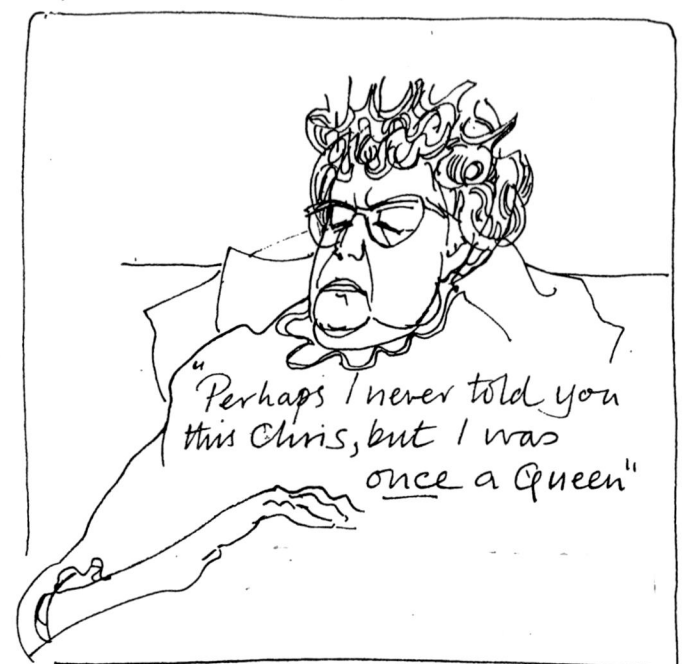

Fig.118 Pen & Ink

Preparations for the Queen's Visit

A selection of pen and ink portraits referring to this theme. The larger crayon drawing was worked on following a day Mum decided to have a hairdresser before Her Majesty arrived later that day. Written thoughts unravel from her 'permanent wave', then gradually fills the space of her 'vision'.

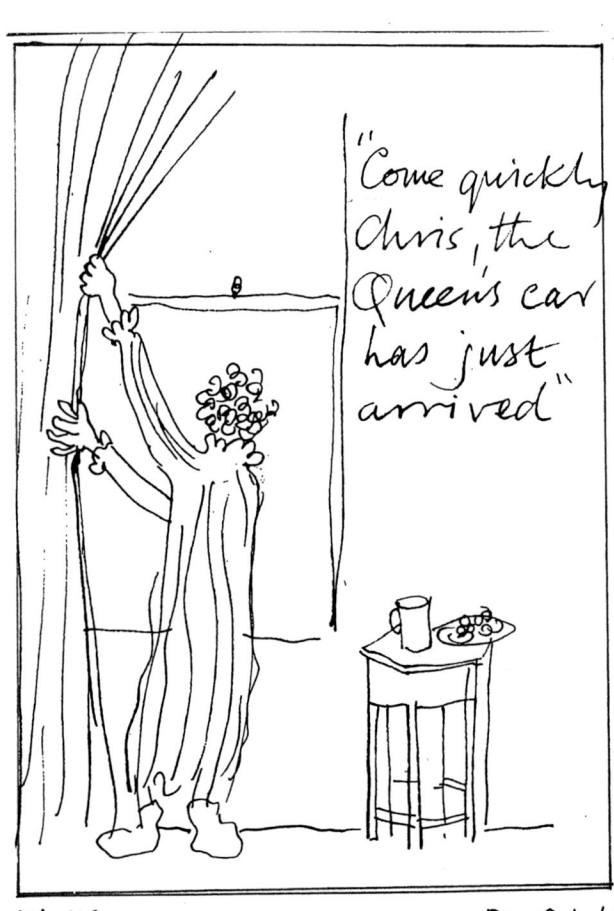

Fig.119 Pen & Ink

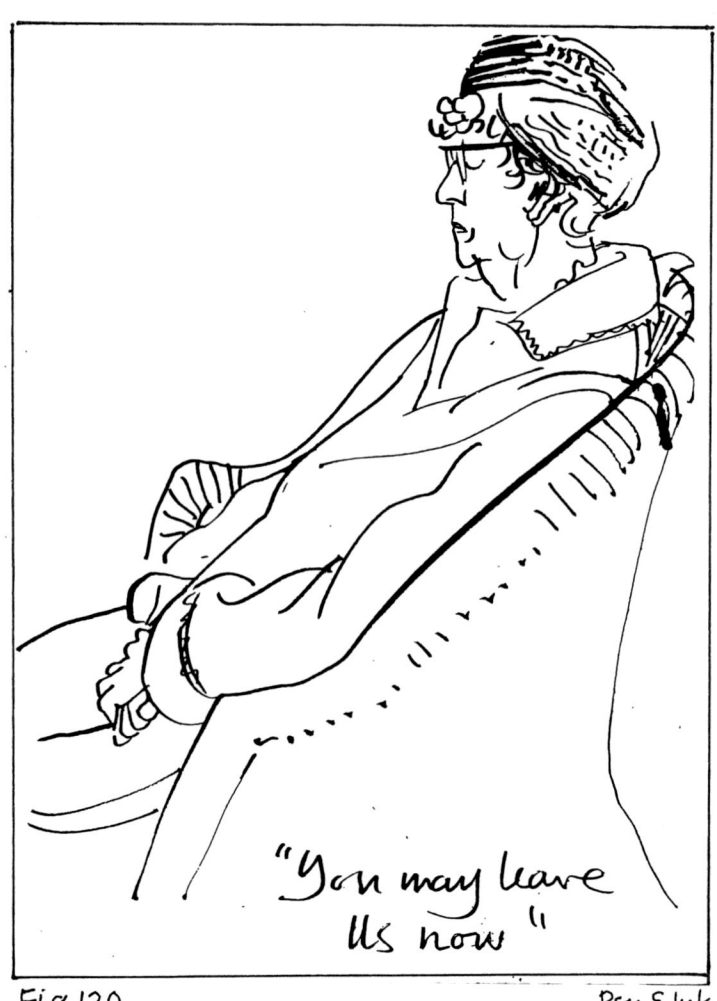

Fig.120 Pen & Ink

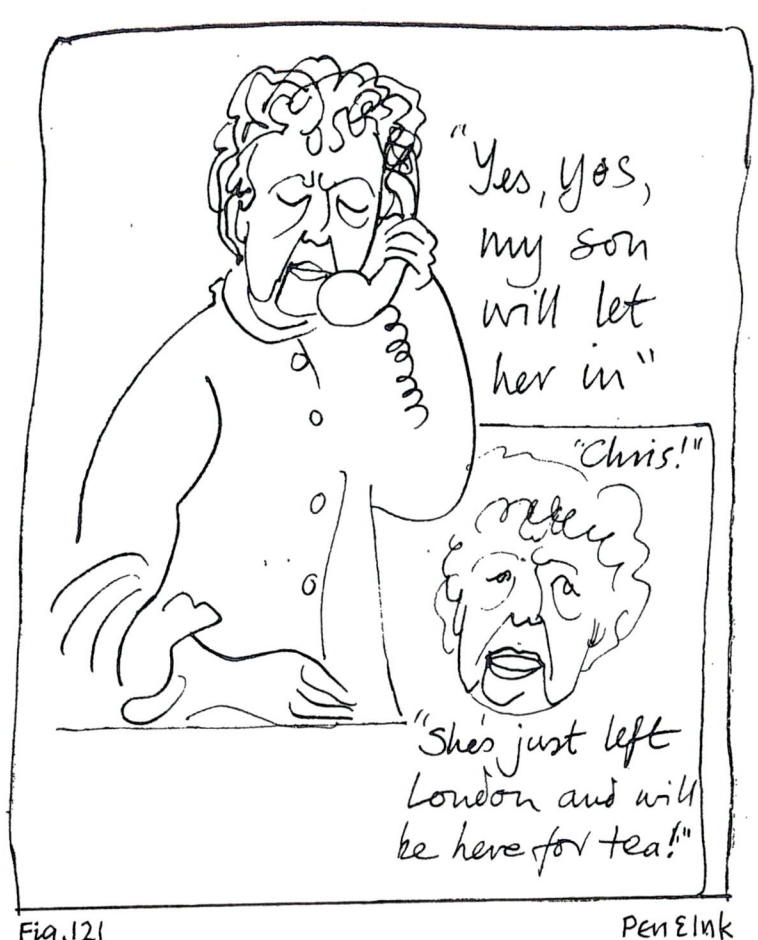

Fig.121   Pen & Ink

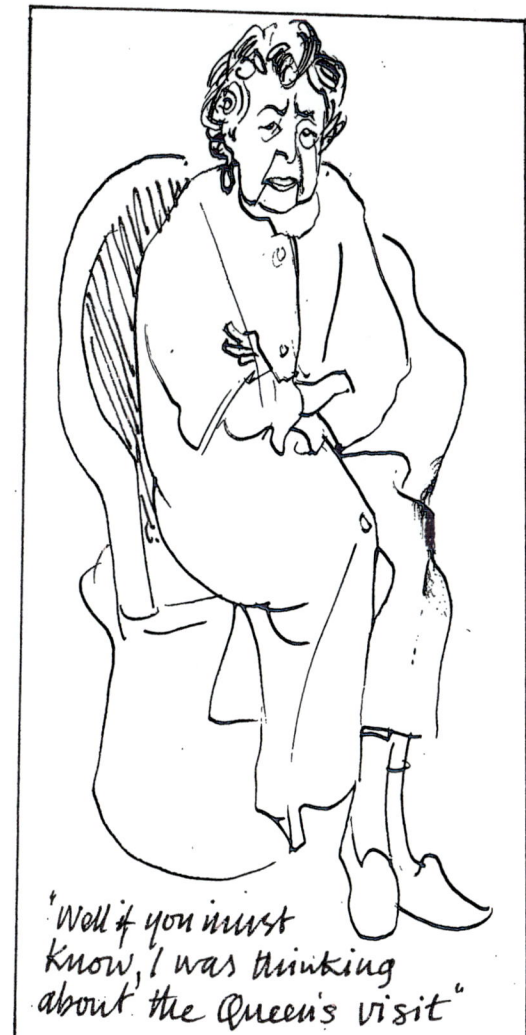

Fig.122   Pen & Ink

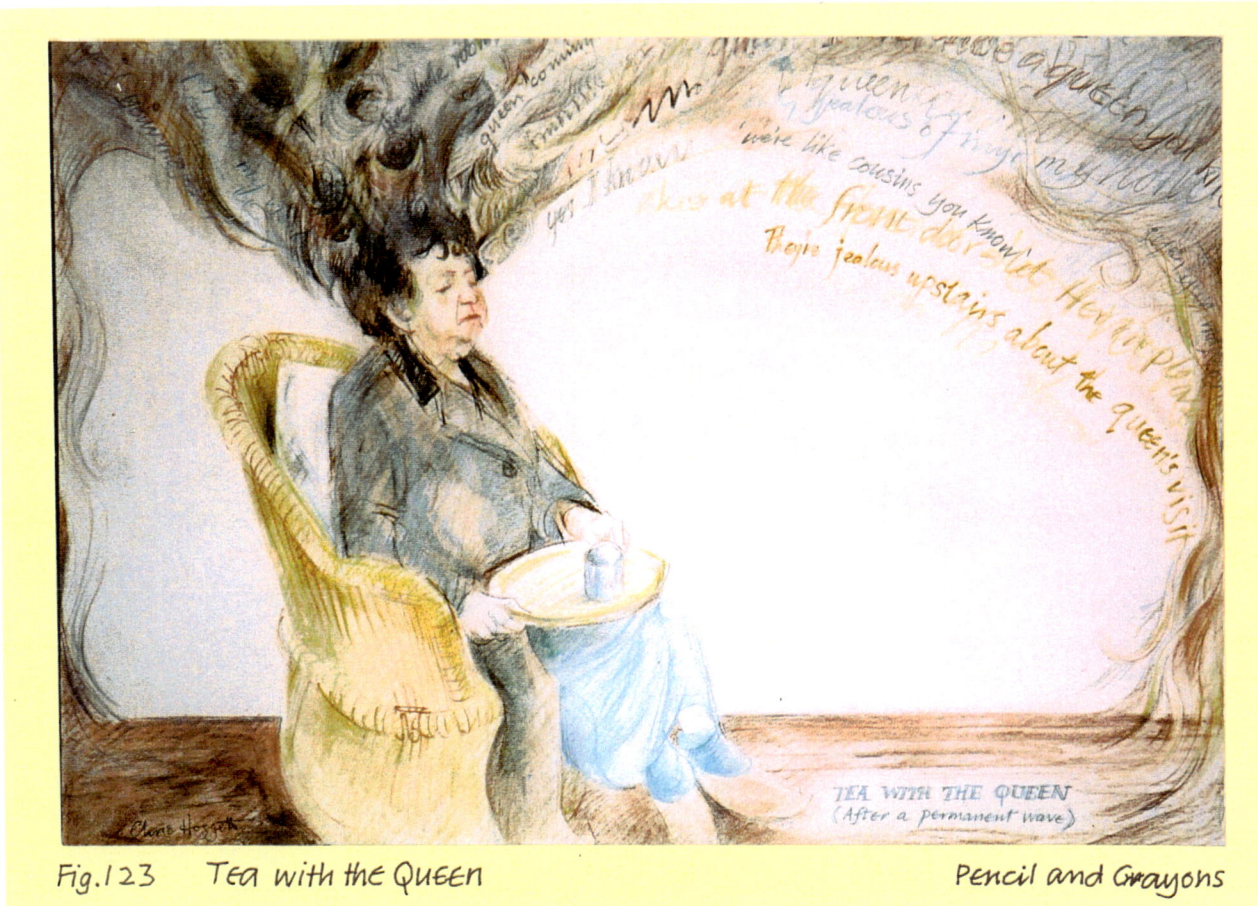

Fig.123   Tea with the Queen   Pencil and Crayons

FEARS AND OBSESSIONS

Left: 'Phobias'

Reputations could be ruined during a phobic spell. Two of Mum's tenants suffered such a reversal one day – from charming to 'lewd and loose' overnight.

Harassed by religious 'condemnation' fears and guilt she had conversations with various church 'leaders.'

Also, for one who loved cats for most of her life, the sudden rejection must have been sad and distressing. Once a stray wandered in and frightened her enough to cause real distress (see text at foot).

The painting 'Phobias' attempts to incorporate these fears or obsessions together: The two girl tenants terrorise Mum by whispering dread thoughts into her ears – one hovers witch-like above, the other sits nude beside her.

Meanwhile two black cats (no doubt 'familiars' to the witch tenants) await, one even on her pillow.

Symbols of Crescent and Cross are at hand to remind her of her lax attitude to the Church's teaching (one of her guilt areas).

Below: Finding a stray cat in the house would lead to a quick retreat with cries of 'Plague'! or "Disease!"

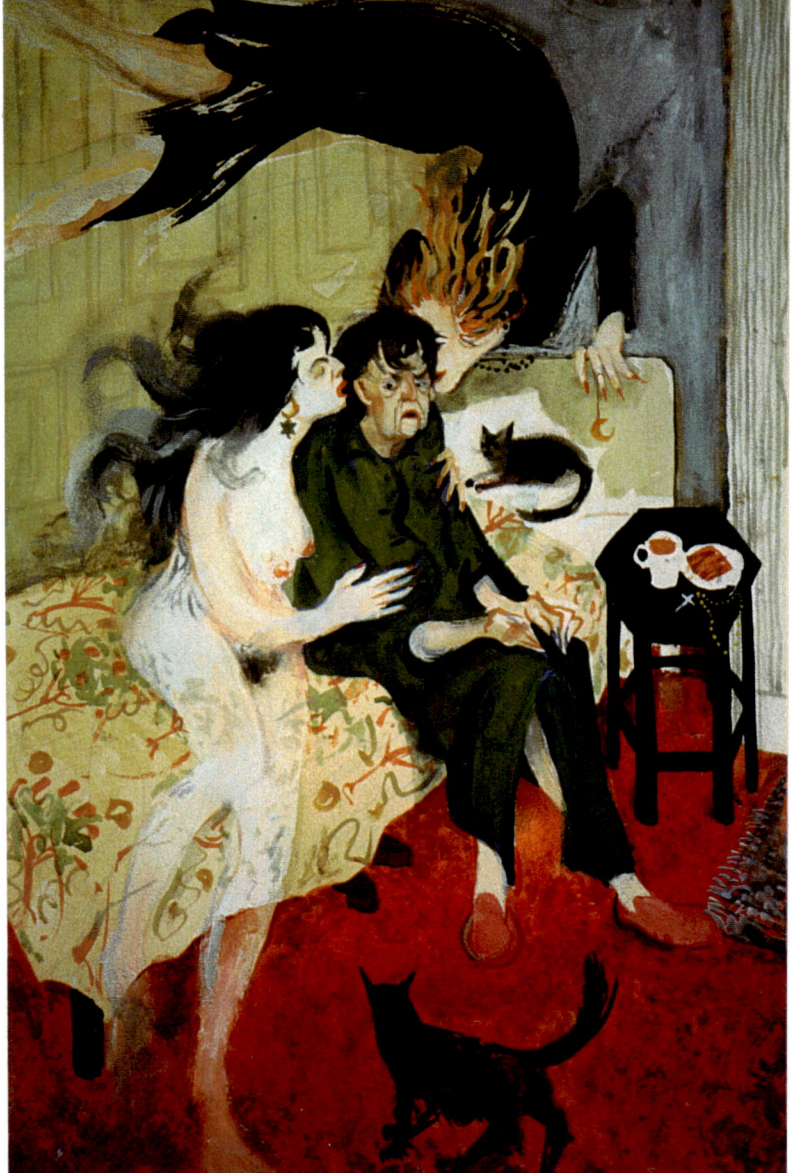

Fig.124 Phobias Gouache

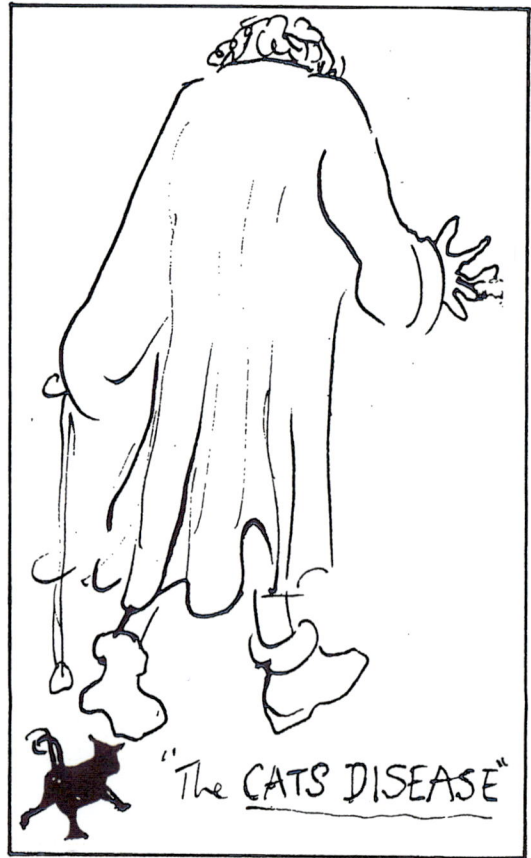

Fig.126 Pen & Ink

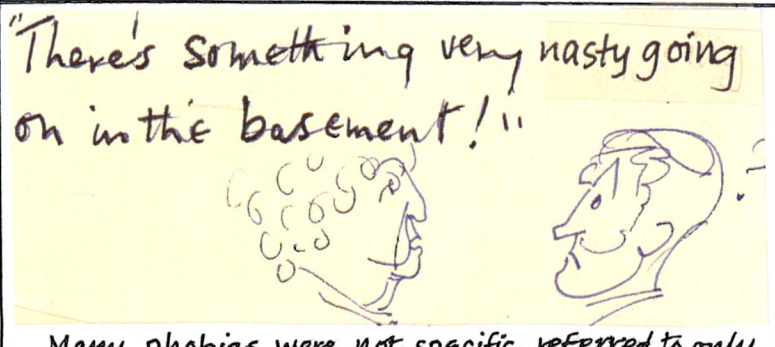

"There's something very nasty going on in the basement!"

Many phobias were not specific, referred to only by a generalised 'something' which was troubling Mum. Of many quotes I can recall, some were often repeated :– "They are out to kill me"; "I've got so many enemies!". Alternatively, the problem is transferred on to me: "I think you are very worried about something".

Fig.125 Pen & Ink

There was a real mystery about the fear of cats. The origins were unknown but lurked always in the background. Mum was troubled by the 'cat plague' which was equated in some curious way with troubles about 'those young girl tenants', usually with sexual connotations. For Mum both carried a label reading 'Contaminated' and 'Beware!' The girls (her top flat tenants) were deemed 'loose' without a shred of evidence and the cats she'd adored all her life were now 'contagious'.

DEATH AND GRAVESTONES

Right: One day Council workmen came to repair the pavement outside Mum's house. Drawing the curtains she saw the men lifting and re-setting the large slabs. Her imagination seemed to quicken and questions on her own mortality arose — were they digging her grave, was one of the headstones bearing her name?

Below: Thoughts of death, of being killed, followed the 'headstone' experience. Mum suggested she move to my house. However this fear quickly evaporated and was never mentioned again.
The sketch attempts to express the shifting thoughts and fears of that particular day. I incorporated writing not as caption, but as part of the linear flow for the first time. This was to be used in later 'free' drawing.

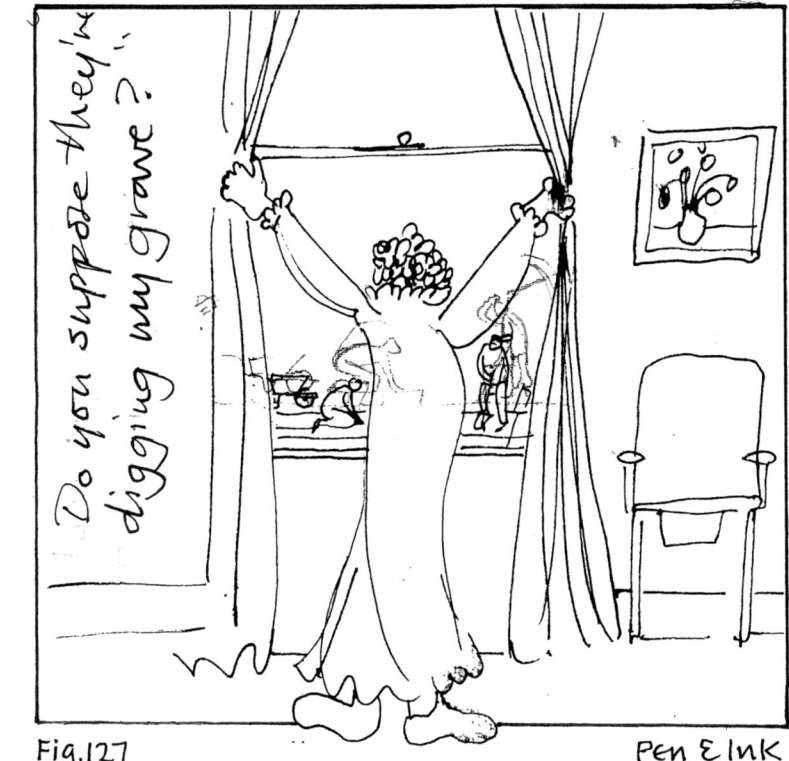

Fig. 127   Pen & Ink

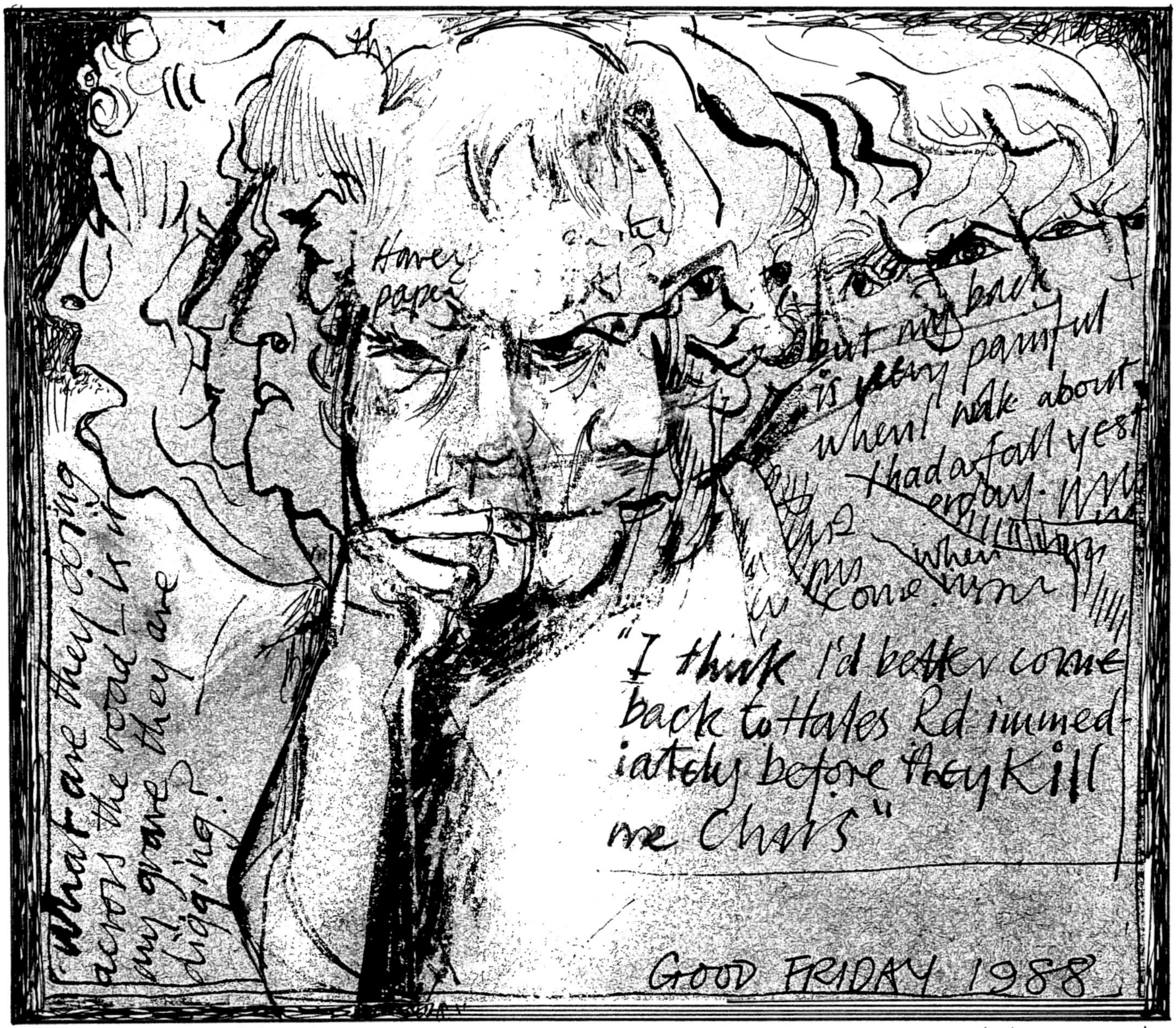

Fig. 128   Good Friday 1988   Ink & Gouache

THE OLD HANDBAG

During Mum's final year one thing caused even greater worry - the imagined theft of her old handbag. A look of rage and despair flickered across her features on certain mornings as I entered her room and I immediately knew the cause.
"Where is my handbag today then?". Knowing all the likely places she could have placed it the previous evening, it usually took only a few moments to retrieve, but on occasion it did seem to wander further afield - once I discovered it in a dustbin.

Mum gave me a smile when I showed her the sketch of her 'Hiding places for a handbag', almost as if knowing the mischief she was causing.

This was not so of course, as her memory loss was something of which Alf and I were becoming only too well aware.

Hunt-the-Handbag

Left: Sometimes the bag was visible when I arrived in the morning but frequently it required a search. Irritated by the constant looking I tried to lift the mood with a touch of humour - I called it the ten most likely positions:

1 The approved position - where Mum always expected to find it.
2 The occasional - amongst her books - position
3 The safe position - behind the pillow.
4 The turned-back-bedclothes position.
5 The slipped-under-the-bed   "
6 The slipped-off-the-table   "
7 The tipped-upside-down   "
8 The back-of-the-bed   "
9 The inside-the-bed   "
10 The 'totally lost' - often an hours search.

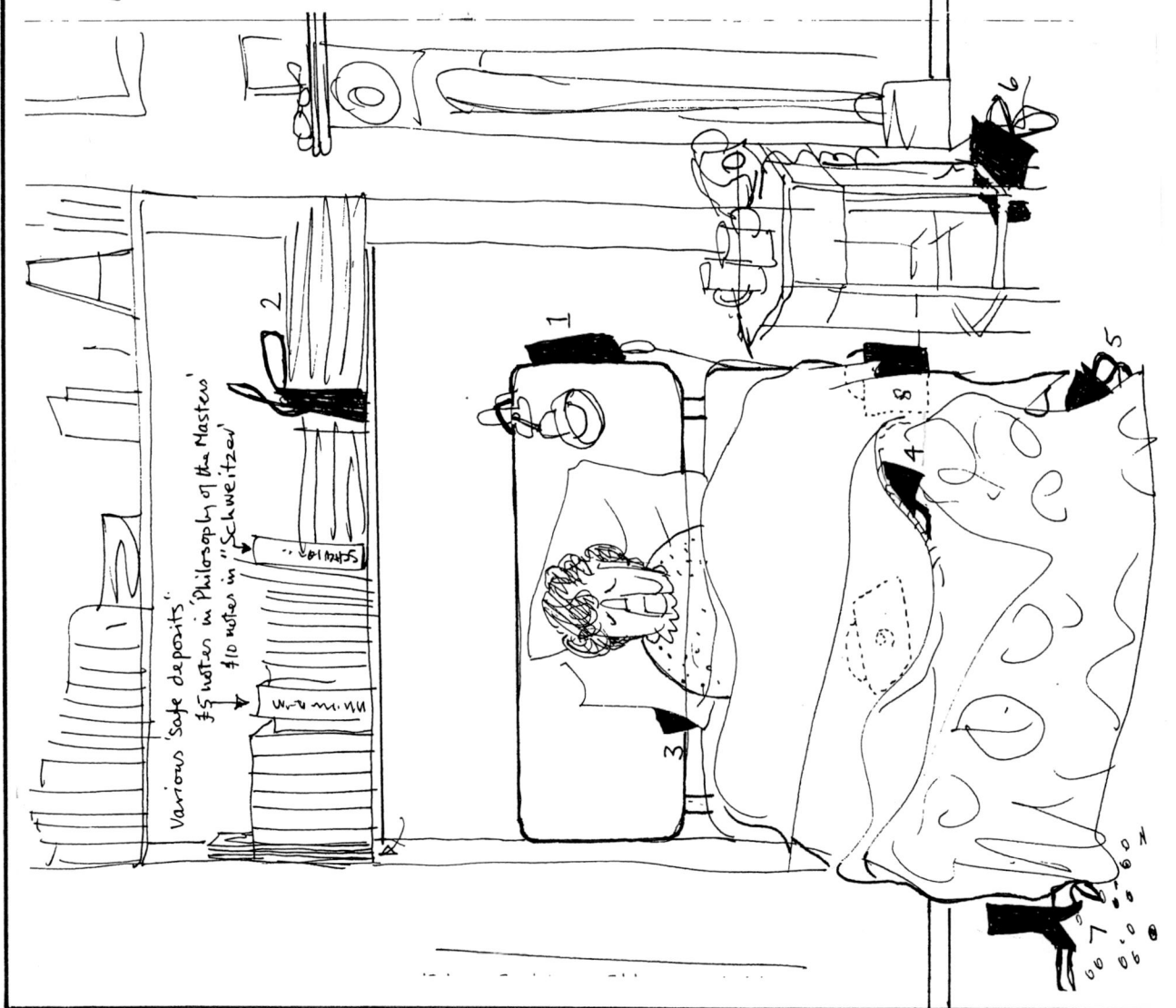

Fig. 129   Hunt-the-Handbag   Pen & Ink

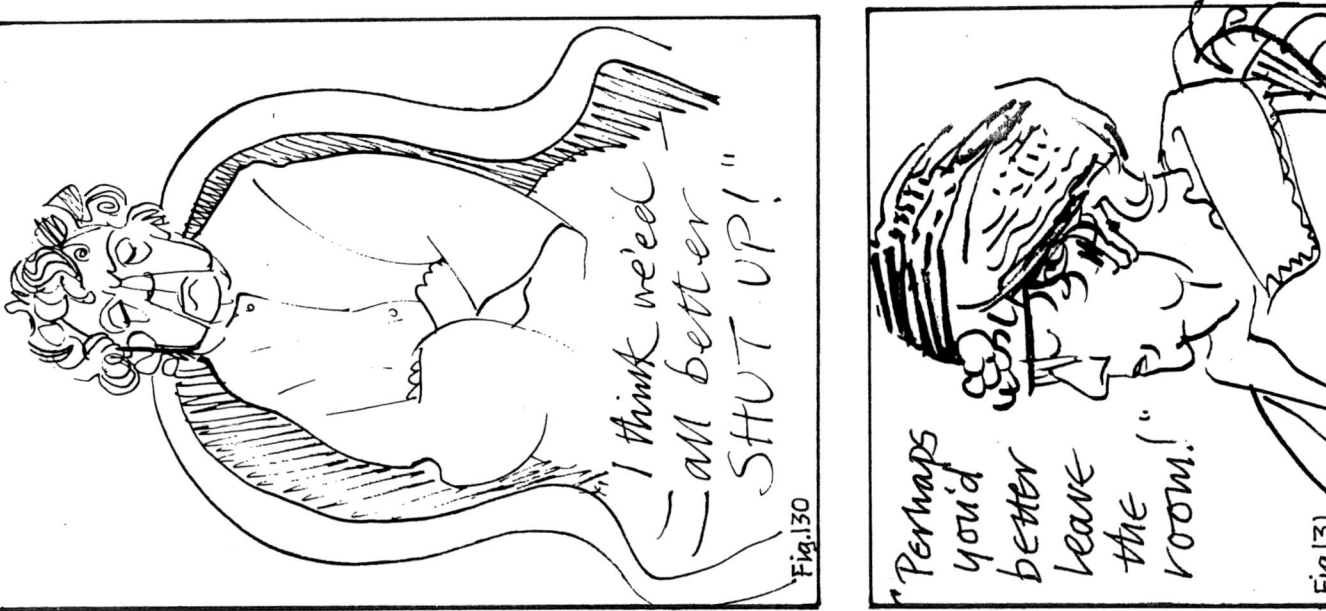

Fig.130 "I think we'd all better SHUT UP!"

Fig.131 "Perhaps you'd better leave the room!"

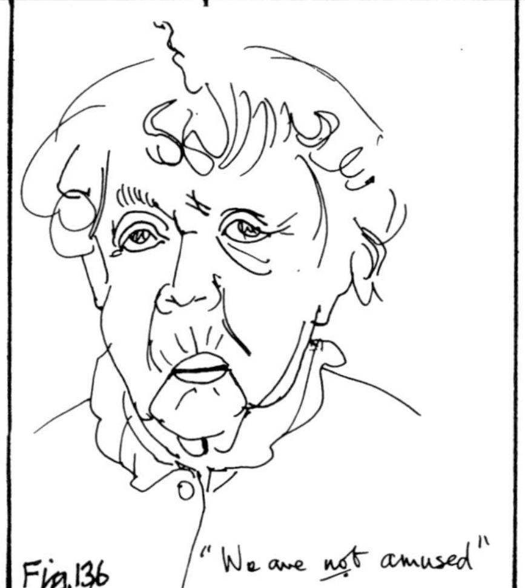

Fig.132 "You may leave us now"

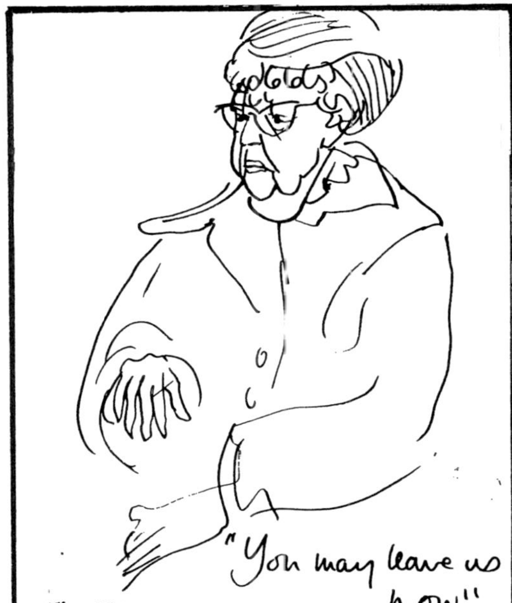

Fig.133 "That's enough of that!"

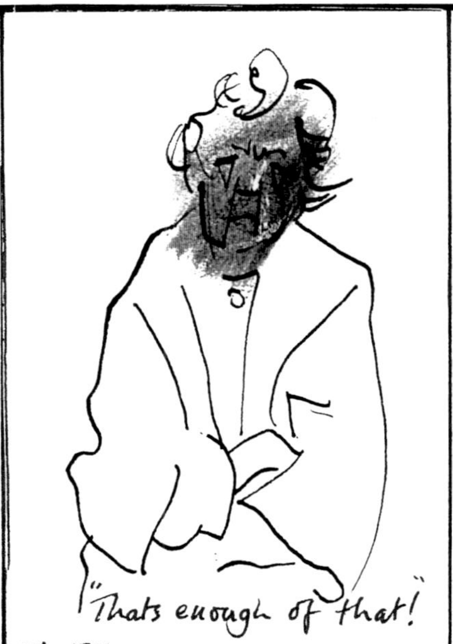

Fig.134 "I am extremely annoyed"

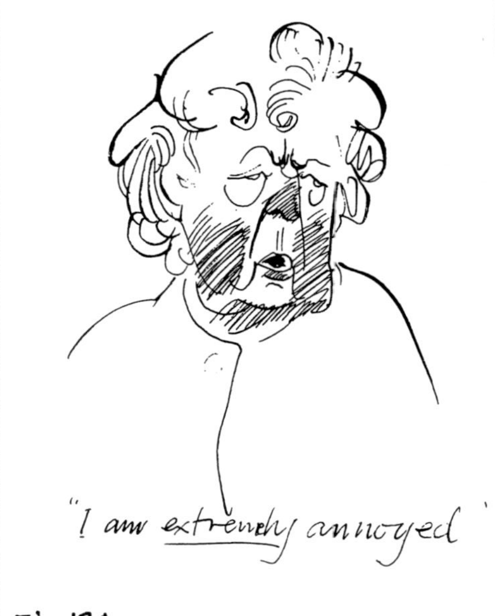

Fig.135 "There's an awful lot of wickedness — AS YOU KNOW!"

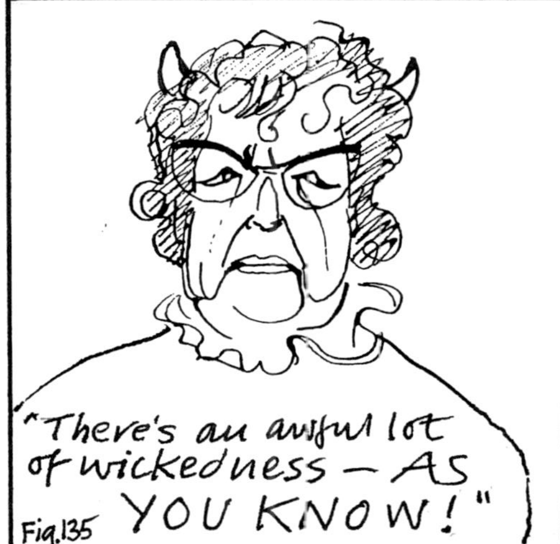

Fig.136 "We are not amused"

Fig.137 "Let's change the subject shall we"

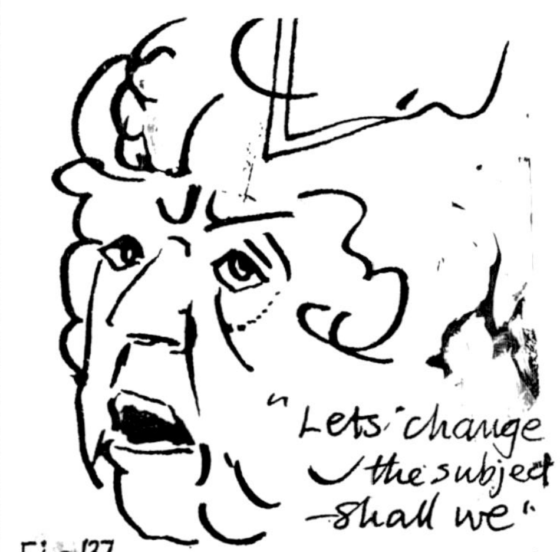

Over our last four years one small group of drawings expressing criticism levelled at myself were especially meaningful. When, in the past, I'd felt inadequate when confronting this kind of confrontational situation and unable to express my own anger, a deep depression soon followed. Now, however, I found that my quick, lively pen drawings came close to a true curative response to her criticisms. Purposely showing them to Mum I was surprised to find that most of them she found amusing. Her positive response had helped heal the former depressions and my retained anger.

65

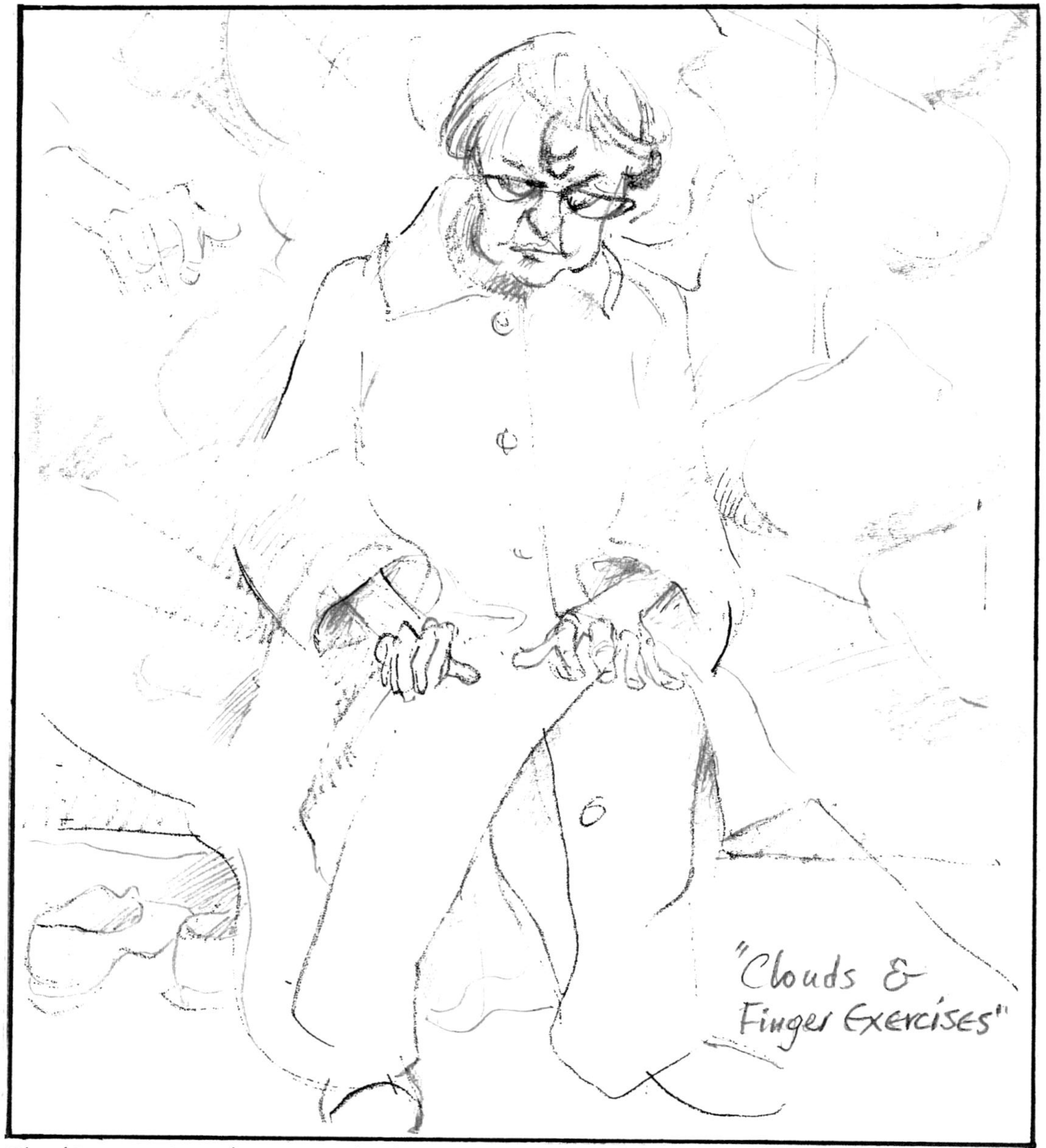

Theodosia
(1896-1989)

Previously our four hand, two
Piano pieces, were conversation enough,
Sharing the Great Composers.

Now the metronome marks ninety-four
Elgarian years, as hands pat out
Personal enigmatic variations.

Rhythmic waves to her friends,
The clouds. Amorphous, shielding
Apprehensions. Dreams of Childhood.

Arthritic thumbs, then fingers
Cease touching the ivories.
Celestial music replaces Debussy.

Theodosia Mary Louise lies
Foetal curved, holding my hand,
Singing: *Where am I?* - Dolce Fine.

FRIENDLY WITH THE CLOUDS

During her final months Mum became fascinated by cloud formations passing by her window (she spoke of 'my friends the clouds').
Left: A pencil sketch of Mum at 93 doing her finger exercises, clouds forming behind.
Below left: Based on this drawing the painting shows Mum surrounded by clouds, with a dove rising above the local church tower.
Below right: Mum, now floating also, 'holds' a cloud form, her face half-takes on the same amorphous substance. Both paintings sub-titled 'In Memoriam'.

Fig.138 Clouds — and Finger exercises   Pencil
"Clouds & Finger Exercises"

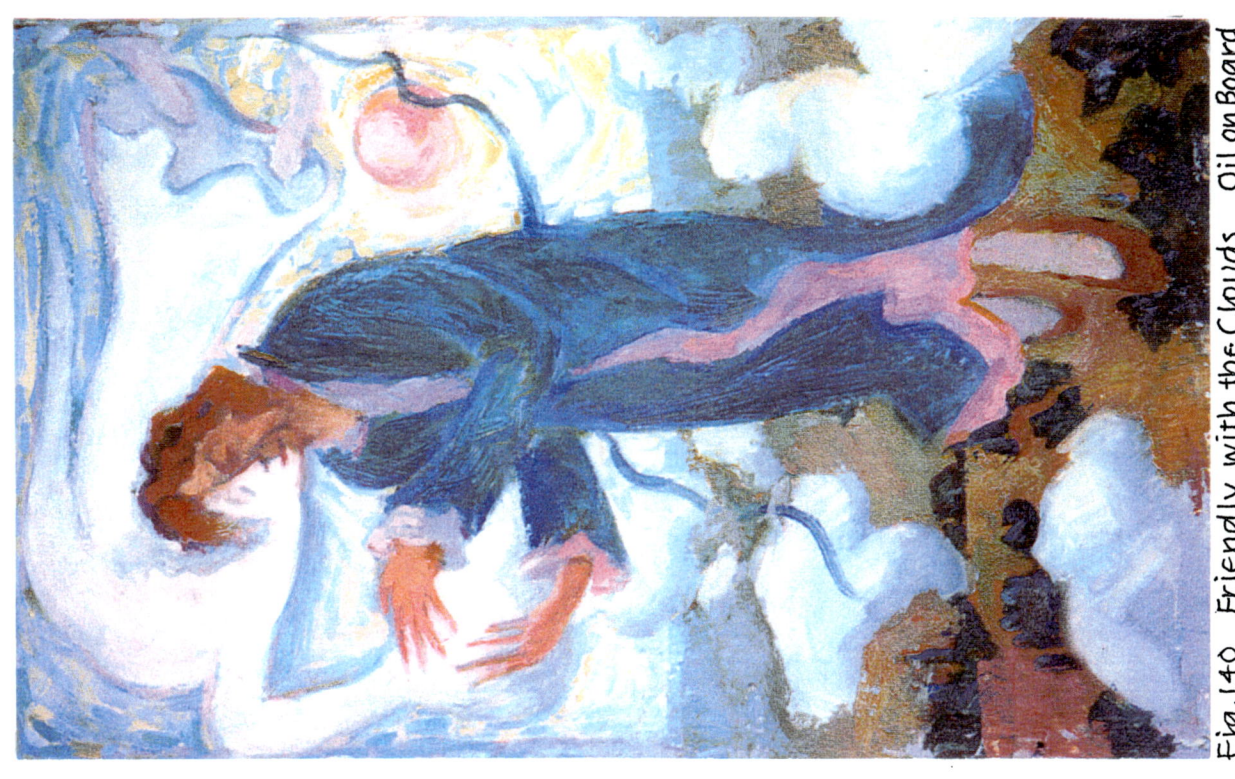

Fig.140 Friendly with the Clouds   Oil on Board

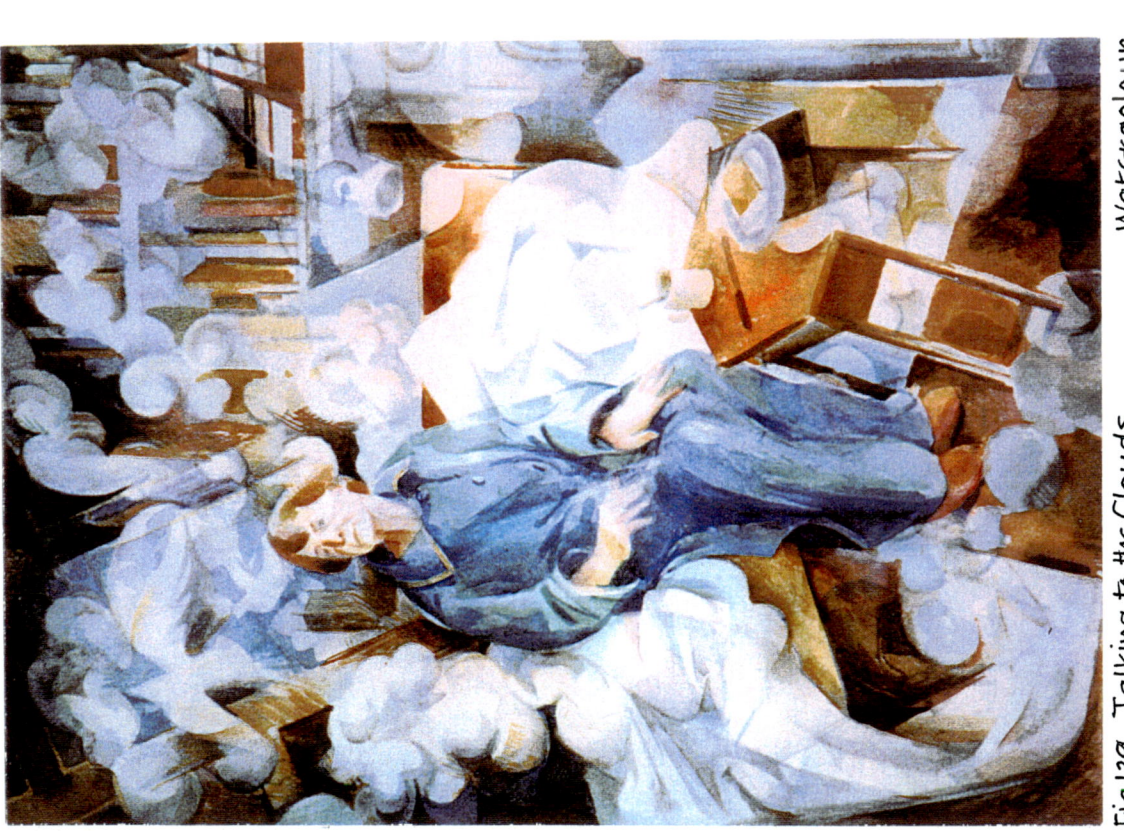

Fig.139 Talking to the Clouds   Watercolour

The real growth in our relationship was brought about by the many pictures of Mum – and simply by 'being there' with her.

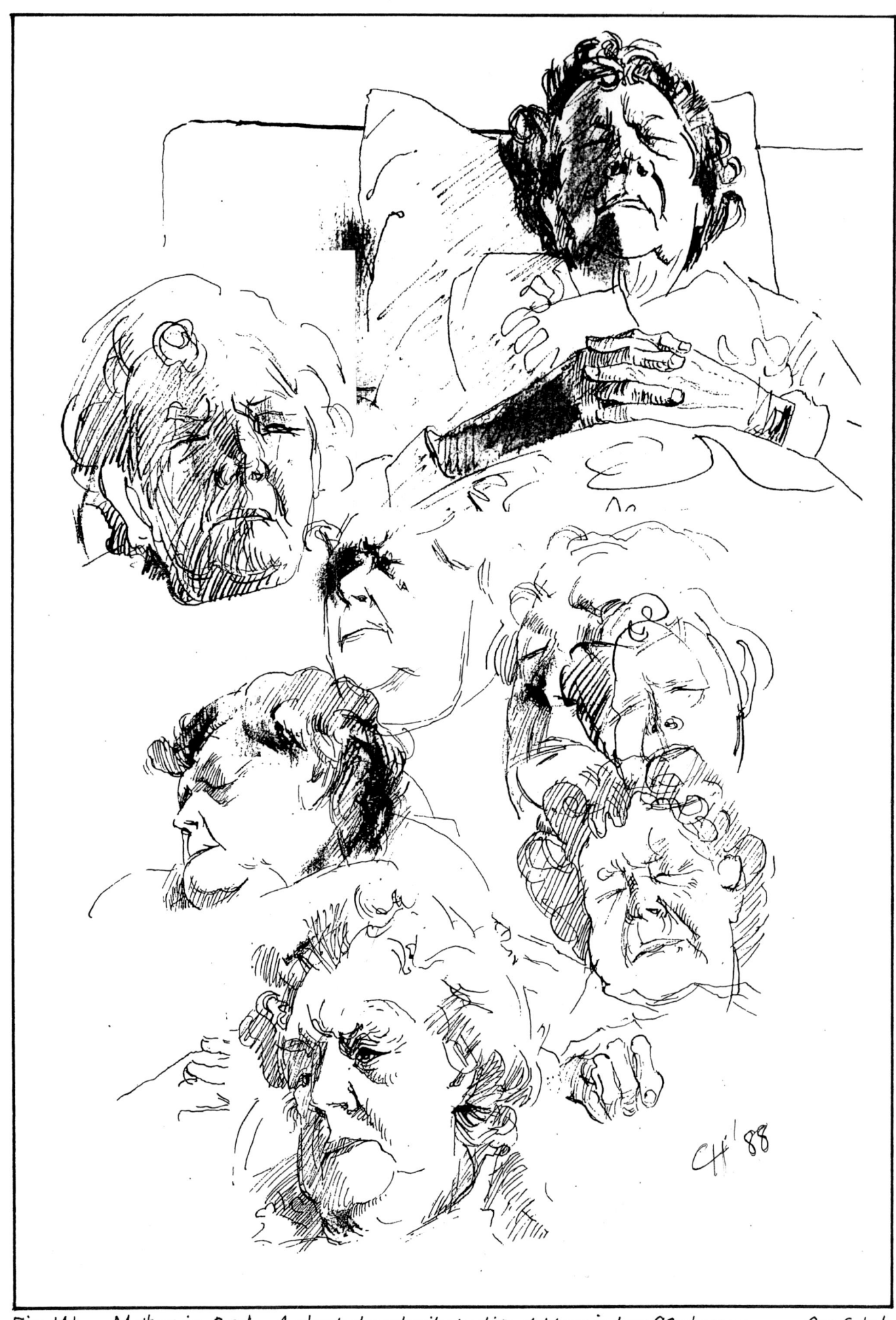

Fig. 141 Mother in Bed – A sheet of portrait studies of Mum in her 93rd. year   Pen & Ink

MIRRORS AND REFLECTIONS 1988-1990

Mirrors have always held a fascination for me, not only for the reflective images of ourselves and our world seen in reverse, but also for the element of chance and fragmentation they can offer.

If unaware of its presence, we walk past a mirror, our peripheral vision may catch that unexpected apparition — a flash of our own passing.

Sometimes one comes across a reflection which startles the senses, makes one laugh or pause for thought, perhaps even strikes fear into the heart. Once at an outdoor sculpture show, an elongated version of myself, Giacometti-like, stared back - a reflection off an ovoid mirrored sculpture (fig 143). This surreal image made me react with amusement and was reminiscent of the distorting ones in a sideshow. A painted mirror distortion shows a six-sectioned head turning through a series of mirror reflections that seem to symbolise the internalised confusion of that time (fig 144). A series of pen sketches expanded this idea with head and features distorted to the limits of recognition: elasticated, split, sliced as if by a cracked mirror (figs 145-148).

Later I used mixed media (plaster bandages, string and plastic filling materials) to make relief pictures - and searched out spatial ideas in which I was interested, in particular that of 'passing through' the surface of the glass. Years ago I'd been enchanted by the film Orphée by Jean Cocteau where Orpheus passes through a watery mirrored surface into the Underworld. Earlier still 'Alice through the Looking Glass' had the same effect. All this related closely to the sense of change which had occurred on the momentous day of the breakdown (see page 73).

While working on the reliefs another strand of interest in spatial effects had begun to unravel. A few painter friends and I were making portraits of each other, using mirrors to introduce side profiles. A close friend, Peter, had a tendency to glance down at his drawing for long periods of time, allowing me to observe his differing head positions which I then fitted together in one drawing (fig.151). Pictures of Pete proliferated from this one study, many showing multiple viewpoints, others a peeling away of features, as if looking behind a mask only to find further masks within. Another diversion was a painted relief of Pete, painting himself, looking into a mirror and then towards the painted image (figs 142, 158).

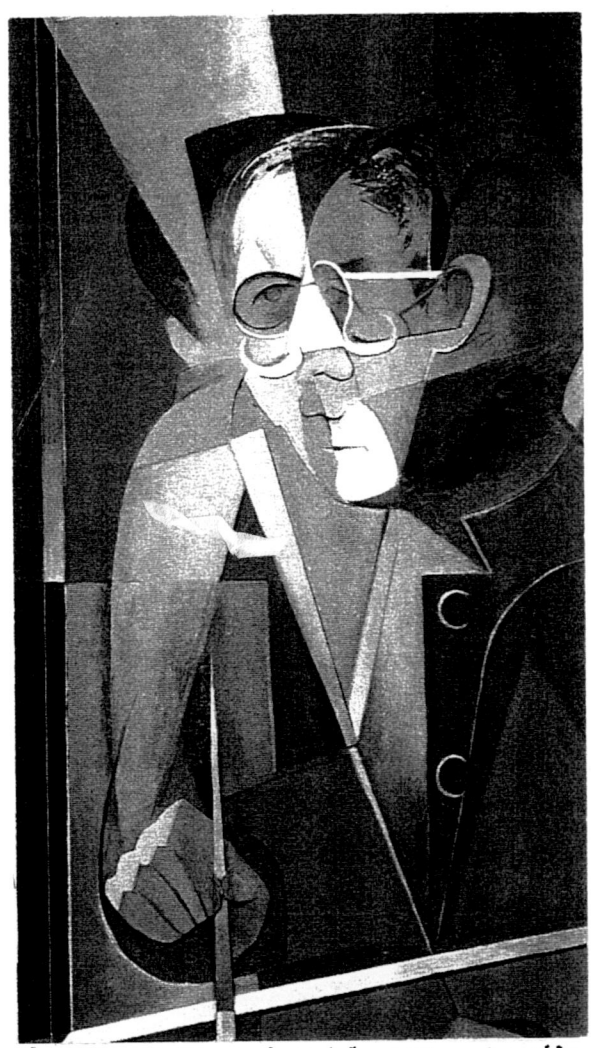

Fig.142   Peter paints himself   Acrylic

In 'Three Studies for a Portrait' the individual gives way to a dual image (fig 159). Intrigued by this infiltration of my own features into the second and third studies, I realised I'd also subjugated my own personality to the much stronger one of my friend.

My friendship with Pete went back many years to when we met at Art College as students in the 1950s, a relationship developed from pictorial ideas in our work.

With hindsight, I now realise that my somewhat indecisive thoughts were often strengthened by his more positive and dogmatic approach and that gradually, through many creative years he had become a father-figure.

These recent portraits I now saw as a way of disguising my own shadow side, of offloading repressions onto my friend's image. I realised that I was surreptitiously hiding behind his profile as if ashamed or fearful of showing my own inner feelings.

It became a game of 'hide and seek' which continued for some time until a feeling of futility arose and temporarily caused a creative blockage.

Aware of a certain timidity, of not often wanting to take risks when aiming for a more imaginative approach to painting was one aspect. Another was my dissatisfaction with 'realistic' work. Something was niggling away just below the surface and I found eventually it was about the hiding aspect: of wearing a persona, a mask, of putting on a performance via my technical skills rather than trying to paint my true feelings.

The imbalance which was recognised in the 'dual' portraits was gradually being adjusted by a new spirit of enquiry, of a search for understanding which was to change this sub-dominant role with my friend.

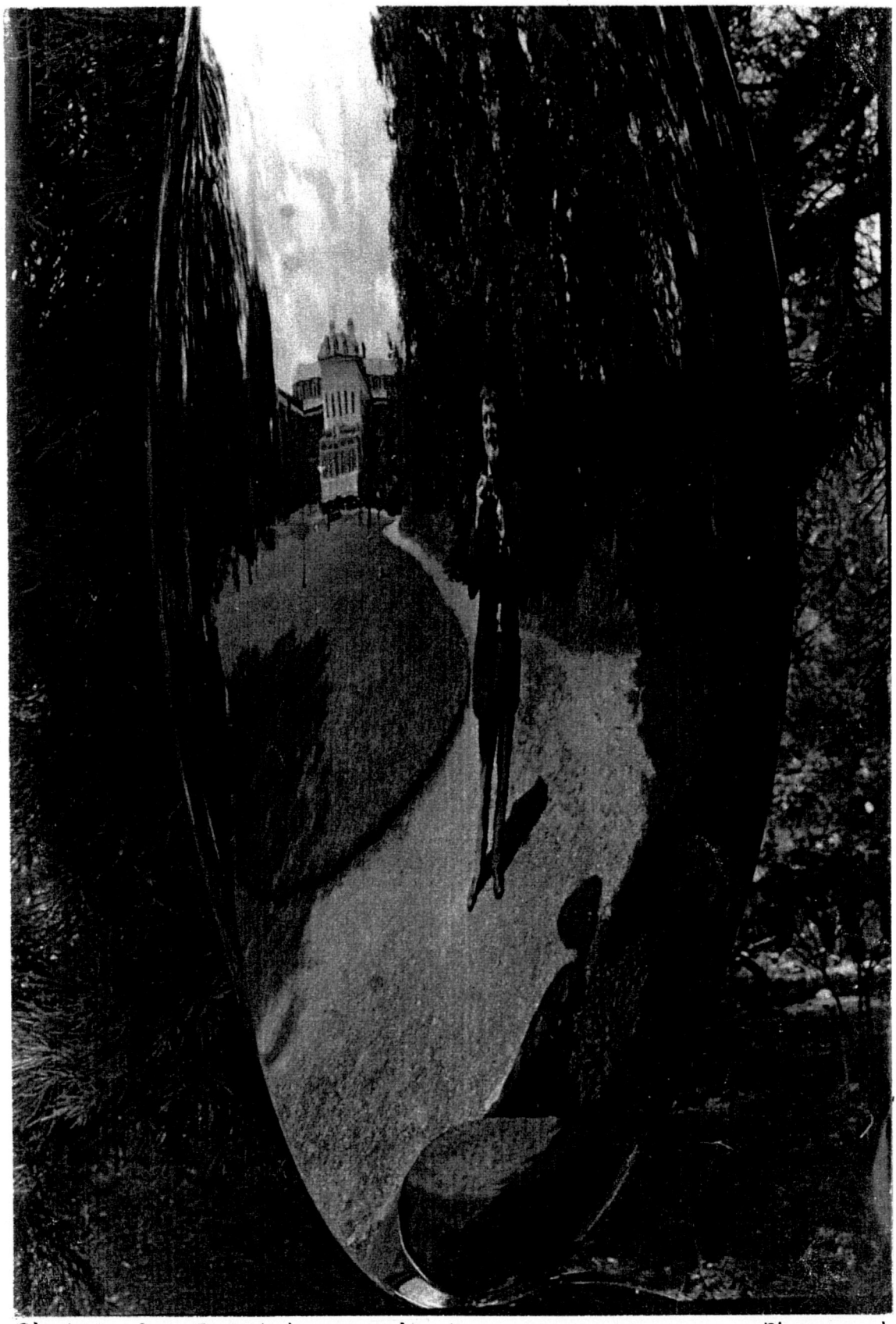

Fig. 143   Self Portrait in an ovoid Mirror   Photograph

An ovoid mirrored sculpture reflecting an elongated self portrait (the camera held at chest height). All the elements: building, sky, figure, shadows are surreal, have their own reality. It is like a painted image rather than a 'real' photograph.

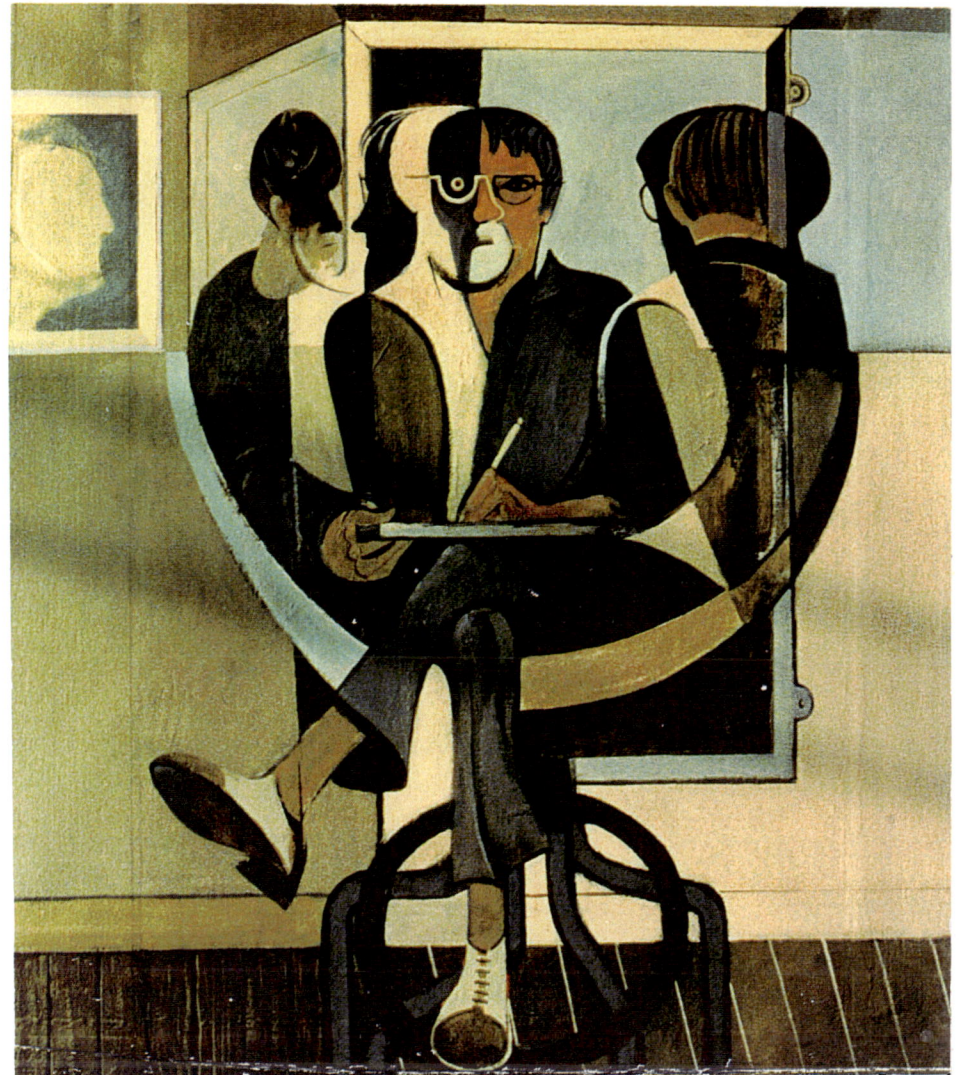

Fig.144   Multiple Viewpoints on a Swivel Chair   Acrylic

Above: A painting from the Swivel Chair series (pages 37-46) concentrating on the reflected mirror image from multiple viewpoints. The many profiles suggest change – of time passing......
Below: Pen studies looking beyond the appearance of the face – again a sense of time passing, the head turning from one second to the next....

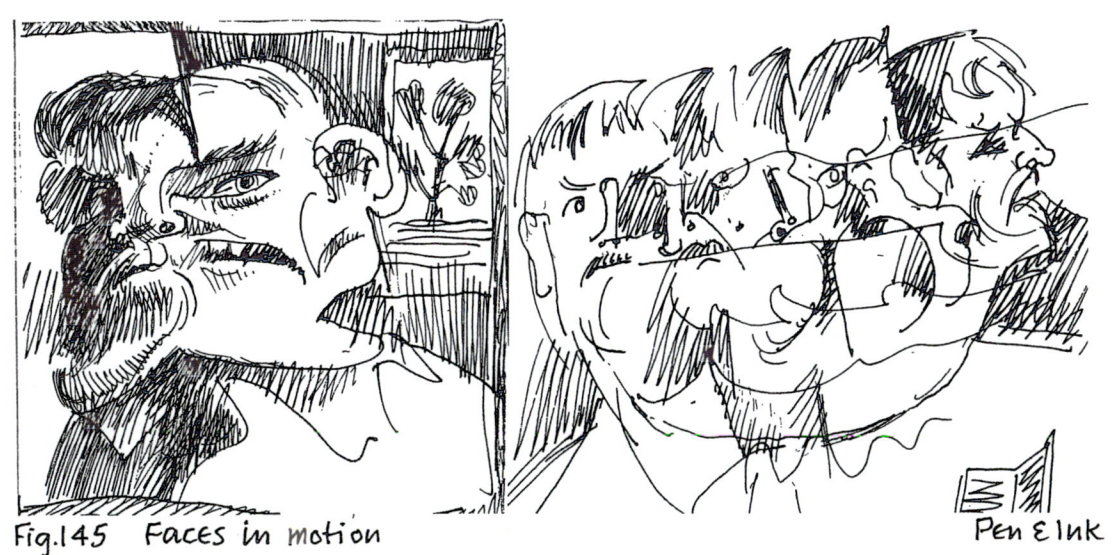

Fig.145   Faces in motion   Pen & Ink

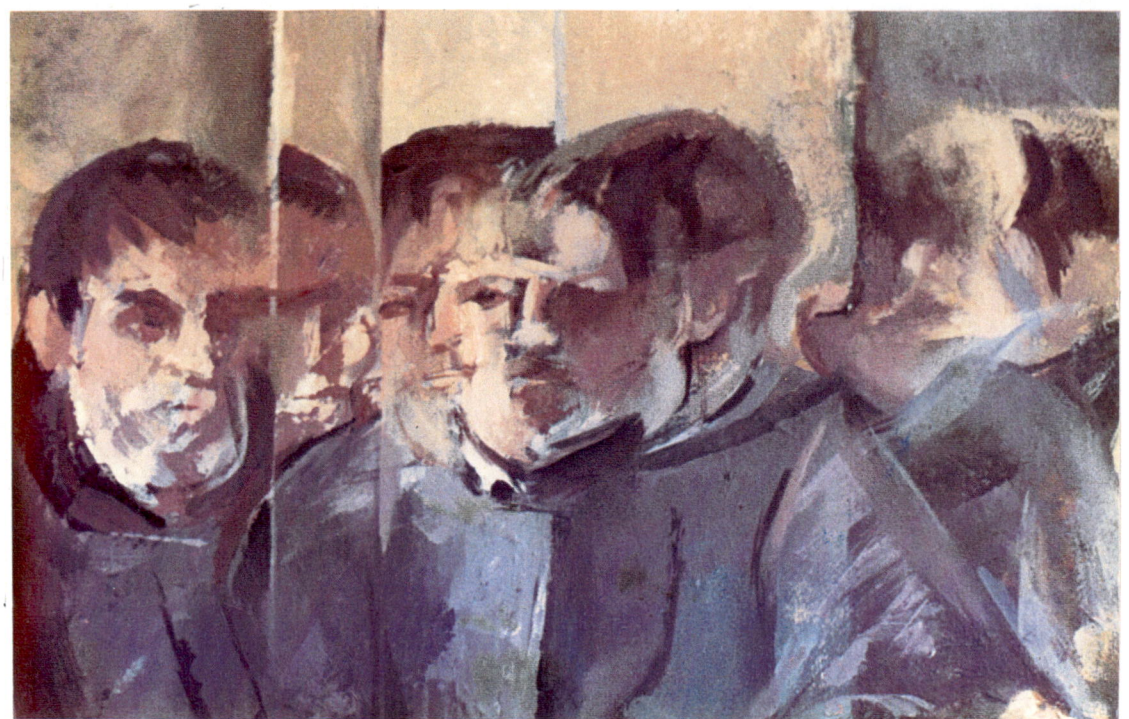

Fig.146 Mirrored Reflections   Oil on Canvas

Above: Interlocking head profiles flowing across the canvas – many mirrored reflections

Below: Sketch and finished portrait. More homogeneous than other multiple viewpoints, the brushwork 'merges' the central group – moments of calm, then restlessness.

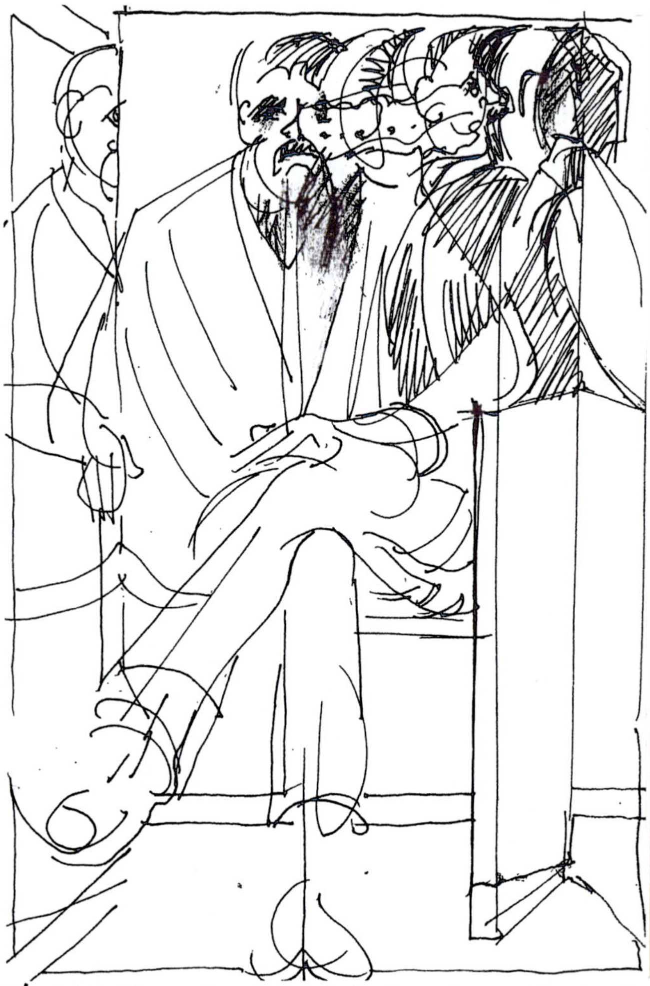

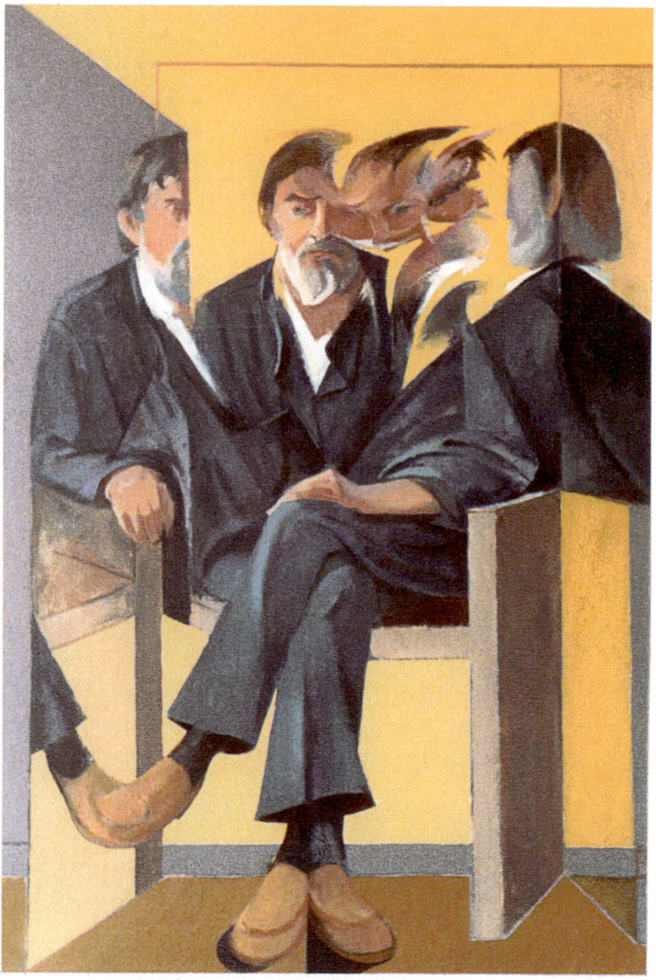

Fig.147 Multiple viewpoints Sketch   Pen & Ink.   Fig.148 Mirrored Self Portrait   Acrylic

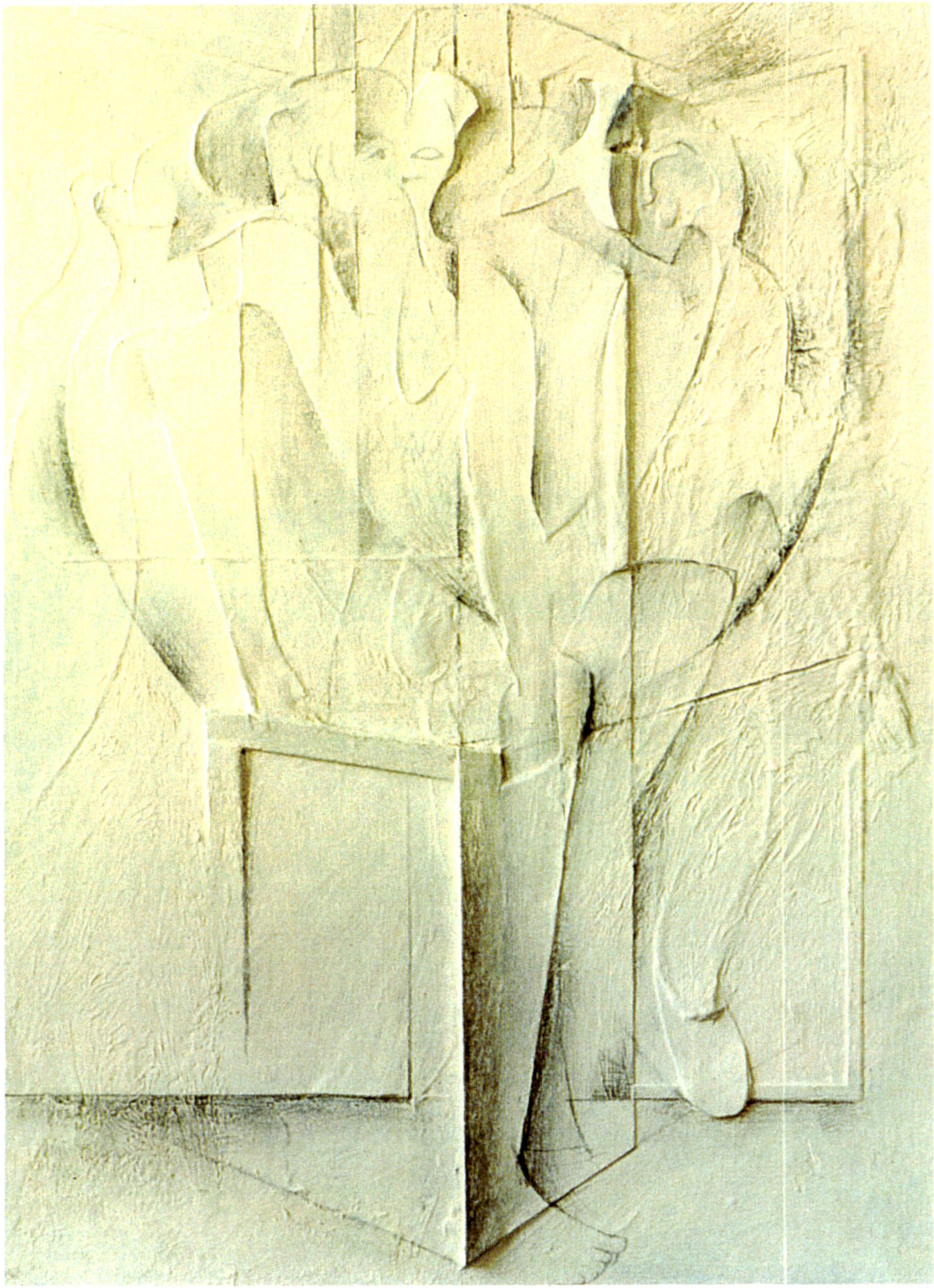

PLASTIC RELIEFS

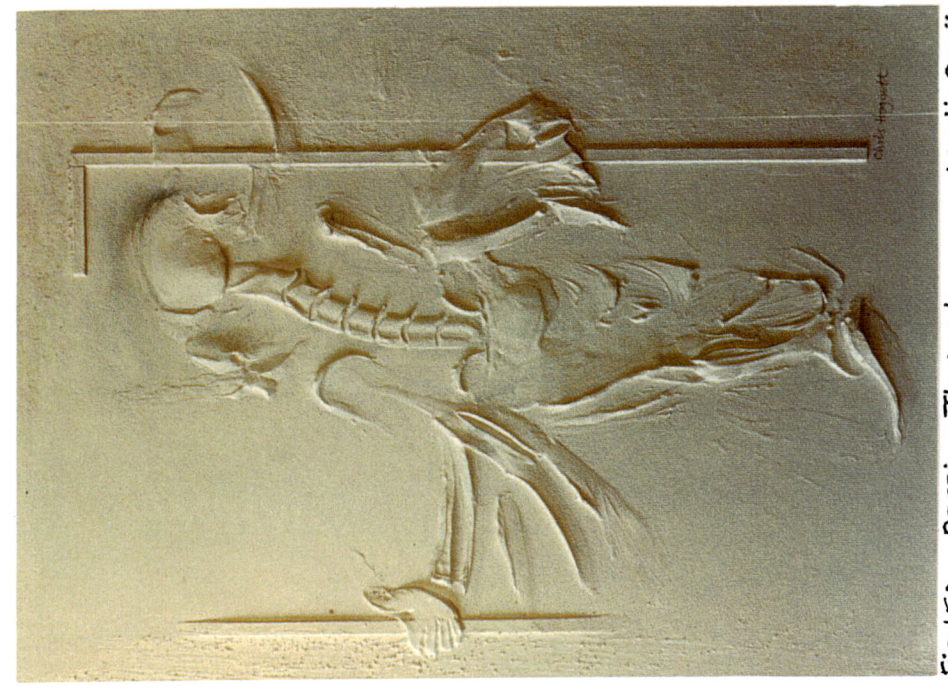

Fig.150 Passing Through Acrylic Caulk

Above: The use of mixed media (in this example Acrylic caulk squeezed from a decorator's gun) allows a more flexible use of materials to express a particular mood or obsession. An echo of the figure in 'Freefall' section (fig 41, page 21), it flows into the interior beyond, part flesh, part skeleton, soon to vanish........

Left: This multi-portrait sits on his stool waiting, as architectural features behind cut through his ghost-like presence. A wavering uncertainty prevails, reflecting his mood and the emotional feelings of instability.

Fig.149 The Company of One Acrylic Caulk

73

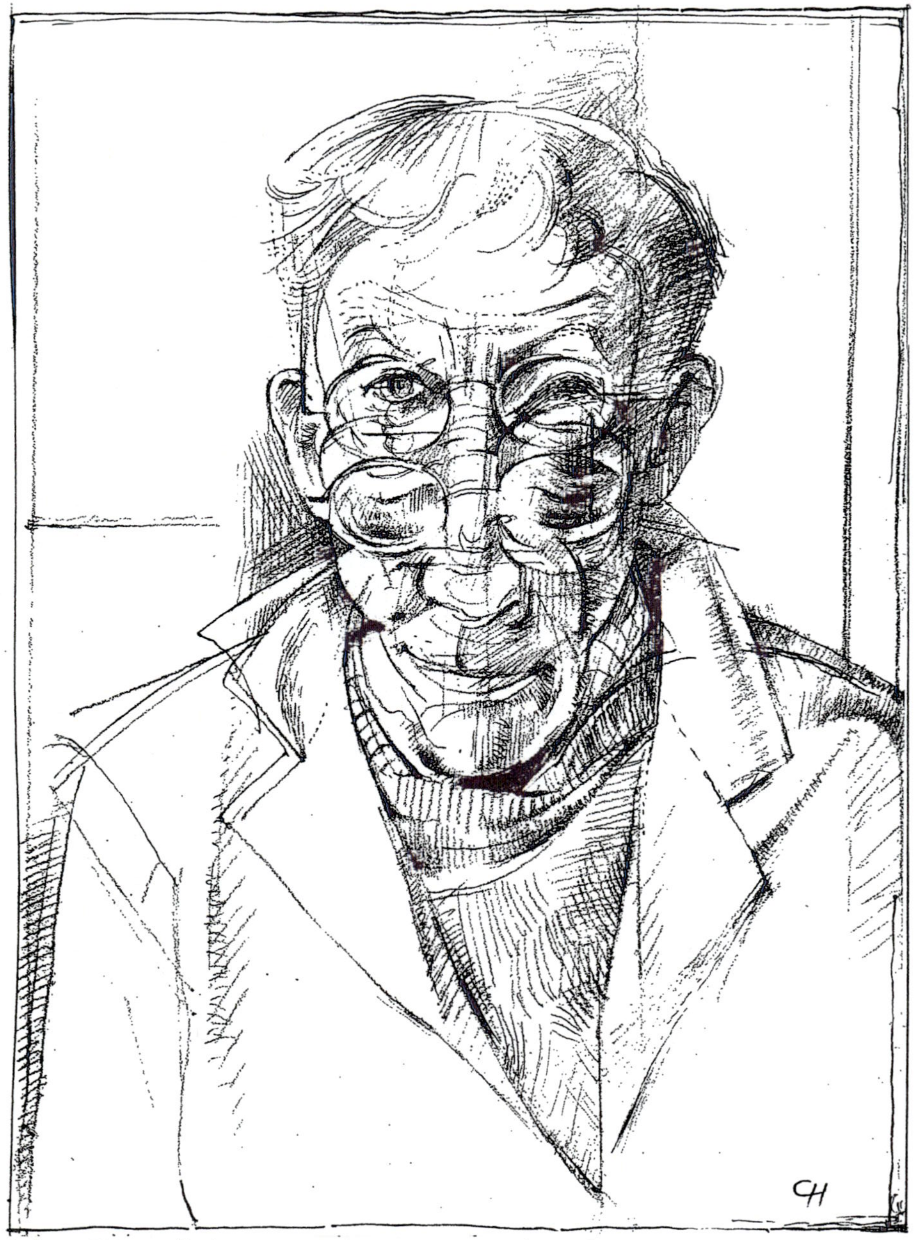

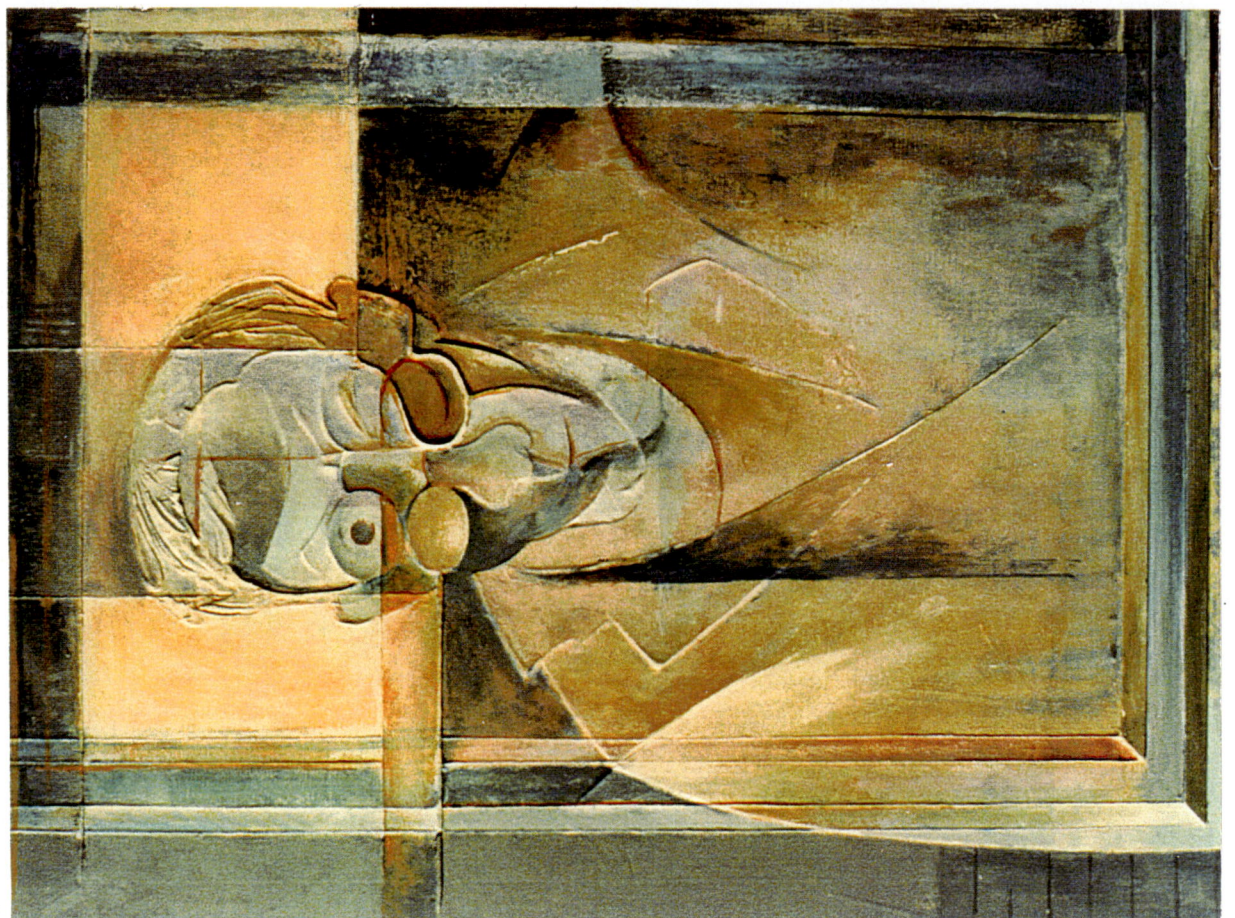

Fig.152 Pete – Mirror Image   Acrylic

Fig.151 Pete – Looking up, Looking down   Pencil

PETE SKETCHING ME, SKETCHING HIM

Above: As my painter friend sketches me, I sketch him. The movement of his head gives me an idea to work on a multiple viewpoint. The painted version is simplified but is less substantial.

Below and Right: Three pen sketches and a painting exploring areas 'behind' the persona. The top right sketch shows a straightforward realistic portrait and those below offer a glance beyond the appearance. By stretching, unpeeling (as an onion), or by combining full and side-face the search is on — not for my friend's hidden aspects but for my own......

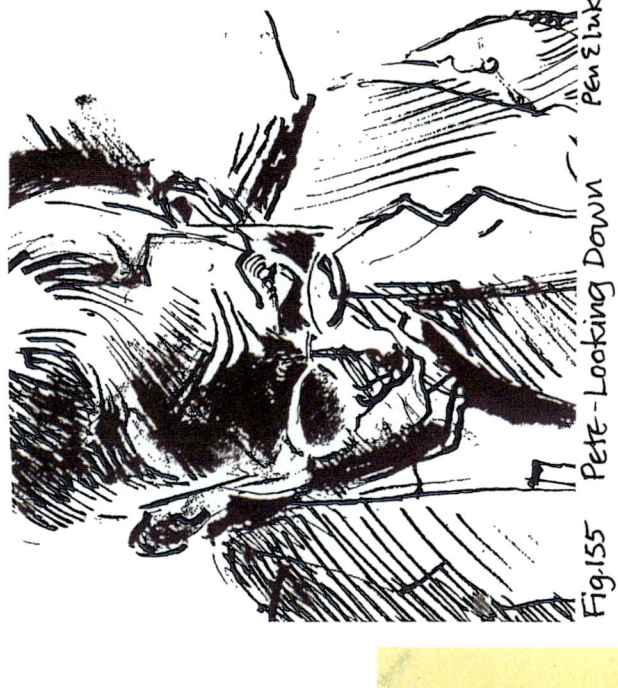

Fig.155 Pete - Looking Down Pen & Ink

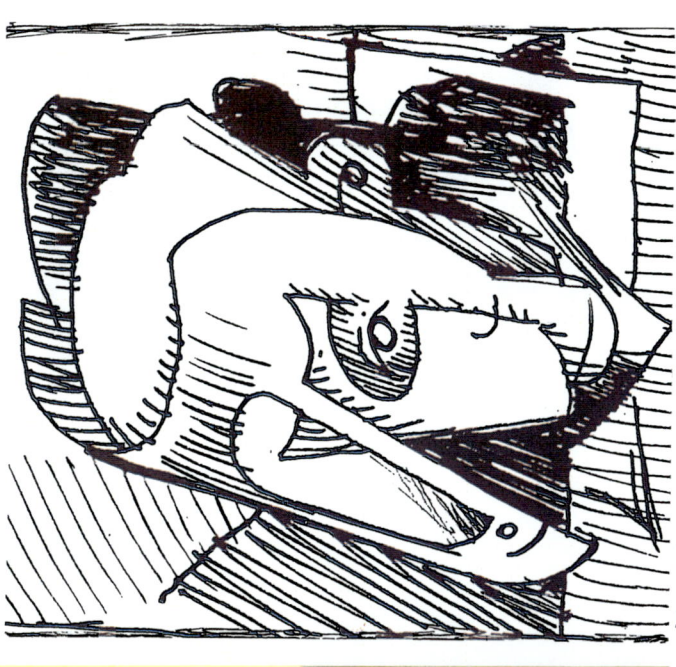

Fig.156 Dismantling the Head. Pen & Ink

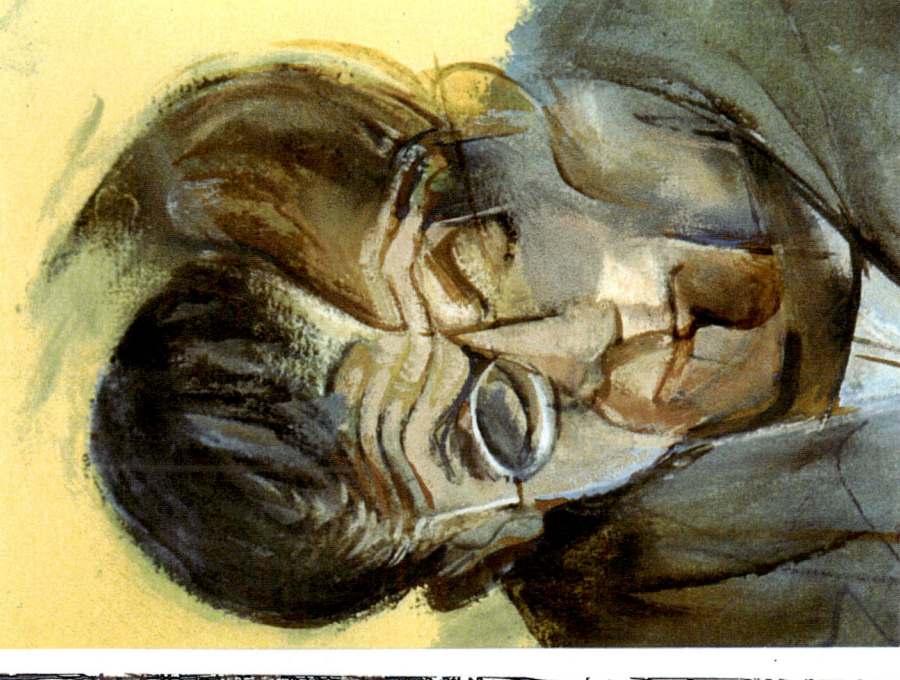

Fig.154 Pete - Multiple view - 2 Gouache

Fig.153 Pete - Multiple view Pen & Ink

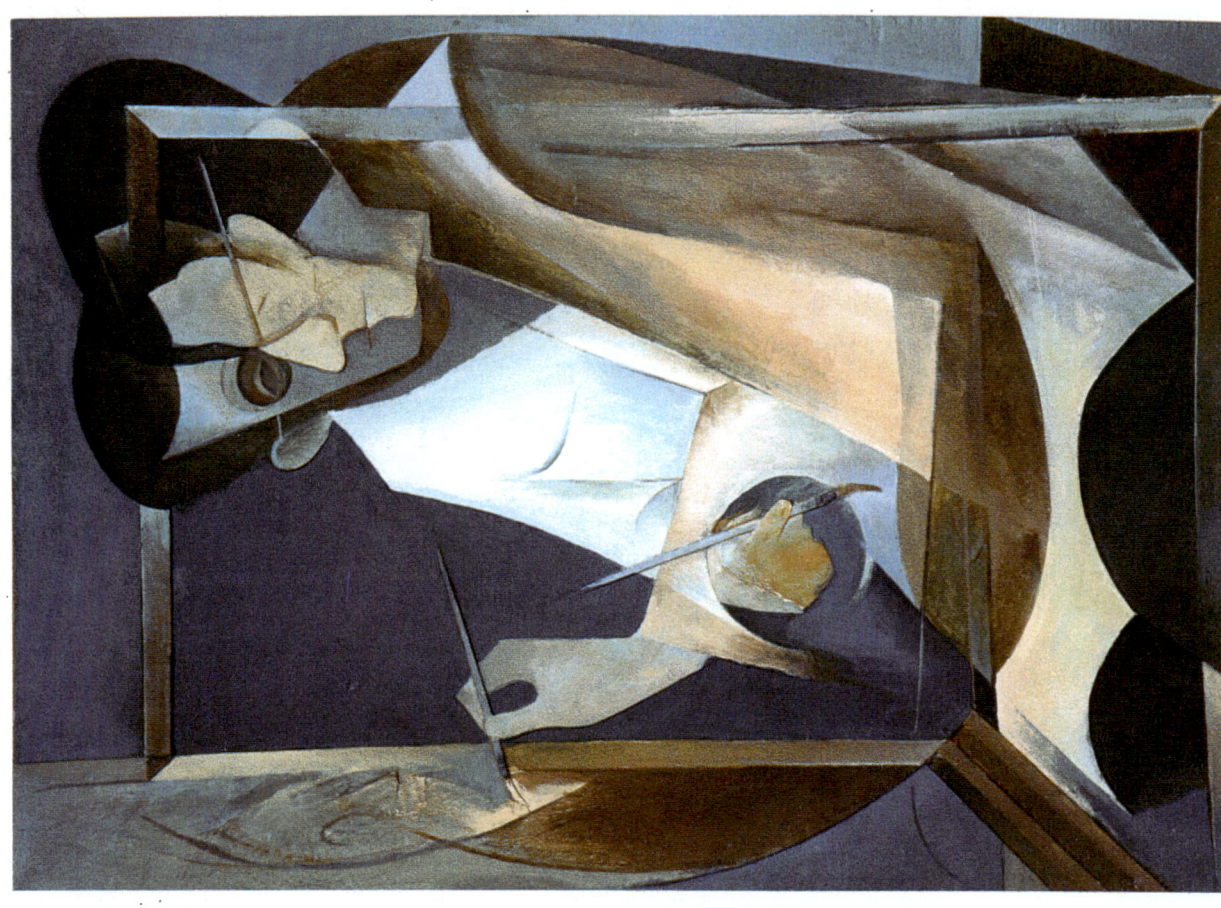

Fig. 157 Pete painting himself – 1   Gouache
The mask-like front face not yet defined (see fig. 158)

Fig. 158 Pete painting himself – 2   Acrylic Relief

Right:: A side profile of Pete painting his self-portrait is superimposed on a masked face looking out to the viewer through the looking glass. This ambivalent mask can be seen either as Pete's front face or as my own persona hidden behind my friends more confident image. I now feel, in retrospect, that I then wished to paint a self-portrait but used Pete's image as a surrogate. The painting could be seen as an act of 'self-effacement'.

Fig. 159 Three Studies for a Portrait – A Triptych – Gouache –

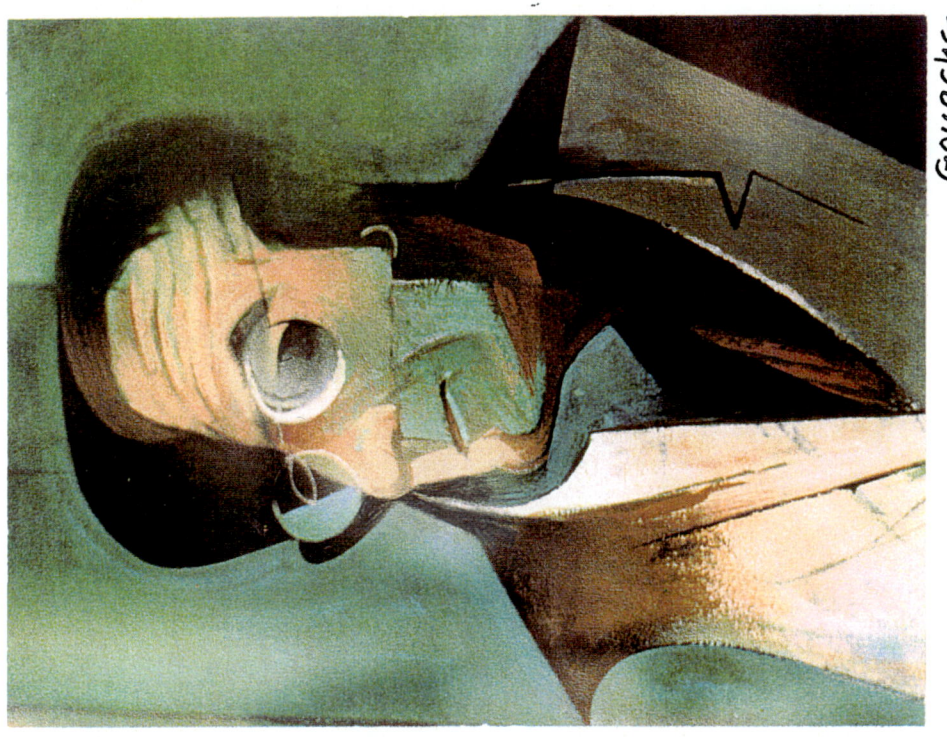

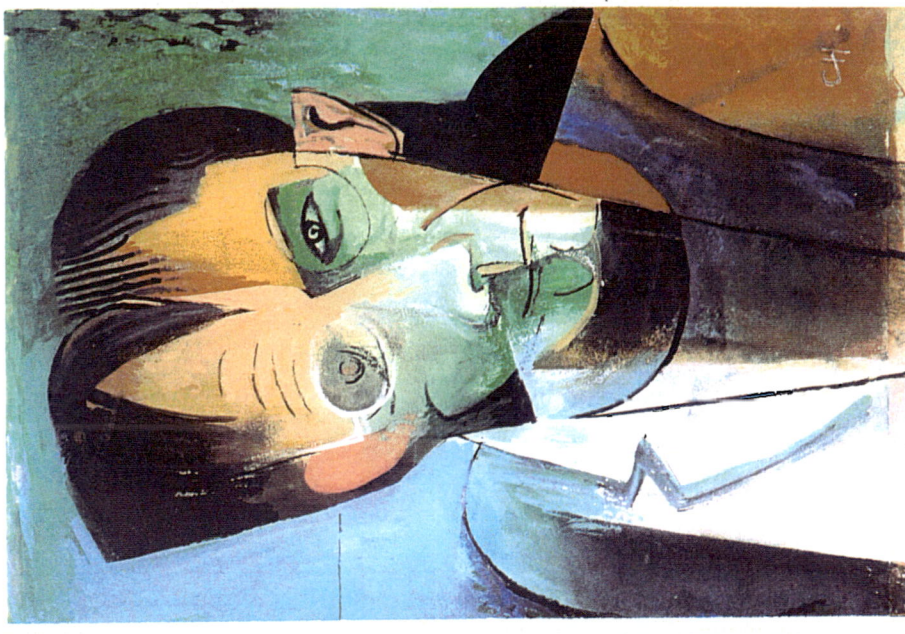

In the 'Three Studies for a Portrait' the individual portrait of Pete gradually gives way to a dual image. The first study (left) is singular and shows a distorted cartoon-like image. In the central study it's still more my friend's face than my own, but the right-hand portrait contains more of my own features.

Finally, in the right-hand study, my own hair and forehead make an appearance. During the first months of the 1990s a degree of certainty and conviction entered into my work. In this study (right) I believe I was beginning to come out of the shadows. The painting overleaf confirmed this conviction.

77

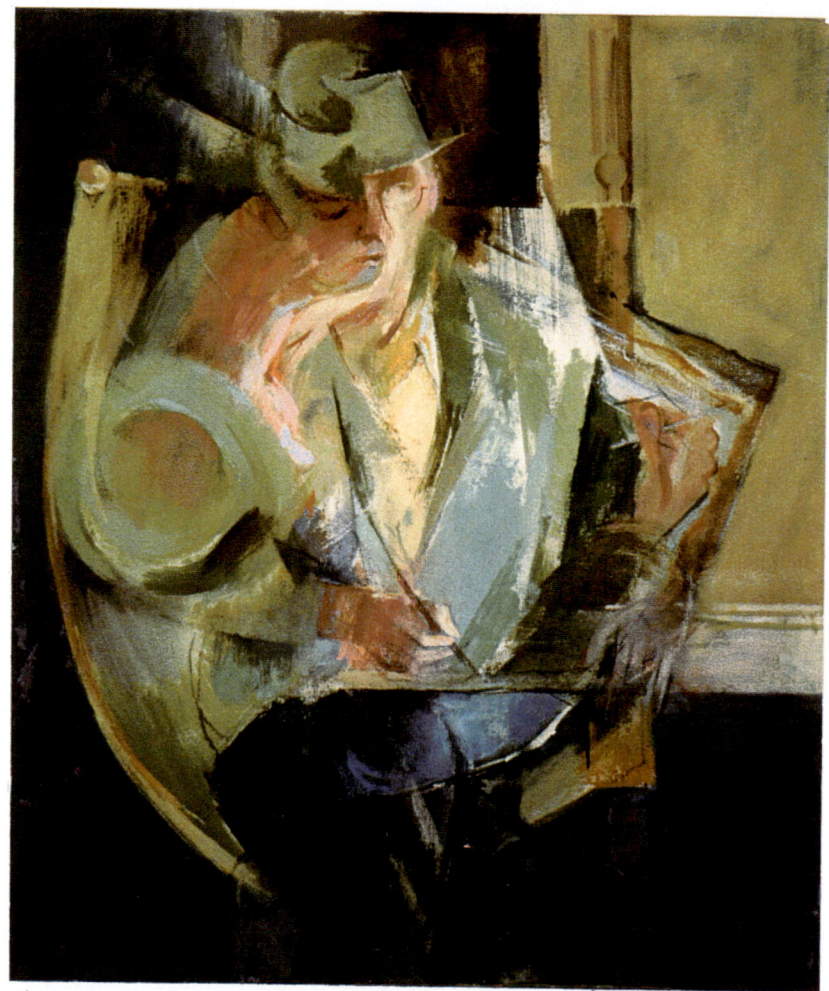

Fig. 160 The Armchair – a double portrait   Oil on board

This painting shows Pete wearing a hat seen from frontal and top (or plan) viewpoints – the final work in the 'Pete' series. Between his two heads my self-portrait is now in a more dominant role, enough to redress the imbalance of the earlier 'hidden' self portraits.

AUTUMN 1990 – GREY MISTS AND BLACK BEARS

Within months of painting this dual portrait (above), I experienced the most severe depression I'd ever known. Interestingly it occurred ten years to the month from the breakdown during the Autumn of 1980. Previous depressions had usually been manageable in that I'd been able to express my feelings through the artwork (as illustrated in these pages).

This time, however, there was an added complication to the condition. I recall a curious grey fog which wrapped itself rug-like around me. It was as if rays of sunlight were unable to penetrate this envelope of doom. Occasionally, while the depression continued it transformed itself from a grey to an altogether darker substance, hanging on like a great black beast (see page 145).

I realised it was time to seek psychiatric help and was soon put on a course of antidepressants and psychology. What was galling – such is pride – was that for all the years of 'DIY' therapeutic artwork, so little was able to overcome the effects of the depression. Again I sought help and was put in touch with an art therapist.

This was to prove the most decisive move taken and was to point the way forward to a breakthrough in understanding the cause of these years of breakdowns and depressions. The Dream Journal which forms Part Two, is the nucleus of the book, the pivotal point between the first ten years self-help and the joint therapeutic work with the therapist and myself. This was to lead to the 'free' and automatic drawing and painting in the final parts and Postscript.

PART TWO

Dream Dominions 1990-1992

THEMES AND VARIATIONS

The Dream as the Theme - The Artwork as Variations	81
1 BREATH AND BREATHLESSNESS - Asphyxia and Claustrophobia	83
2 A TUMULTUOUS RUSH - Confusion, Excess of Feeling	85
3 AUTOMATONS - Institutions and Conformity	91
4 A PROPHETIC DREAM - Clay as Therapy	101
5 UNMASKING THE MONSTER - Facing the Fear	123
6 AN ABSENCE OF LIGHT - The Shadow Side	145
7 METAMORPHOSIS - Growth and Transformation	153
8 CONFRONTATION - Conflict and Reconciliation	171
9 MASQUERADING - Hiding and Seeking	183
10 DECAPITATION - Death and Regeneration	191
11 VICTIMS AND SACRIFICES - Acceptance	195

THEMES AND VARIATIONS

The Dream as the Theme   The Artwork as Variations

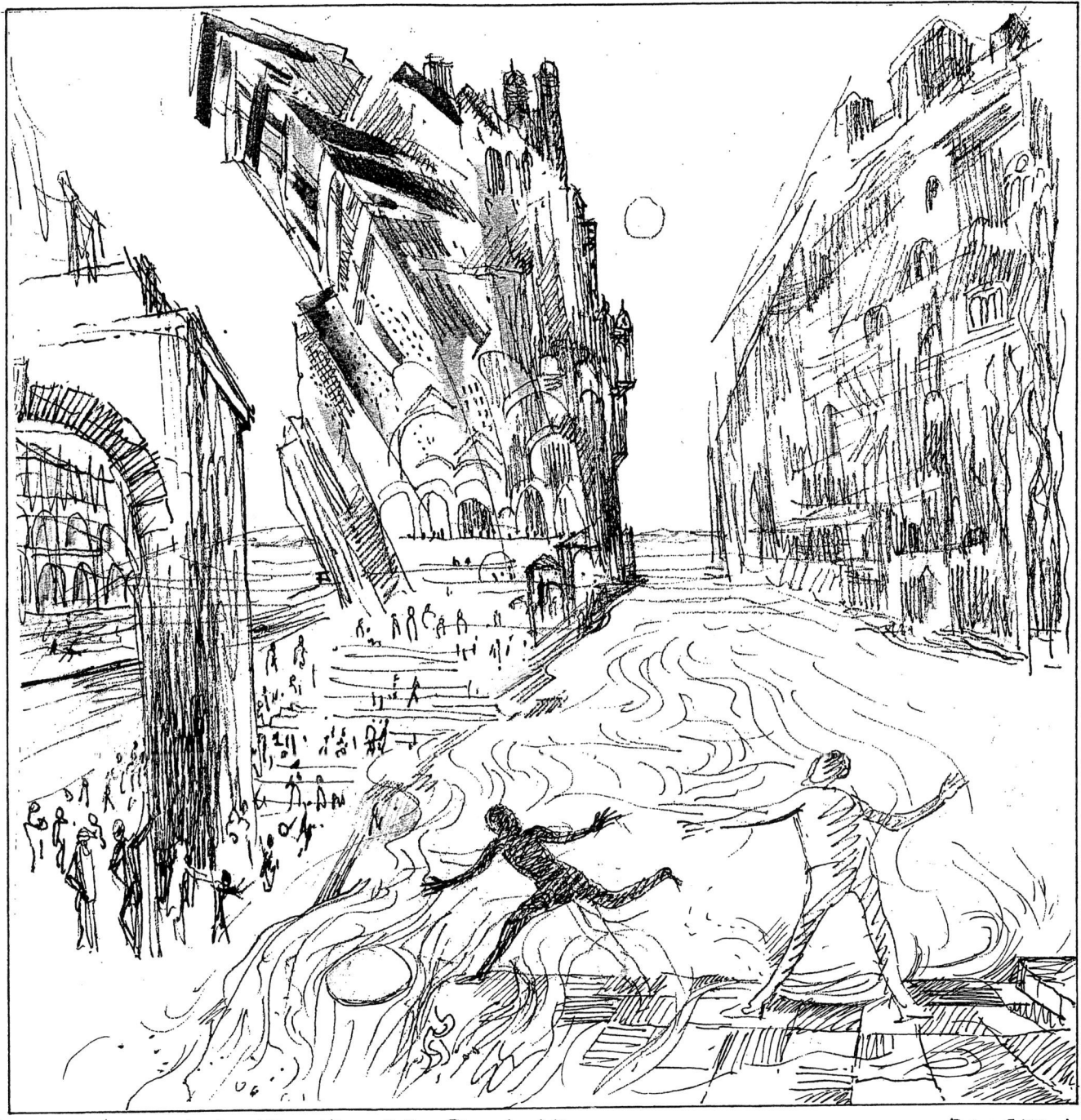

Fig.161 Dream 102 'Duality of the Psyche' *   Pen & Wash

In retrospect, the second breakdown during 1990 was the catalyst for seeking some professional help. Frequent depressions and occasional manic phases had developed to an extent where I felt I had less and less control over my life. A solution or 'cure' of some kind seemed essential, provided I could avoid the medication which had proved so negative following the 1980 breakdown.

* from 'An Illustrated Dream Journal' by Claire Skailes, based on a sequence of 170 dreams from 1990 to 1992 by Chris Hoggett. In preparation.

I was fortunate this time to find a therapist who offered the assurance I was now seeking. During our introductory meeting she emphasised that the purpose of our sessions would be to help form a relationship of trust between us; that it would be difficult and entail much hard work, and that it would take some time to develop and reach an understanding of the root causes underlying these emotional breakdowns.

I had yet to commit myself to the therapy, but a suggestion was put forward at the end of the meeting, 'You might attempt writing down any dreams you can remember.'

I was sceptical about this, having never recorded a dream before, but this parting remark must have made some impact, for within a few weeks four dreams had been written down with a few sketches added. The advice that I should be prepared beforehand had helped: a blank notebook, pen and pencil, a bedside lamp. Then an excess of drink on going to bed to ensure getting up in the night, plus a determination to stay awake on returning to bed. Very soon these simple preparations produced results, and gradually the brief notes, sketches or diagrams demanded more and more attention.

My older parental voice was highly critical of the 'crude and childish' sketches, but slowly a new expressiveness in the drawings silenced these internal reproaches and, after three years, a sequence of 170 dreams had filled up the blank book. 'A Dream Journal - 1990-92' then stopped as abruptly as it had started, not by design but rather by some natural 'dying away', as if everything that had needed to be said, had been said. (Later many scattered dreams were recorded but never as a continuous sequence, and these were written on separate sheets of paper for later discussion during our therapy sessions.)

Twenty-seven of the original 170 dreams from the Journal make up 'Dream Dominions', each selected because of the subsequent series of artworks engendered by them – all of which deal with particular territories of fear, anxiety or prophecy. Some of the fears, such as Claustrophobia and Darkness, were so compelling that the later drawings could be seen as conscious extensions, trying to comprehend the subliminal material – the dream the theme, the artwork the variations around it. Dreams 38 and 161 about the 'Shadow Side' stimulated some dozen strands of illustrative and freestyle variations on the theme of Darkness, gathered together under the heading 'An Absence of Light'.

'Confrontation' (Dream 65) conjured up a young boy having to confront approaches by a crippled youth – figures symbolising the self facing his 'monster' – his inner fear and 'stunted' growth caused by the fear of change. The subsequent artworks are probably attempts to reconcile the wish for change with the fear of 'growing up', acts which accept the challenge of the dream imagery.

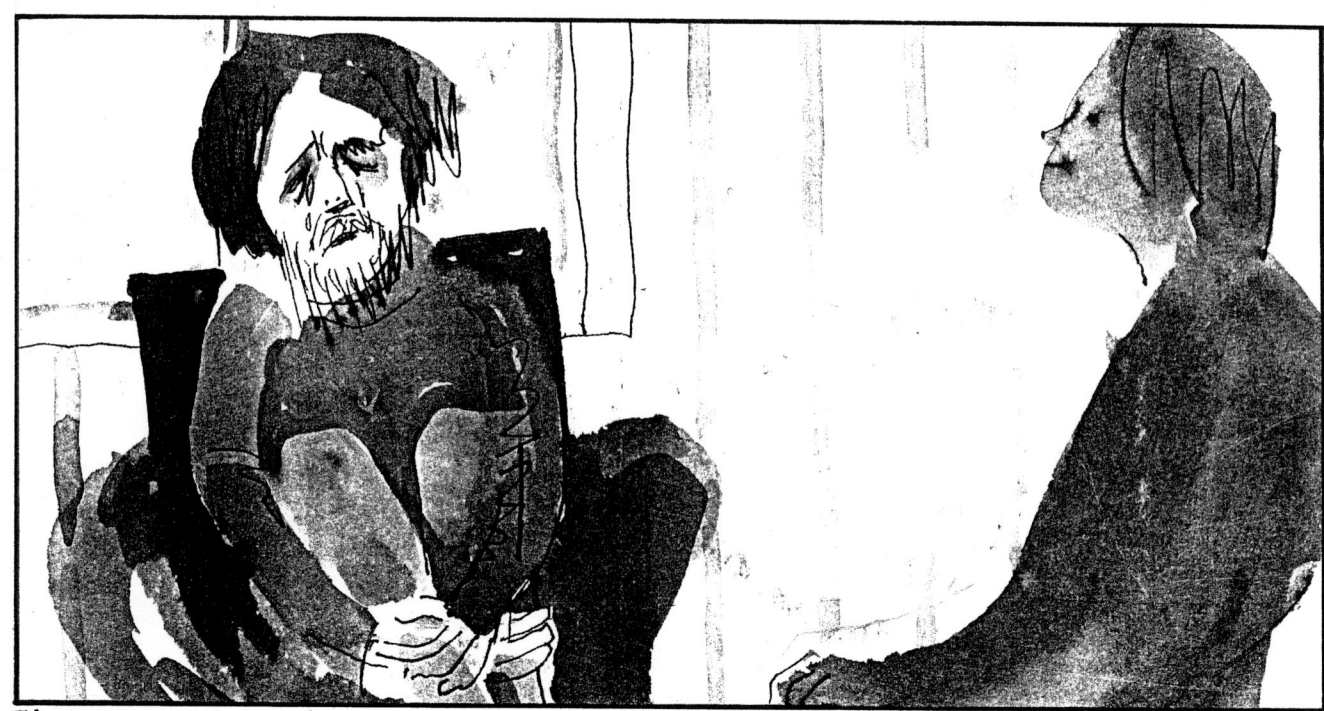

Fig. 161A   A Session with my Therapist (from A Dream Journal 1990-92)   Watercolour

1 BREATH AND BREATHLESSNESS

Dream 2   Asphyxia and Claustrophobia

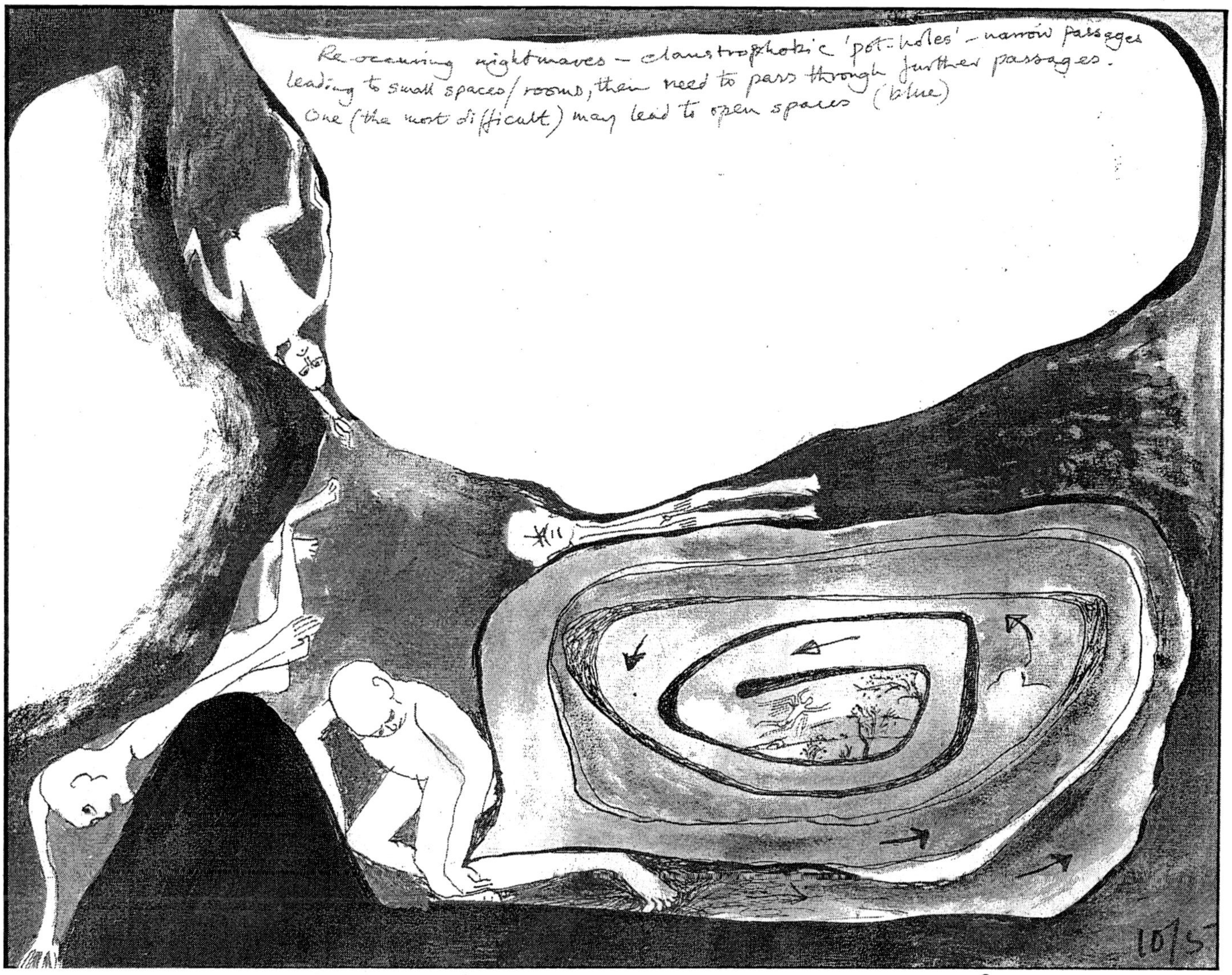

Fig. 162   Claustrophobic Journeying   Pen & Watercolour

Re-occurring nightmares — claustrophobic 'pot-holes' — narrow passages leading to small spaces/rooms, then need to pass through further passages. One (the most difficult) may lead to open spaces (blue)

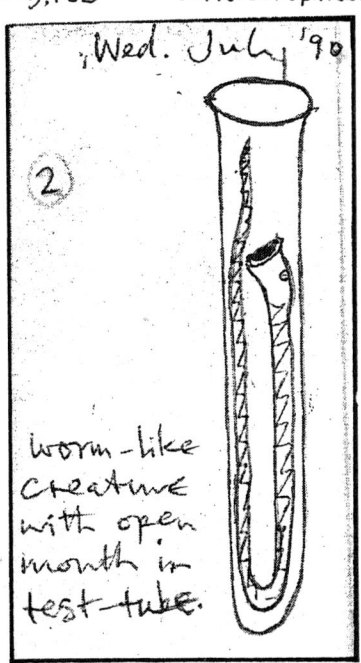

Fig.162A   Dream 2   Pencil

Top: Later freestyle painting relating closely to dream N°2, where the figures are struggling and forcing themselves through very narrow tunnels, en route for......... a birthing?
The dreamer felt he had little hope of survival, rather a slow strangulation before reaching desired end of the tunnel. Yet frequently he squeezes through to another open space giving some hope. Was the garden paradise ever to be reached? Would there be enough air to breathe?

Left: Dream 2   July '90 'Worm-like creature with an open mouth in a test tube.'

Comment: This small drawing is fearful in the extreme summing up in a simple image many other claustrophobic dreams when I awoke gasping for breath.

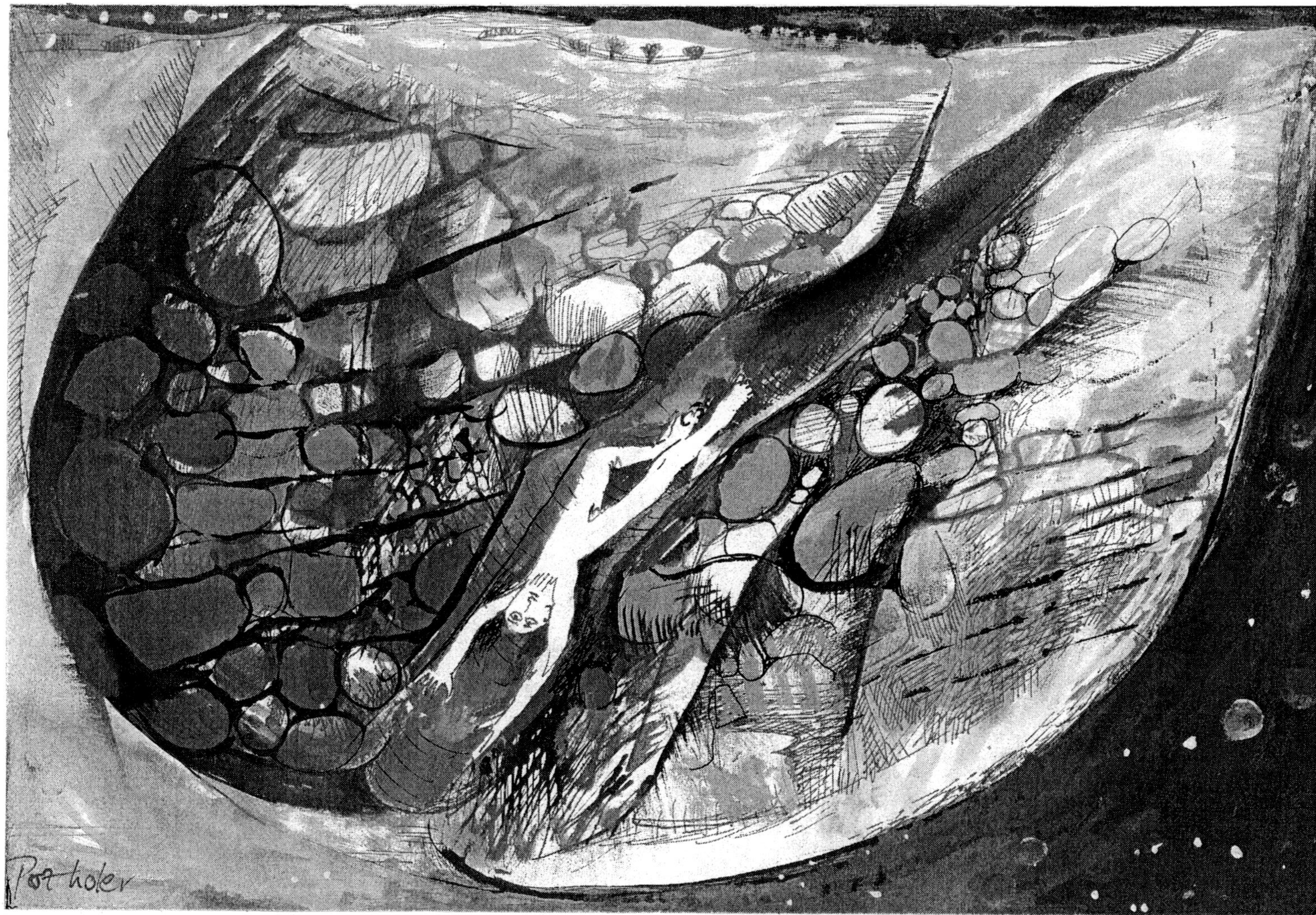

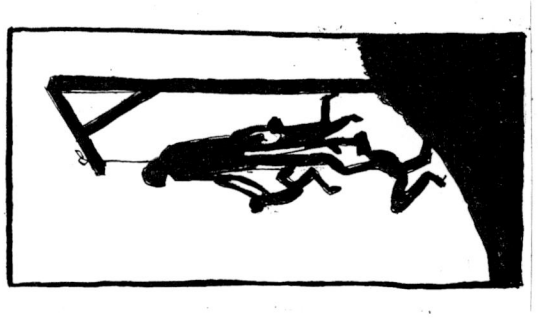

"... my companions help me fulfil this wish, swinging me down into darkness."

Fig. 164 Gallows Humour*   Ink

Above: '96 dream in New Zealand. Here the dreamer is suffocated. He has moments of fear & panic about giving up the power of his head (on North Island).

There is a desire for a more spontaneous approach to everything and so my intuitions (companions) grant me the opportunity to explore a new way of living with my feelings, by throttling me on a gallows.

Tomorrow's destination on New Year's Day, is South Island.

*This dream is recorded in full in 'Land of the Long White Cloud' on page 250 - second panel.

Fig. 163   The Pot-Holer   Ink & wash

Unlike fig 162 (overleaf) the sense of asphyxiation is lessened in the 'Pot-Holer'. A single exit from the 'underworld' offers easy access to the air.

There is no struggle to squeeze through the tight turns of this earlier imagery. It looks like a much easier birth.

A late dream (following completion of Dream Journal). I have to go through the smallest of doors to enter a compartment. Foreknowledge about squeezing through makes me hesitate, but then I decide to enter and claustrophobia overwhelms me until I manage to struggle along a narrow passage onto a bogland where rain is falling.

Compared with the pot-holer, this is a difficult birth.

2 A TUMULTUOUS RUSH

Dreams 5, 12, 14   Confusion, Excess of Feeling

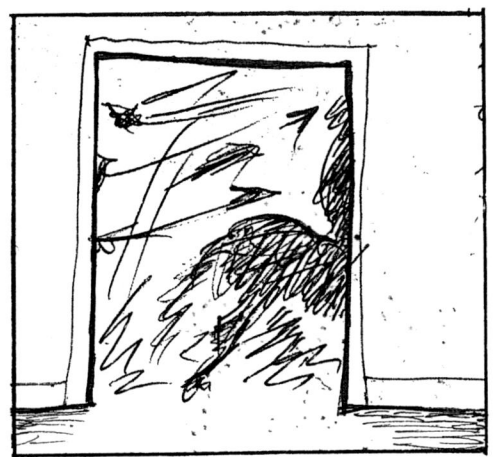

Dream 5: July '90. A flurry of activity seen through a doorway: a horse with rider, general confusion.

Comment: Blurred images are fascinating – why? By looking indirectly at the object · by clicking a camera as the object flies past a blurred image results. The painter Francis Bacon's portraits possess this quality, especially the heads, suggesting movement within a static pose – an un-nerving sensation. The dream shows arrows flying towards the horseman – a medieval battle possibly, with an army in retreat.

Fig.165 - Dream 5   Pen & Ink

Dream 12. Aug 13 '90.   No image recalled – no illustration, but a remembrance of chaos, of many voices with masses of figures flashing past. Related to Dream 5 – the essence of the dream was about movement.

Right: Fig.166

This pencil and chalk drawing followed the two dreams 5 and 12 above. Reminiscent of the figure passing through a doorway in the 1980 work (see page 20)
The repetitive flowing lines recall rhythms on stringed musical instruments.

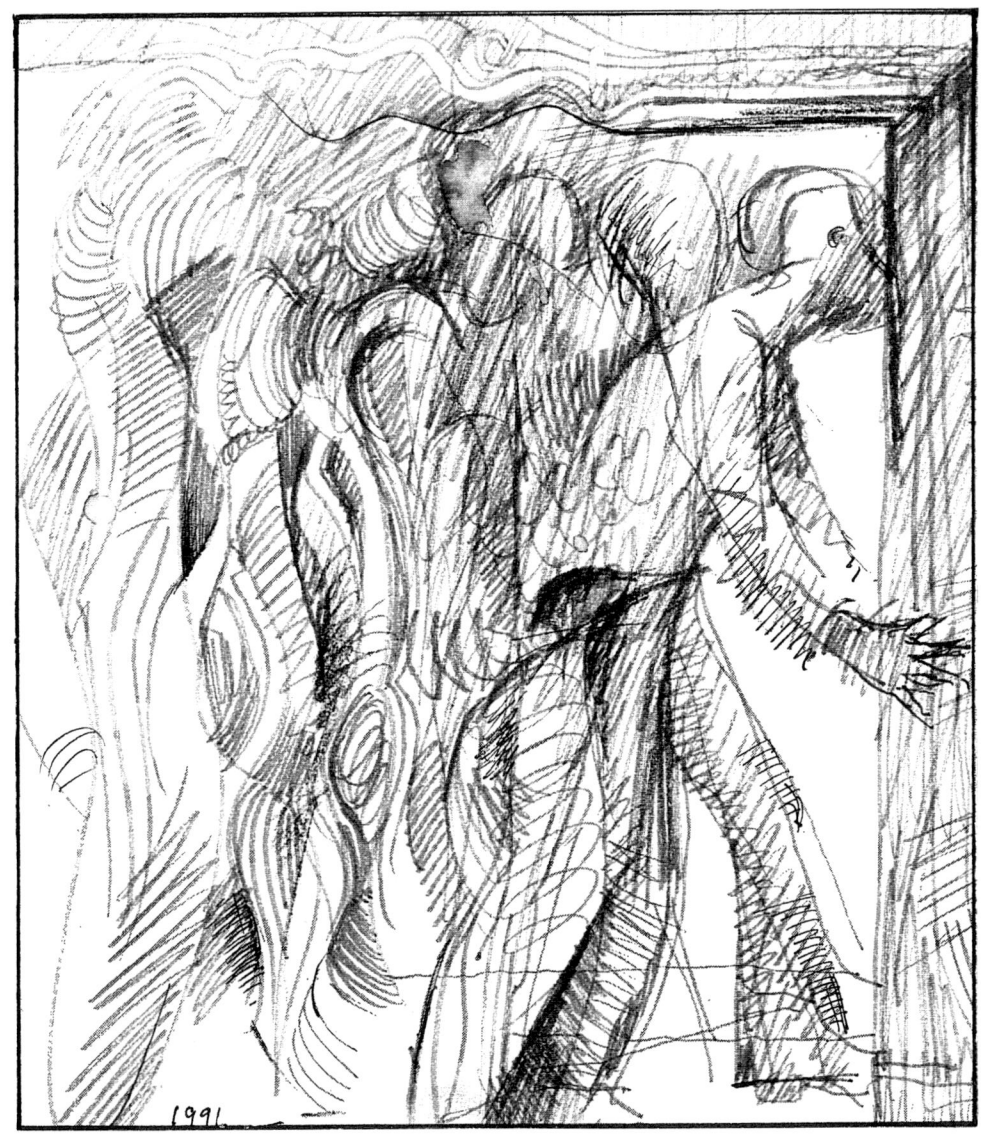

Fig.166 Untitled
Pencil & Chalk   1991.

Dream 14. 14 August 1990.

A very crowded auditorium in semi-darkness, a hush of expectancy. Then an Opera Group surges across the hall from the main entrance, intensely coloured in hot reds and oranges with vivid cool and creamy white. The group now begins to differentiate into the principal singers in front, who burst into song. There is little space for the cast who occupy the centre of the hall – it's a kind of Theatre-in-the-Round. It's all like a great tidal wave, colour and music dominating.

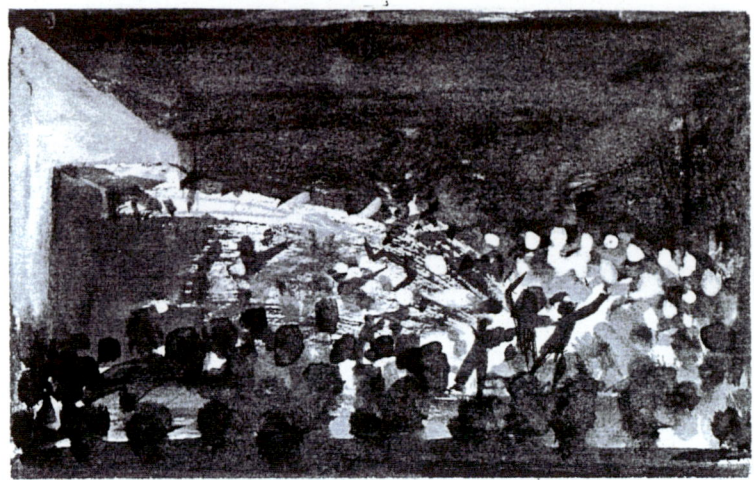

Fig.167   Dream 14   Gouache

My orientation from a close position by the singers seems now to move to the far end of the hall. I find myself looking at the lower part of a small cottage whilst the Opera continues, my attention focused on the entrance area near the front door. I examine the ground and scrape away some surface material (soil, gravel?). Underneath I find, to my surprise, a new paving-stone, and a person to my left exclaims 'how interesting', offering me a couple of Mars bars. The opera finishes with a final flourish as I exit with my generous companion, only to note that he is a VIP of the Festival. We remark on the success of the attendance figures as we negotiate a narrow cliff top path with a deep space to our left side.

Comment

For me the visual imagery shouts SPONTANEITY, a need to act more openly, to 'let go' of inhibitions – the self saying Wake Up! The surge of heat and the strong vigorous movement into a drama space shows an emotional out-pouring of a passionate red and white-hot intensity.

It seems to strike a balance with my cool and retentive reactions to any confrontations during my waking hours. Then the second part of the dream seems to concentrate on the clearing away of long overlaid cover-ups (the soil and gravel) to reveal the new possibilities from the inner, hidden away paving or, perhaps, mosaics, hinting at the need for a fresh start (before entering the door into the 'cottage'?).

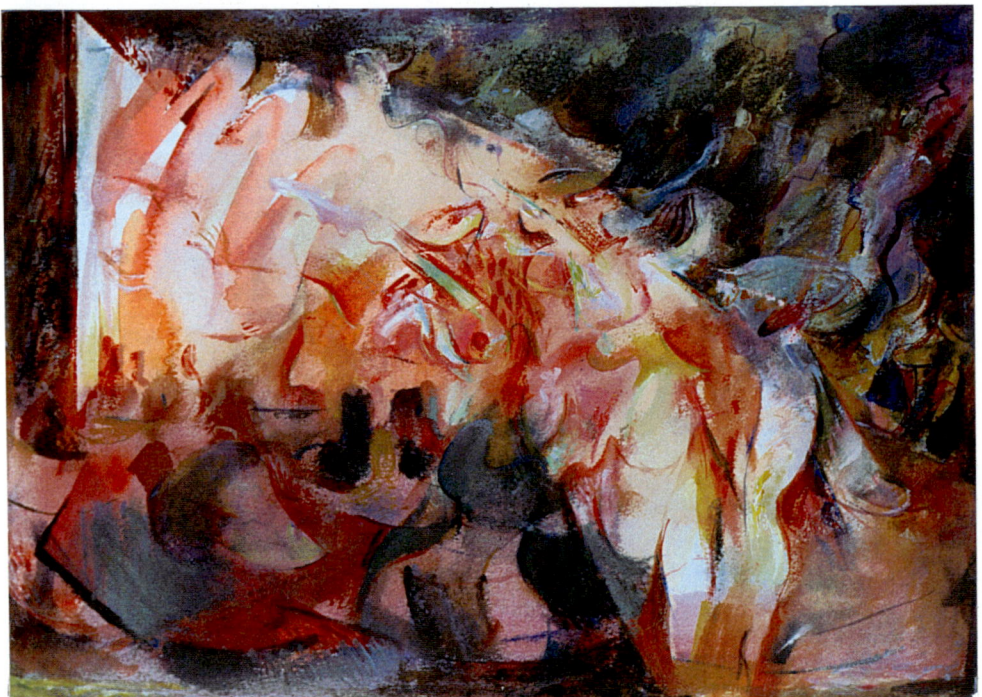

Fig.168   Night at the Opera   Watercolour

Reinterpretation of the dream, the wave of performers blurs across the 'stage'. The audience sit in the reflected light from the Opera cast. A study in contrasts: active, dynamic performers bathed in light and the passive, relaxed viewers in the shadows.

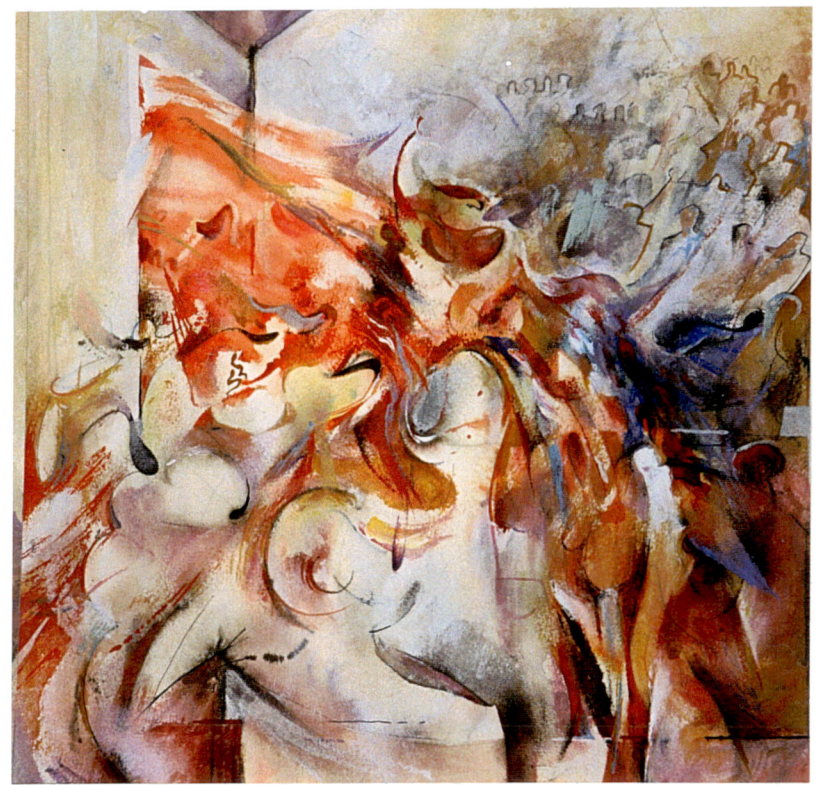

Fig.169   Opera – A Theatrical Dream   Watercolour

Further developments: The cast more clearly defined, yet still largely amorphous. A Joker (or Harlequin) makes an appearance to the right of the group.

Below: The above painting developed further, the Joker's presence is emphasised (and not improved either). This picture is an example of how not to develop something which was already 'satisfactory':- had sufficient form to be left alone. This picture I finally destroyed, but a record is retained through the photographic print conveying something of the original feelings on Dream 14.

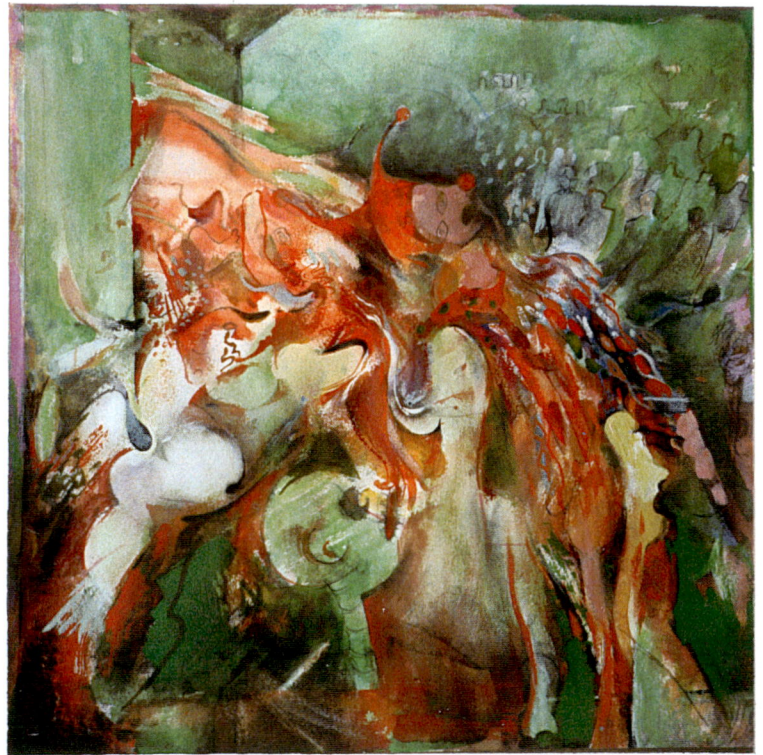

Fig.170   Development of Fig.169 (later destroyed)   Gouache

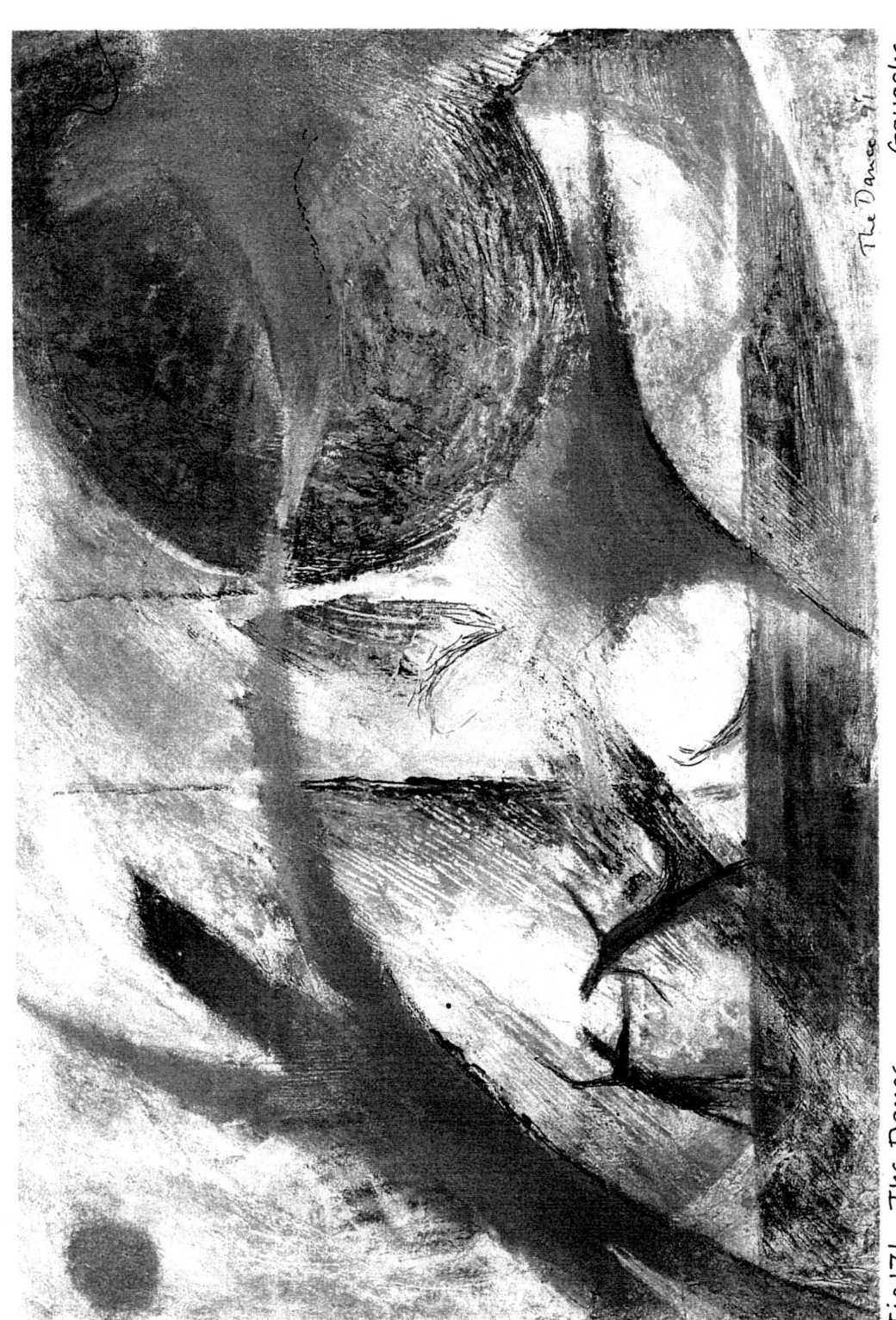

Fig.171 The Dance

Above: 'The Dance' - a freestyle painting of leaping dance into space.

Below left: Fig.172 'Falling Figure'. Reminiscent of the fragmented pictures of the 1980s (page 21, fig.42) but more soft-edged and blurred. Again, it shows a sense of rush, an inability to stay quiet or still......

Below right: Fig.173 'Figure Ascending a Staircase'. An obvious reference here to Duchamp's 'Nude Descending a Staircase', although the movement of the figure developed from the shape of the staircase itself, with its tight, winding curve. (See also pages 176 & 177 for further developments of the staircase).

Overleaf: Fig.174 'Dancing on Stage' - A hectic, twirling movement of figures on stage. Using a dragged paint technique, with a piece of cardboard cut as a comb pushing thick gouache across the picture.

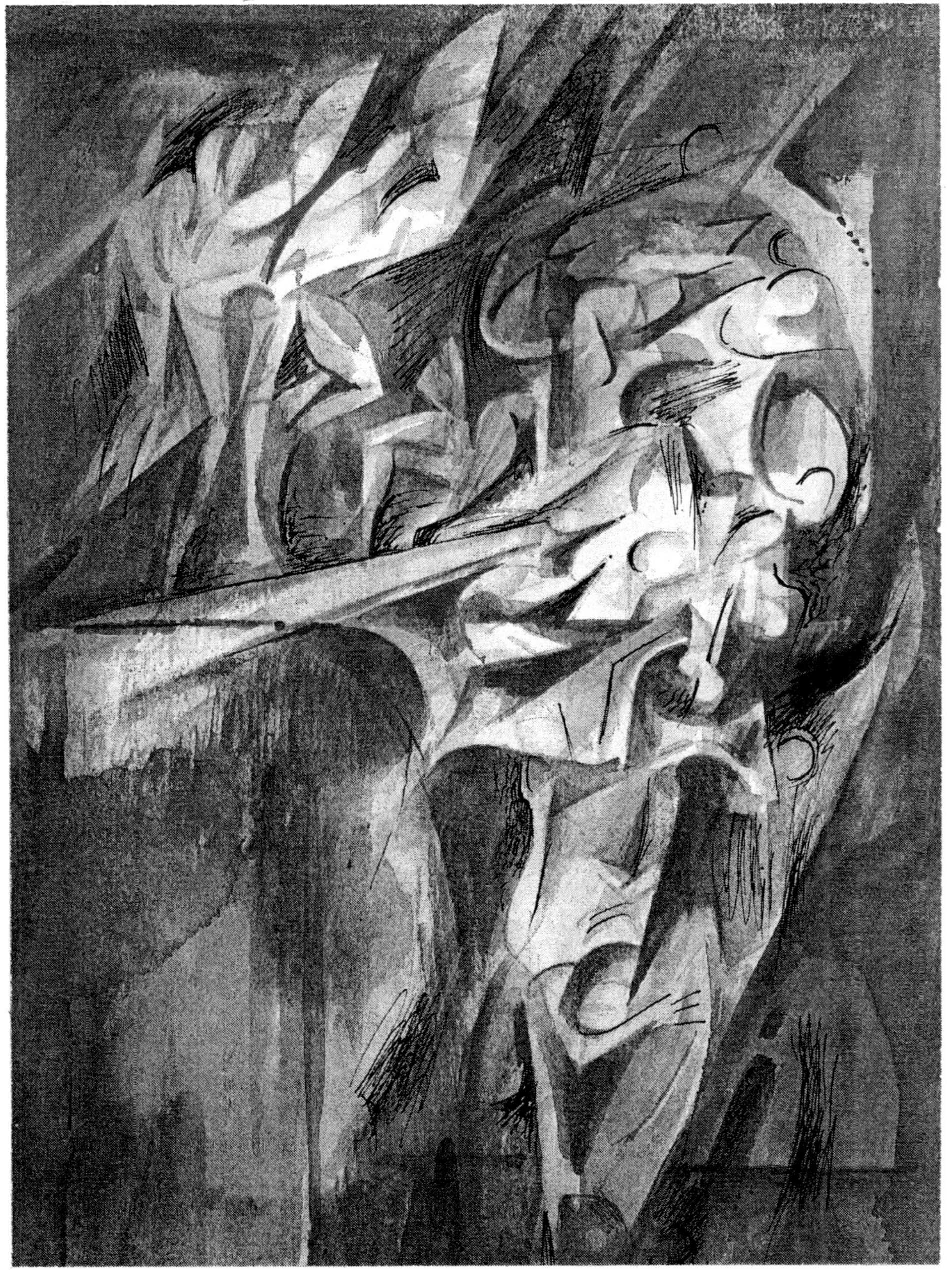

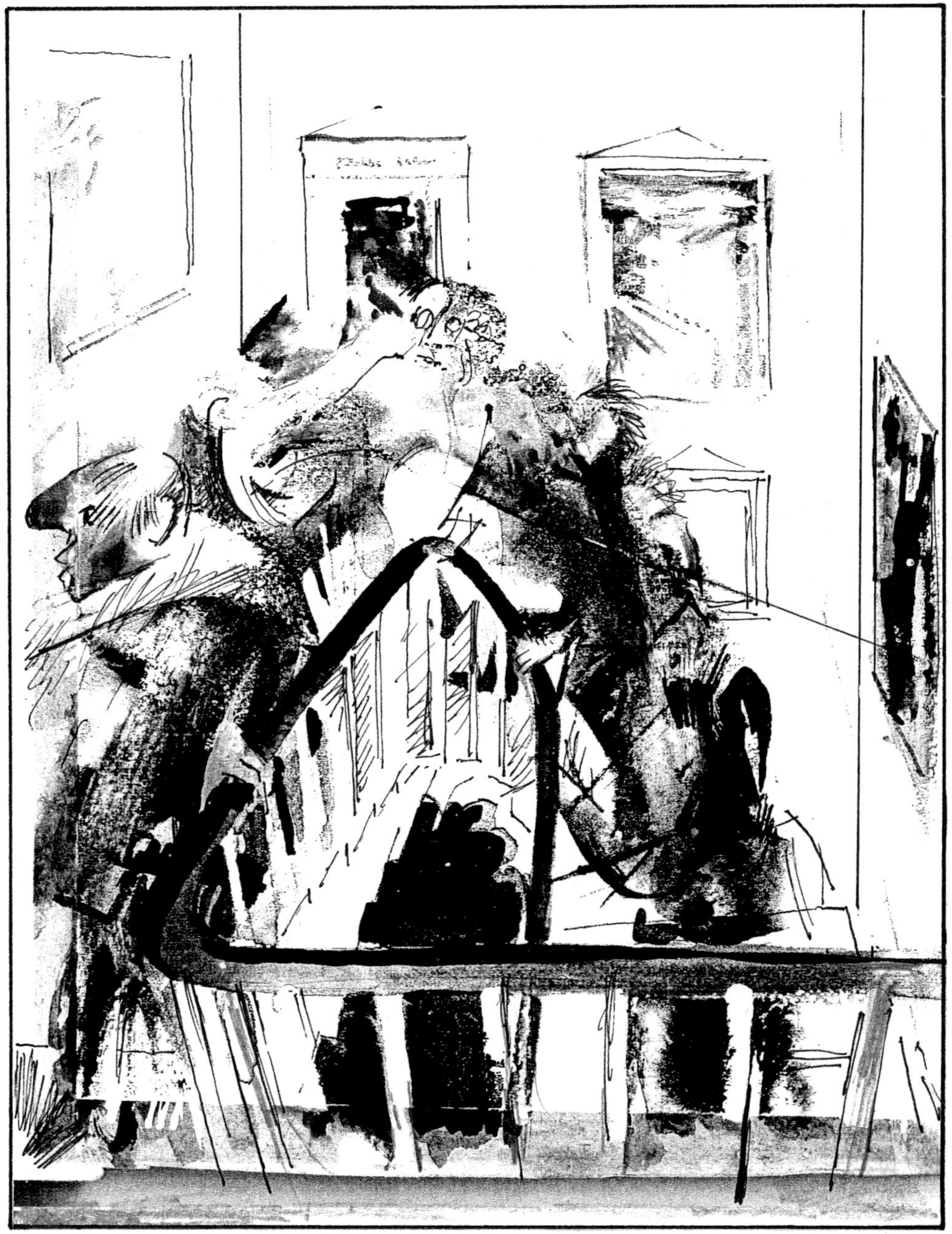

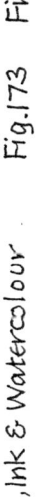

Fig.173 Figure ascending a Staircase   Gouache

Fig.172 Falling Figure   Pen, Ink & Watercolour

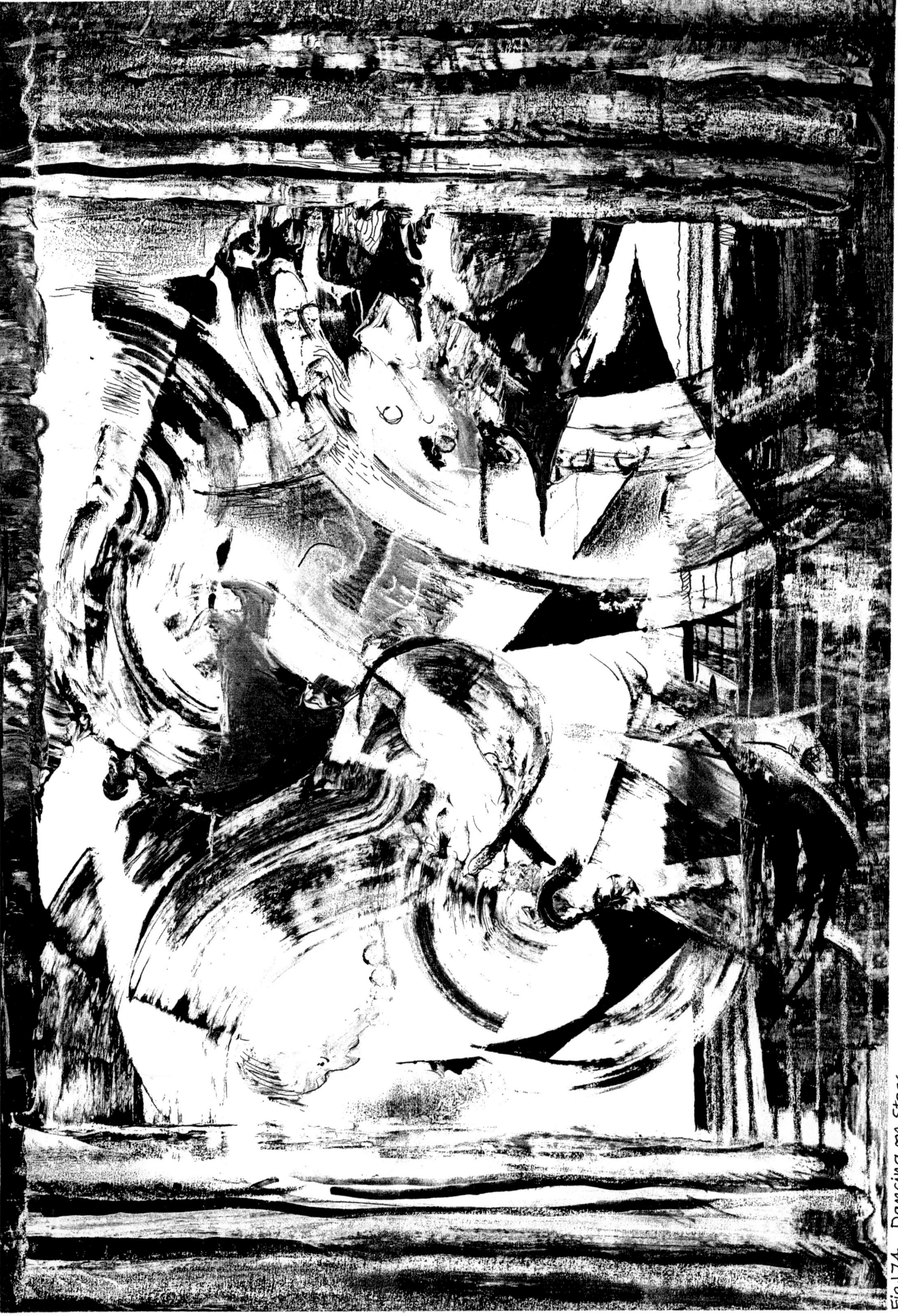

Fig.174 Dancing on Stage   Cardboard Comb - Dragged Paint

3 AUTOMATONS

Dreams 7, 20, 27, 33, 80   Institutions and Conformity

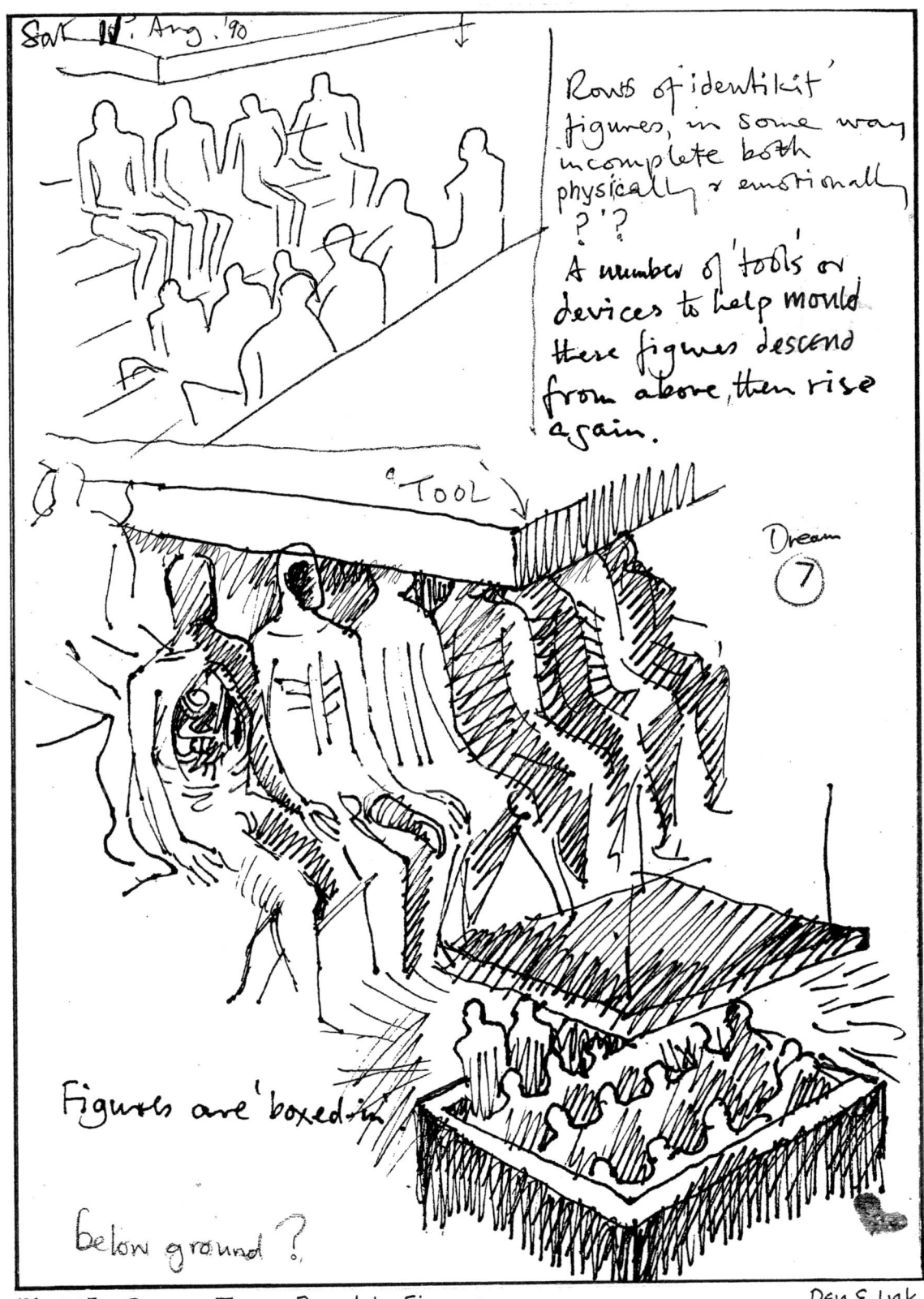

Fig.175 – Dream 7   Boxed-In Figures   Pen & Ink

Dream 7 – 11.Aug 1990 – Scenes of regimentation and conformity, of men 'moulded' into a system, which reflects the realities of my early years – submerged by rules, regulations and dogma. This is the first dream which depicts what I call a mechanised 'restraint' device, designed to restrict the freedom of expression, turning the individual's independent spirit into an automaton.

Looking again at dream 7 with its press moulding 'tool' I see the cloned figures, like androids from a sci-fi fiction. The image of all these identical seated figures seems to offer a warning — 'DON'T BECOME LIKE THIS'. All independent thought, uniqueness, can so easily be stamped out if I allow it to happen. It reminds me not to follow blindly rules and regulations without close scrutiny; reminds me of a tendency to believe 'hype' without close questioning.

The dream seemed to challenge some internalised conformist who depended on certain structures in order to survive. The institutional rules couldn't be reconciled however with this inner creative voice, causing more and yet more anguish. More and more other voices seemed to be swamping my own, as if I was being dragged towards goals I no longer recognised as my own. Why, for example, was I teaching along formulaic lines when I really believed in more experimental approaches? All too often I found I was working with 'received' ideas rather than my own, of not finding I was able to strike out into more original thoughts.

What the dream did recall was a group of technical drawings I'd done during WW2, whilst working in an aircraft component factory, 1942-1945. I'd retained a few of these old draughtsman's illustrations and started to make connections between the 'now' and the sixty-year-old work.

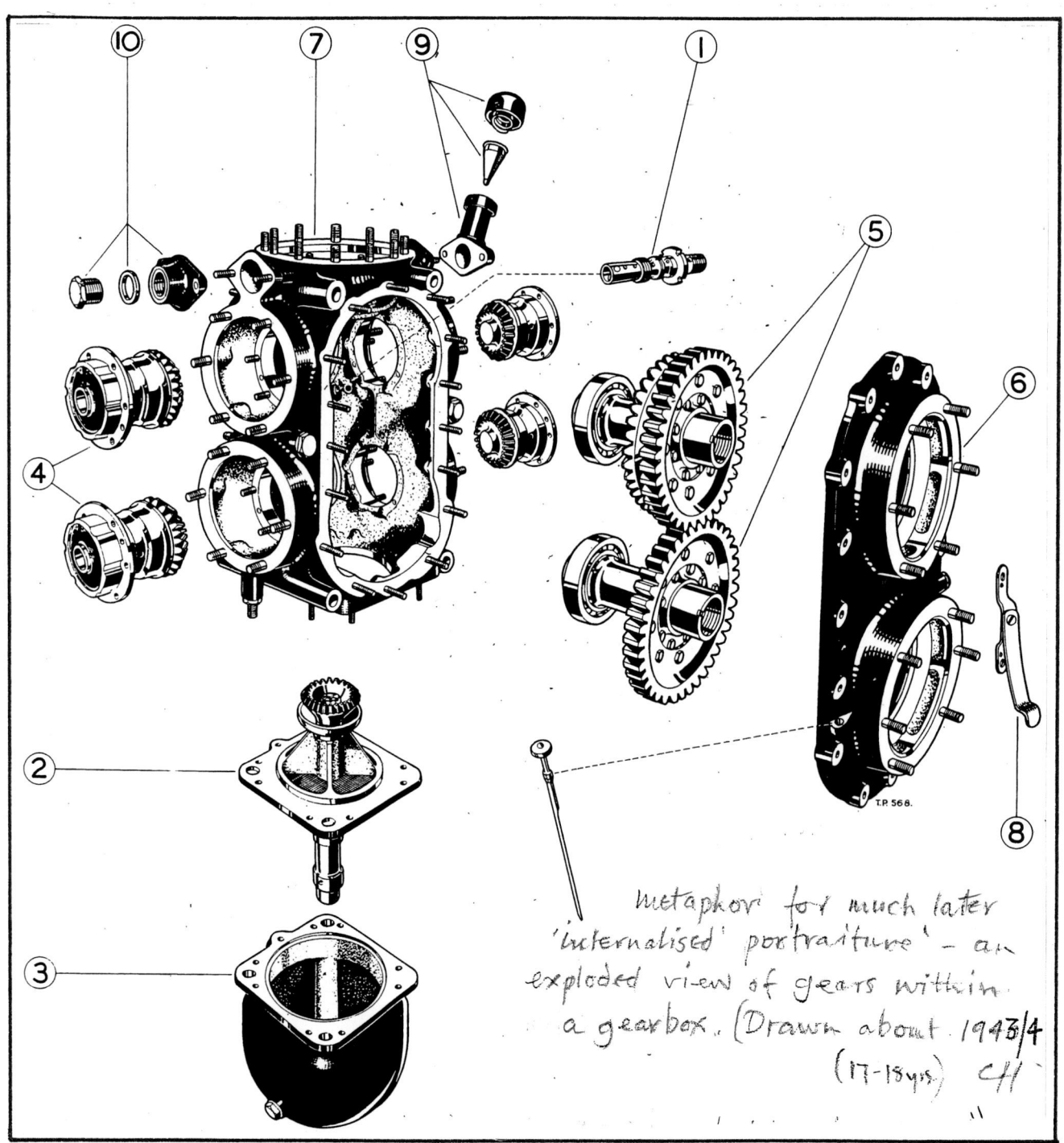

metaphor for much later 'internalised' portraiture' — an exploded view of gears within a gearbox. (Drawn about 1943/4 (17-18yrs) CH

Fig. 176 Exploded view of Gearbox   Ruling Pen – Perspective Projection.

As a technical illustrator I was entirely dependent on mechanical means to make technical drawings – rulers, compasses, T-squares and set squares and so on, with no direct hand contact with the drawing surface. Also it was necessary to be subservient to the 'G.A.' (mechanical plan views) from which to work out projections of the various machines. These drawings for use in aircraft manuals had to be accurate enough to be fully understood by mechanics and engineers who used them for dismantling, repairing and re-assembling machine parts in often emergency circumstances.

All these controlling elements – instruments for drawing, copying others' plans, extreme accuracy and detailing were in complete opposition to everything I was now doing, and, at first sight seemed to bear no relationship to the 'freestyle' line and brushwork and often non-subject matter.

And yet what was now so intriguing were the connections between these oppositions. There were obvious connections between looking inside an engine to view its many cogs, spindles, etc., and the internalised, reflective 'viewing' of the interior of my own superficial appearance. What was happening behind a steel engine casing could be as unknown as what was occurring behind my skull, skin and tissues – until I started to 'open' it up. (see page 100).

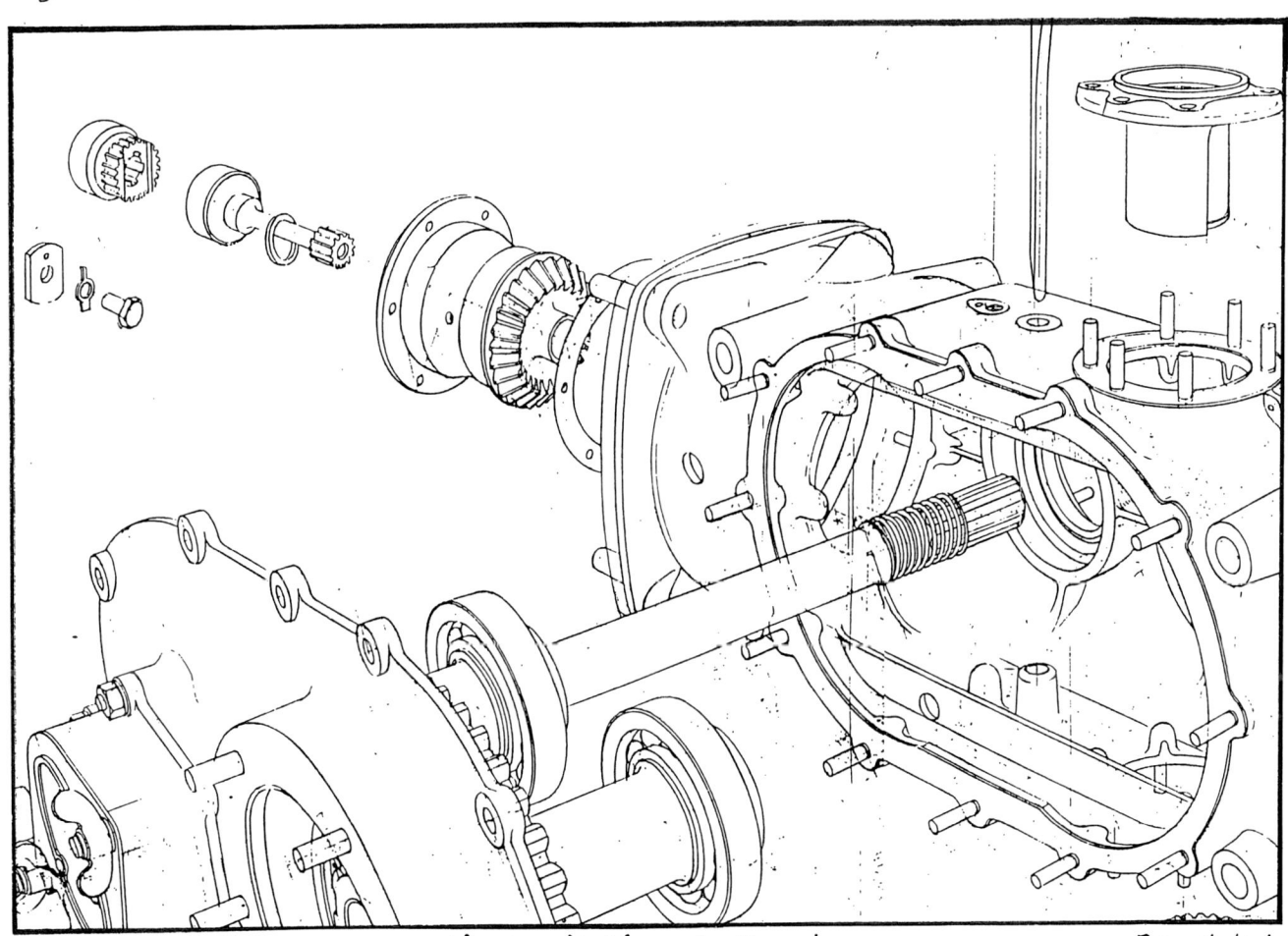

Fig.177 Detail from a perspective projection of a Gearbox   Pen & Ink

The most practical way to show the 'insides' of a machine, keeping the correct arrangement of parts, is to project the parts outwards from the central casing (or body) in an exploded manner, using perspective or isometric projection. The result, as in this technical drawing above, is often more than 'the sum of its parts'. In art history terms, the Futurists had a great interest in the metaphorical possibilities of the machine, and Dadaists like Picabia treated the machine with irony. I could imagine Picabia re-entitling my drawing of the gearbox detail (after adding watercolour or oil paint) "That's the couple who don't know when to stop", making what he would call a symbolic portrait of machinery.

This drawing and the one opposite both revealed, I feel, a close connection with the oil painting completed in 1996 entitled 'Hello, Everybody' (fig.178 overleaf). The intention of the latter is entirely different, concerned as it is with the final 'letting go' of repressions and retentive attitudes, but it shares a common ground of projection or 'explosive' means of expression.

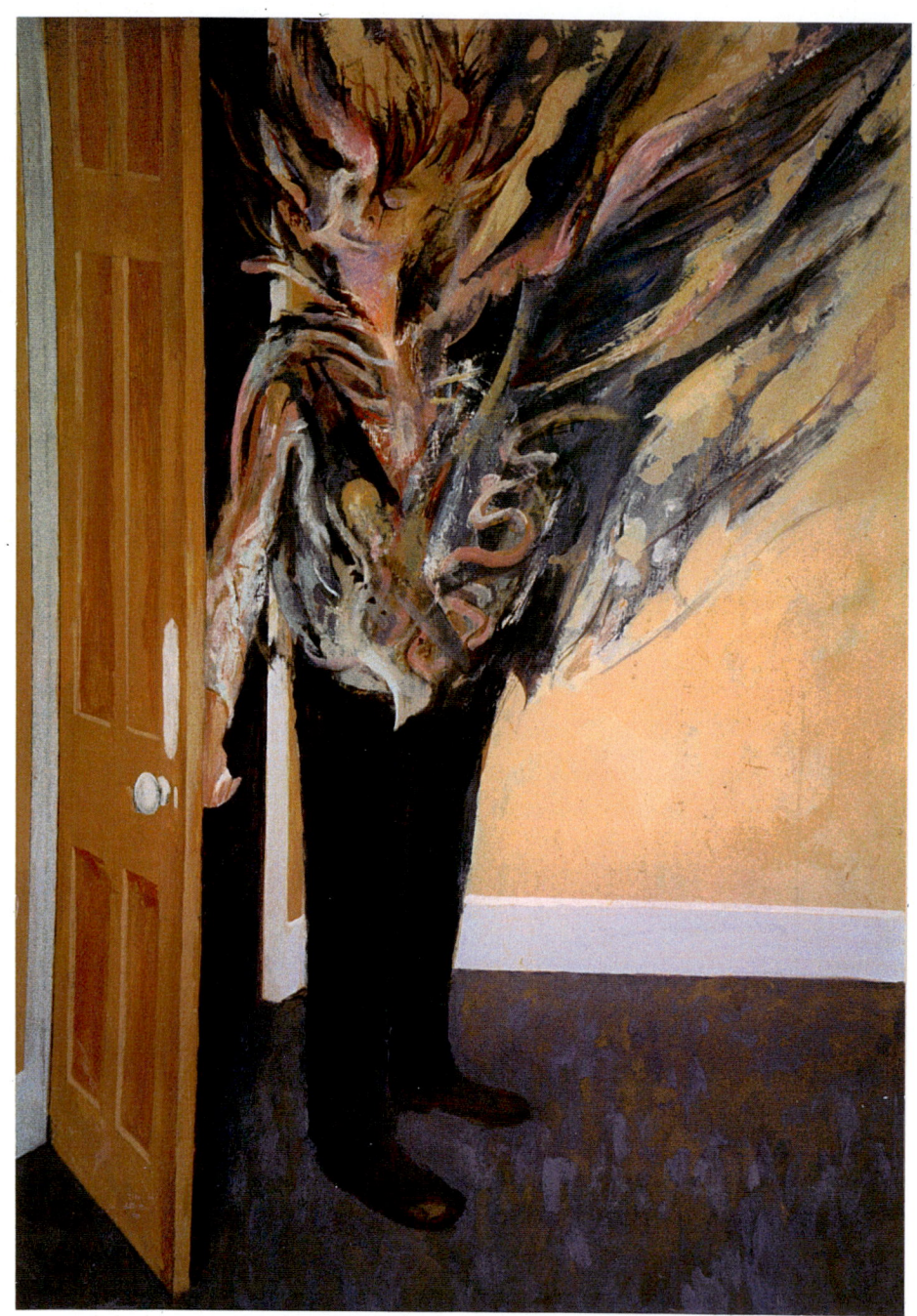

Fig. 178 'Hello, Everybody' Oil on Board

'Hello, Everybody' shows a projection of the self. An attempt to 'open out', with a wish to communicate more directly with people without feeling encumbered by the embarrassment if asked questions on any topic in public gatherings.
 At the time it was only a wish, not a fact. It was as if one might effect a change by advertising the event in advance - like a preview for a forthcoming film saying, 'Look out for this strange happening - soon!'

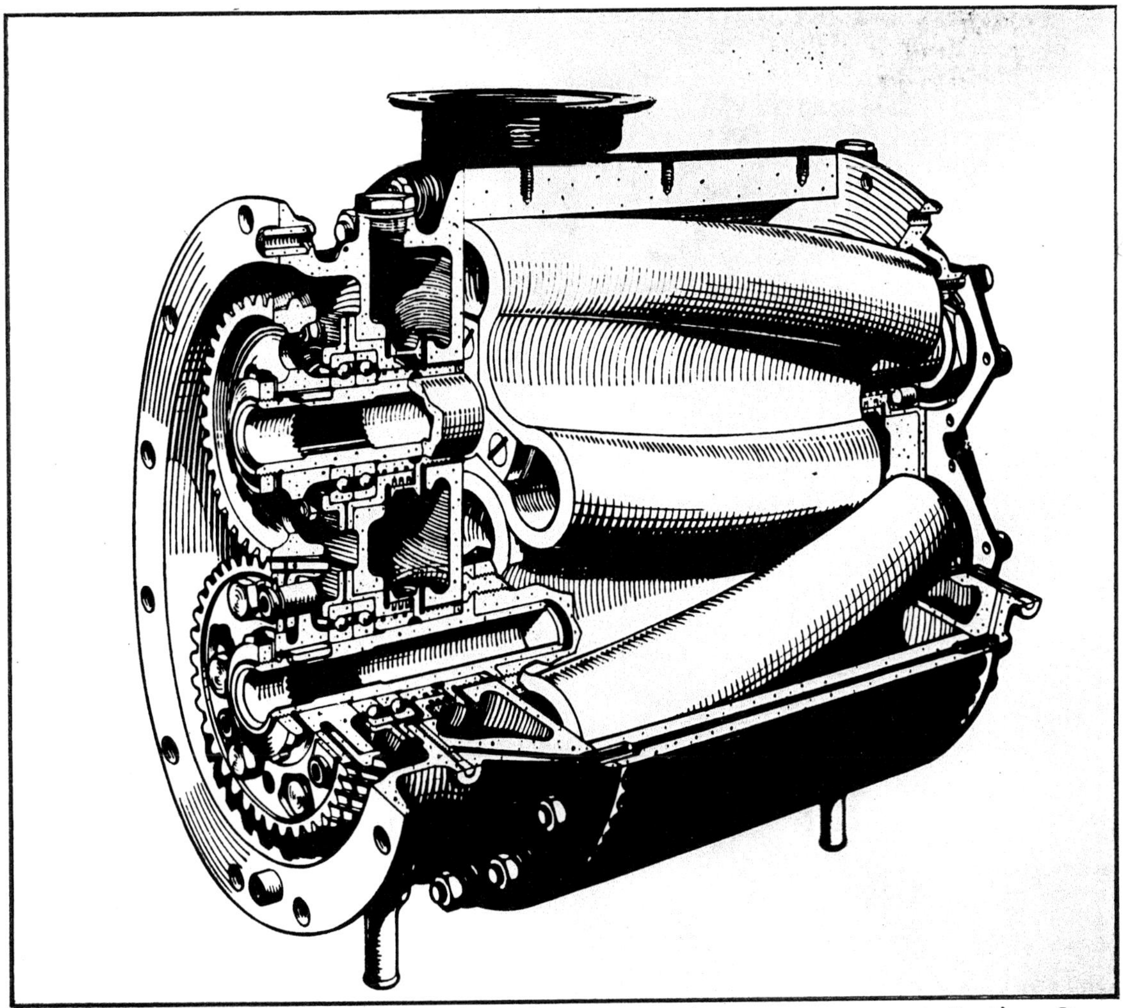

Fig. 179 Perspective 'Cut away' drawing of Gearbox.   Ruling Pen

Another type of technical illustration required all parts 'in situ', and revealed, by removing part of the casing to show each part in relation to the others.
This is containment, everything in its place, compared with the breaking out of the exploded views, and relating more to the dreams on page 97 (figs 183 & 184).

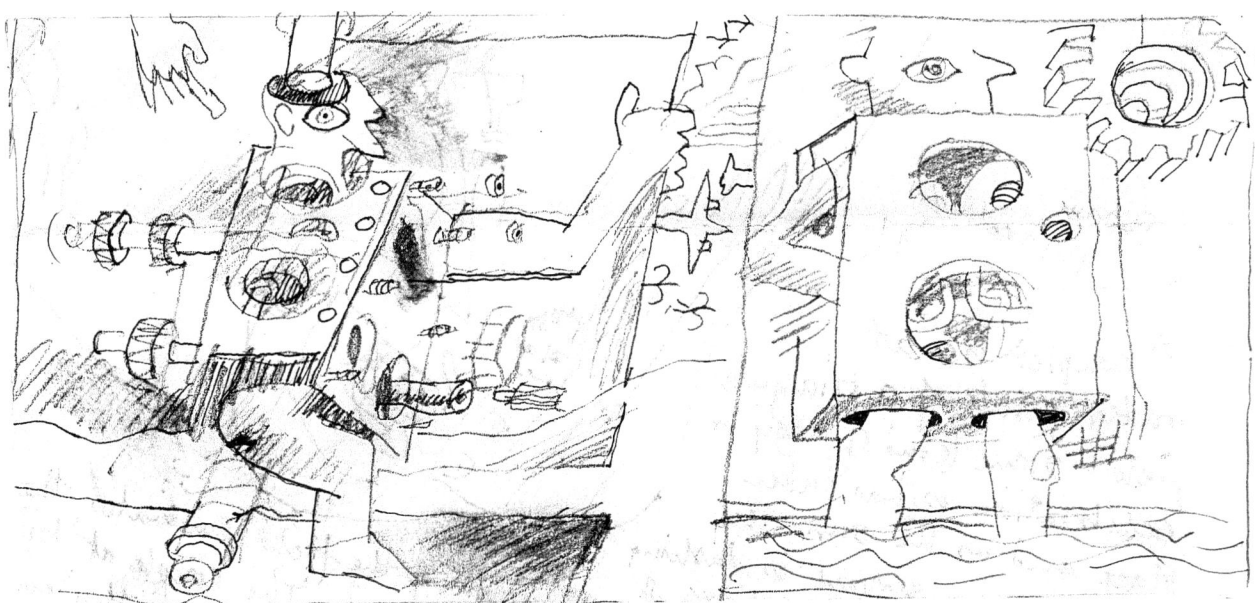

Fig. 180 Doodle sketches of 'Machine Men'   Pencil

Two machine-men 'doodles' combining dream imagery with some of the technical drawings shown here. The right-hand sketch has something in common with the central left figure in the dream 7 illustration, showing his interior plumbing.

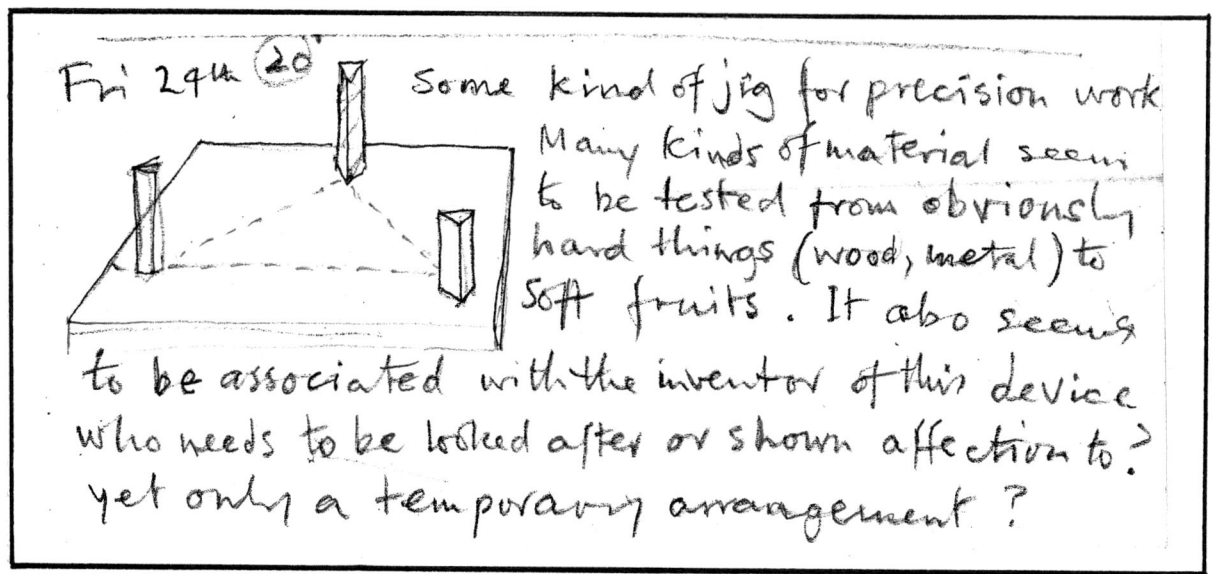

Fig.181   Dream 20   Pencil

Dream 20 24 August 1990

To be 'shown affection' in relation to this metal device seems obscure until I recall other holding devices — they hint at imposed control.

Having gained some independence from constraints perhaps the self was suggesting that occasionally a temporary 'prop', support or guiding system could be useful at moments of self-doubt — until ready to move forward independently again.

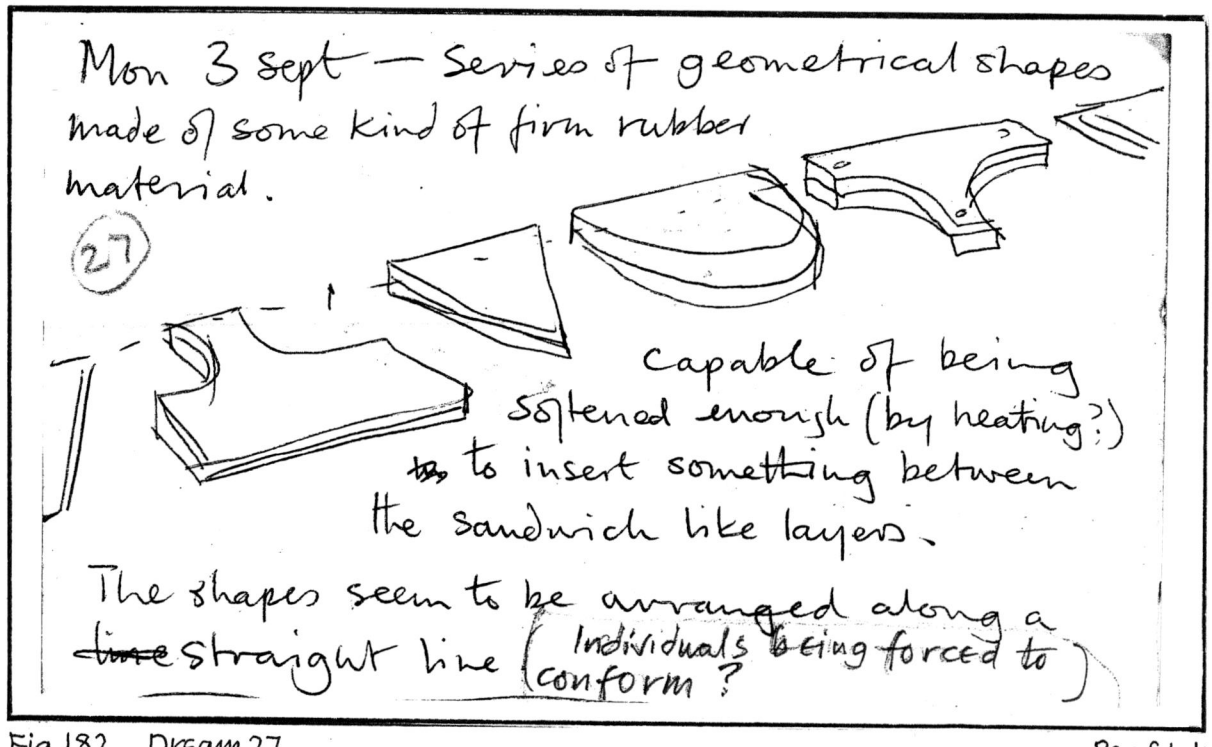

Fig.182   Dream 27   Pen & Ink

Dream 27 3 September 1990

I see this as an assembly line. Even if the shapes are not uniform, they seem to relate to some kind of hidden conformity. The feeling is of the creative intuition being stifled by received opinions. Perhaps it is nothing more than an arrangement along a straight line which causes unease.

These two dreams relate to controlling or containing devices. Dream 20 relates to a clamping and, perhaps, a guiding device. Dream 27 suggests the conforming rigidity of the assembly line.

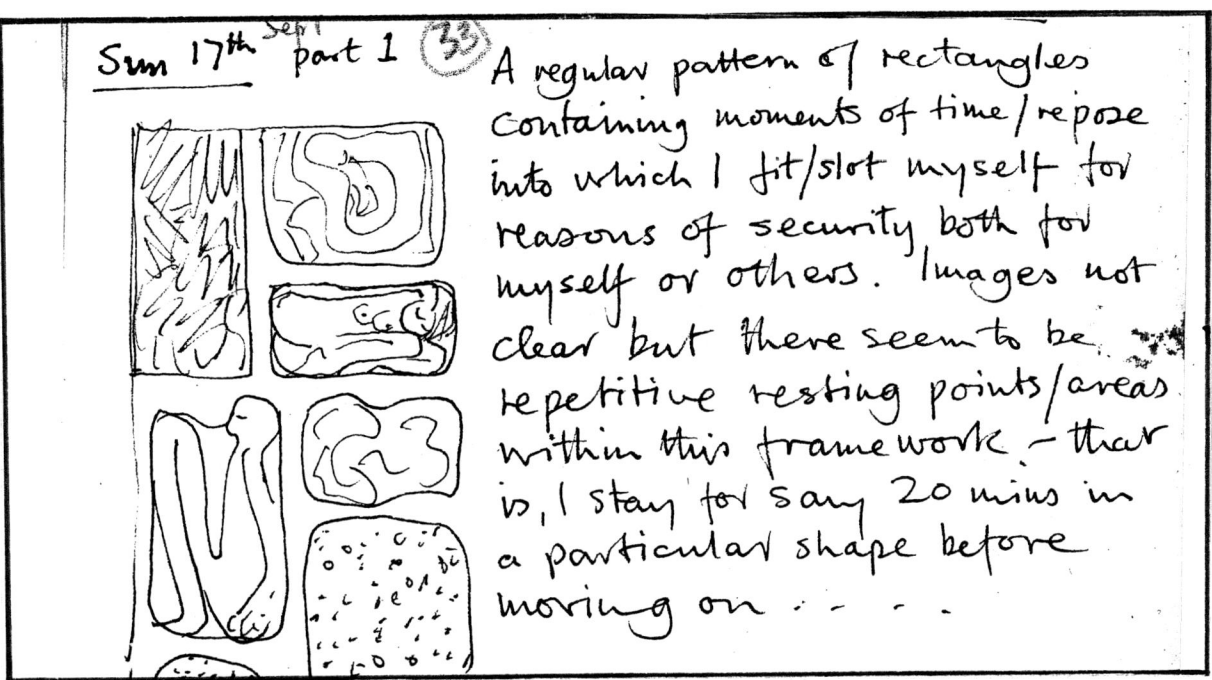

Fig. 183   Dream 33   Pen & Ink

Dream 33 17 September 1990

Is it easier to feel 'safe' inside a rigid harness or a box, or quartered in a small space rather than being free to do as one might aspire towards? Probably.
 So the dream may be throwing up symbols of past patterning and asking "Is this what you want?", or, "Do you still wish life to be like this and make something positive out of it?"
 Or, "Can you accept a degree of conformity?"

Dream 80 28 May 1991

This dream seems to re-inforce the sense of confinement and claustrophobia, relating quite closely to dream 33 above
 Is this a womb or tomb place?

Dreams 33 and 80 take conformity to claustrophobic levels, where figures are cramped into tight containers or very close quarters with others.
 What isn't clear is whether I seek or reject these conditions. Are these places of security and conformity but also subconscious 'warnings' of what can be expected if I refuse to meet any life enhancing challenges offered?

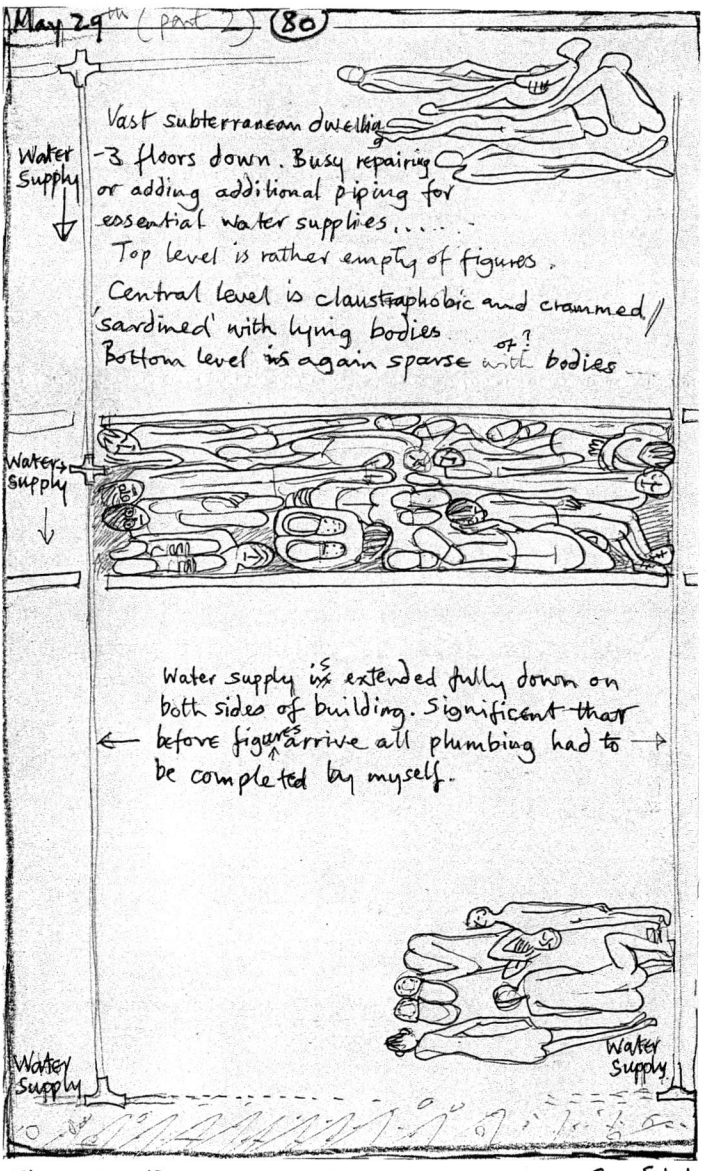

Fig. 184   Dream 80   Pen & Ink

A part-organic and part-mechanical machine with an operator who looks glum at the prospect of walking behind this tracked apparatus for the spreading of retentive 'muck'.

This freestyle drawing recalls a memory of staying in hospital (when ten years old) for severe constipation for a three month period.

Drawn in 1996 I feel it was influenced both by this early hospitalisation and the interest in technical drawings I had been doing during my teenage years, and dreams dealing with 'machined conformity'.

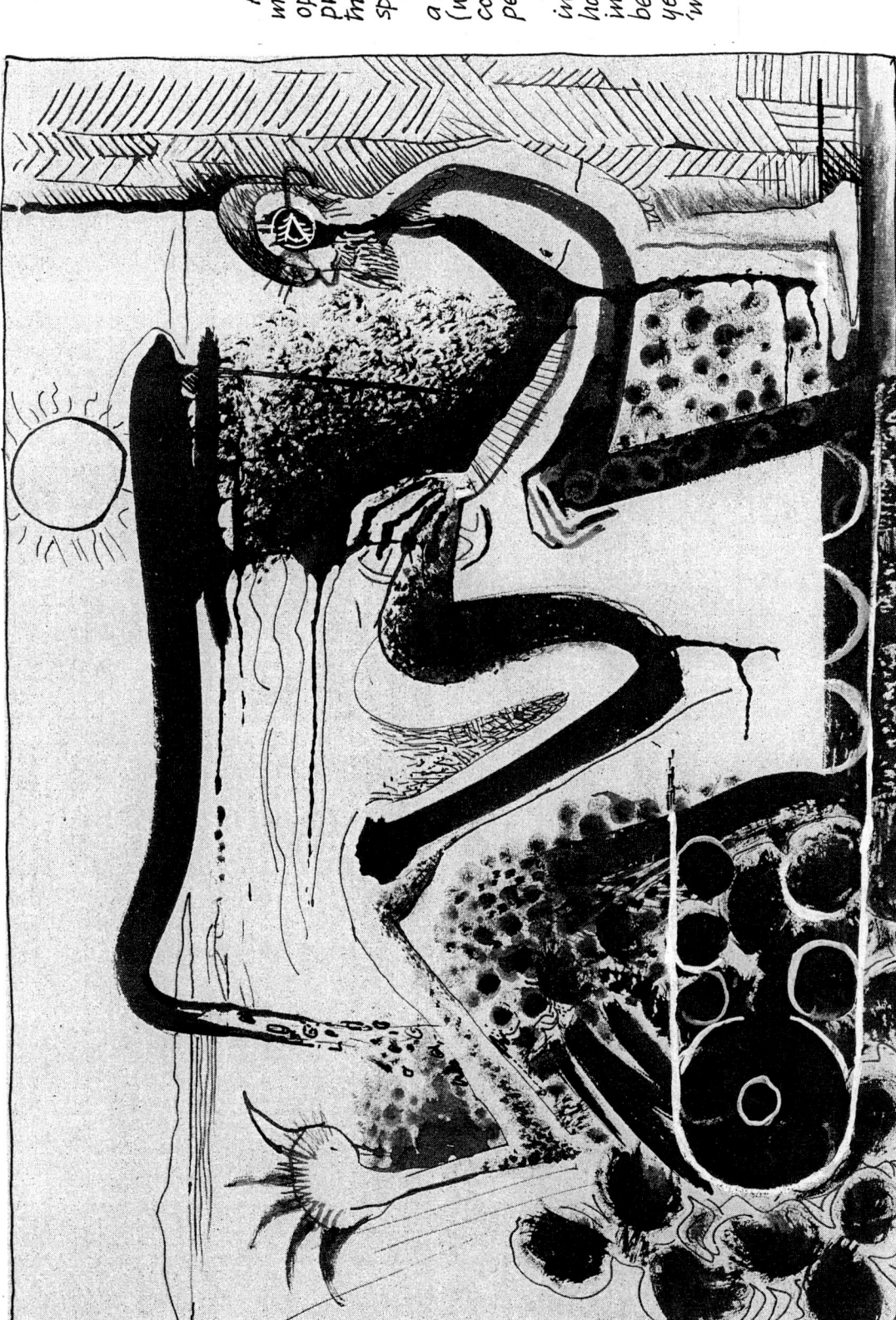

Fig. 18.5 The Muckspreader   Pen, Brush & Ink

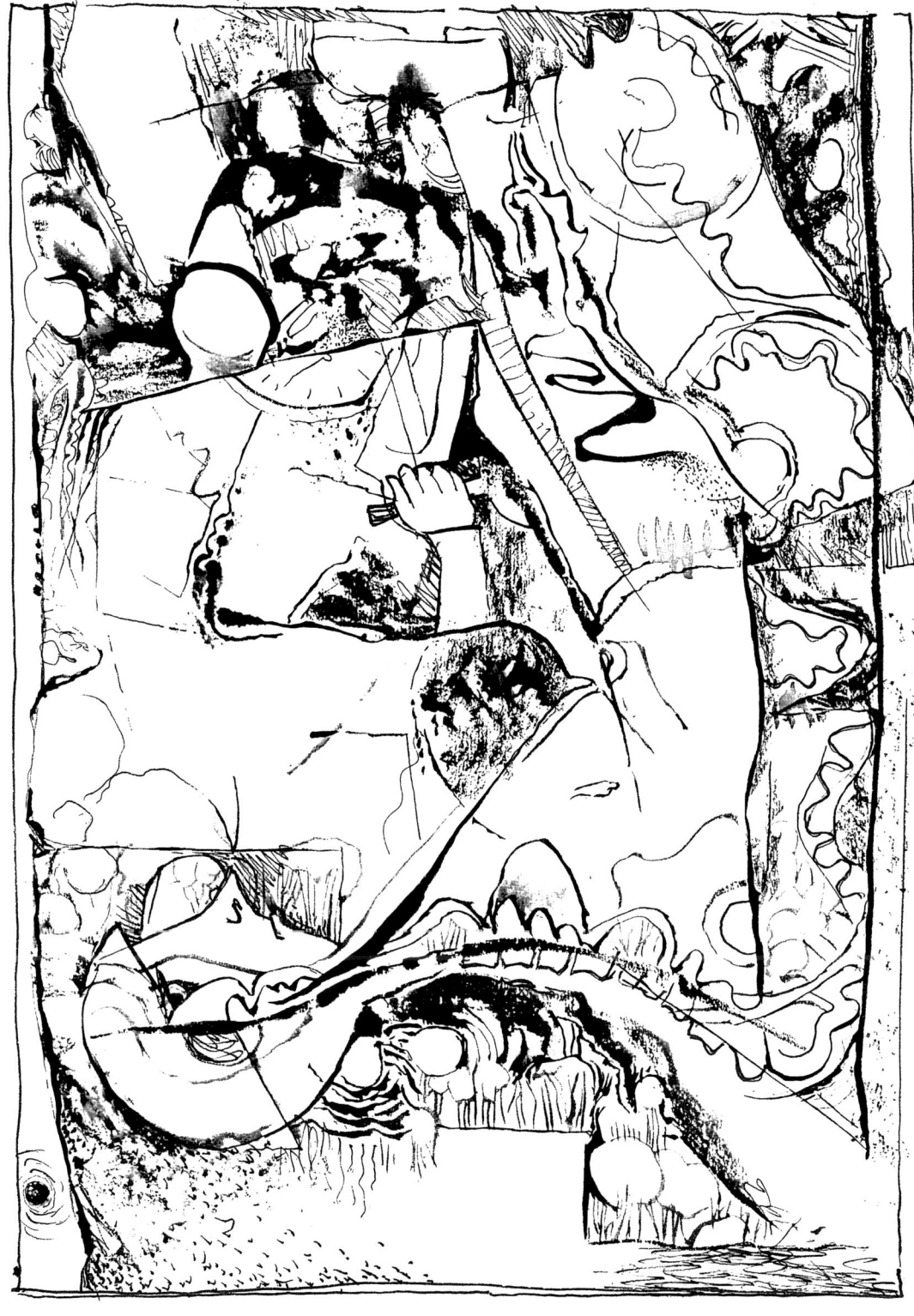

Fig 186 The Quarryman   Pen, Brush & Ink

The quarryman, both human and machine, his spinal column transforming en route towards a caterpillar track system below.

He drives a destructive engine, out to inflict as much damage as possible. The feeling is of 'letting go', but with a vengeance — out to destroy everything which formerly controlled and held him back……..

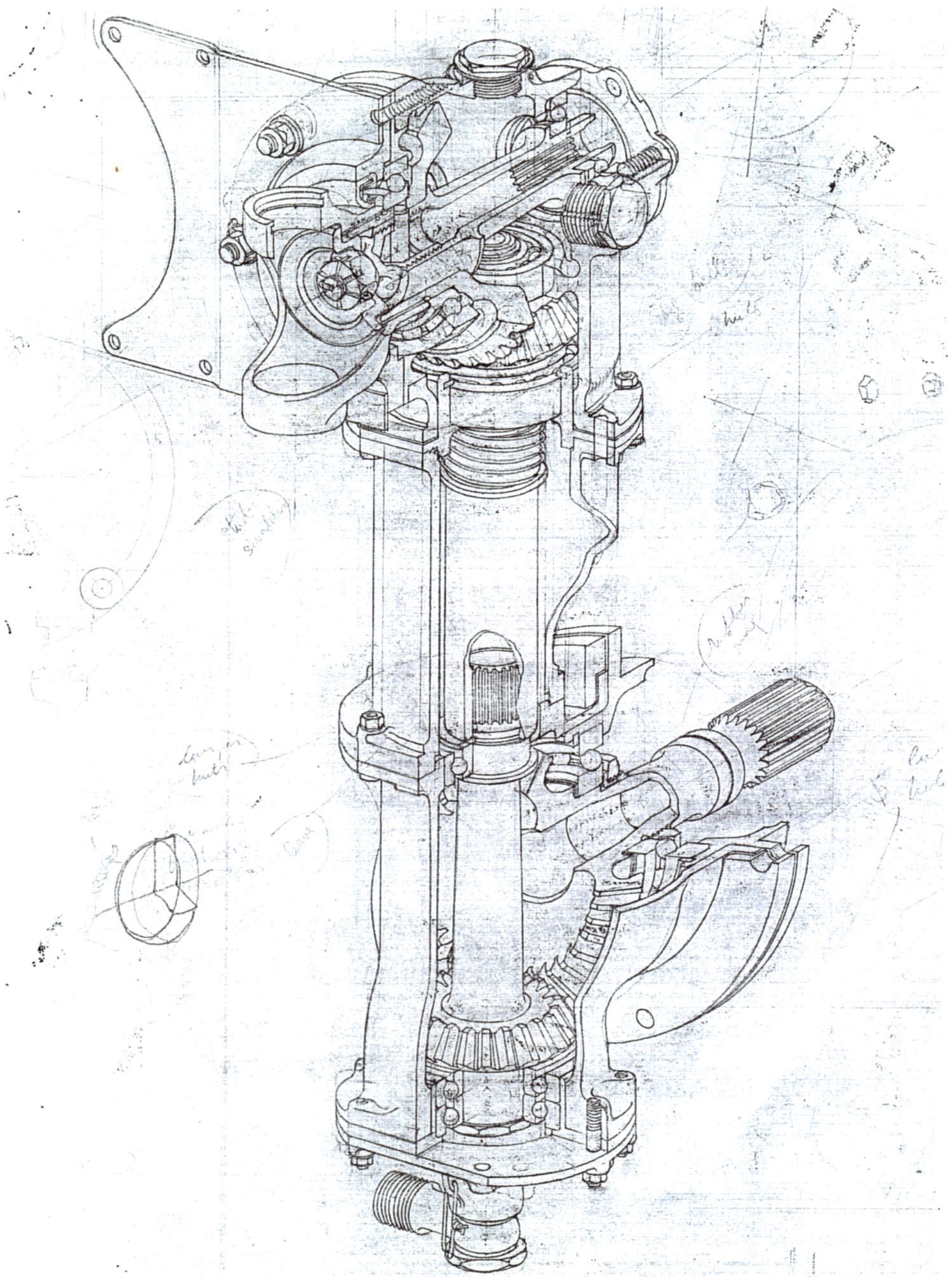

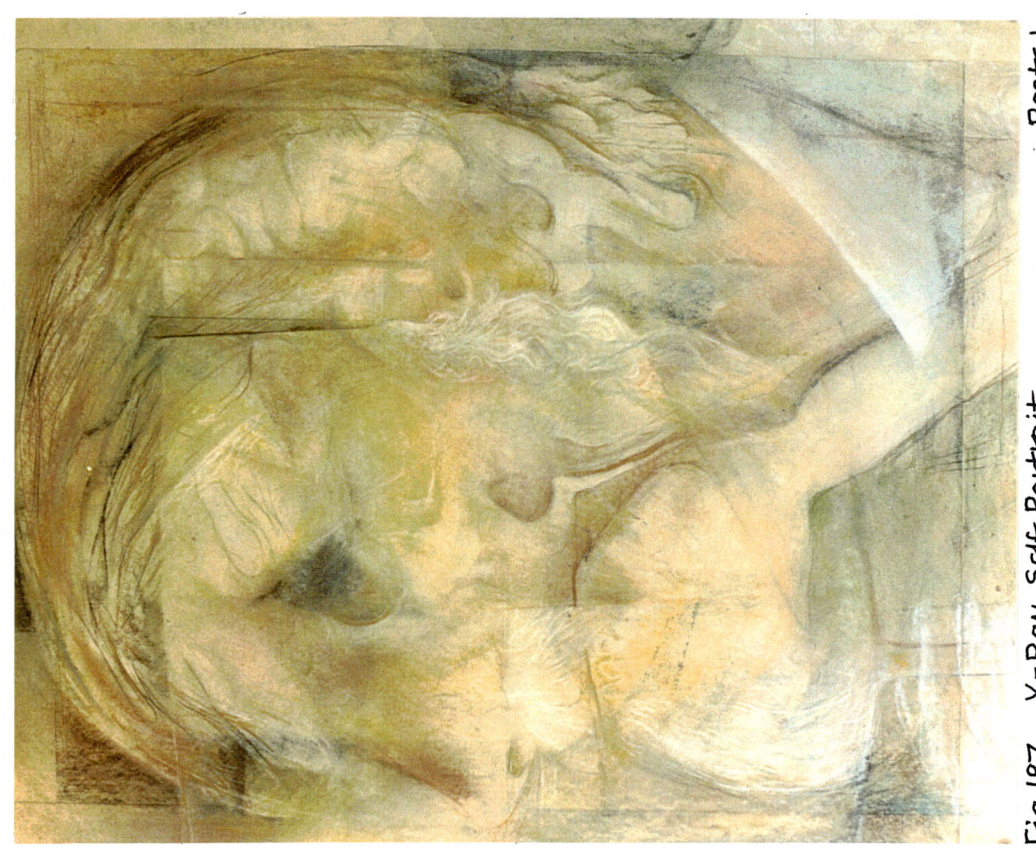

Fig.187   X-Ray Self Portrait   Pastel

Both drawings have a common aim — to reveal the interior behind the exterior casing. The machine drawing clarifies for mechanical information where — as the portrait offers a psychological insight.

Fig.188   Cutaway Section of a Gearbox Arm — Ruling Pen   1943

4 A PROPHETIC DREAM

Dream 17   Clay as Therapy

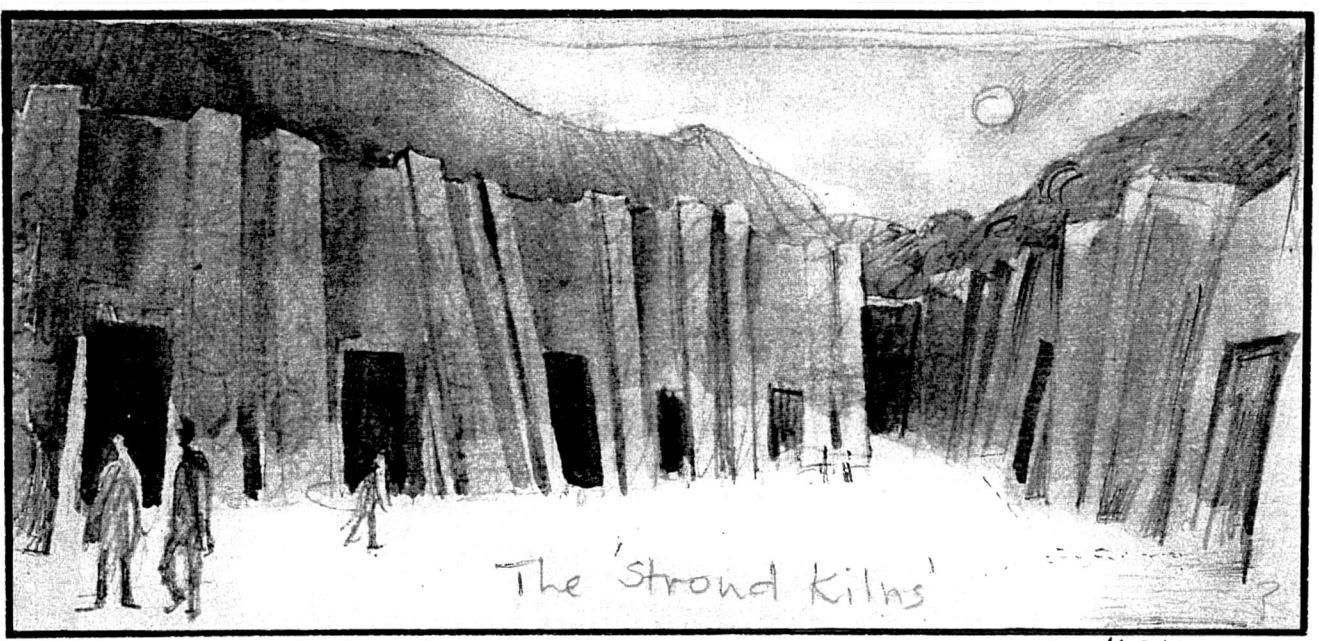

Fig.189 Dream 17 The Stroud Kilns   Pencil & Watercolour

Dream 17   (from 'A Dream Journal') 21 August 1990.
'I'm now entering a narrow valley in an undulating landscape. There are man-made structures of strange shape and proportion which support the sides of the valley, leaning slightly into the earthen banks behind. The huge slabs appear to be made of some dense metal mesh, not unlike the texture of a car radiator. Large open doorways lead into the interior of the hills, and a few figures stand outside. As I puzzle about what this place could be used for I hear a loud voice proclaim, "These are the famous Stroud Kilns"!'

Knowing the town of Stroud and the (un-related) purpose of kilns was of no help towards an understanding of the imagery and vocal expression of the dream. Only after what happened later did I come to feel that the dream possibly carried certain prophetic elements. It seemed to 'know' the dreamer's future in which a severe blockage in creative work was soon to occur. Within a year I'd enrolled onto a part-time ceramics course at Stroud College of Art, working with clay, a material I'd not used before, which gave me a new lease of creative life.

Another aspect of the dream seems now, in retrospect, to make a connection with the clay itself. This soft malleable material, eroded and decomposed from ancient rock can, after reworking in the potter's hands, be transformed back to its former rock-like hardness through the fire of the kiln.

I thought again about the dream's juxtaposition of kilns and Stroud and now clay, and wondered how far the subconscious could foresee what the conscious self was, as yet, unaware of. Only the next several years would clarify these speculations.

DIGGING UP THE PAST

When, in 1992, some two years into a ceramic course, I started to take an interest in shards, I realised how these pottery remains may have helped us to reconstruct our human past. And then, by association, I saw how these pieces of pottery and my own sense of fragmentation at this time, made connections with Archaeology and the therapeutic process. There seemed much between these two, each dealing with deeply embedded material which needed exhuming and examining before any reconstruction could begin.

WATER - Waves and Surflines

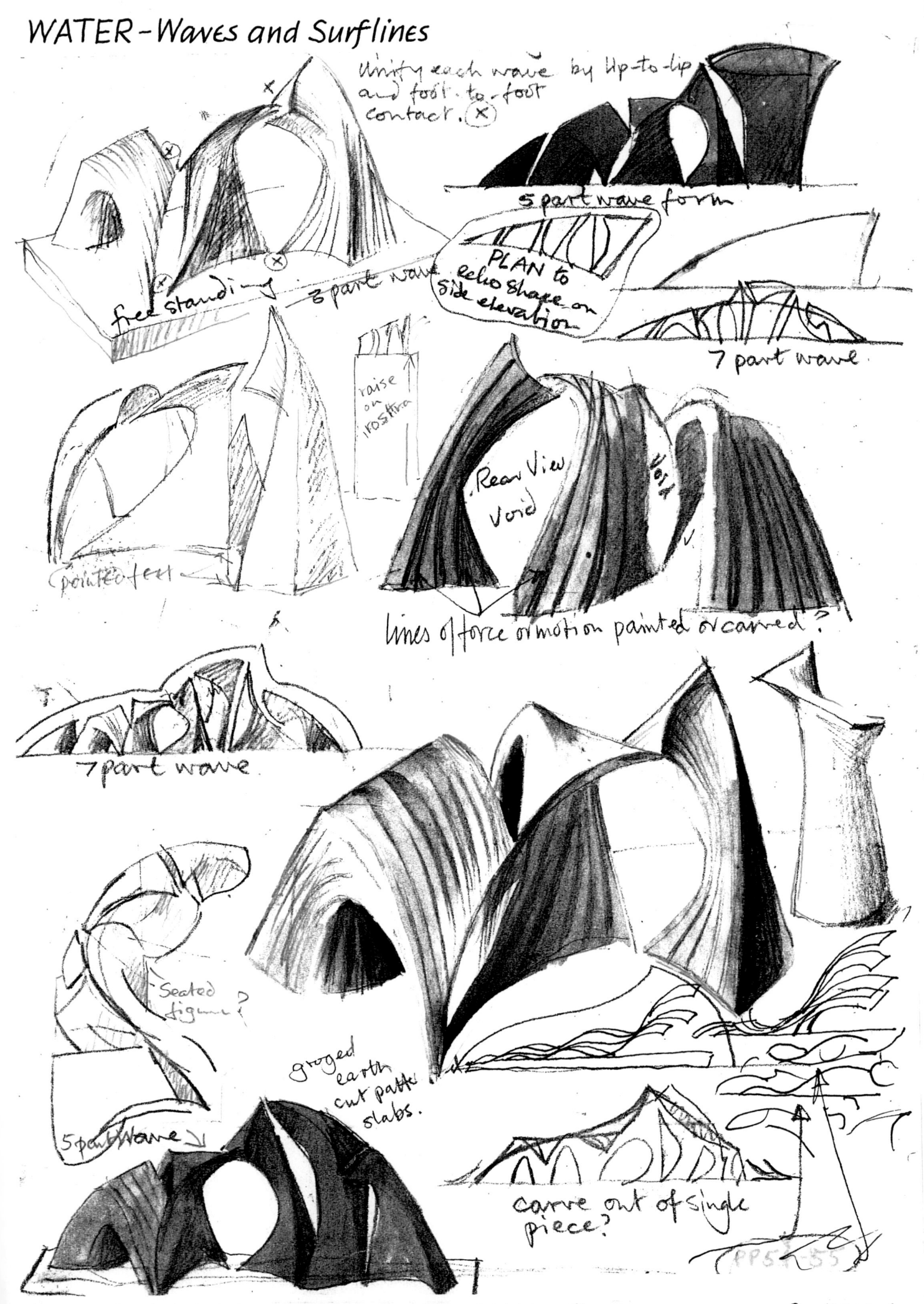

Fig. 190 Sheet of Studies - 'Wavelets', Wave Shapes   Pencil & Wash.

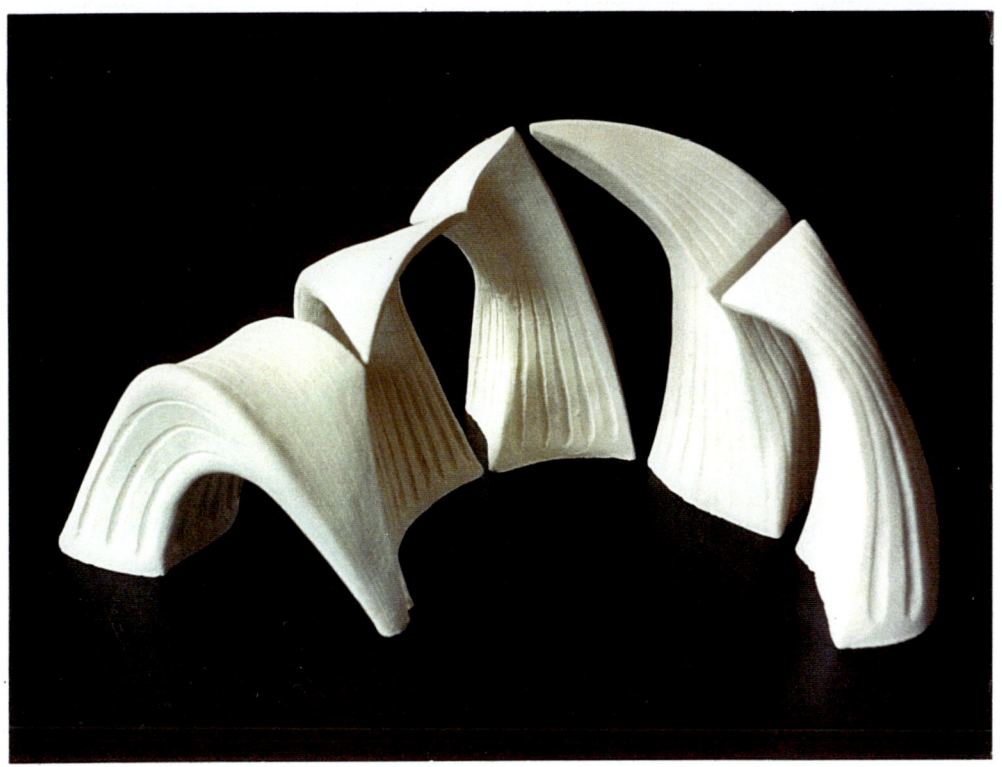

Fig. 191   Set of five Wavelets   Biscuit Fired Clay

Once started into clay, an old obsession reared up again. A fascination with the seashore and the movement of waves and surf needed to be expressed in this new medium (see the sequence from Clover Cliff, page 3).

Whereas painting, like the sea itself, can be constantly transformed, clay is pliable only up to the moment of hardening (decisions need to be finalised with more certainty). Yet fascination with wave forms and lines of surf tempted me to try modelling and making waves in three dimensions.

The intangible, ever-changing movement of water became a challenge. Even knowing that this insubstantial form was never likely to work as sculpture, the attempts to design something increased the interest in drawing — and scores of sketches tried to disprove this awareness. One way to design the shape was by linking the tops and bases of small wavelets to form a larger wave (fig. 191).

What seemed a more successful venture was the use of surf lines as a decorative element to define the surface of pots (fig. 192).

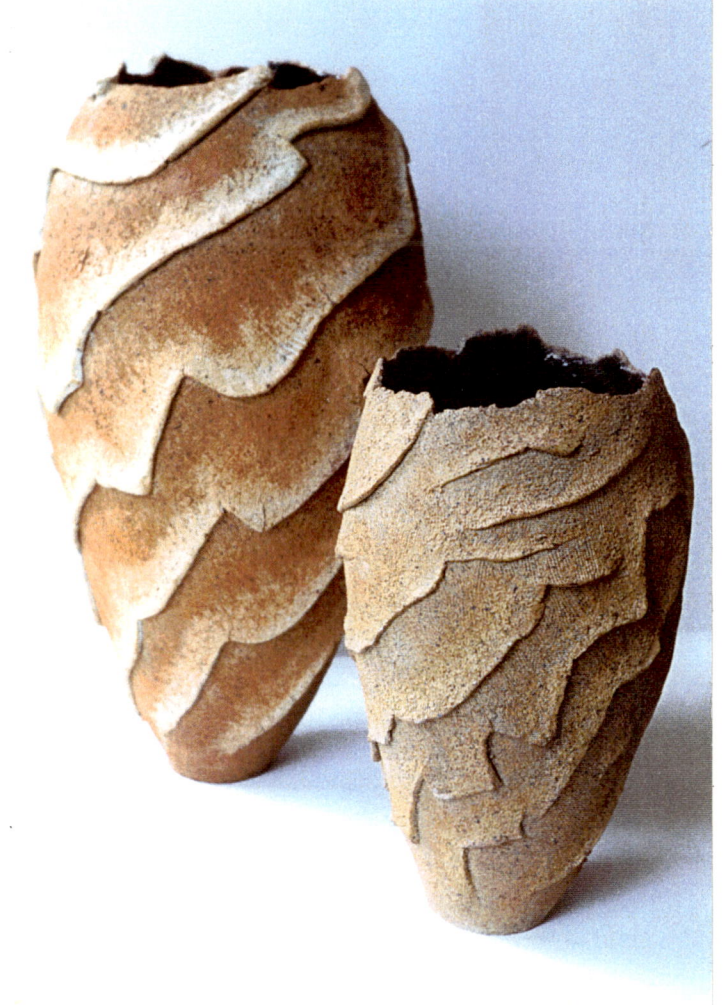

Fig. 192   Coiled Surflines   'Cranks' Clay

103

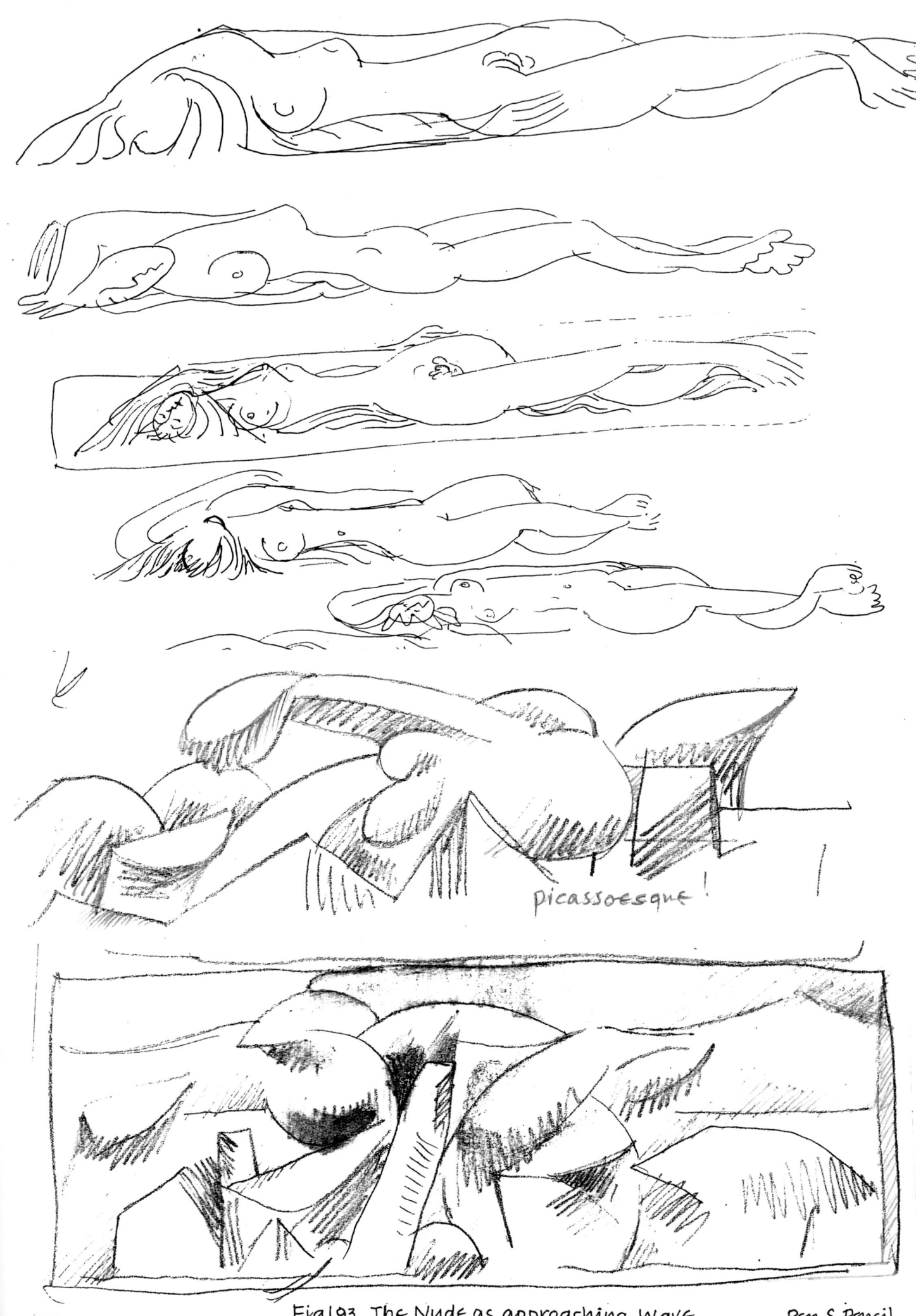

Fig.193 The Nude as approaching Wave

THE NUDE AND WING INCORPORATED INTO WAVES

Opposite page: Fig.193. Sequences of surf lines incorporating the reclining nude and abstract variations never reached the ceramic stage.

Other wave drawings which had high-rising winged forms led into more unexpected directions – one sketch became the model for a range of bird pots (inset A below). Another, (inset B) towering even higher reminded me of an earlier interest – a costume for Neptune (overleaf).

Left: Fig.194. Slab-building for wave movement – edges heightened with Lustre glaze.

Below: Fig.195. Wave drawings transform into birds and a model for Neptune.

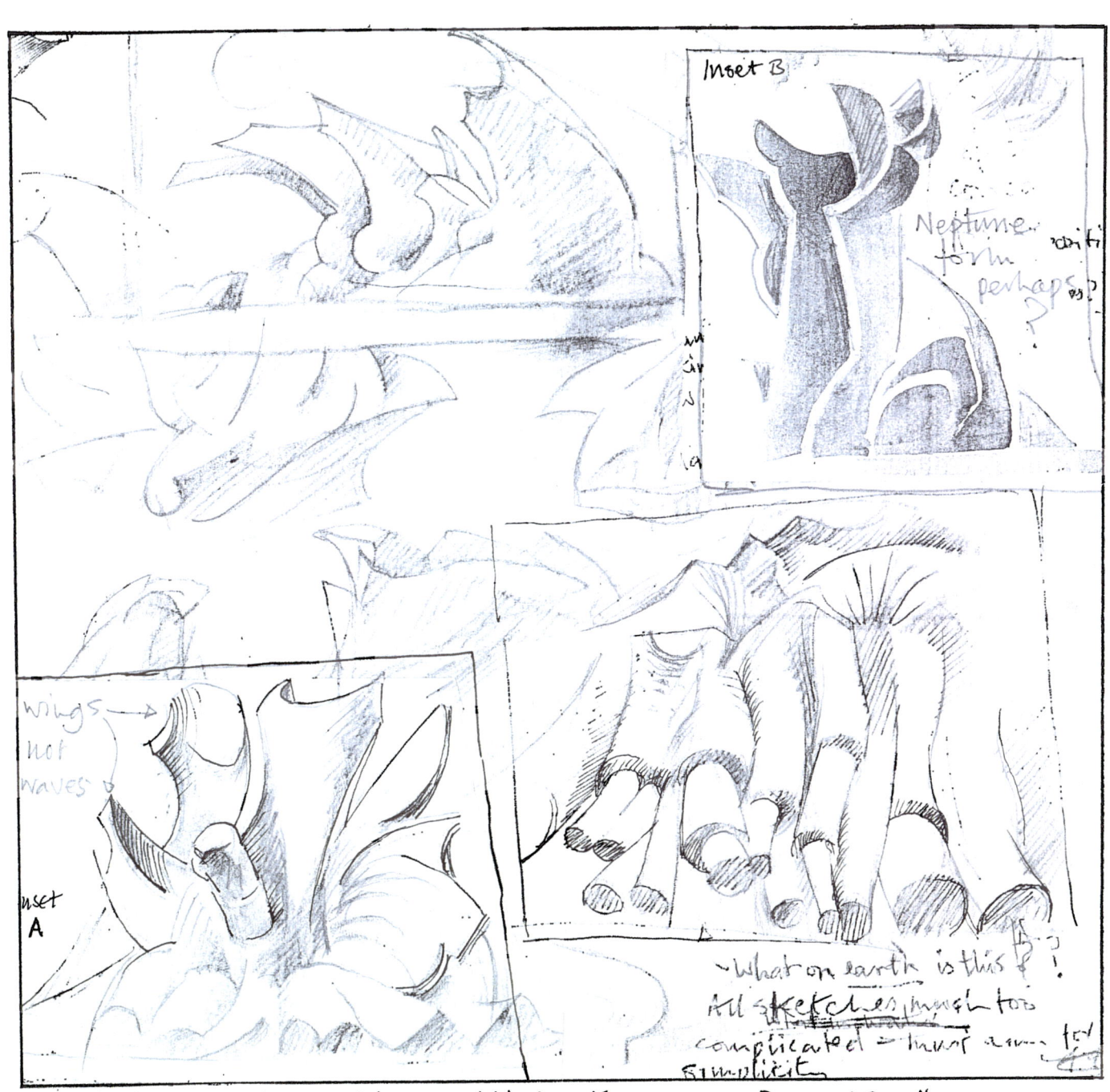

Fig.195   Page of Sketches – Waves and Neptune Form.   Pen and Pencil

DESIGN DRAWINGS FOR NEPTUNE

During the late 1970s I designed a costume for a dance drama based on Joan Aiken's 'Kingdom under the Sea' for a school production. The costume was made from plastic scrap and silver painted paper sculpture for the mask which shimmered like sun-lit water under stage lighting. The drawing (inset B, overleaf) and a photograph of the costume stimulated me enough to resurrect the Sea God in this new medium. Using a number of slab built pieces of clay I constructed two forms using this technique.

Either the kiln firing or my method of construction was faulty, for both of the Neptune pieces collapsed. Fortunately the drawings allowed for future efforts.

Right: Original Neptune Costume.

Below: Two drawings for the clay model which disintegrated.

Opposite page: Sheet of studies for a ceramic sculpture of Neptune.

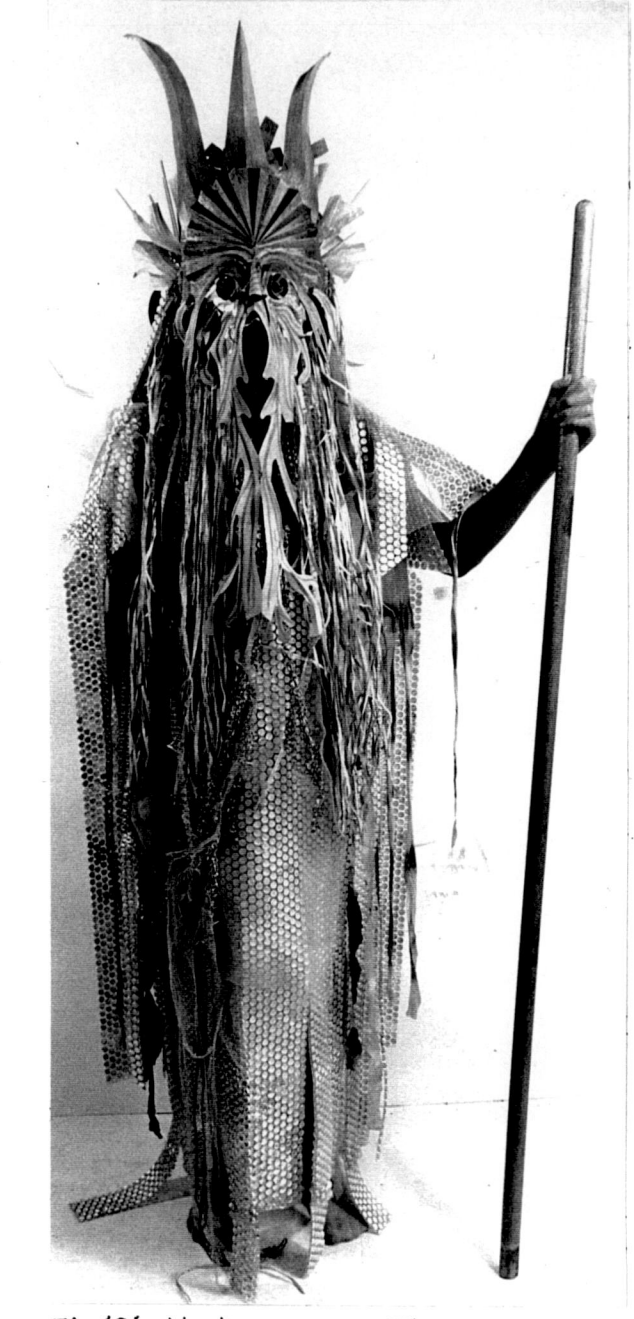

Fig. 196 Neptune — Theatre Costume

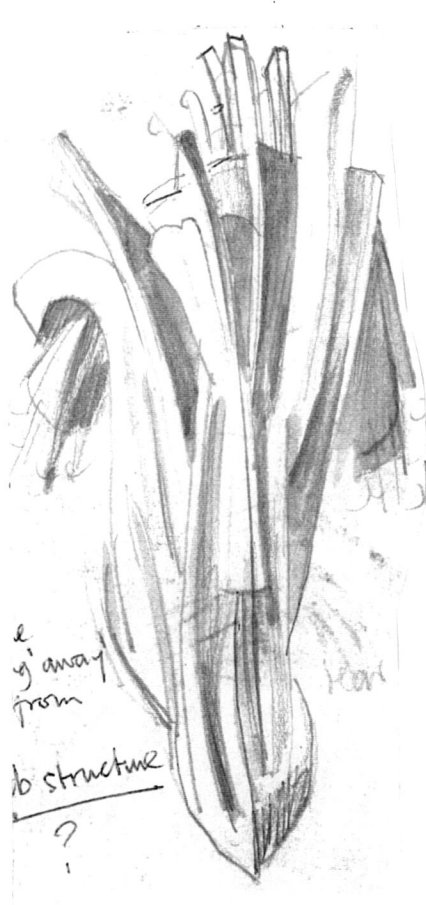

Fig. 197 Neptune — Rear View

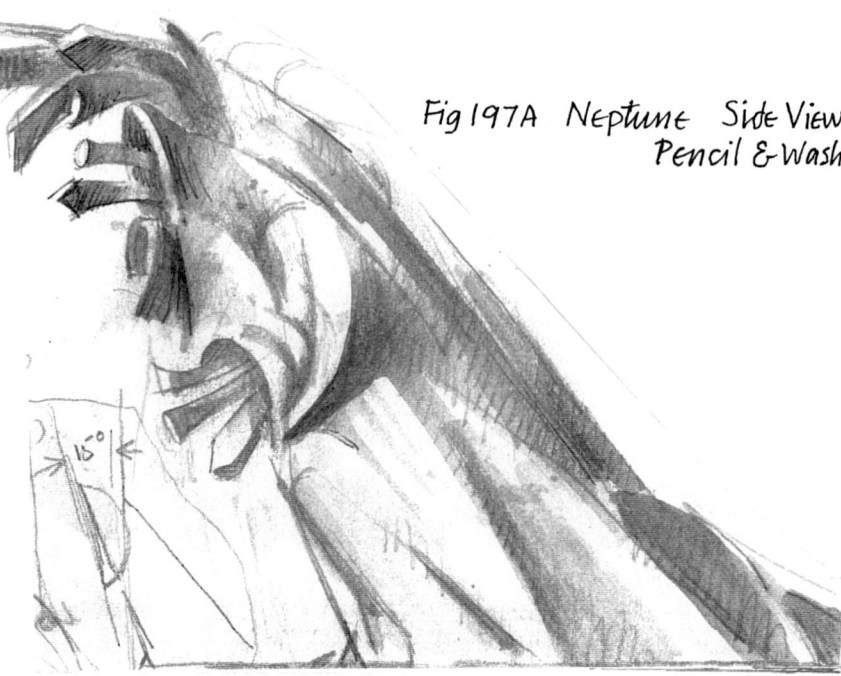

Fig 197A Neptune Side View Pencil & Wash

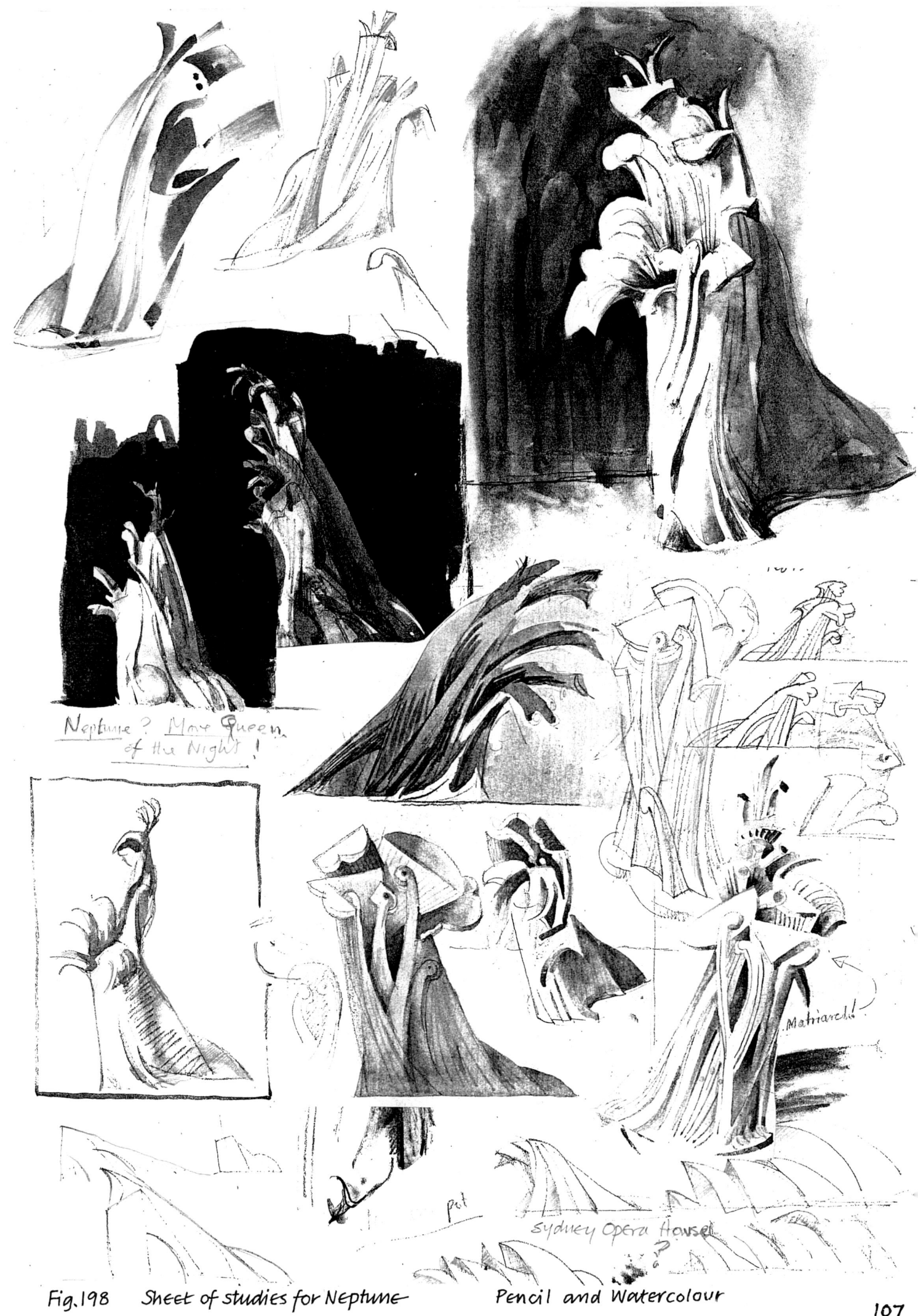

Fig. 198   Sheet of studies for Neptune   Pencil and Watercolour

DESIGNS FOR AN EAGLE POT

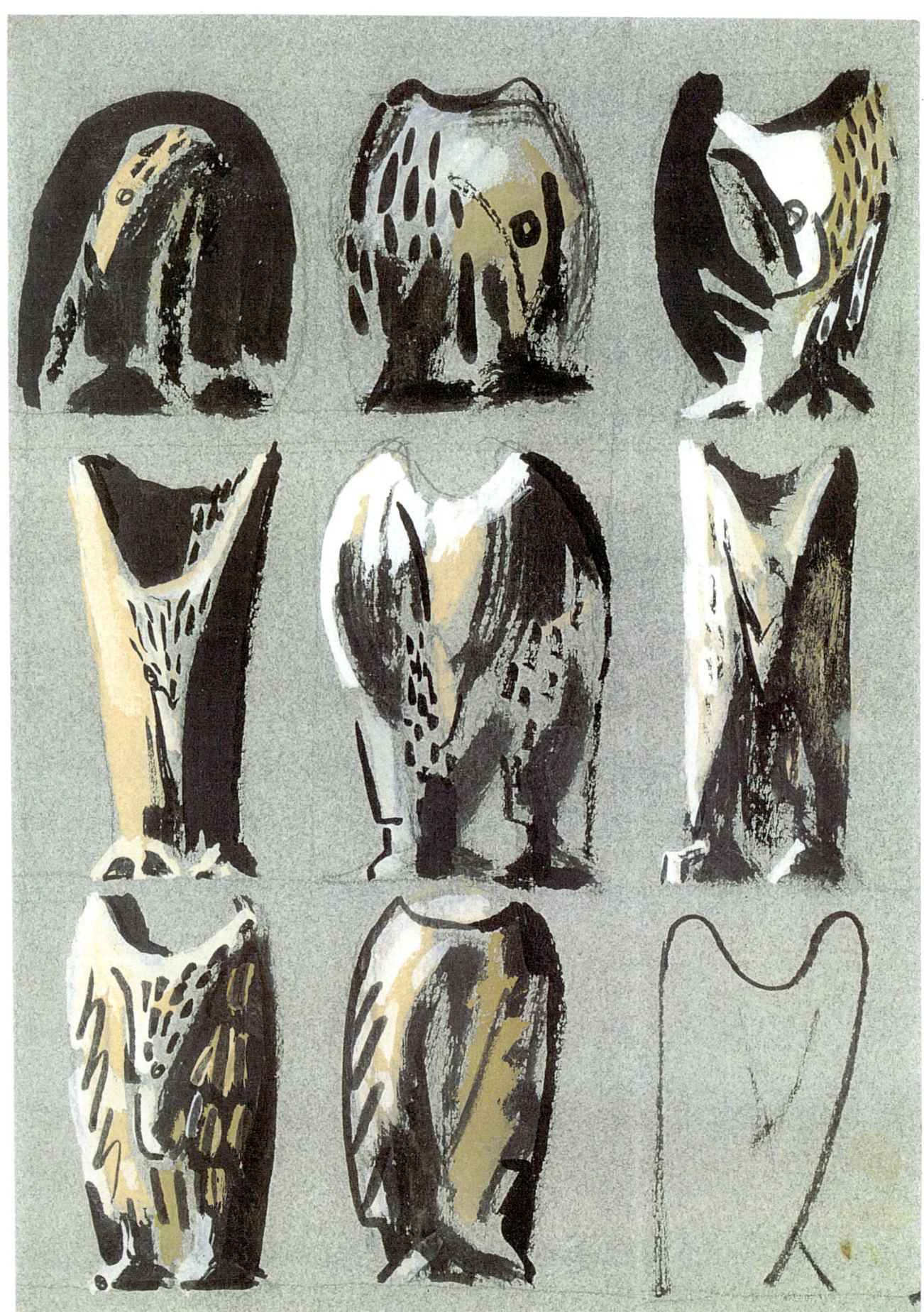

Fig.199 Sheet of studies for an Eagle Pot — Gouache on a Toned Ground

BIRD POTS: Perched, Flying and Pecking

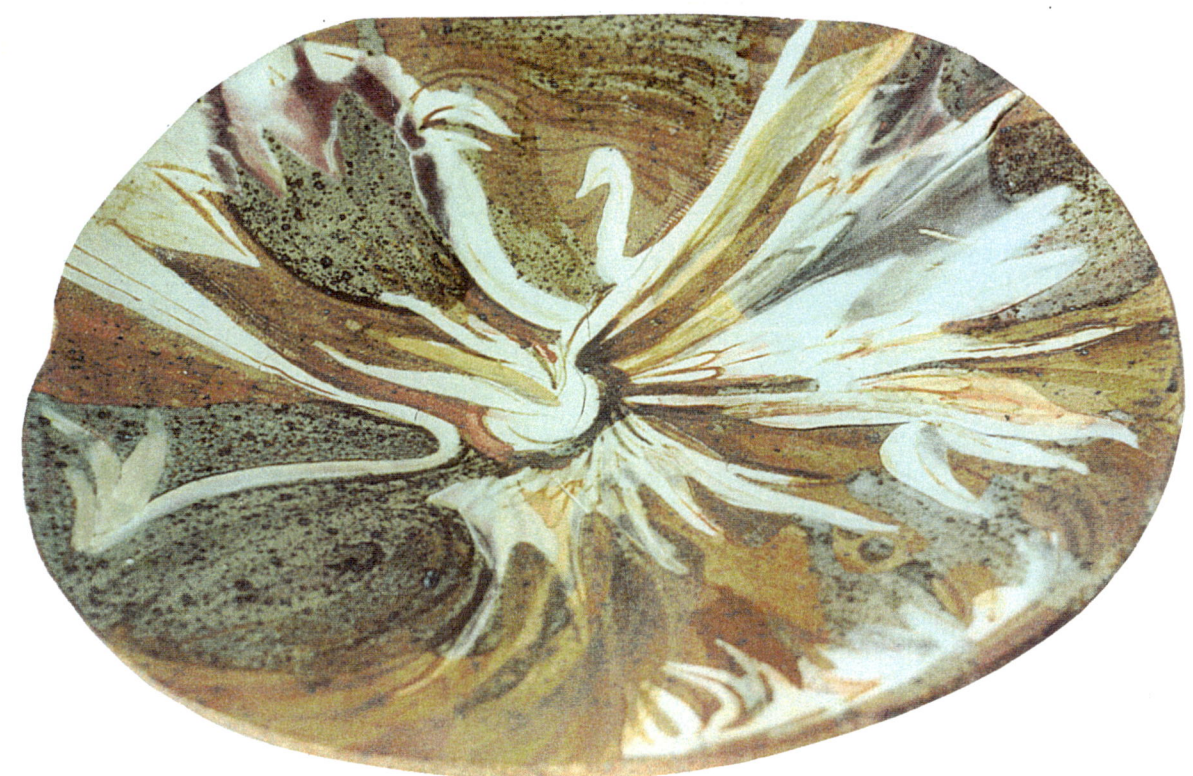

Fig. 200 Platter decorated with spreading wings

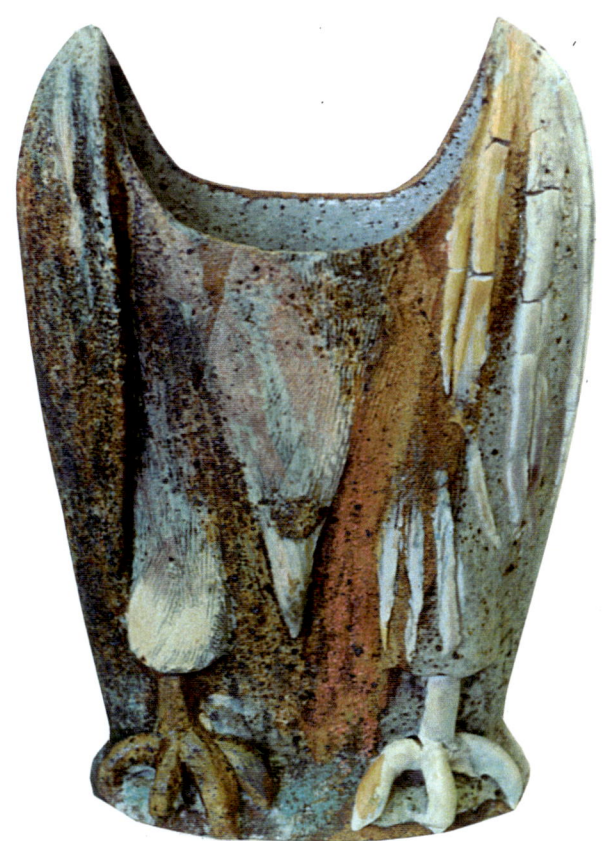

Fig. 201 Eagle Pot

There was the feeling that some of the wave drawings (like inset B on page 105) were fragmenting and moving skywards – the wave 'took wing' and the bird was born.
A series of bird vessels developed and became the dominant theme during months of ceramic work.

In retrospect I now realise that this group of pots was the precursor for a wide range of freestyle drawings and paintings of birds from 1995 onwards. These were later assembled into the section 'Stretching the Wings' in Part Three (page 215)
Unlike waves, which by their amorphous nature, didn't transform easily into sculpture, the bird was an ideal subject. With its compact form and transformation through flight it lent itself to many ceramic designs.

When the wings opened out, these offered excellent decorative shapes on flat dishes, plates and platters (fig. 200 above). Sometimes a series of drawings suggested a pot form (figs 119–207).

VARIATIONS... ...ON THE BIRD THEME

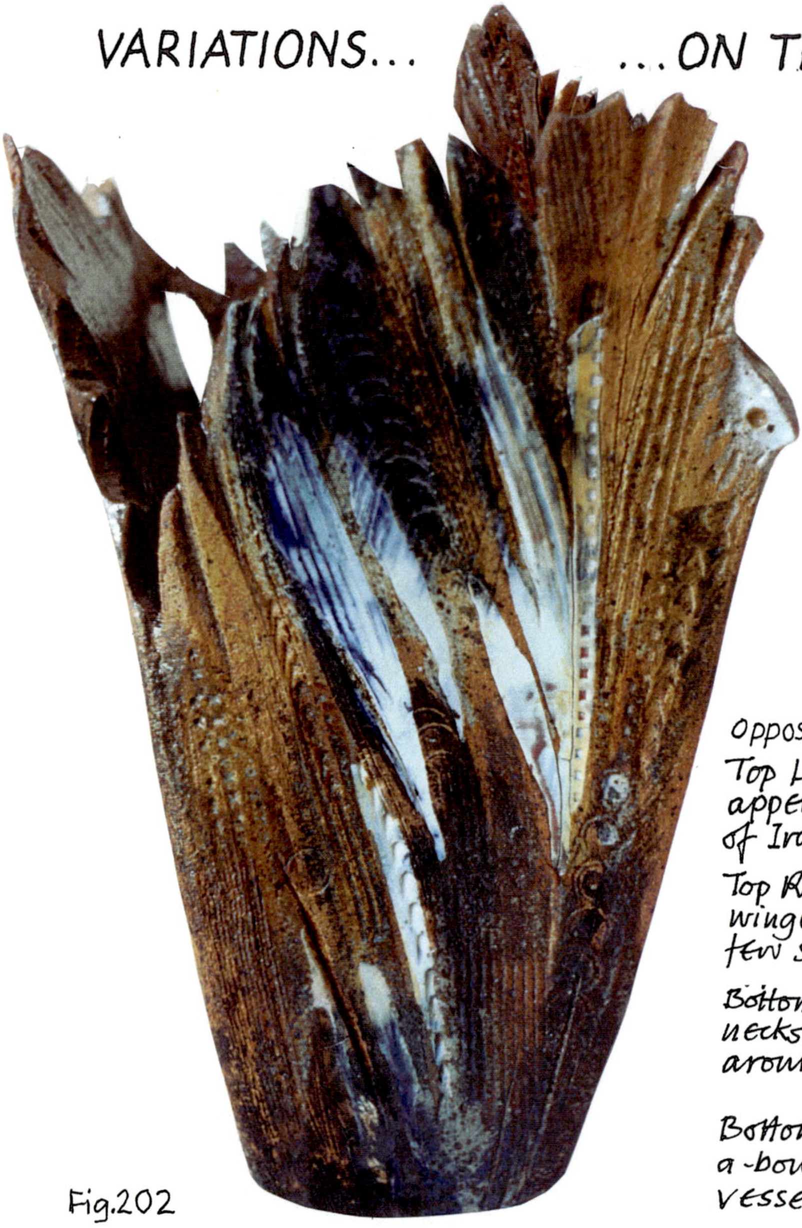

Left: Fig.202. Winged Planter. The wings alone when sufficiently spread apart and arranged vertically could themselves become the chief component of the pot.

Below: Fig.203. Pecking Birds. Another arrangement was to angle the bird's body into a pecking pose, the tail feathers forming the rim of the pot.

Opposite Page:

Top Left: Fig.204. Ethnic influences appear in some pots — a small owl of Iranian origin

Top Right: Fig.205. Bird Bath. Using an winged, open-palmed 'hand' with a few small birds on the rim.

Bottom Left: Fig.206. Birds with long necks and beaks can wrap themselves around the 'tail', rising above the head

Bottom Right: Fig.207. A Bird Roundabout based on Nigerian Nupe vessels

Fig.202

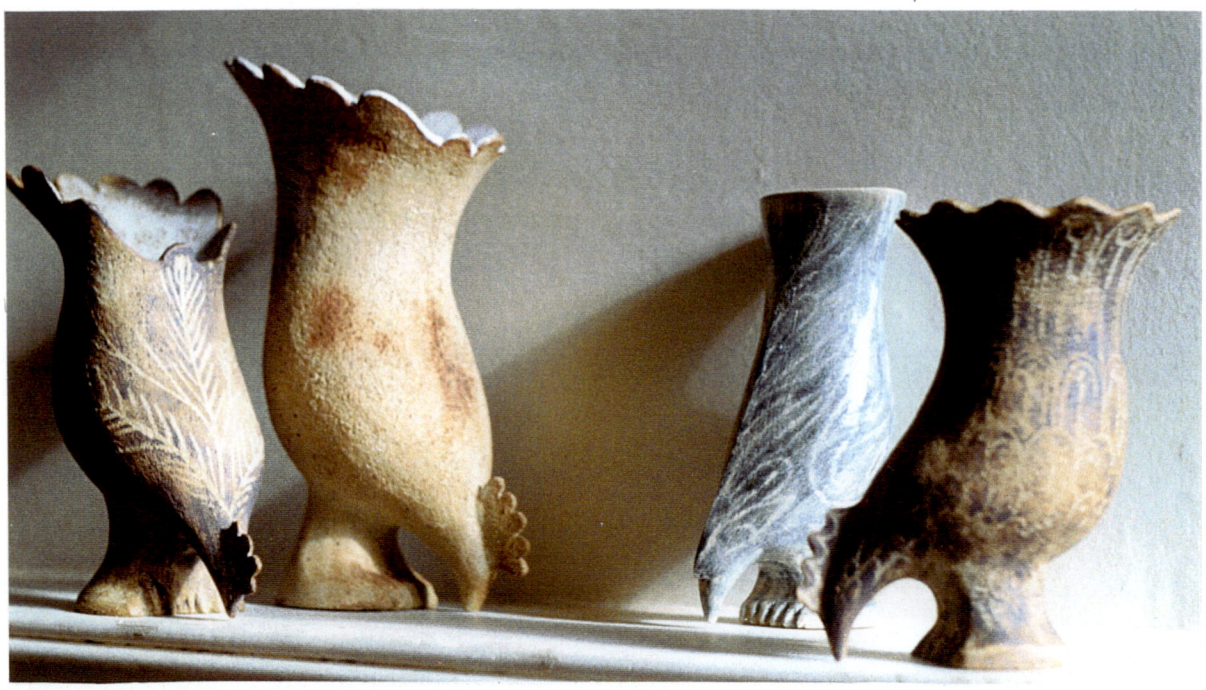

Fig.203   Four Pecking Birds

110

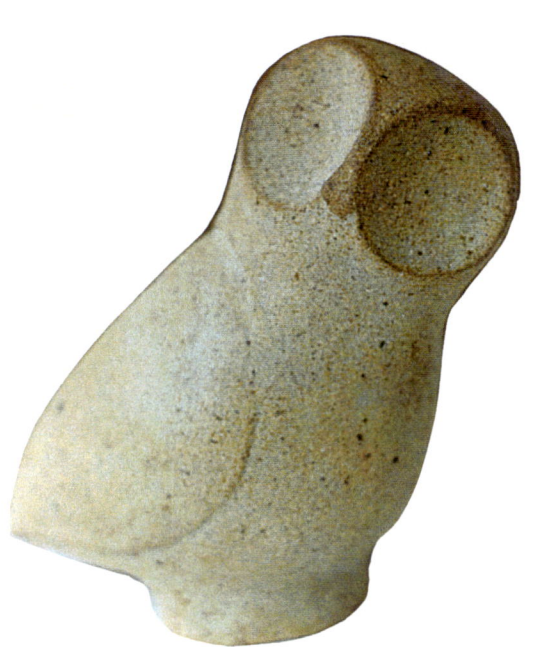

Fig. 204 Little Owl

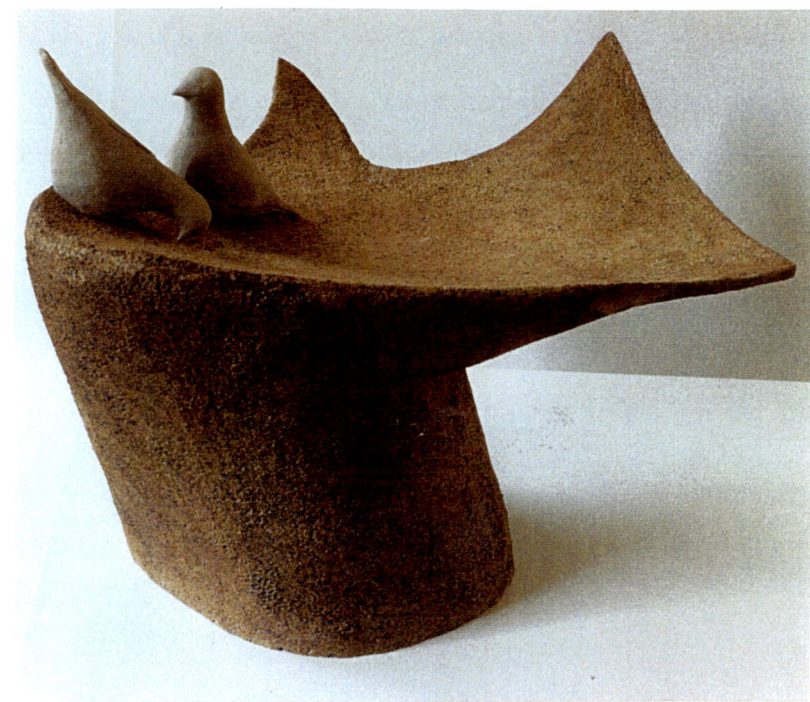

Fig. 205 Bird Bath

BIRD POTS AND SCULPTURES

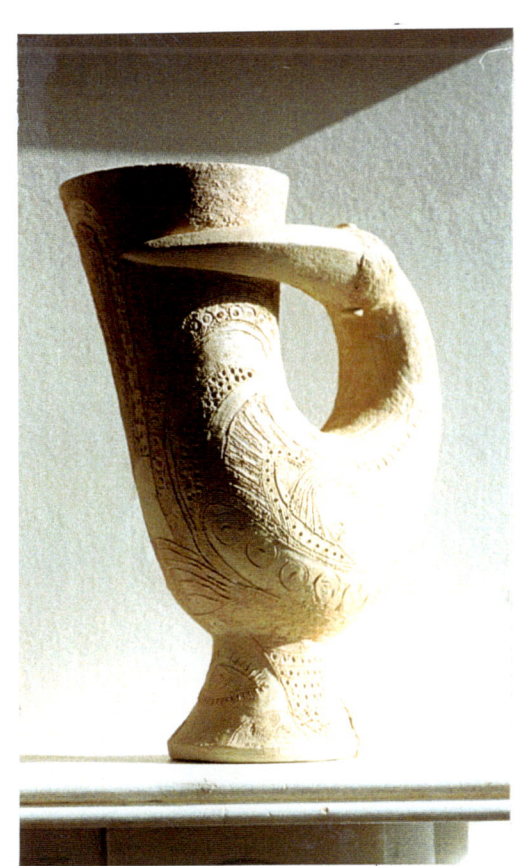

Fig. 206 Bird Vase

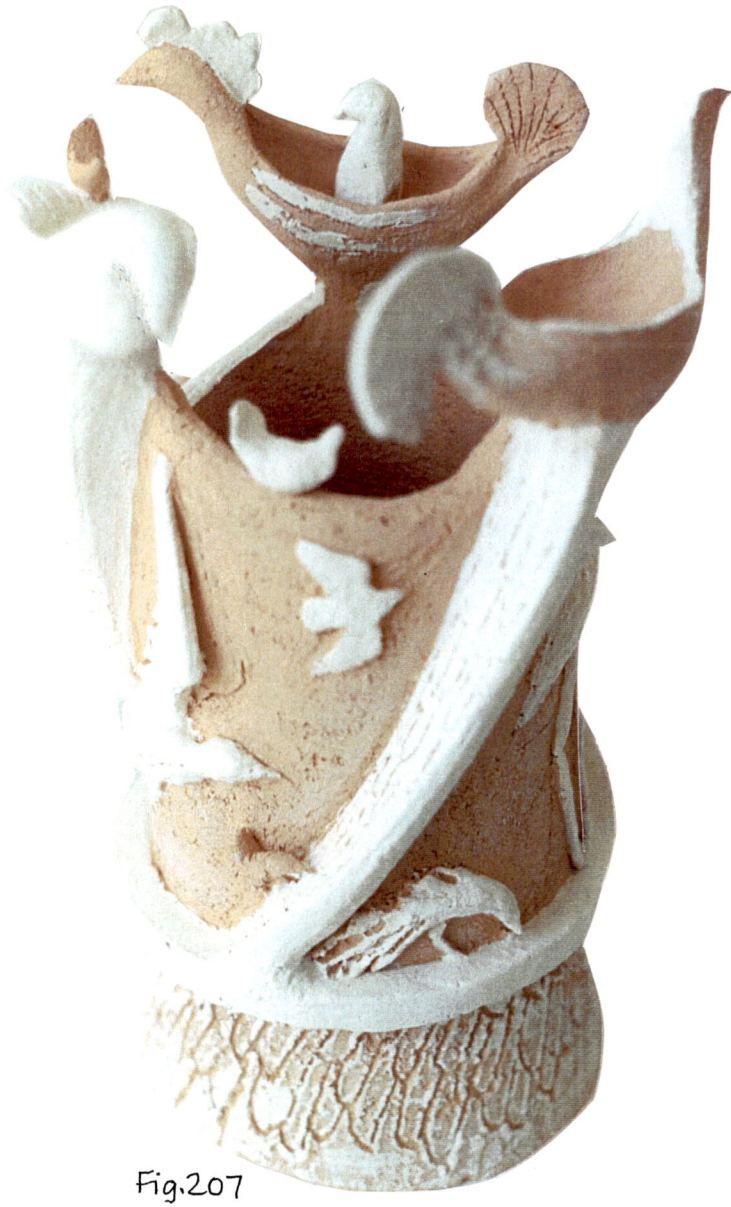

Fig. 207

DESIGNS FOR WINGED CREATURES - SLEEPING & FLYING

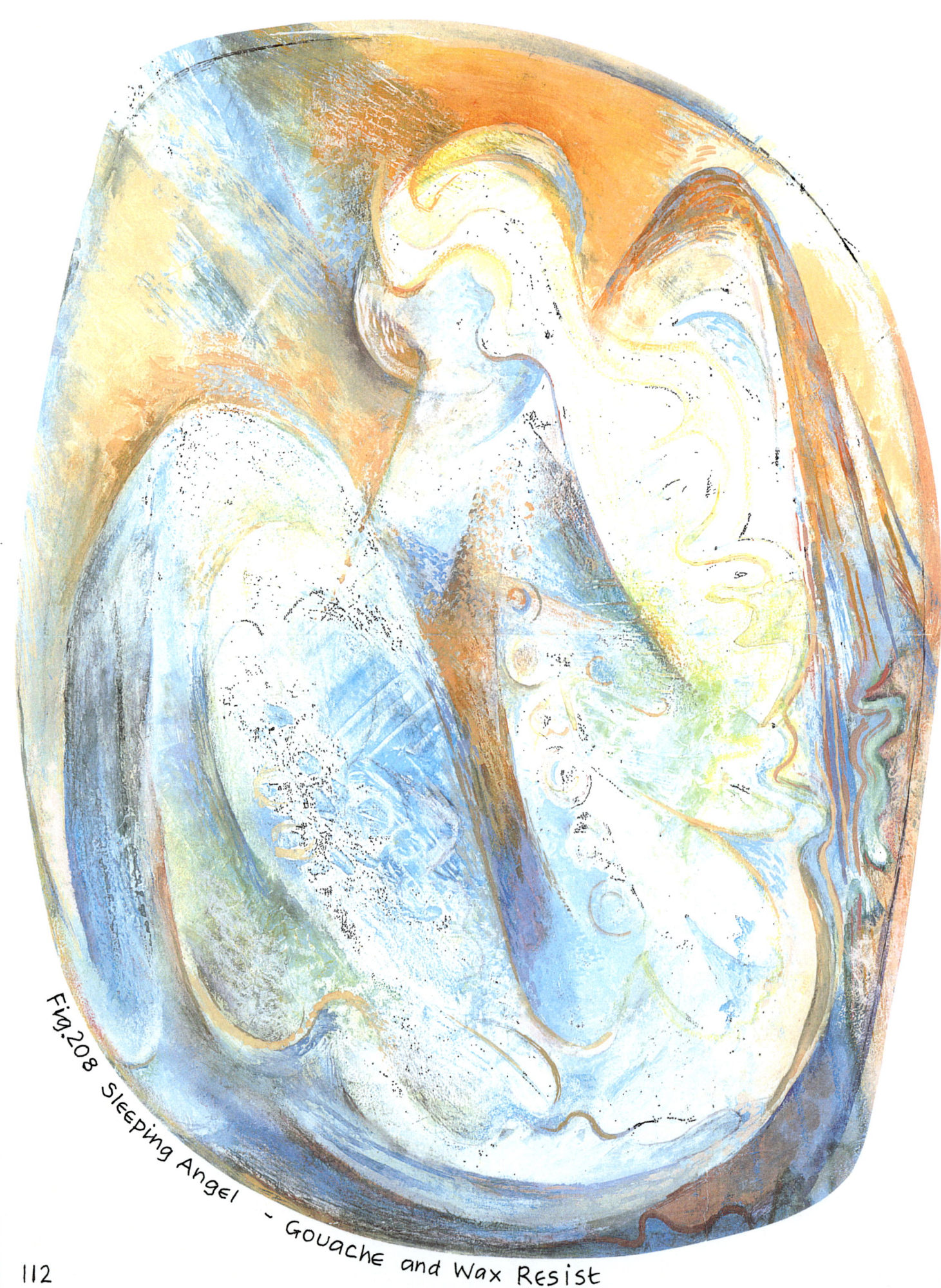

Fig.208 Sleeping Angel - Gouache and Wax Resist

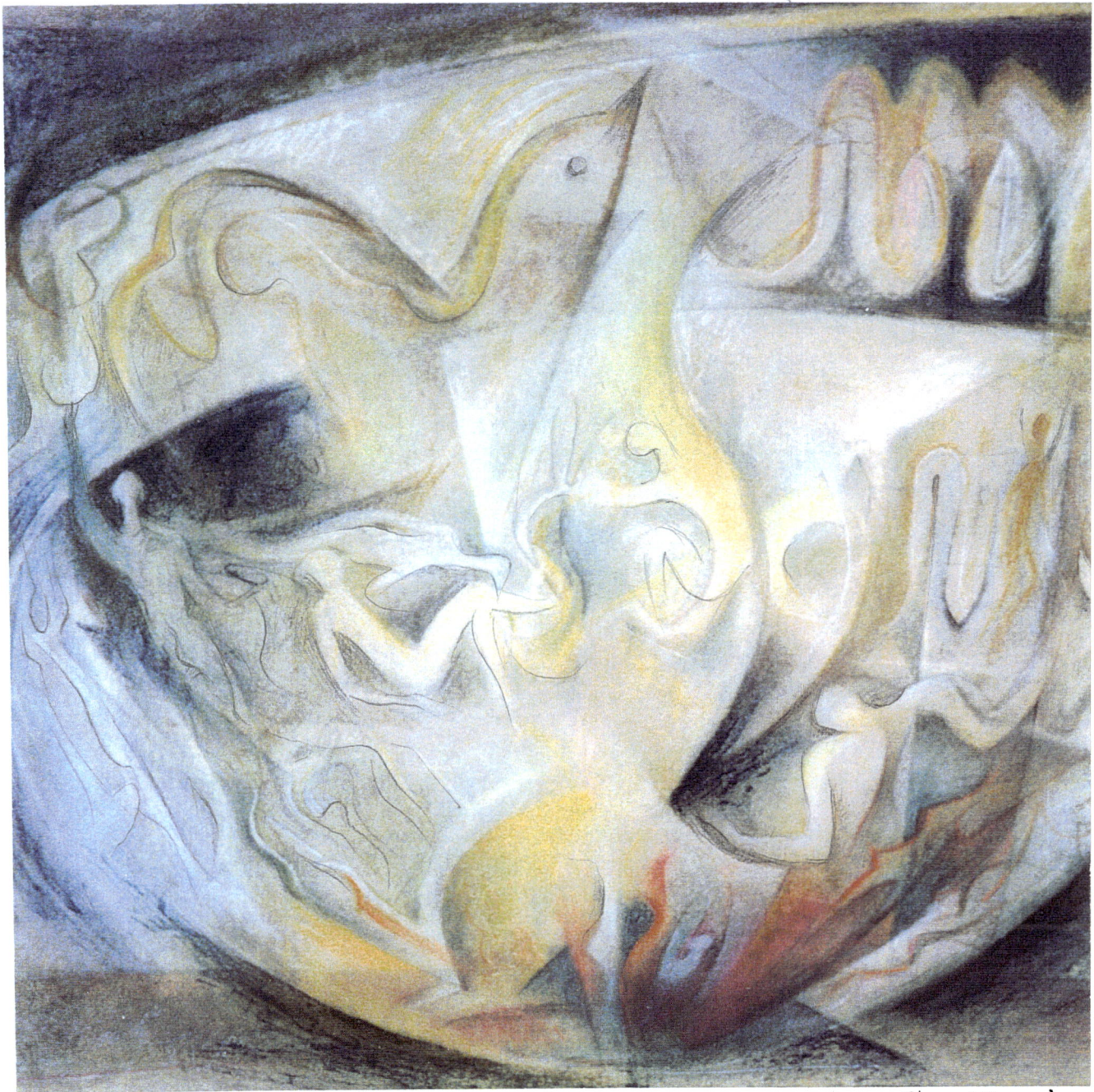

Fig. 209　Life Vessel   Design for a Large Bowl　　　Pastel Drawing

My enthusiasm for making watery and flying forms eventually waned but the ideas continued on paper. A few drawings developed into clay but most never went beyond the pictorial idea. But I was still influenced by forms and thought of transposing wings onto other creatures. One example was of a sleeping angel, curled within an oval shape to fit a platter but this failed to transfer successfully, as I never learnt enough about translating pigment colours into glaze colours after firing — the glazes turned into an anaemic disaster.

Another picture never reached beyond the design stage. 'Life Vessel' (fig. 209) was a pastel drawing arranged to fill the inside of a large bowl, representing birds and human forms flying and floating up from the base to the rim.

What did arise from these two designs was the renewed interest I felt for drawing again and also for the introduction of human and then animal forms as subject matter for ceramic sculpture.

FOUR PSYCHOLOGICAL SELF-PORTRAITS

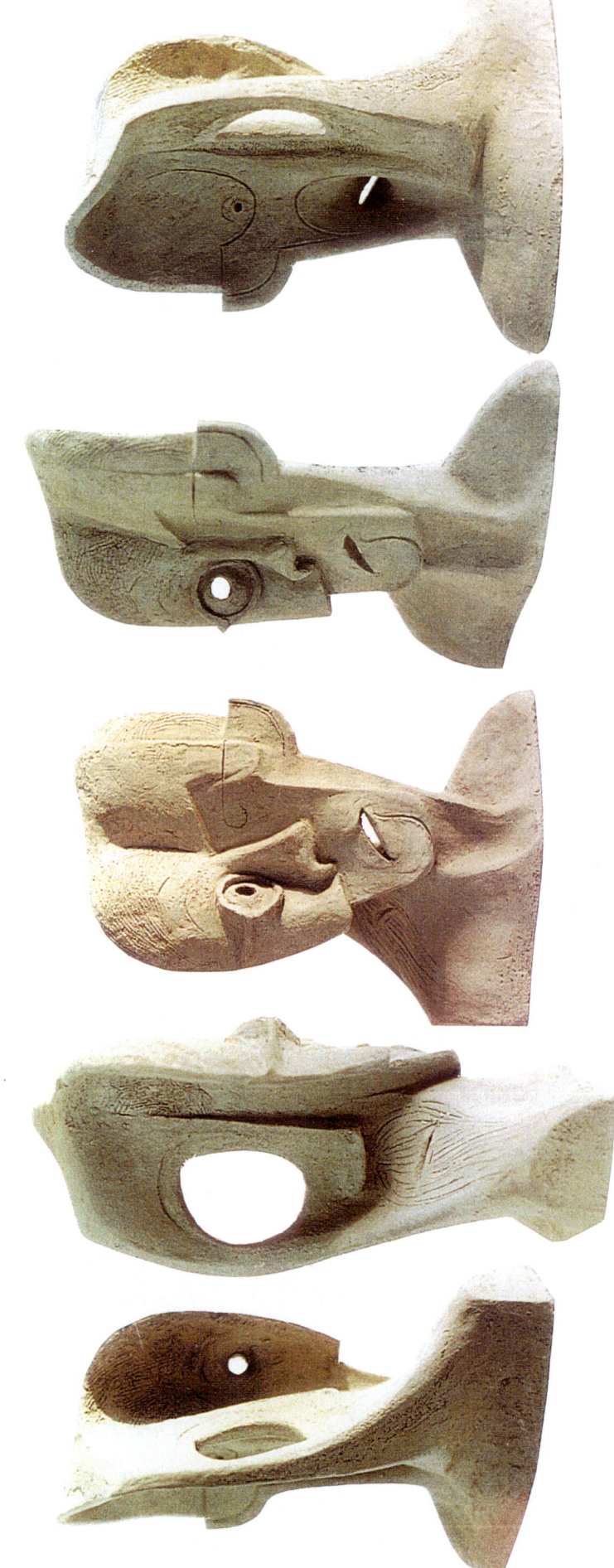

Fig. 210 One Portrait — Five View-points

Deciding to take an exam in Ceramics, I was attracted by many of the coursework projects. One in particular resonated for me. The project paper read:

"As things fall apart or rot, they may provide unusual or interesting effects of form, colour and texture. Make studies of objects at various stages of disintegration or find examples of decay in your surroundings. From your studies produce forms which explore the aesthetic elements using construction (form), decoration or colouring methods."

Although the project description was specific about external observation — 'your surroundings' — I felt it also applied to metamorphosis in psychological terms — 'Calmness leading to Anxiety', 'Hardness into Softness', etc. Thus the idea, based on my own experience, of using an emotional breakdown seemed a possible area of research. The first studies were related to some earlier 'fragmented' self portraits which now became the main source of inspiration.

The many-faced three-dimensional portrait above, shown from five viewpoints (fig 210), was one of the first attempts in clay. Others followed, including those below (figs 211–213).

A self portrait by Francis Bacon (1972) seemed an elegant painterly solution to the disintegration of a face through vigorous sweeping brushstrokes. This encouraged me to explore my own 'internalised' features, but in clay.

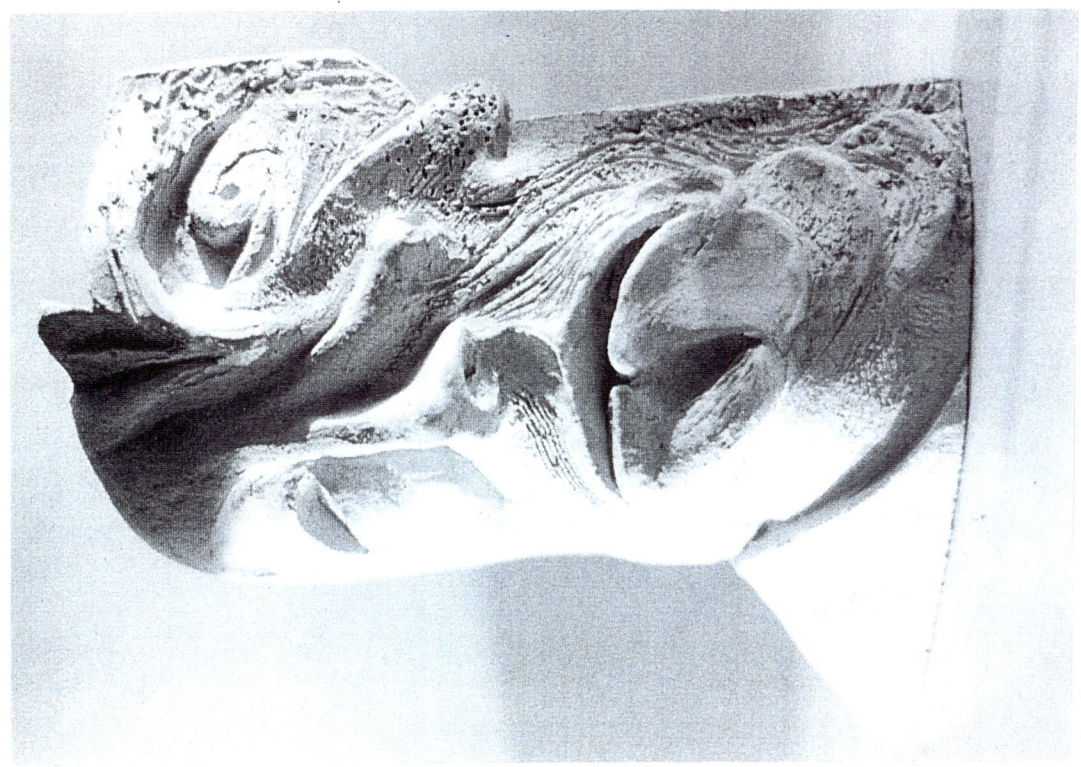

Fig. 213 Self Portrait 6   Biscuit Fired

Fig. 212 Self Portrait 5

All portraits biscuit-fired without later glazing. Portrait 3 closely followed Bacon's 1972 Self Portrait.

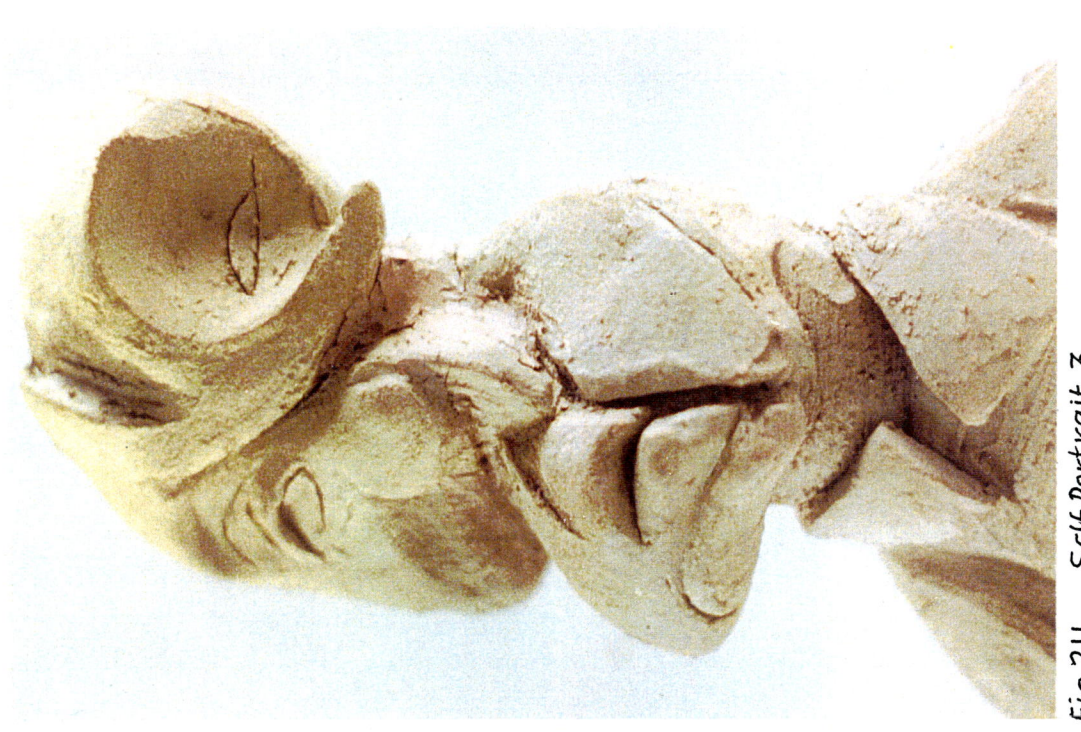

Fig. 211 Self Portrait 3

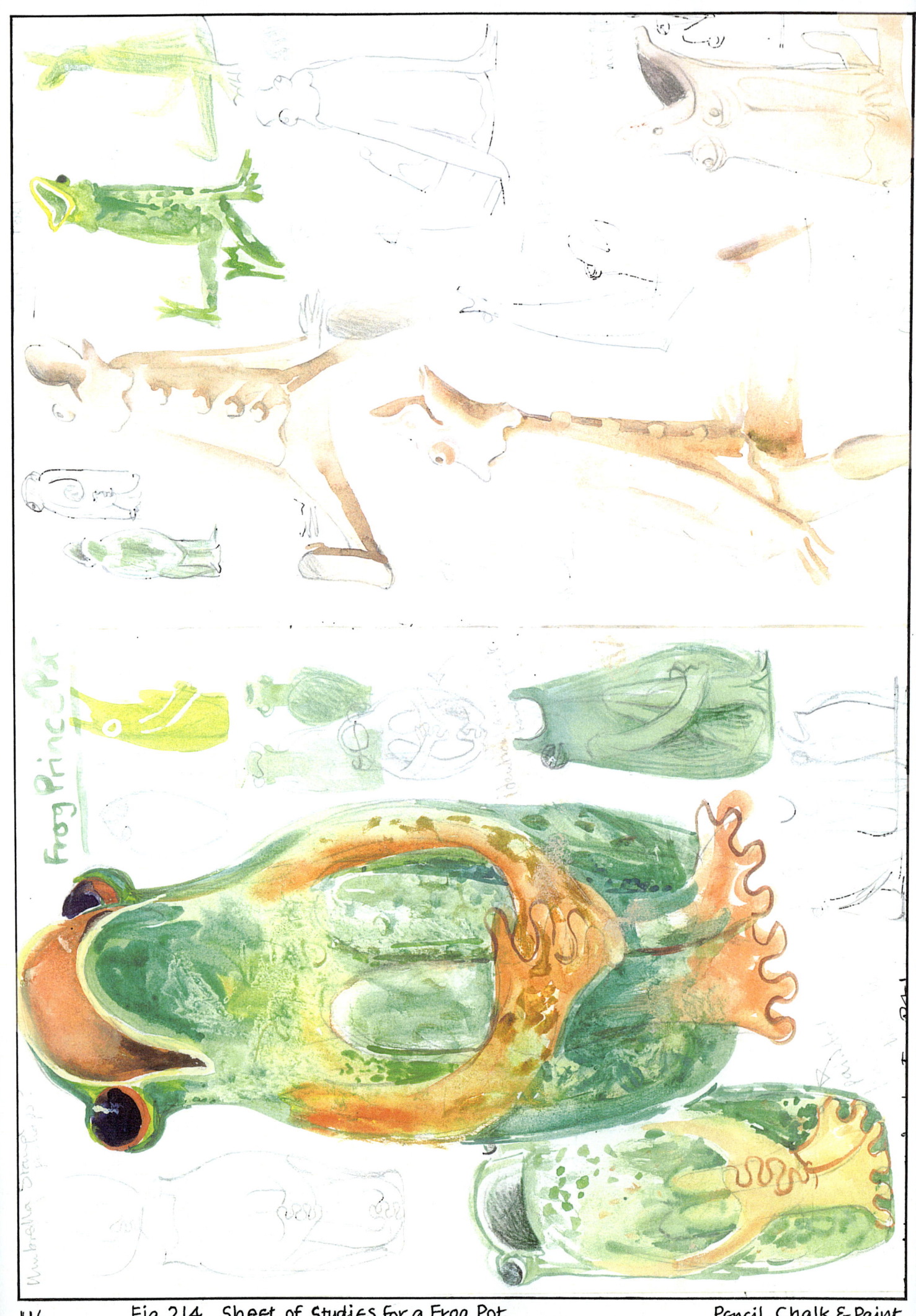

Fig. 214 Sheet of Studies for a Frog Pot

Above: A sheet of studies (fig.214) for a Frog pot based on the "Frog Prince" ended up with a clownish figure which related more to my conception of the Joker (see fig.218 below and fig.578, page 345)

Birdbath Lady (fig.215) & Yoga Posture (fig.217) both show an Indian influence.

Little Horse (fig.216) shows the Cypriot influence.

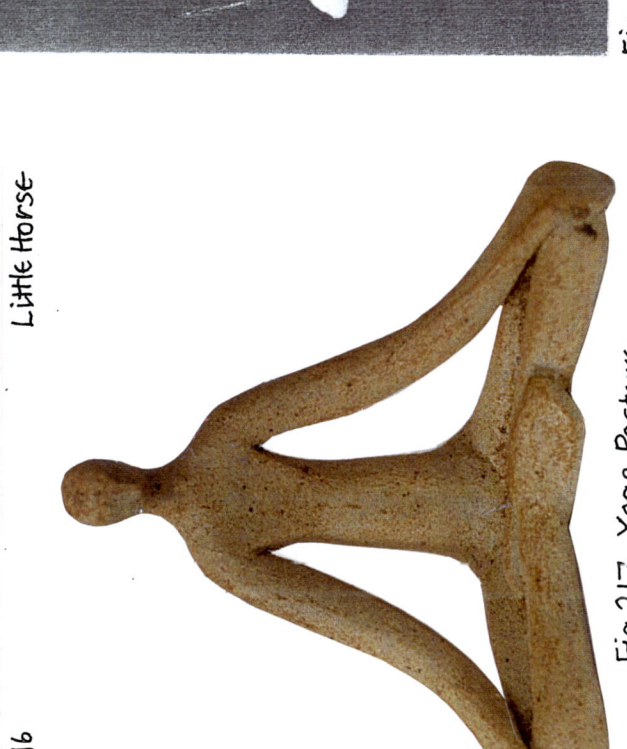

Fig.218   Frog Prince (aka Joker)

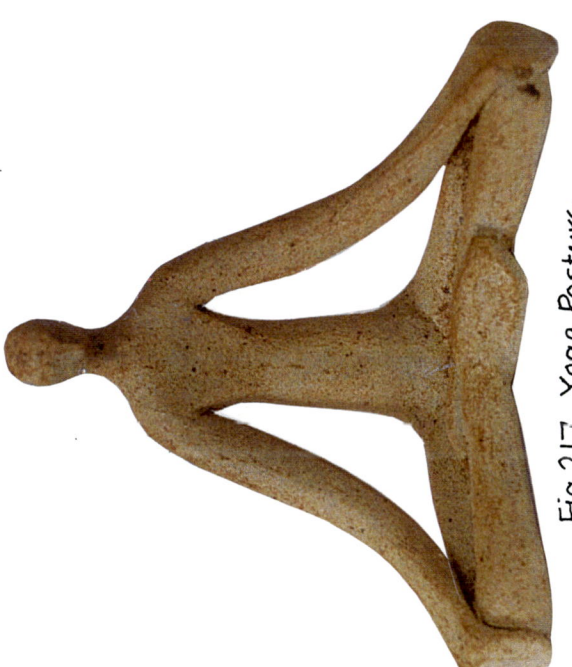

Fig.216   Little Horse

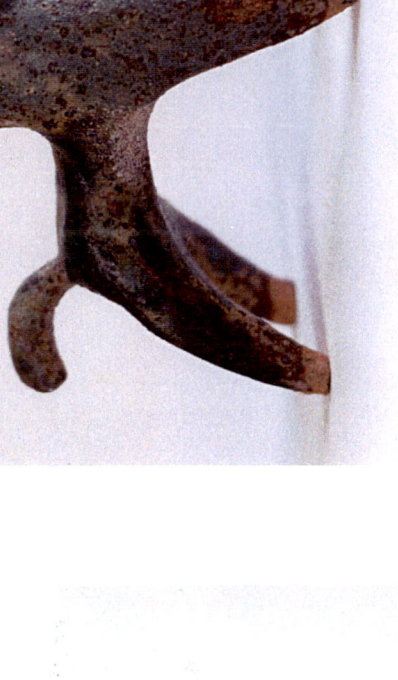

Fig.217   Yoga Posture

ETHNIC & FAIRYTALE FIGURES

Perhaps inspired by the figurative drawings for the large bowl (fig.209), small figurines and statuettes developed, mostly relating to Fairytale and Ethnic characters.

Fig.215   Birdbath Lady

117

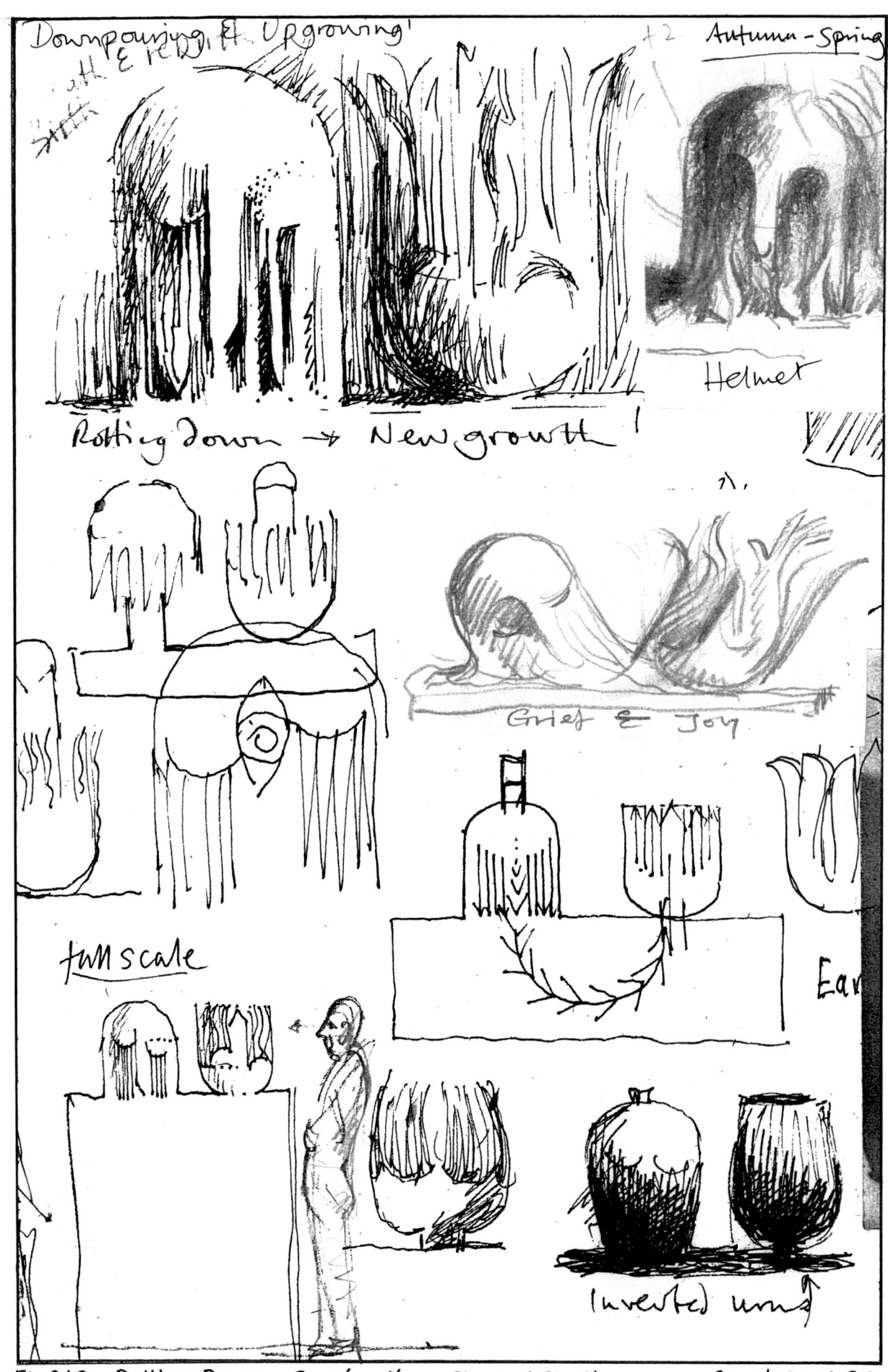

Fig. 2.19 Rotting Down – Growing Up.   Sheet of Studies   Pencil, Pen & Ink

BREAKDOWN – BREAKOUT

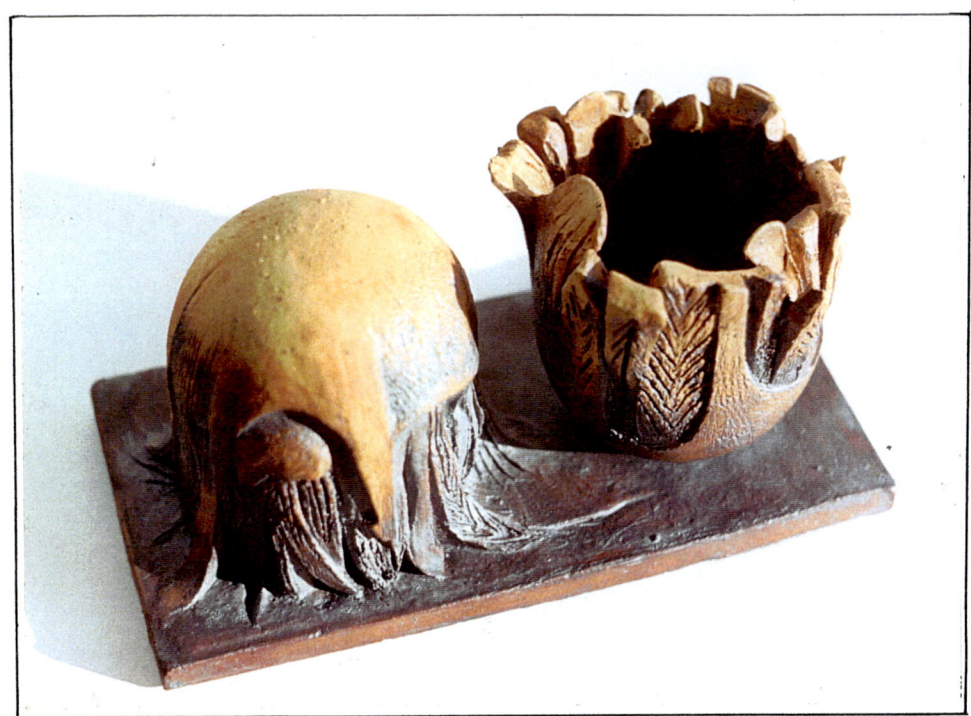

Fig.220   Breakdown – Breakout. Top View

Just as things disintegrate, change and cease to be, so new growth flourishes, in the act of 'becoming'. The portrait exam project led to the idea of showing both a breaking down and then a breaking out to parallel what I sensed was beginning to happen internally. Using the portrait head again, this time partially concealed within a helmet, I tried inverting another head alongside the first, trying to convey this metamorphosis.

The sheet of sketches (fig.219) shows some variations on this theme. Figs.220 and 220A show two viewpoints of the sculpture.

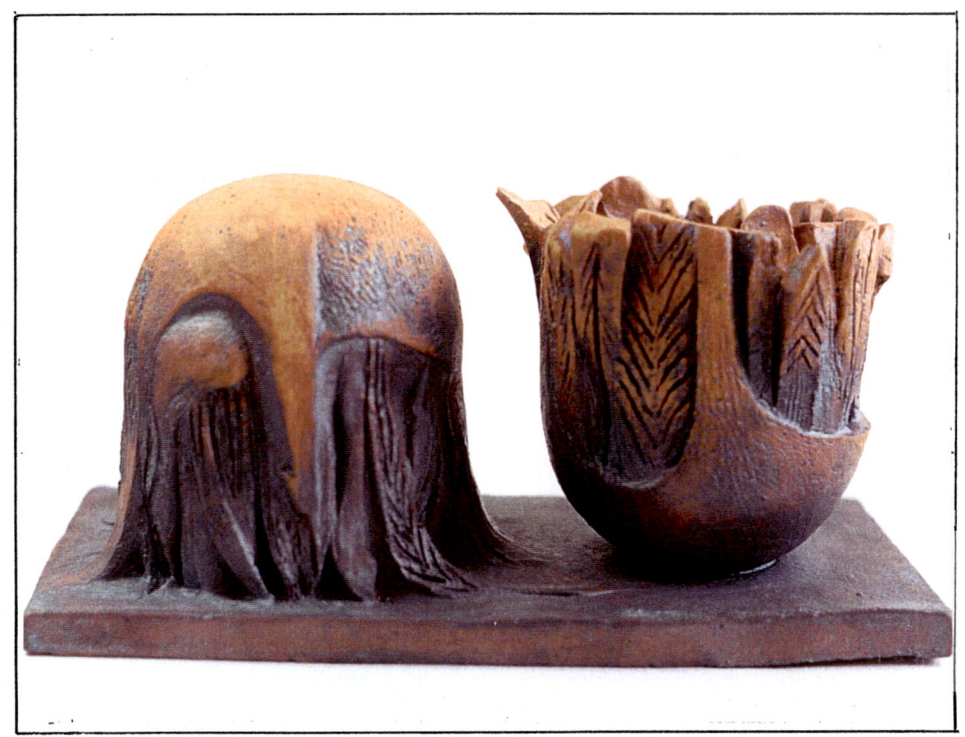

Fig.220A   Breakdown – Breakout – Front View

119

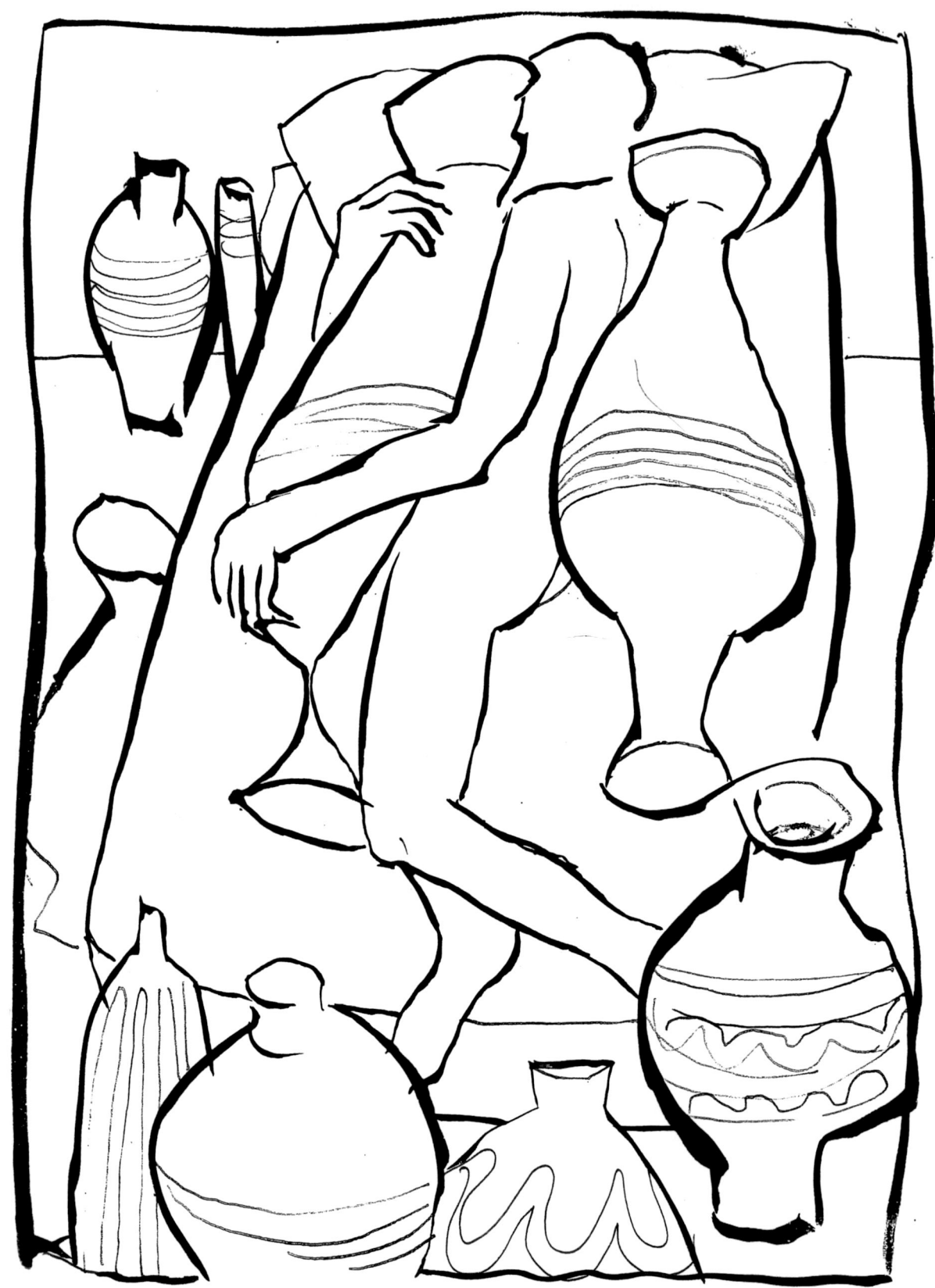

Fig. 221   Potter and his Pots   (from a dream in 1993)   Calligraphic Brush

As the designing and making of pottery slowly waned after working for four years with clay, so drawings about its effect on me increased, stressing the empathy with this 'energising' material.   The dream 'Potter and his Pots' (fig. 221), reflected the feelings of containment with clay.

Other paintings stressed other aspects of pottery: 'Close to Clay' (fig. 222) emphasised my close empathy working with clay whilst the 'Looking at Pots' (fig. 223) showed a more reflective attitude towards the pot.

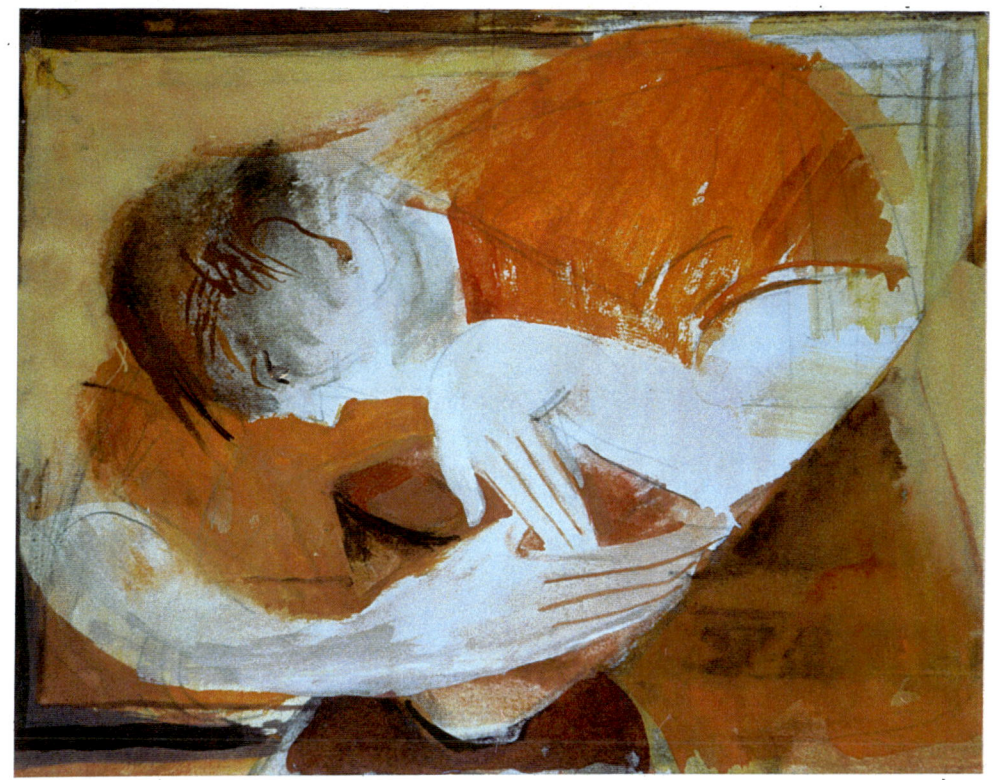

Fig.222 Close to Clay Watercolour

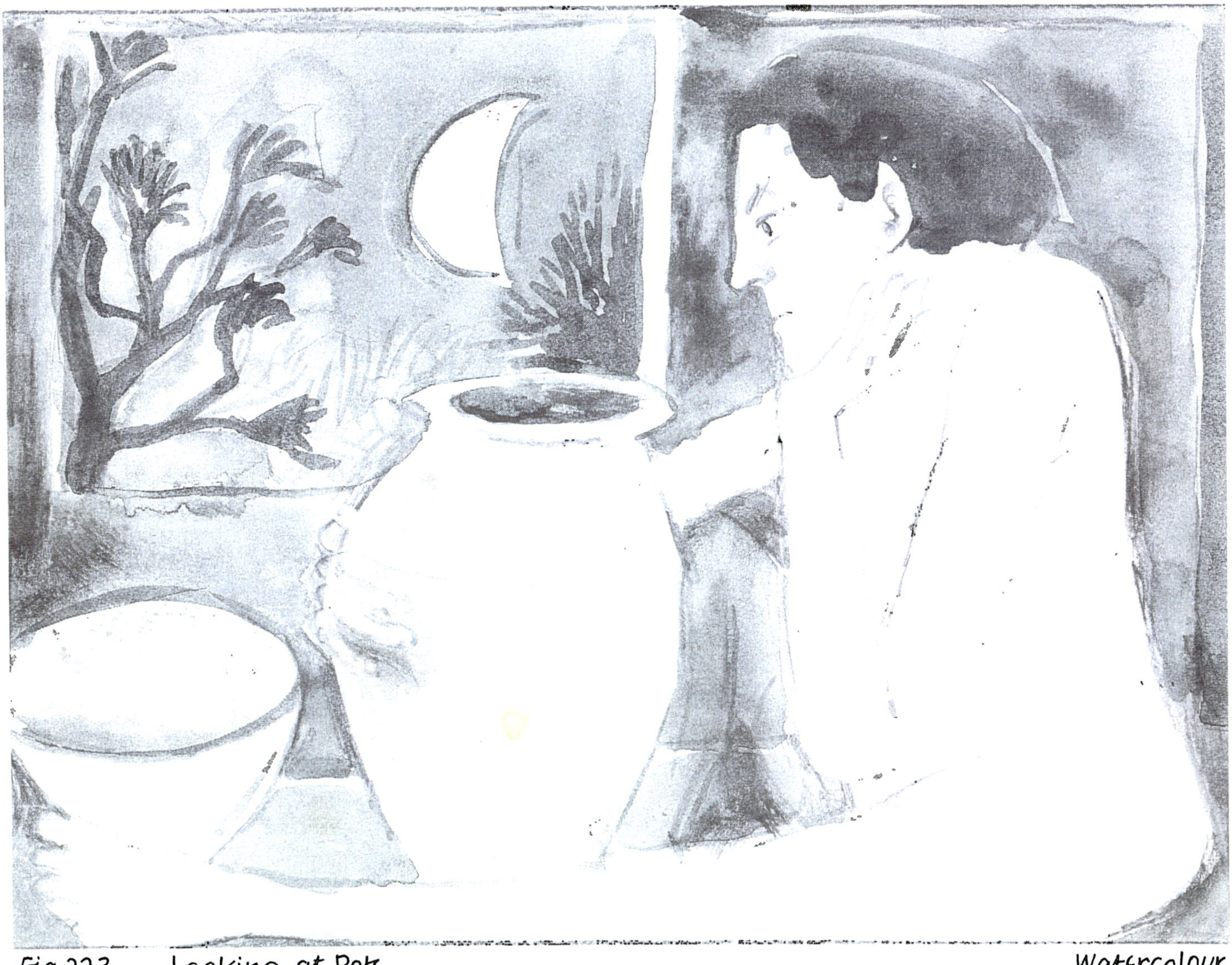

Fig.223 Looking at Pots Watercolour

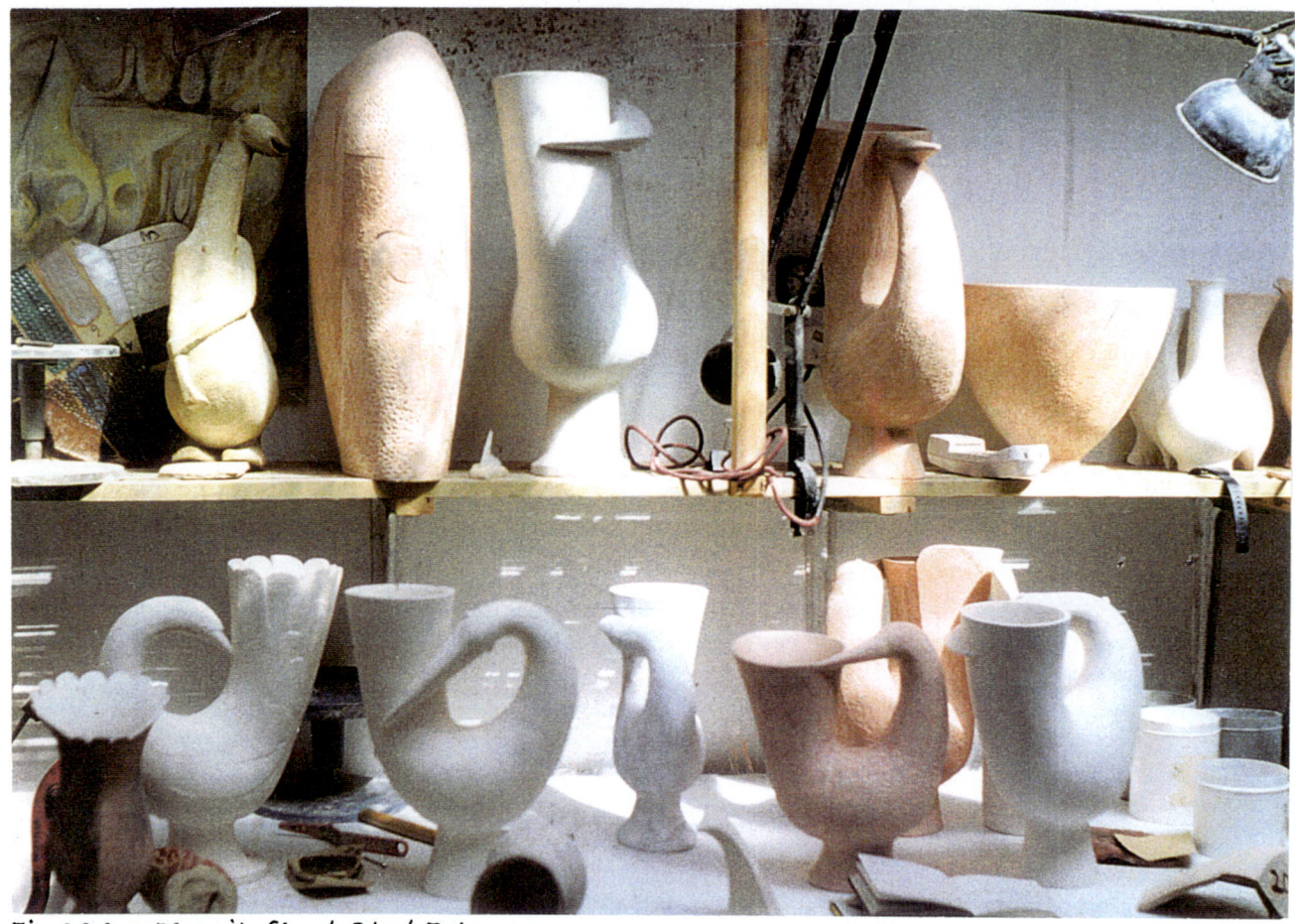
Fig.224   Biscuit-fired Bird Pots

THE FINAL FIRING

Towards the end of the Ceramics course at Stroud I purchased and installed an ancient electric kiln in the garden studio and started potting at home. There was also a return to more painting and drawing and a renewed interest in bird forms which led to many more variations on this theme. But there was also an undercurrent of something else happening.

If the dream about 'The Stroud Kilns' had been the harbinger for the following years of pottery, then a surfeit of designing and making pots may have been the reason for a gradual decline of interest.

Shortly after photographing the group of biscuit-fired bird vessels in 1996 above, the impetus and desire to 'pot' quickly declined and the bird influence transferred into a more expressive sequence of 'freestyle' artwork (see Stretching the Wings, page 215).

The lessening of interest may have been of subconscious origin. Certainly it felt as if some subterranean preconceptions were at work with this change of interest rather than any conscious decision making. The final kiln firing was a glaze-firing of the set of pots above.

5 UNMASKING THE MONSTER

Dreams 23, 30, 46, 108   Facing the Fear

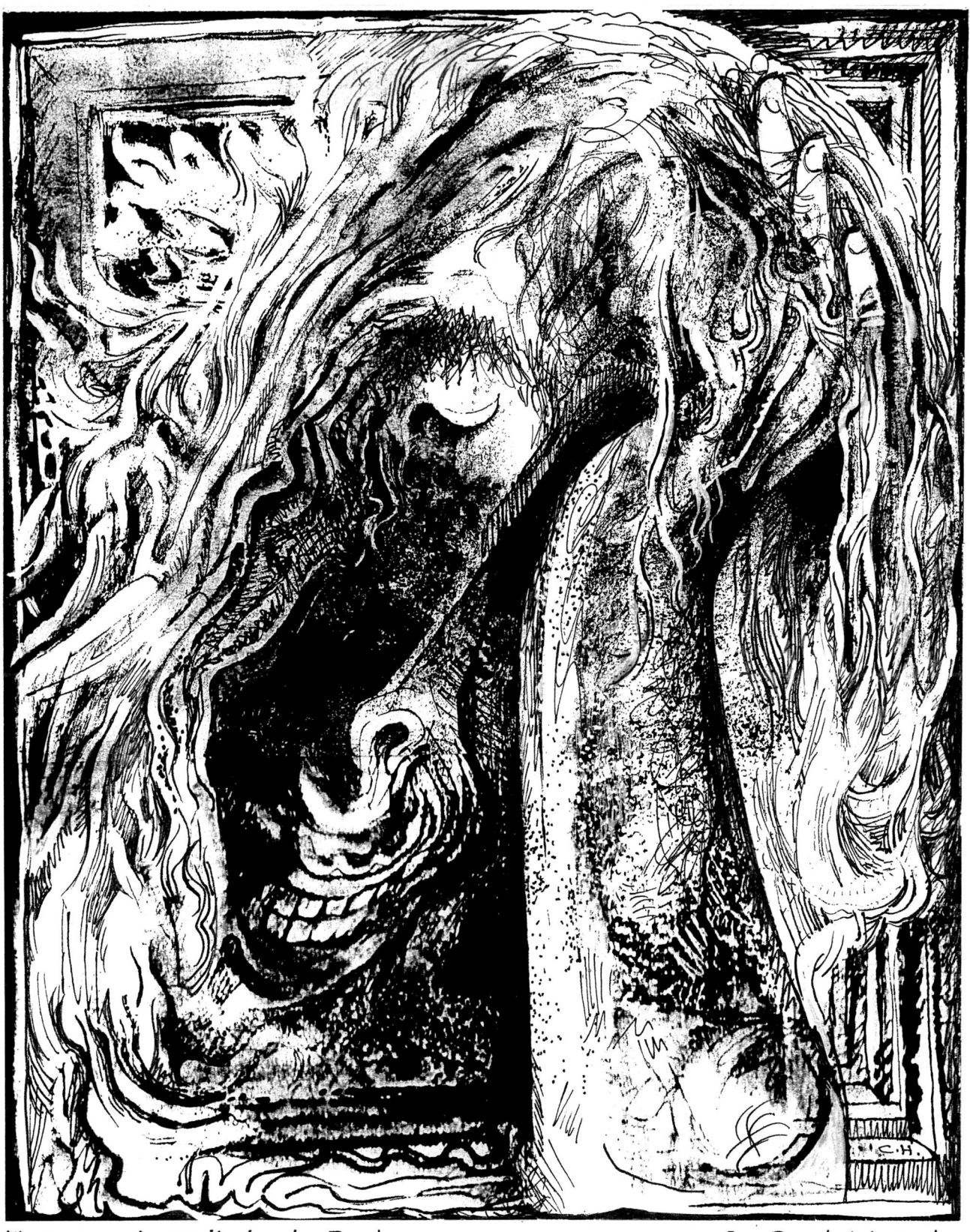

Fig. 225   A smile in the Dark   Pen, Brush, Ink & Paint

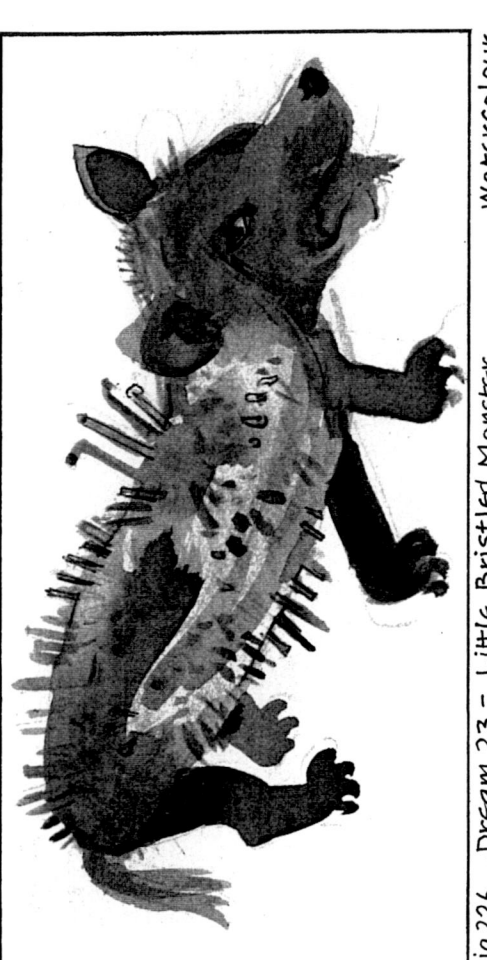

Fig. 226 Dream 23 - Little Bristled Monster   Watercolour

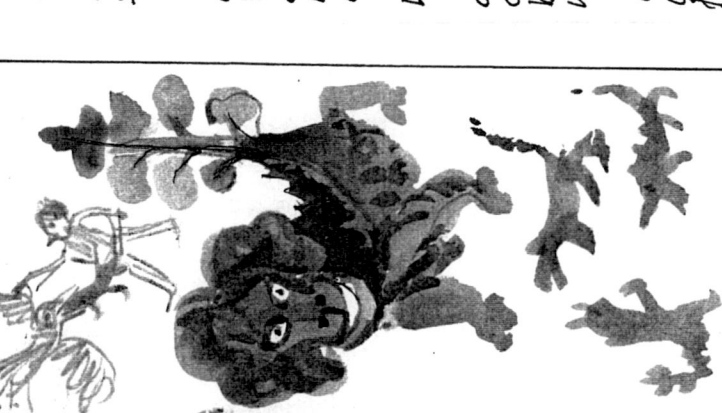

Fig. 227 Dream 46 - Plant-tailed Monster.   Watercolour

Above: **Dream 23** 27 August 1990
This creature walks by. It has a carapace-like back, is green and shiny with hard metal bristles.

I felt this dog-like 'monster' was offered up as a benign companion. Was it my animal-child spirit offering encouragement during the more traumatic dream material elsewhere?

Left: **Dream 46** 20 October 1990
I meet this green creature with a decorative tail and its four young, one of which is caught by a large bird. I rescue it and return it to its mother, who is constantly smiling.

Unlike many other dreams, the sub-conscious seems to offer a respite from more probing and trouble-some images with these two benign and peaceful 'monsters'.

In 1990 I'd become aware of an encroaching danger - the shameful discovery that a lifetime's pretence of playing the strong, silent type, able to cope with life's tribulations, was about to collapse, exposing a self-centred creature loaded with fear and anxiety. It seemed that this insight could have been the aftermath of the struggle to deal with the 1980s breakdown. A breakout appeared imminent.

As a result, after starting the art therapy and deciding to compile the dream journal, I became aware of a surprising new development in the dream material - the appearance of some strange creatures which I termed 'little monsters'. The only monsters I'd been involved with previously were those of my own making - costumes for drama, when staging productions of fairytales or myths for children in schools. (pages 130, 131 and 184-187).

Of these dream images, two were dog-like with odd appendages (right), another was of a 'larger than life' spider (below) and one other was a particularly fat hen (fig. 231, page 127). These four creatures became, for me, the precursors of a wide range of grotesque and fabulous monsters during the following years.

I shunned any kind of publicity for this new self-revelatory drawing, fearing imagined ridicule or contempt from outside and also from embarrassment within. The very idea of up-setting, let alone shocking, any of my more conventional friends and neighbours was, at the time, too unnerving for my withdrawn and depressive nature. Yet gradually these concealed images demanded an outing' - they needed to materialise into the real world, wanted to be exhibited. Unmasking these monsters took time because my mind lagged so far behind these intuitive markings.

Attempting to understand the imagery also caused me to dwell more frequently within the shadow side of the depressions. I realised that some of my friends advocated a more 'optimistic' attitude, as if there were a contradiction in looking into the darkness to find enlightenment. Perhaps it implied a pessimistic tendency, yet I found that seeking out the more obscure aspect of the psyche a totally positive pursuit. The outcome veering always towards an emotional 'uplift' and, more to the point, the lessening of heavy depressive moods.

The illustrations follow no apparent sequential among-ement as the other sections do (as I rarely date anything). Each image appeared (in the usual 'freestyle' method) out of amorphous textures, smudges, marks and lines with-out any connection to anything else.

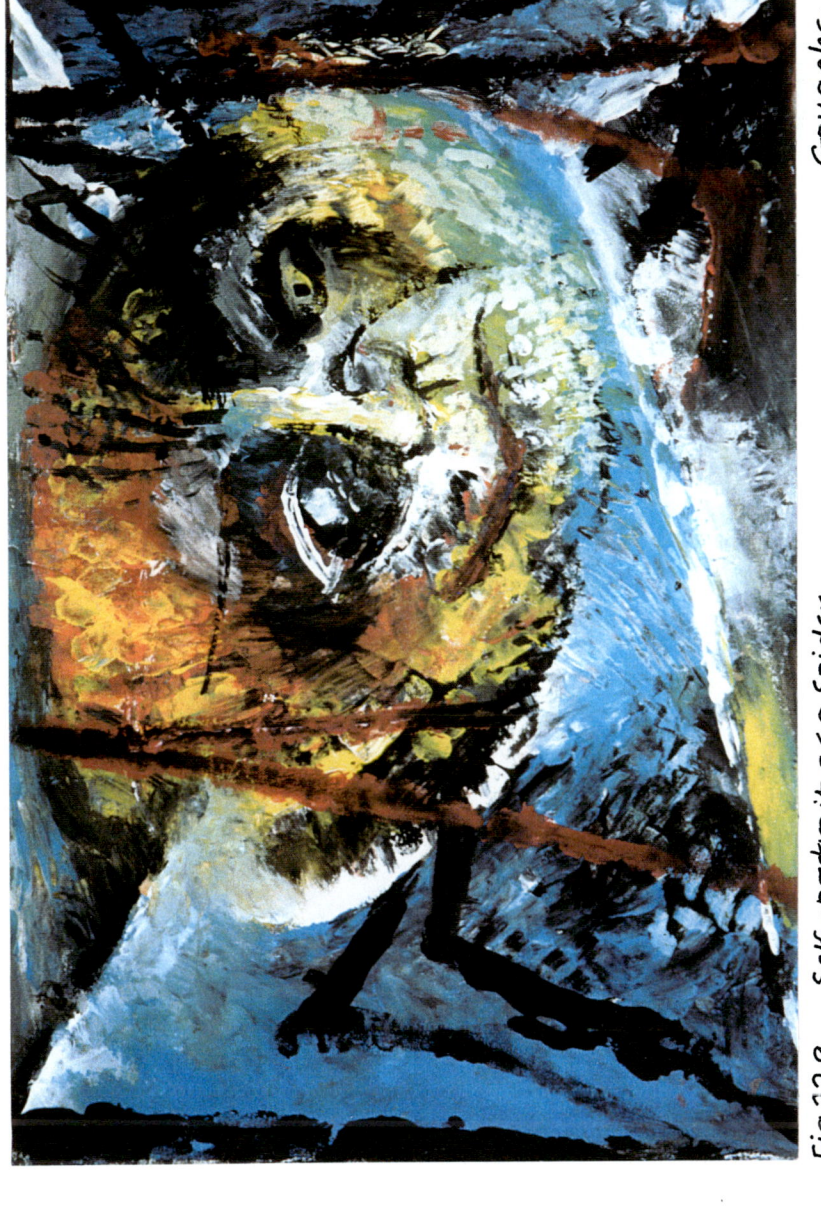

Fig. 229 Self-portrait as a Spider   Gouache

Fig. 229 Spider Head (Self-portrait as a spider).
Long after dreaming about the spider (dream 30, left), the painting above, like a Odilon Redon nightmare, appeared from under my brush. No longer showing the aggressive stance of the dream, this spider is in retreat, holding a posture only likely from some threatened species.

The apprehensive expression, the scuttling retreat of its legs, the 'boxed-in' corner. Here was a creature fearful of imminent oblivion, of being stamped out by a big boot of self-loathing — the beginnings of self-awareness aren't palatable.

Fig. 228 Dream 30 – A Spider Dream   Pencil, Watercolour

Spider dream.
Young friend of mine has a pet Tarantula & is assuring me it is quite friendly — somewhat anxiously I back out towards door ......

One part of me — the 'young friend' – was quite at ease and enjoyed his spider. Another part, the anxious dreamer, was not at all relaxed and was in retreat.

VORACIOUS MONSTERS

Creatures with greedy appetites, Id-monsters whose needs cannot be easily supplied, the hidden desires of the inner child are imagined here. The Goya-like painting below is a double image:
1 – A singing, shouting figure strides forth, arms out-raised disc playing a multifaced cloak.

2 – Turning the picture through 90°, a voracious monster lunges forward, devouring everything in its path – perhaps a symbol showing the enormous physical energy expended consuming the many internalised dissident voices threatening my 'retentive self-preservation.

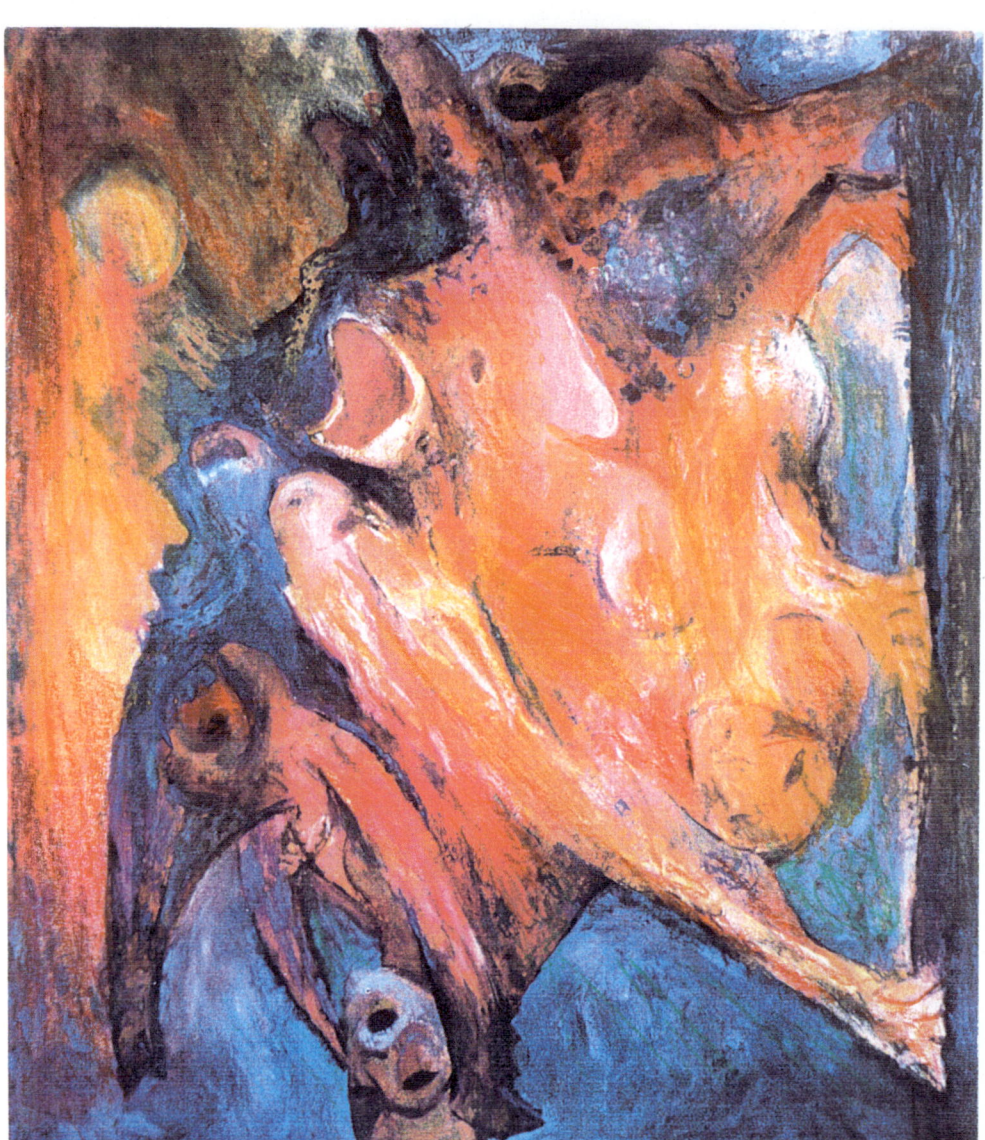

Fig. 230A   A Carnivorous Monster   Oil on Board

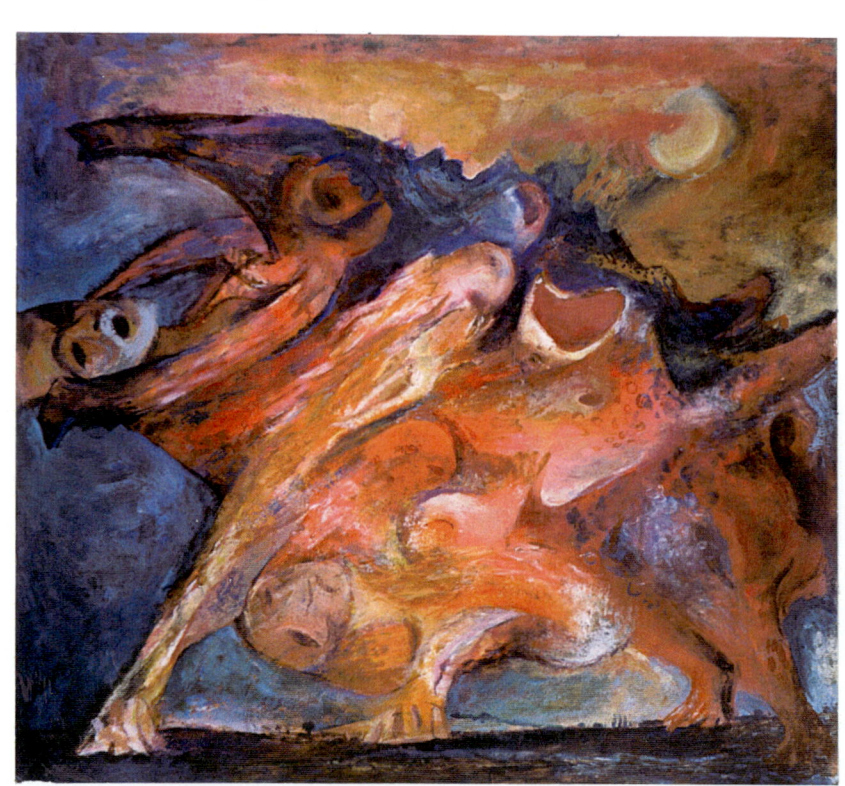

Fig. 230   A Goya'esque Fantasy
A painting which can be seen from two viewpoints

Fig. 230 Striding Figure

126

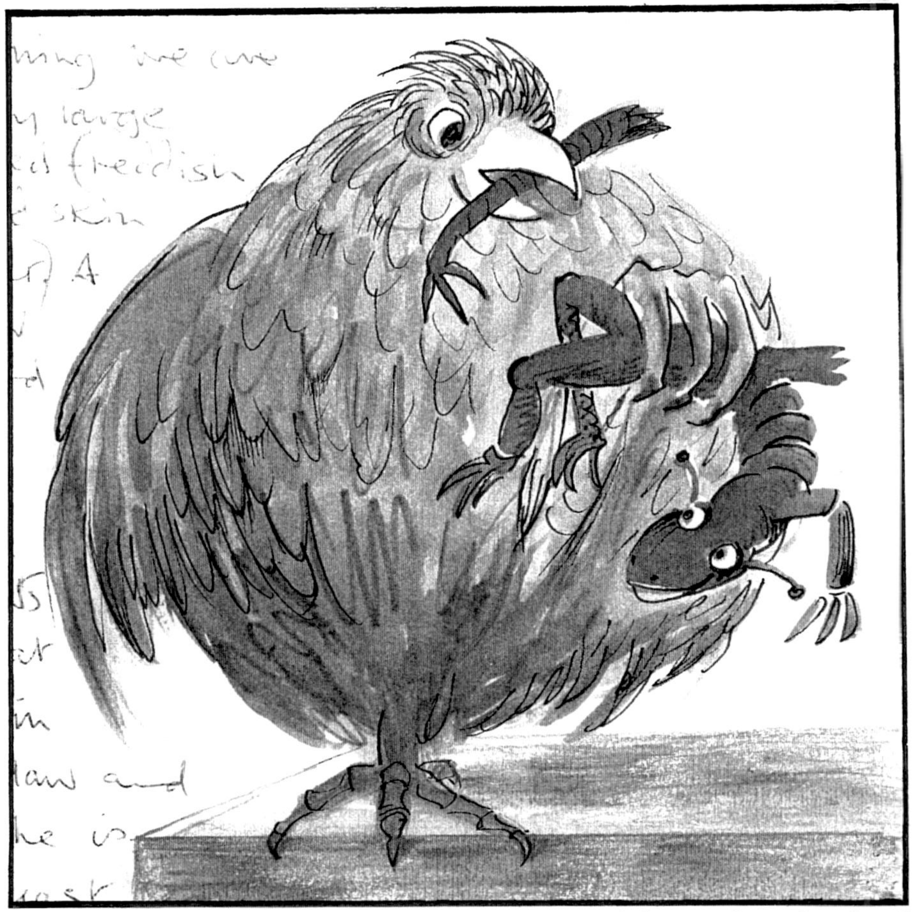

Fig. 231   Dream 108   Watercolour, Pen, Pencil

Above: Spherical bird eating a Lizard. I'm reminded of a 'Monty Python' sketch in which a duellist constantly challenges his opponent to continue the fight despite the progressive loss of each limb by the sword.
Both bird and lizard are oblivious of the pain of dismemberment — some mysterious activity is in progress — of one part of the psyche challenging another?

Right: Another creature with clawed hands, holding scraps of flesh, demanding flesh, blood or bones

Fig. 232 – Flesh Eater with Sun Glasses –   Watercolour & Gouache

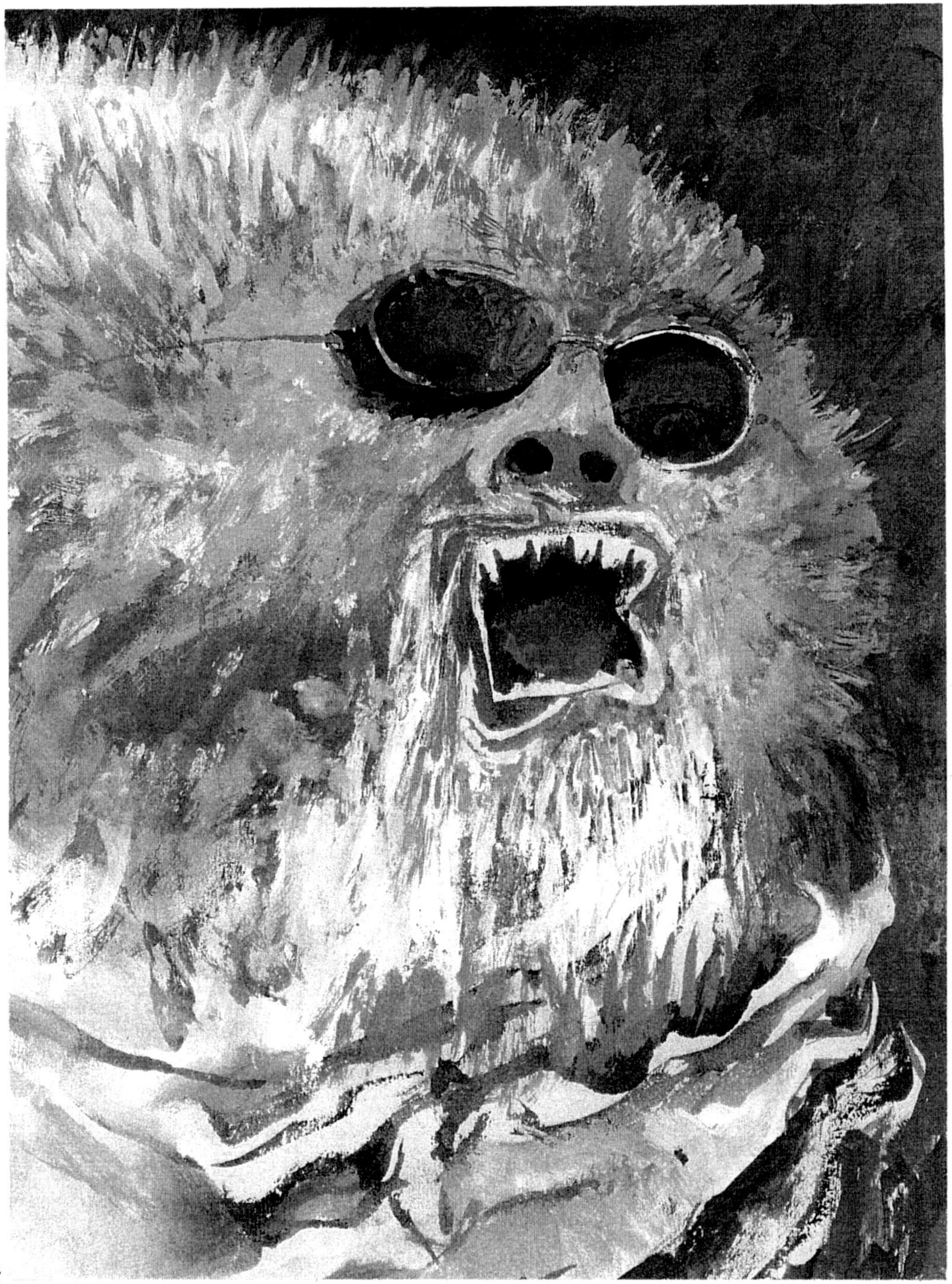

127

LAND OF ENCHANTMENT

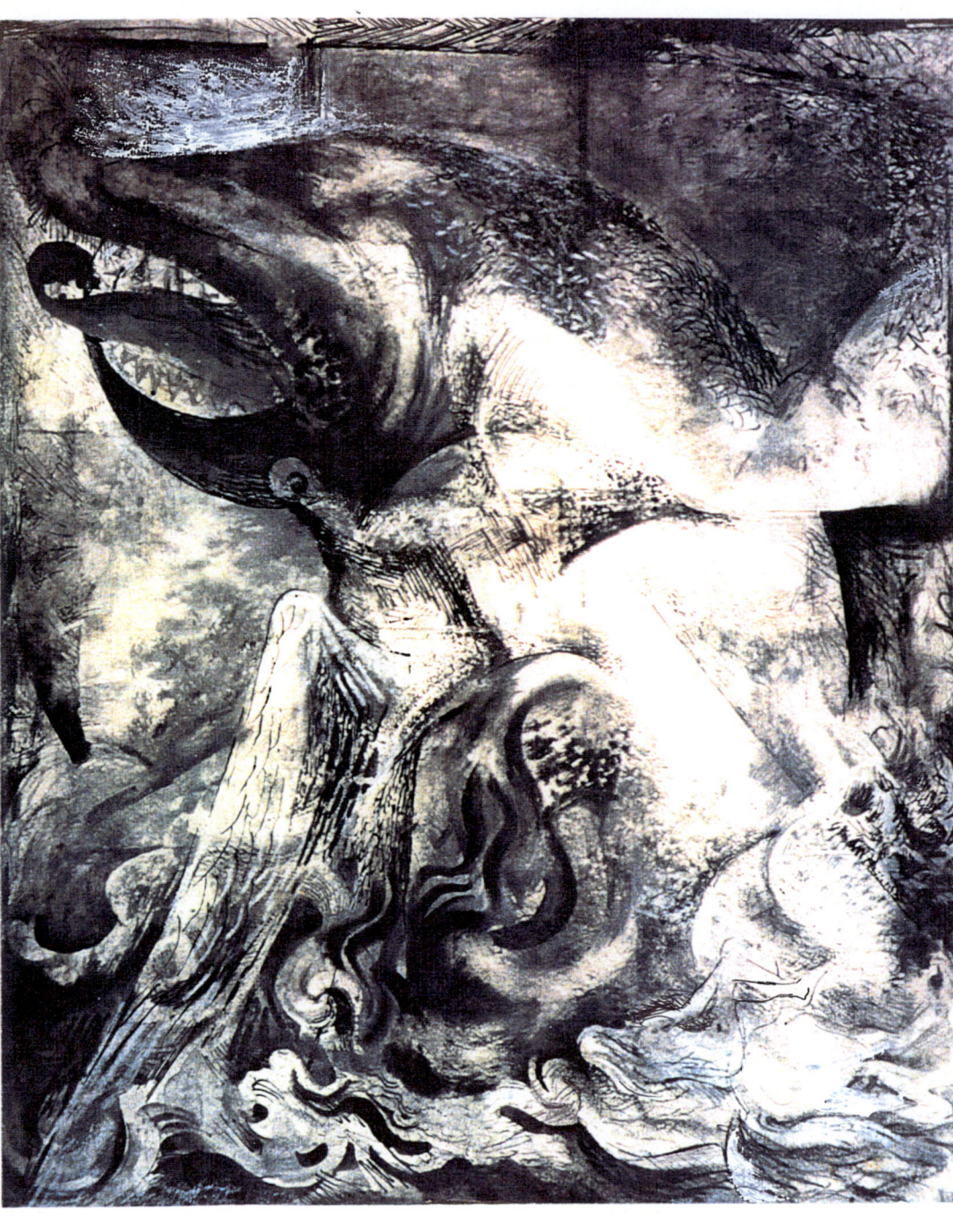

Fig. 233   Untitled Fairy Tale   Pen, Ink & Gouache

Right: Fig. 233 'Untitled Fairy Tale'. The possibility of being consumed by the unknown, during spiritual explorations into 'shadowlands' is, perhaps, the implication. The young couple (Prince and Princess?) ride into some mysterious land of 'faery', oblivious of the dragon's speculative eye.

Below: Fig. 234 "The Witch and the Manikin".
A double self-portrait. The little chap is plainly scared that his feminine side is overwhelming his once 'macho' attitudes — thoughts which stem from the witch's determined stride, her apron and her 'stirring' staff, suggesting that the manikin is destined for the stewpot.

Afterthought: Has she inadvertently skewered herself through the head, giving the manikin the hope that he may yet survive?

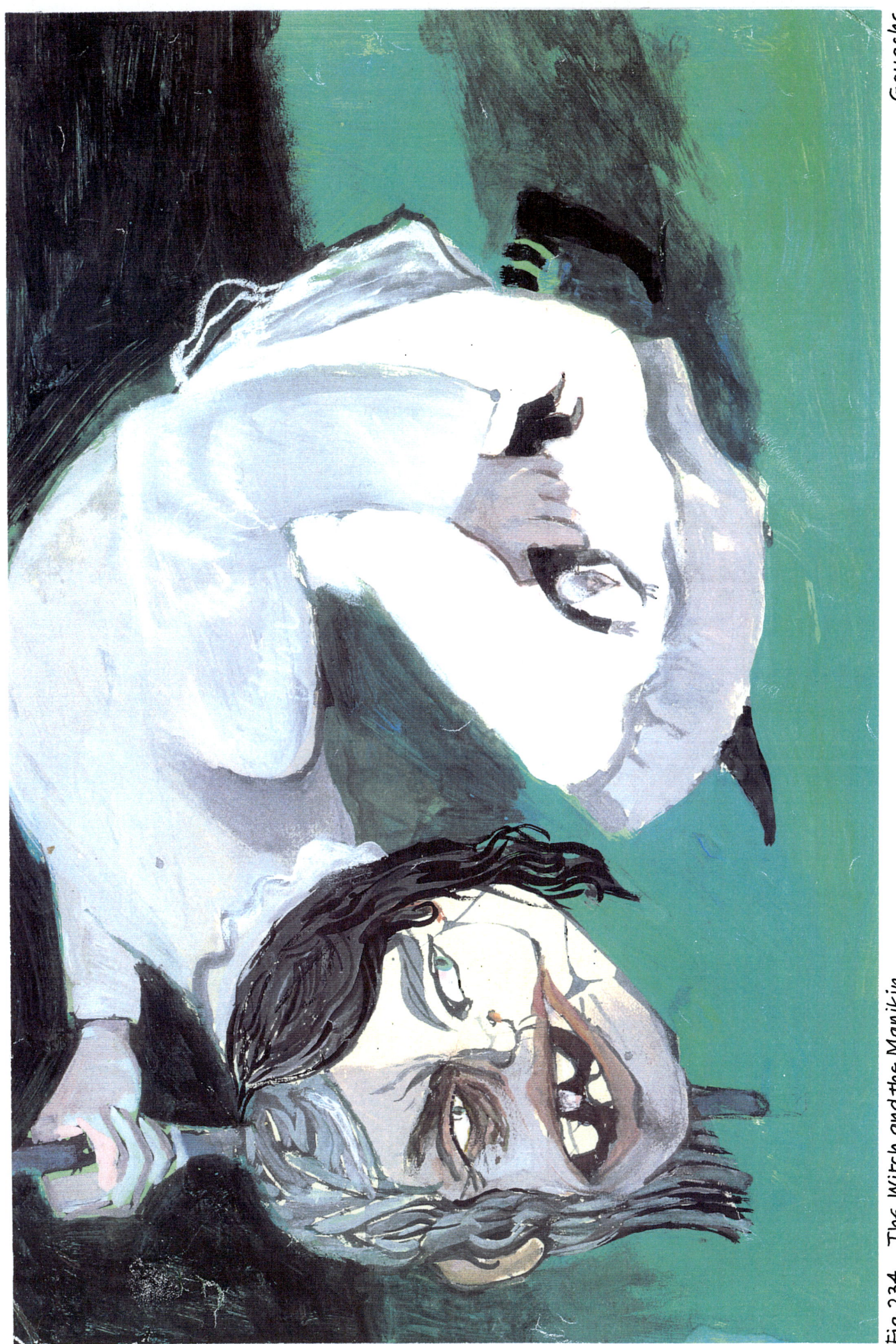

Fig. 234 The Witch and the Manikin Gouache

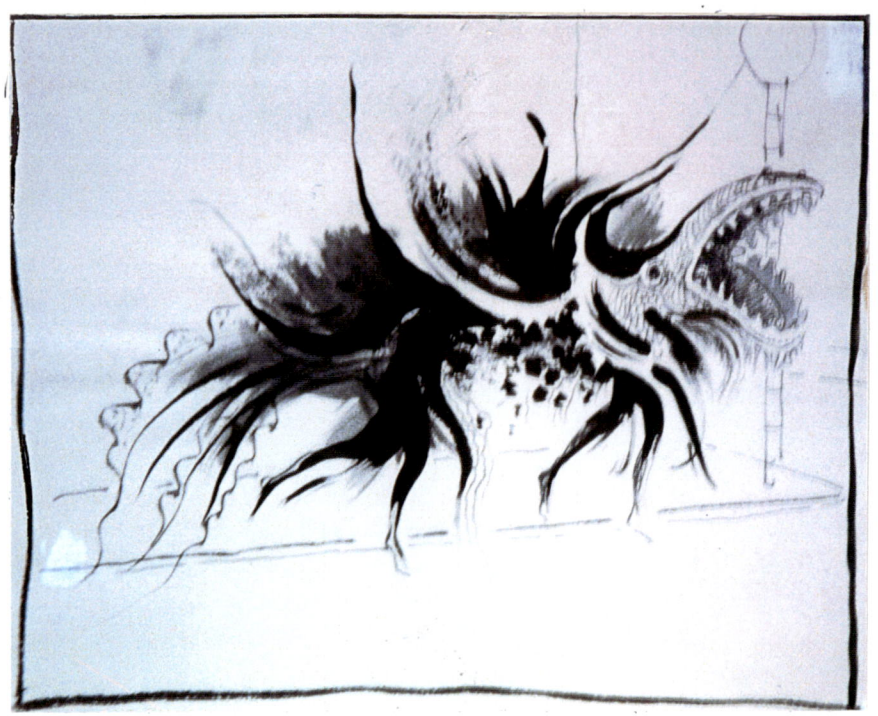

Fig. 235 Sketch for a Carnival Dragon   Pen & Brush

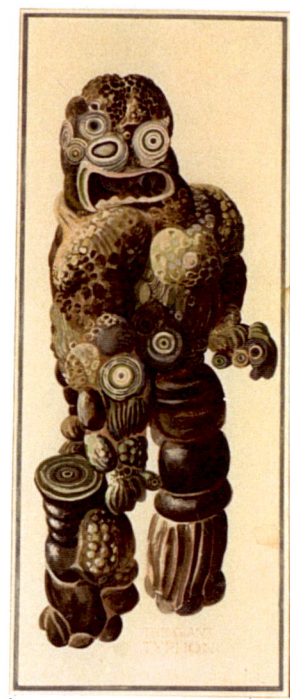

Fig. 236 Design for the Giant Typhon — Gouache

THEATRE MONSTERS

I was making stage costumes in the 1970s mainly for dance drama productions in schools. These were fantasy outfits for fairytale and myth adaptions — Gods, Goddesses, Dragons or Giants and alien monsters. The designing entailed thought and some introspection about the nature of 'abnormal' shape and form (see also page 184). These ideas could well have contributed and influenced the later 'freestyle' creatures shown in this section.

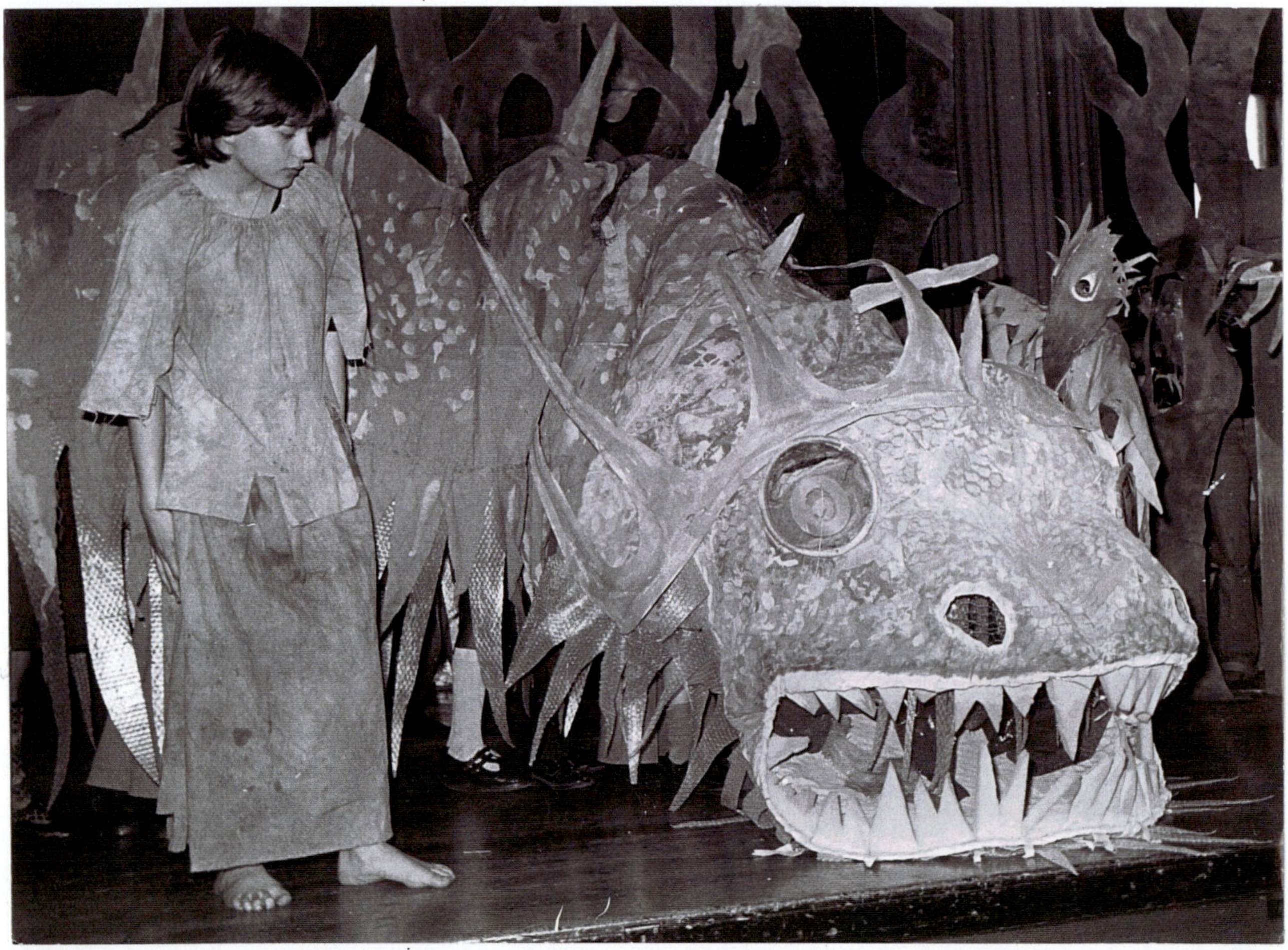

Fig. 237 Giant Sea-Dragon (from a production of Joan Aiken's 'Kingdom under the Sea)   Photo

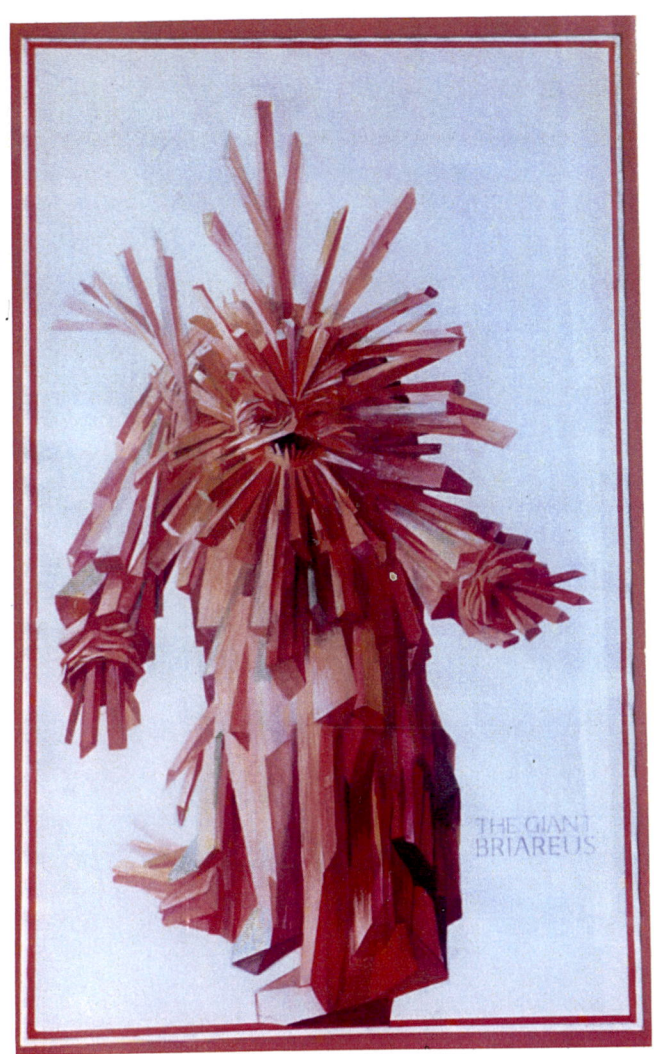

Fig. 238 Design for the Giant Briareus – Gouache

Above: The Giant Briareus. A costume design for a production of 'Persephone'. The construction of the costume is shown on page 186.

Top Right: Lobster Monster costume made from old blankets and various scrap items. Standing seven feet tall the actor looked through eyeholes cut at neck level (A rear view of this can be seen on page 185).

Right: Design for an alien creature for a 'Sci-Fi' production. (See also page 184). The young performer stands centre back manipulating wires to move the long head and neck to and fro. Made over a cane framework with sheeting and felt.

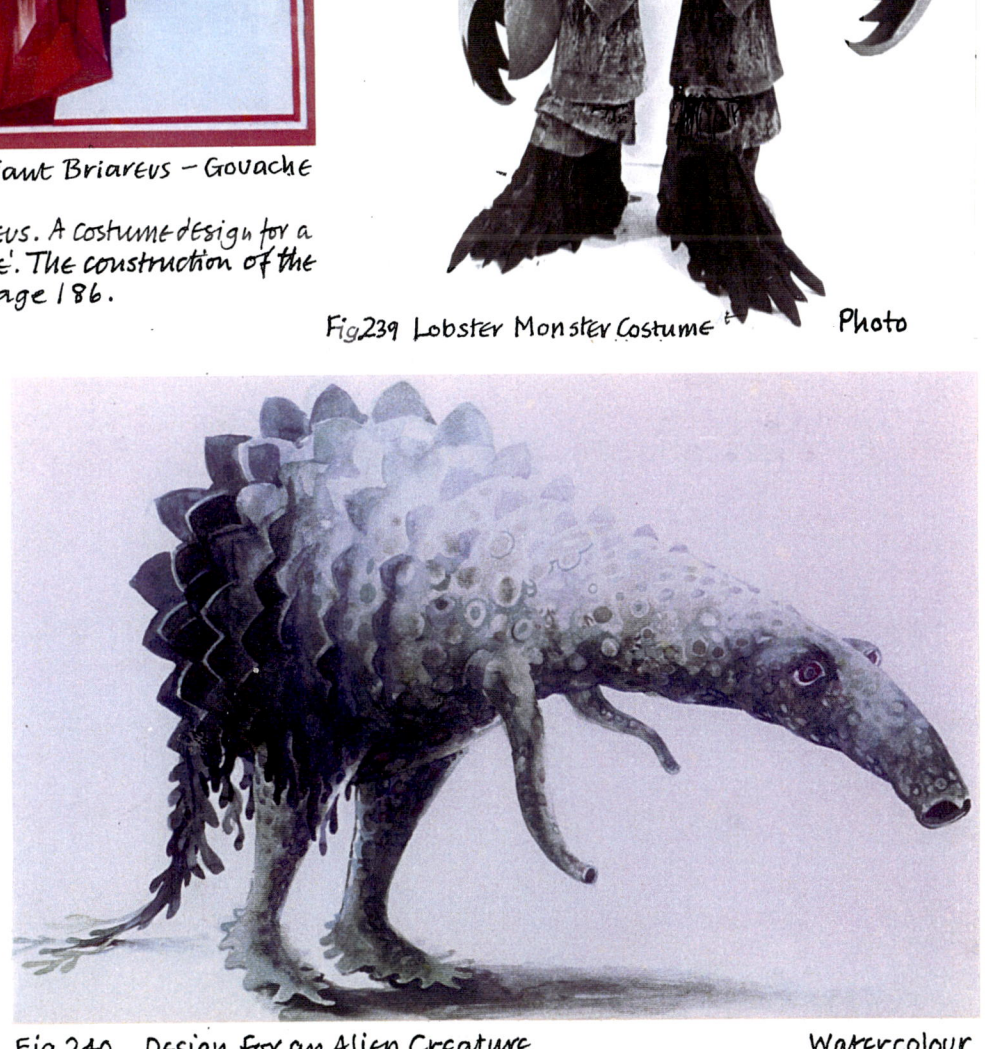

Fig. 239 Lobster Monster Costume — Photo

Fig. 240 Design for an Alien Creature — Watercolour

131

HATEFUL MONSTERS

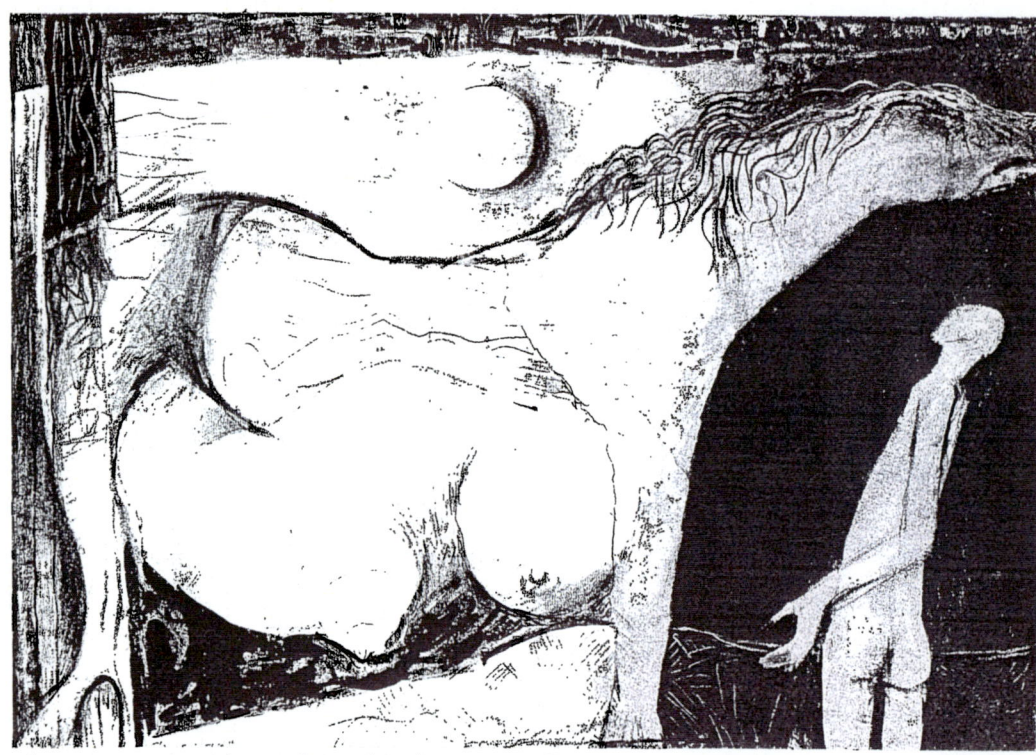

Left: 'The Plea', the final variation based on the Uffington White Horse from 'Visionary Landscapes'. See pages 289-296.

Fig.241   The Plea (Variation on Uffington White Horse)   Ink, Chalk, Paint

Below: Fig.242 'Snake Woman'. A loathsome image of a predatory monster ready to devour any man foolish enough to engage with her rapacious needs. A symbol of the unease and apprehension towards those I scarcely knew or understood. A final retentive and repulsive image which needed to be expelled from a hidden misogynistic past.

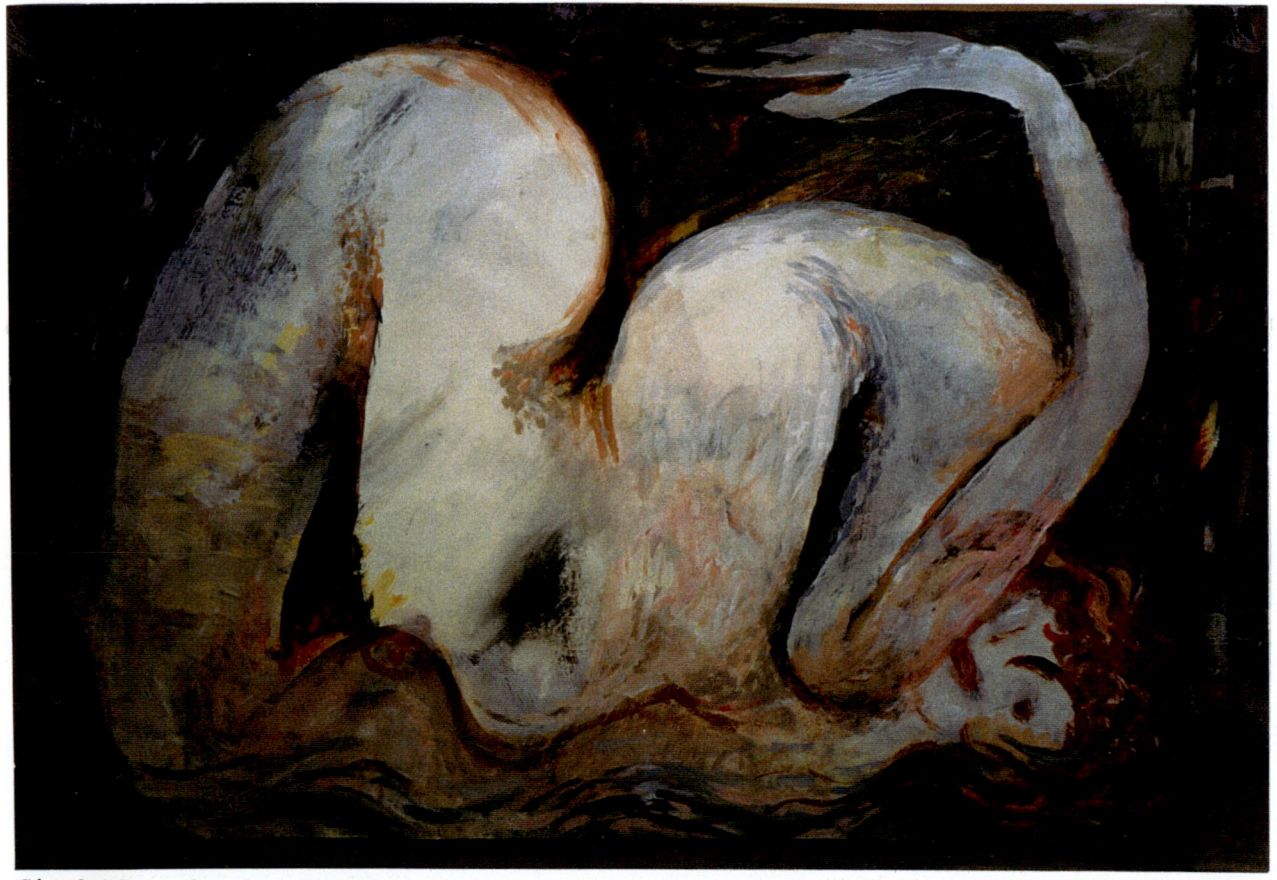

Fig.242   Snake Woman   Acrylic

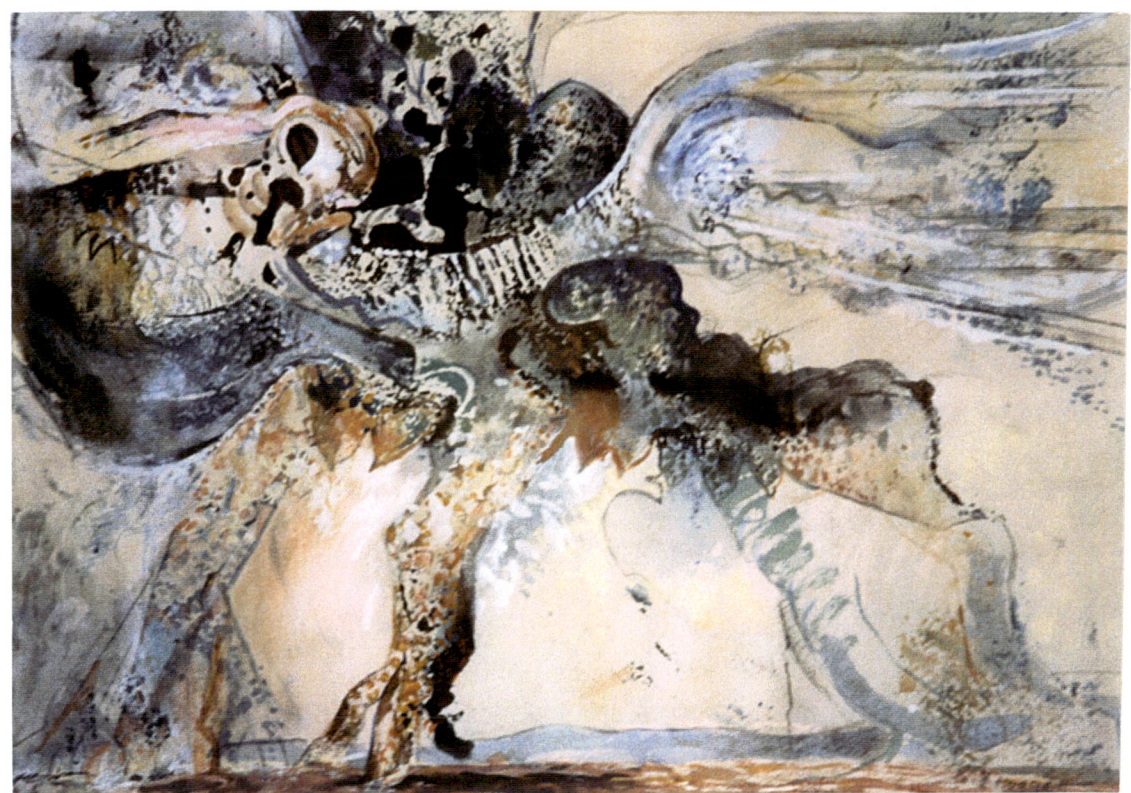

Fig. 243   Gale Force Twelve   Watercolour & Gouache

Above: Fig. 243. A violent aspect of Gaia, seen as a vast storm force, dominating the land.

Right: Fig. 245. Originally 'A Spectre' - (see page 55) the creature's head and left arm were emphasised making a more yawning and insatiable mouth.

Below: Fig. 244. The fear of capture by this un-nerving creature is not helped by the treacle-like substance underfoot impeding escape......

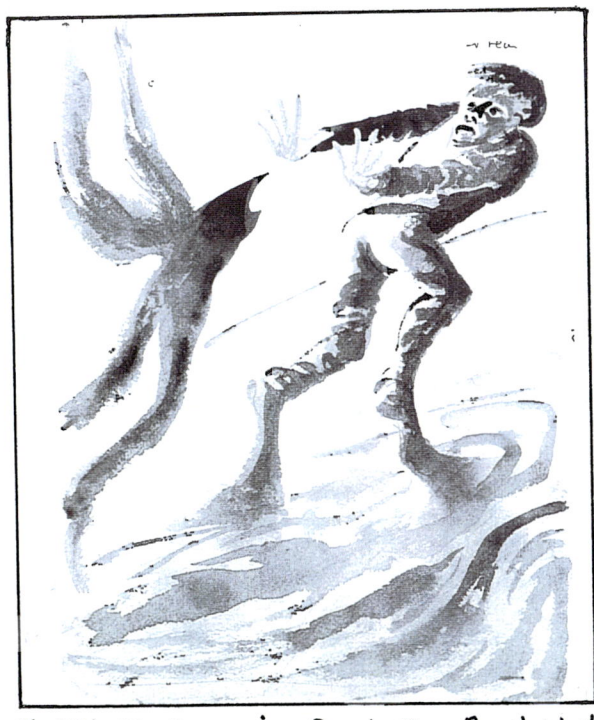

Fig. 224 The Un-nerving Creature – Brush, Wash

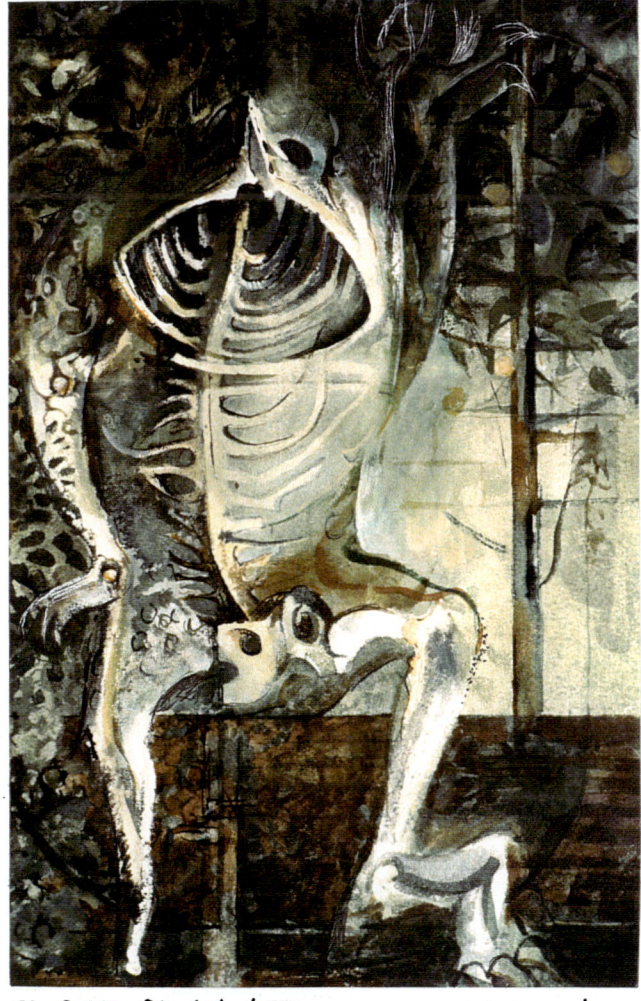

Fig. 245 Skeletal Figure   Watercolour

HOPEFUL MONSTERS

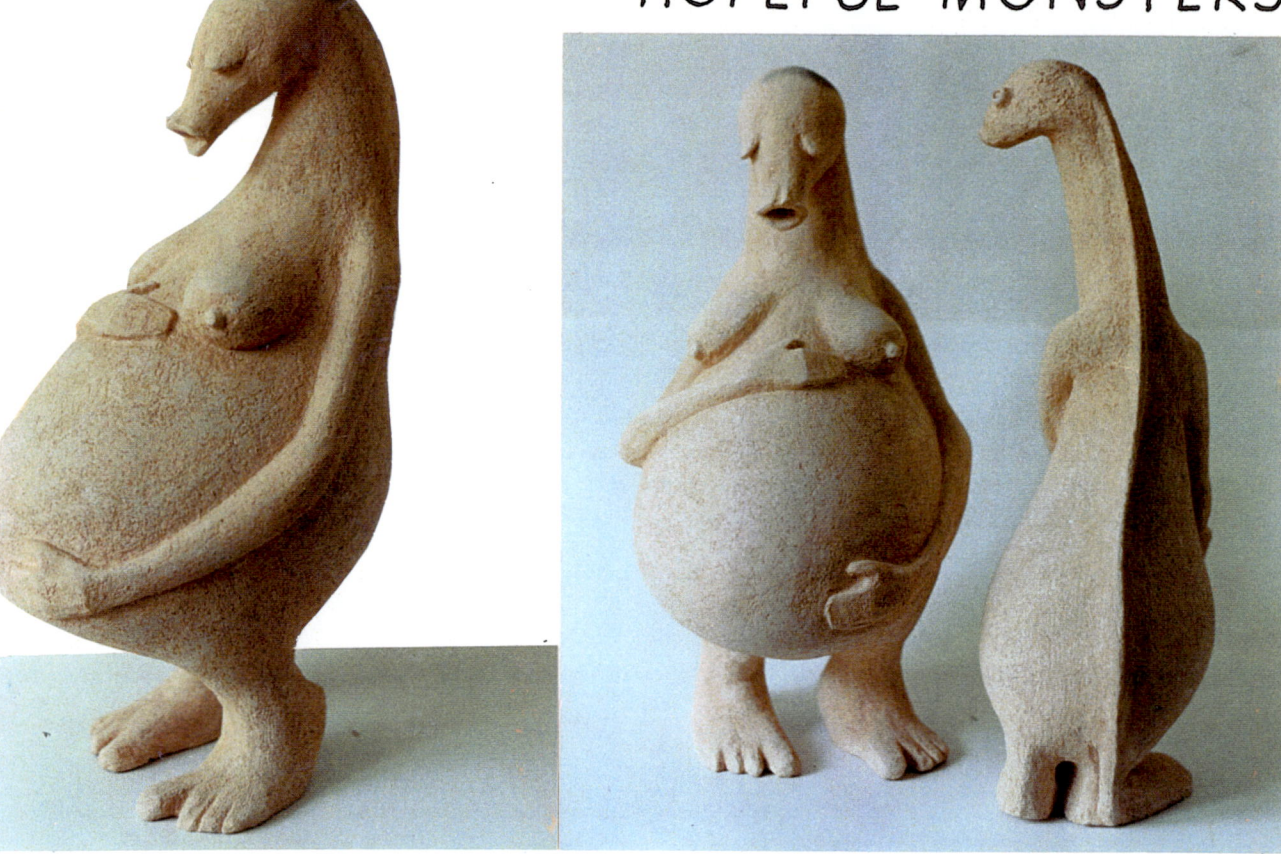

Fig. 246   Pregnant Dinosaur and Friend (two viewpoints)   Ash glazed Ceramics

Above: 'Pregnant Dinosaur and Friend' I felt exorcised the ghost of 'Snake Woman' and similar dark imagery with its strong maternal forms.
Below: 'Dinosaur Family'. This group confirmed an even more positive state of mind — a sense of the future and the consolations gained from the family group.

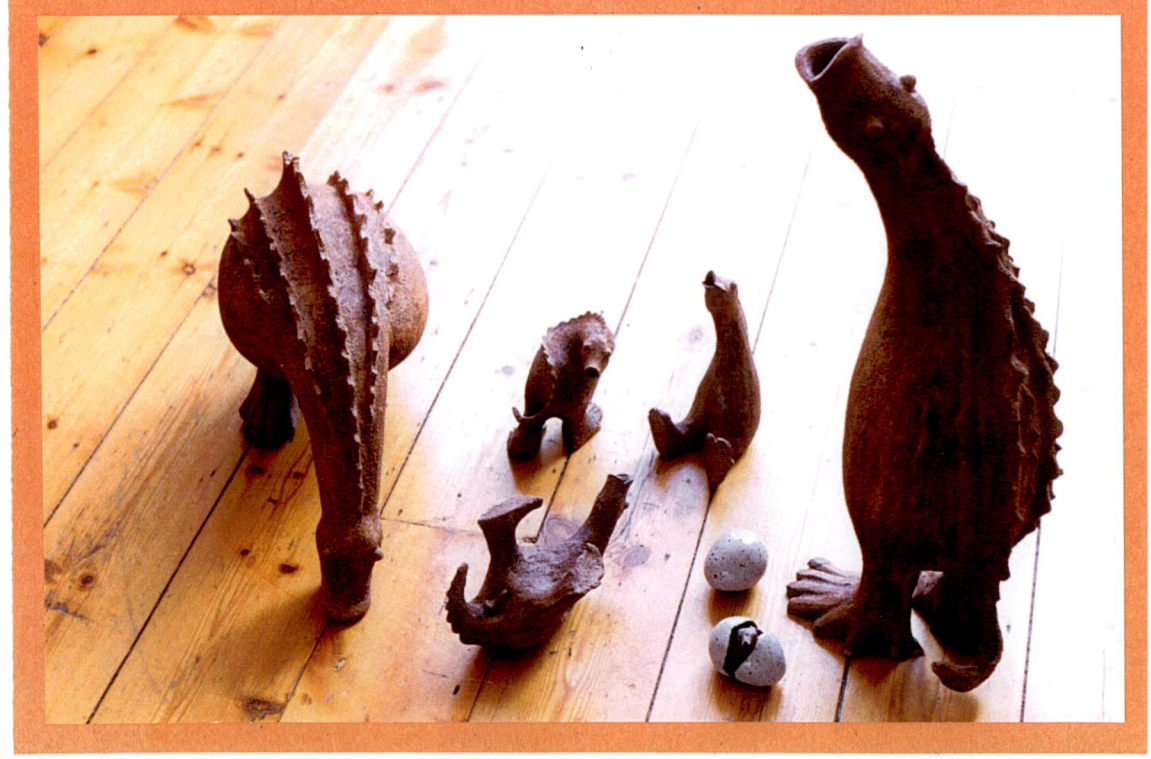

Fig. 247   Dinosaur Family – Seven-piece Group   Iron Glazed Ceramics

Towards the end of working with clay there had been an increasing interest in making fantasy birds and animals.

These final pieces I later thought of as 'hopeful monsters'; a series of creatures, dinosaurean or prehistoric in form, which displayed a fundamental optimism. They were certainly an antidote to the images on pages 132-133.

Alongside these 3-dimensional pieces were more recent paintings which emphasised in various ways an expectation of success, of feelings of confidence or, at the very least, a desire for some change for the better.

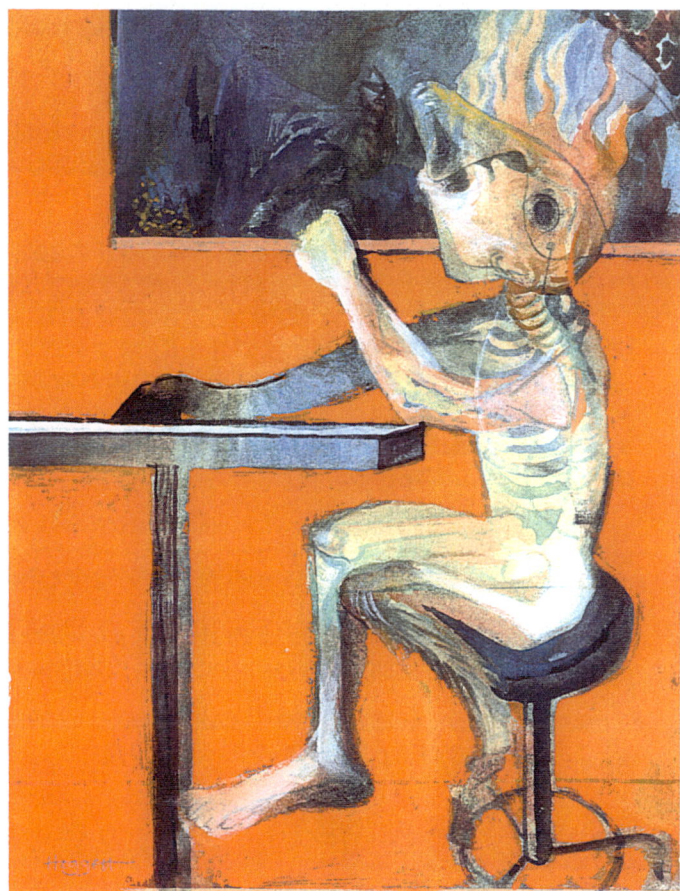

Fig. 248   Rage against the Dark   Gouache

Above: Fig. 248 is a later version of the painting 'Claustrophobic Burial' on page 56.. 'Rage against the Dark' offers a more challenging aspect of hope; the spirit of struggle; a way of sloughing-off old and decrepit ideas of the self as victim, trapped in 'worn-out' outfits. The idea of fighting one's way out of a skeleton certainly suggested a resurrection.

Anger and rage were soon to play an important role in the therapeutic recovery shown and discussed in 'Thinking the Unthinkable' (see page 201).

There were also a few paintings which anticipated a change of attitude between the internalised father and son. Fig. 249 'The Gentle Giant' shows the self getting close to the father/giant with a feeling of an understanding or consoling movement. This was a dream image from a later period than the dreams recorded in this section, occurring during the final months of completing this book.

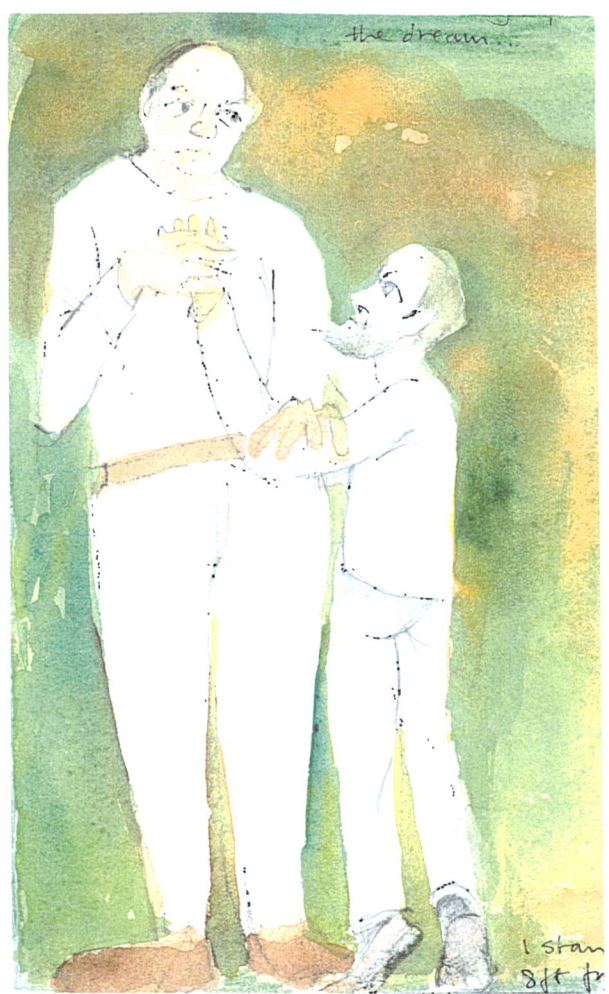

Fig. 249   The Gentle Giant   Watercolour

135

AMBIGUOUS MONSTERS

Below: Fig.250 'Tittle-Tattling' or 'The Censors'

Interior voices gossip and censure one's attempts at 'letting-go', of seeking freedom from fear, of restrictive practices or beliefs of the past.
  Overcoming these voices required patience. 'You can't do that! You can't do this!' they exclaim. 'Any hope of a passport is futile!' they cry, determined to keep me imprisoned inside my own historical patterning.
  Only when faced directly, do these monstrous visions of principle, dogma and internalised authority begin to fade, as chimera will, when confronted with the desire for change.

Top Right: Fig.252 A Little Woodland Creature

  His leap conveys his sense of release from various constraints. He 'lets go', pees on the undergrowth. The arc of his movement shows his first taste of freedom.

Bottom Right: Fig.250 The Dragondog's Plea

  This little monster, rather like a temple statue, pleads for attention and affection from the girl. On the left a patriarch gestures his disapproval, whilst just behind him another figure, perhaps an old crone, looks on with a sour expression. But the animal spirit of the young dog ignores these negative signs.

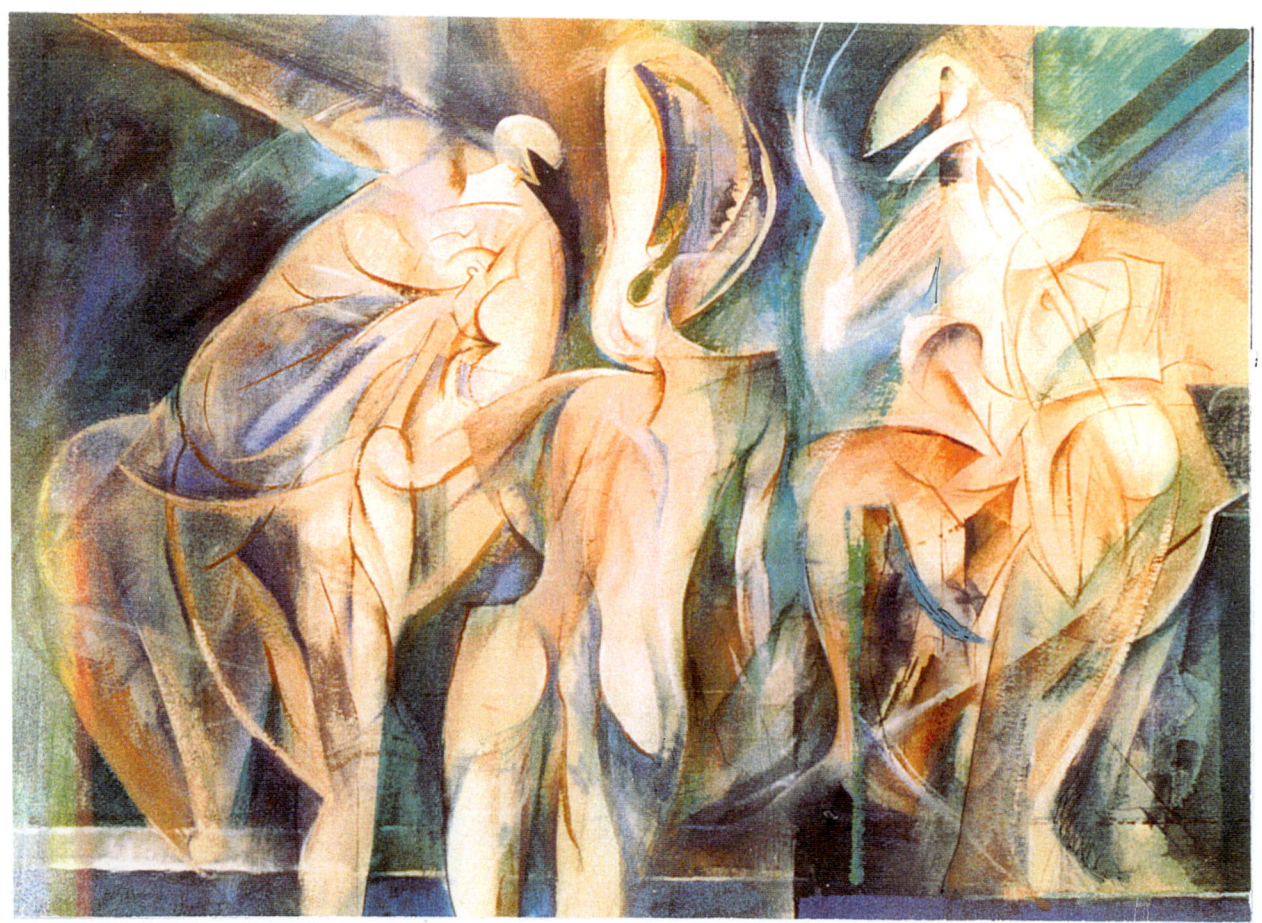

Fig.250 Tittle-Tattling or The Censors   Chalk, Watercolour, Gouache

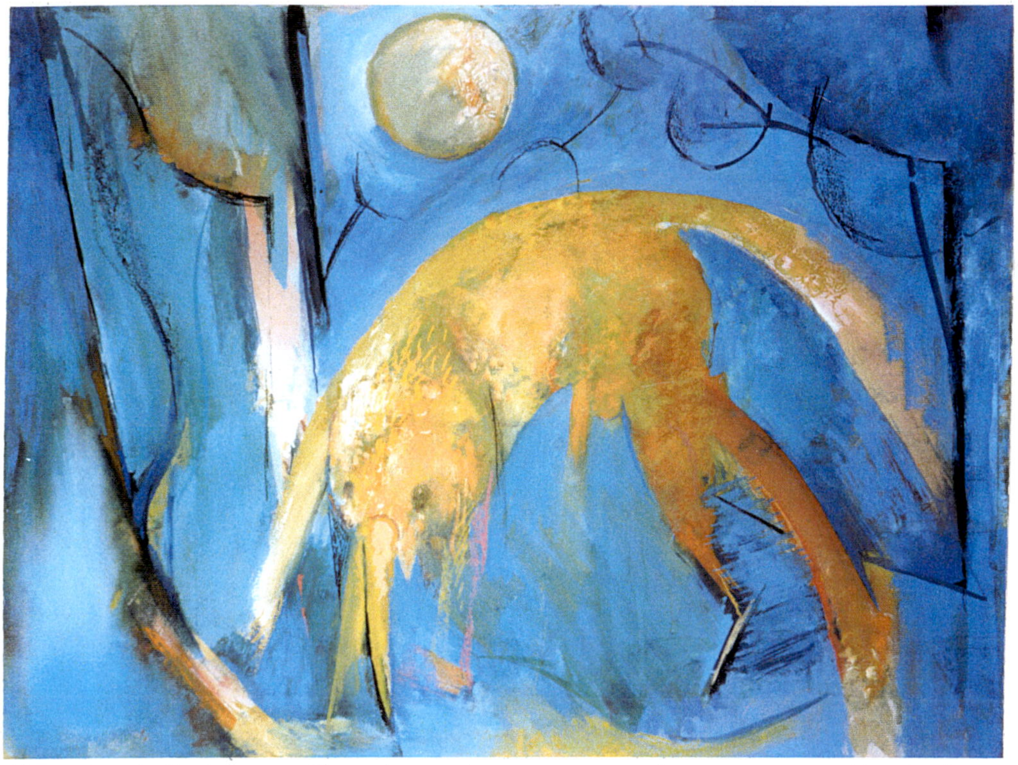

Fig.251   A little woodland creature   Gouache

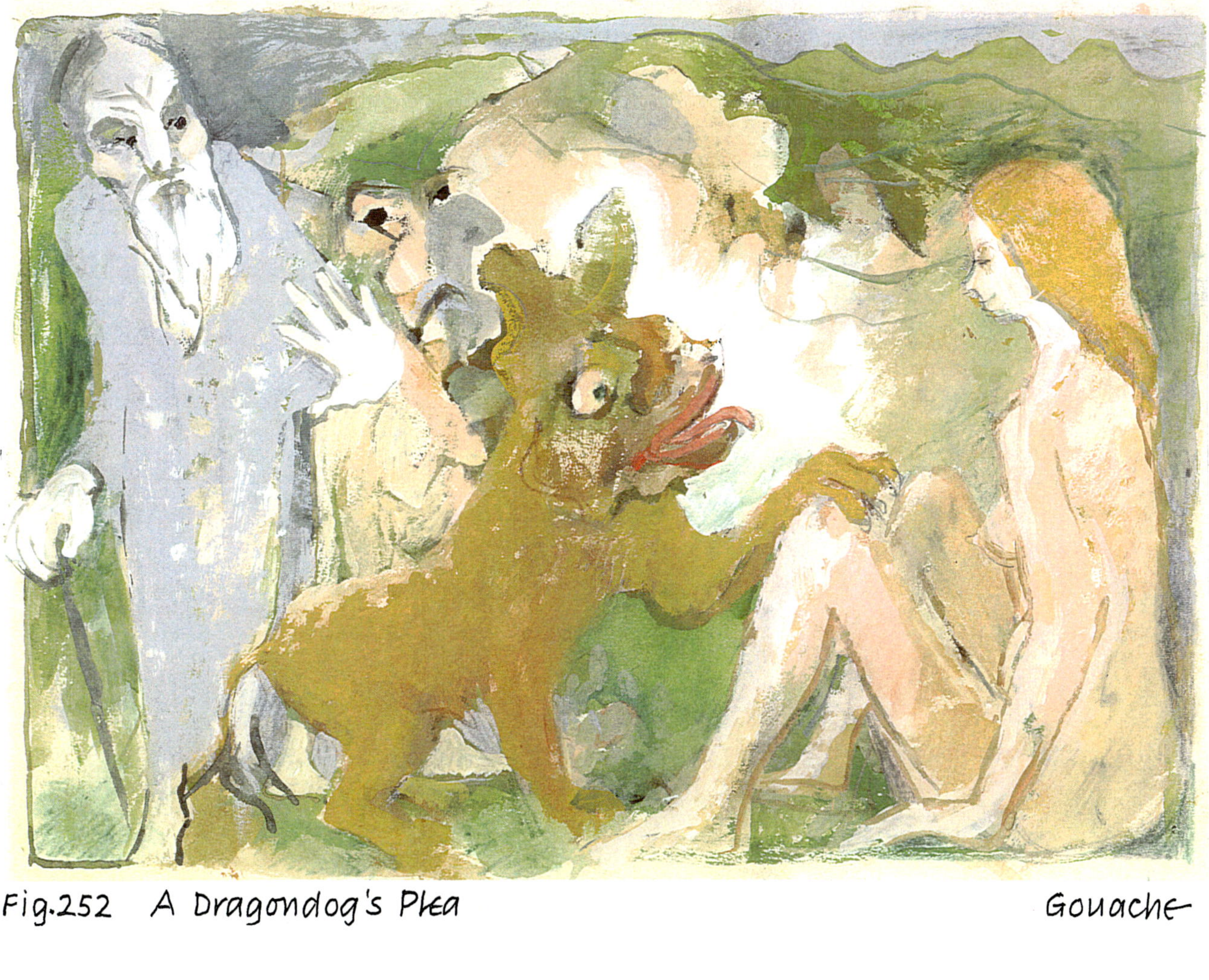

Fig.252   A Dragondog's Plea   Gouache

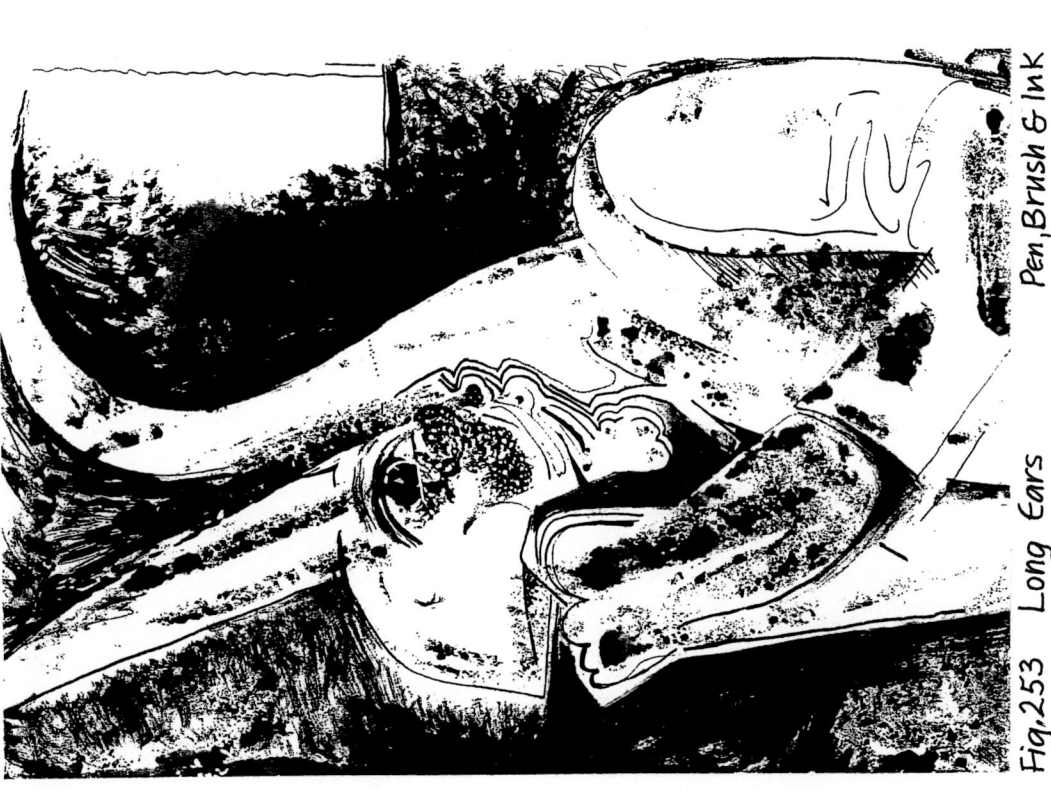

Fig.253 Long Ears   Pen, Brush & Ink

The drawings on these and the following pages seemed more spontaneous than usual, perhaps as a result of using a Chinese calligraphic brush used in decorating pots. It responded so readily to the lightest touch that it became the ideal tool for drawing.

Right: Fig.254 Long Trunk, Thinking   Pen, Brush & Ink

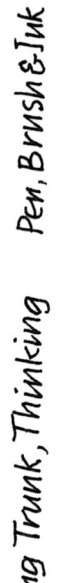

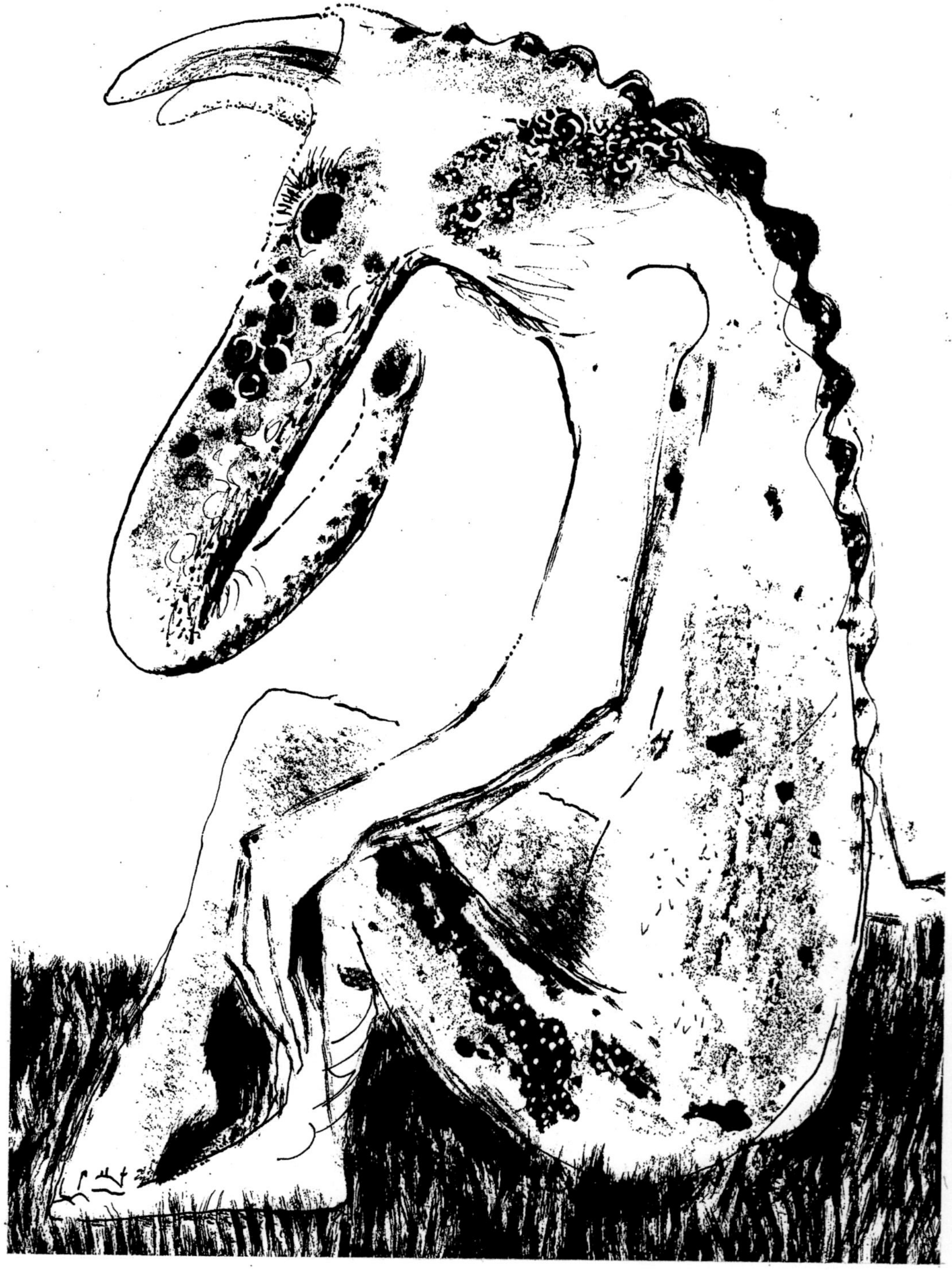

Noses or proboscises appear to predominate in this group of creatures, as if they are 'scenting' or seeking something.

Top Left: Fig.253 'Long Ears', like a sleuth, tentatively scenting out a mystery.

Top Right: Fig.254 'Long Trunk, Thinking' Seated monster, contemplating the nature of change.

Left: Fig.255 'Little Worrier — Anxious — or melancholic?

Bottom Left: Fig.256 'Hangdog' An attitude of resignation, the proboscis-like nose sniffing the ground. Its anatomy has a slight affinity with Aboriginal painting — except this is purely decorative. 'A dejected mood predominates.

Below Right: Fig.257. The garb of a giant shields a traveller from the heat of the sun (and perhaps his own feelings of smallness before the face of nature).

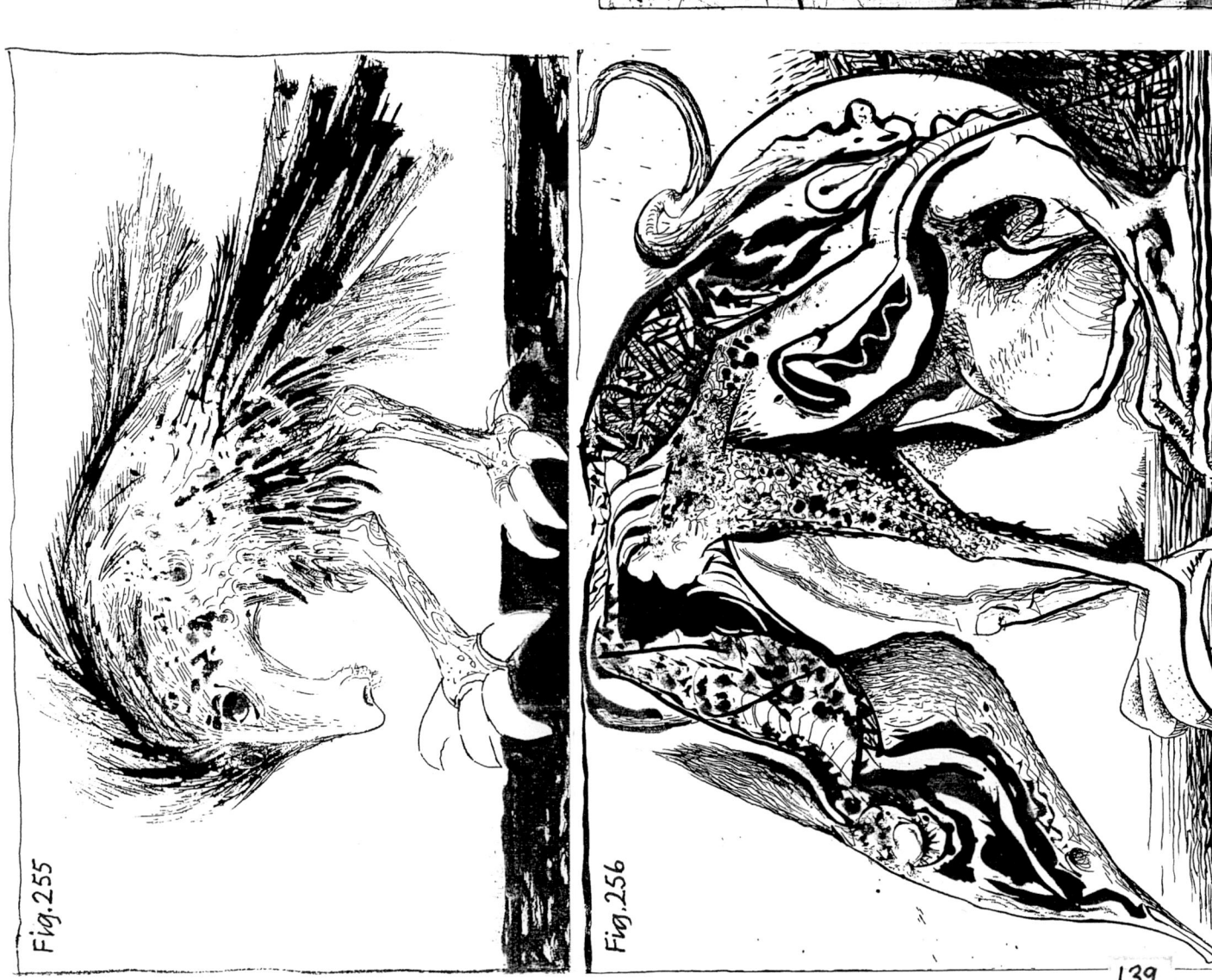

Fig.257

Fig.255

Fig.256

139

HIDDEN HATES, DESIRES AND A CONFRONTATION

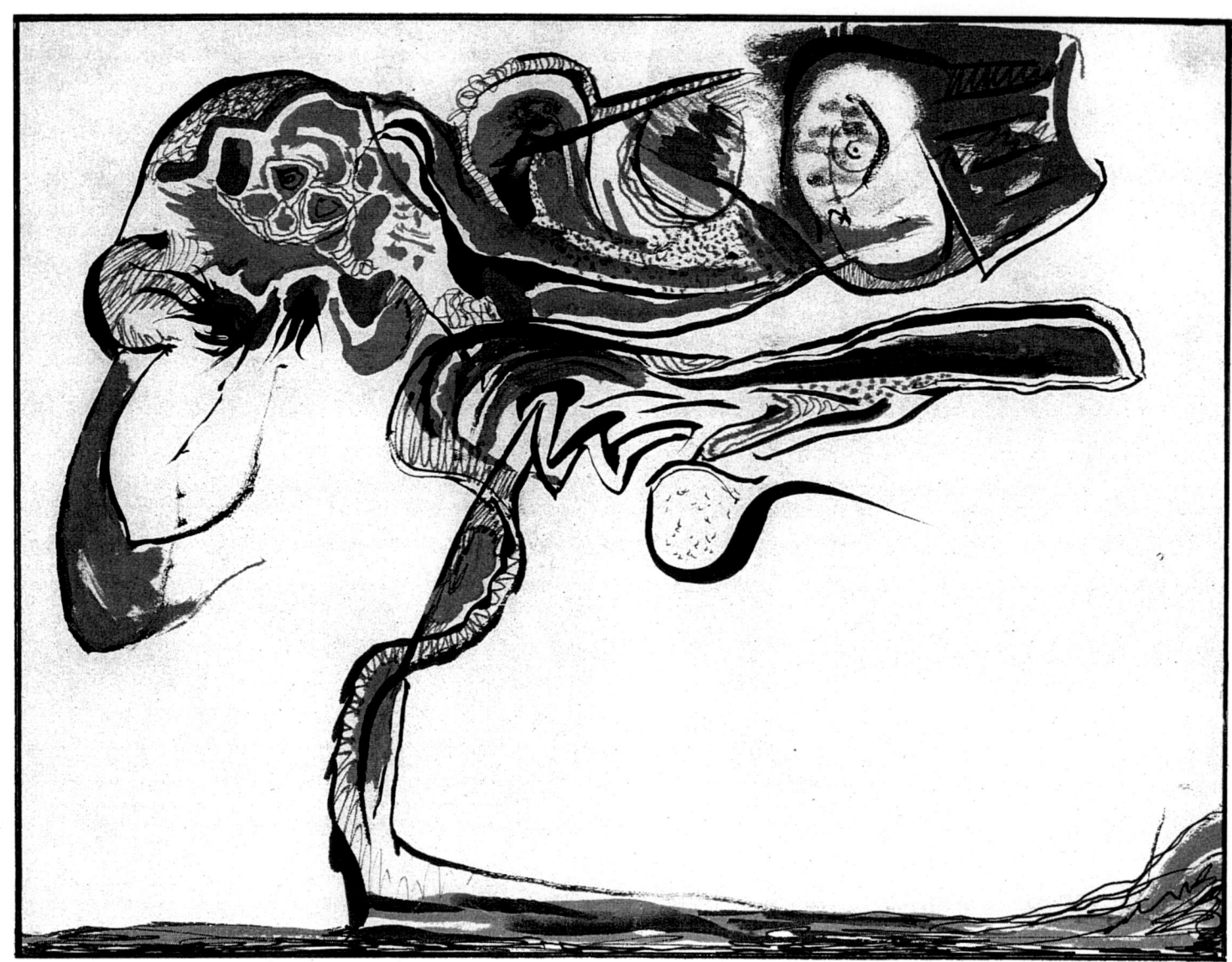

Fig. 258   Cock-a-Snook   Calligraphic Brush, Pen & Wash

Above: Fig. 258 'Cock-a-Snook'

This little 'tinpot' monster, in a posture of defecation, shows the animalism of the outraged child. This is the outpouring of defiance and contempt towards the former retentive nature.

Top Right: Fig. 259 'Flower Face' — Calligraphic Brush, Pen & Sponge.

Behind the charm of a petalled display lies the grimace for a smile. The hidden desire of an underdog?

Bottom Right: Fig. 260 'The Dragon and the Serpent' - Calligraphic Brush & Pen

The internalised struggle for survival and change. I take on the form of a serpent, suspicious of the dragon's intention. Its aggressive stance challenges my complacency. Now it's a confrontation for survival, change — or death.

Top Right: Fig. 259 - Flower Face.   Bottom Right: Fig. 260 - Dragon and Serpent.

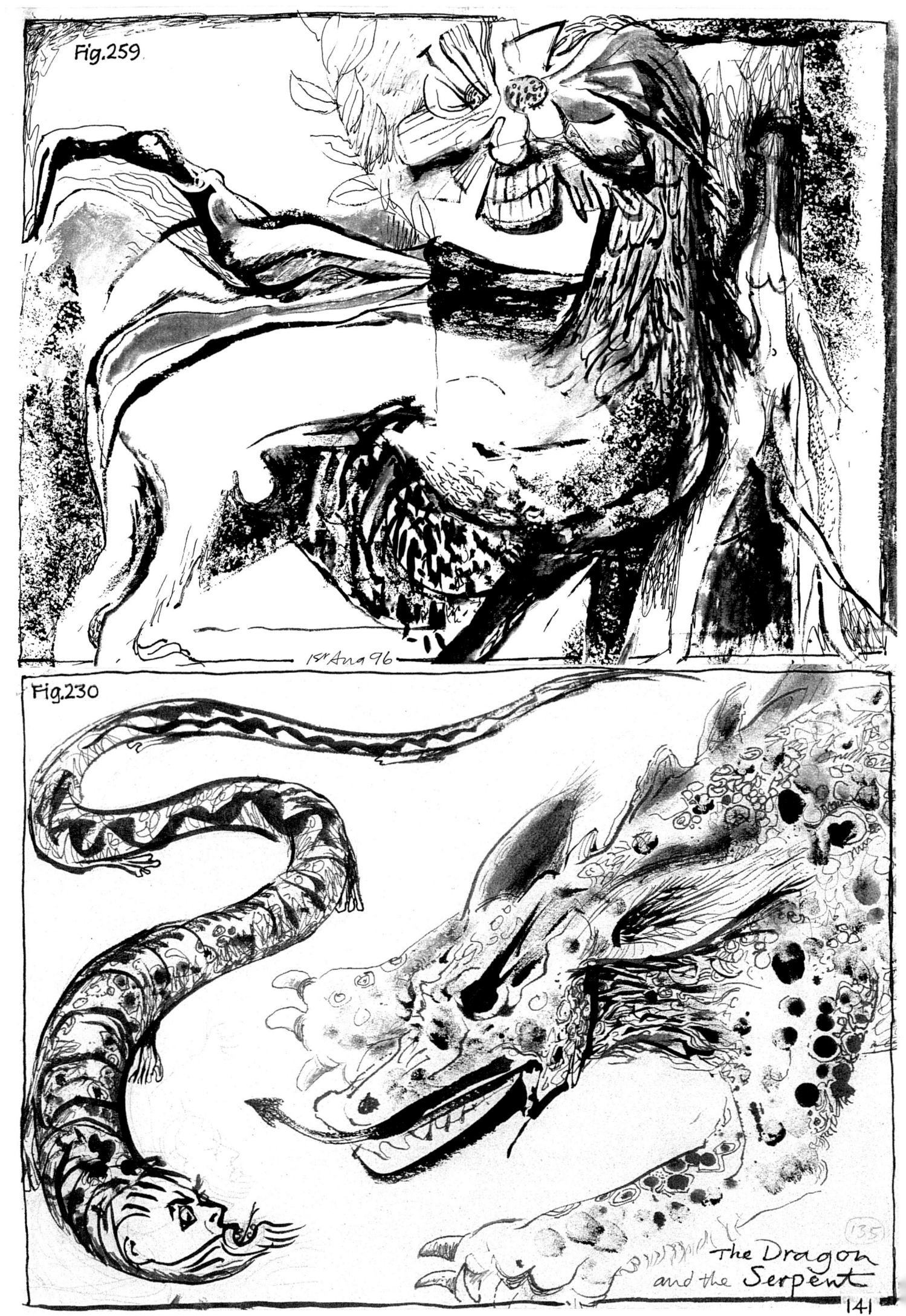

Fig.259

1st Aug 96

Fig.230

The Dragon and the Serpent

141

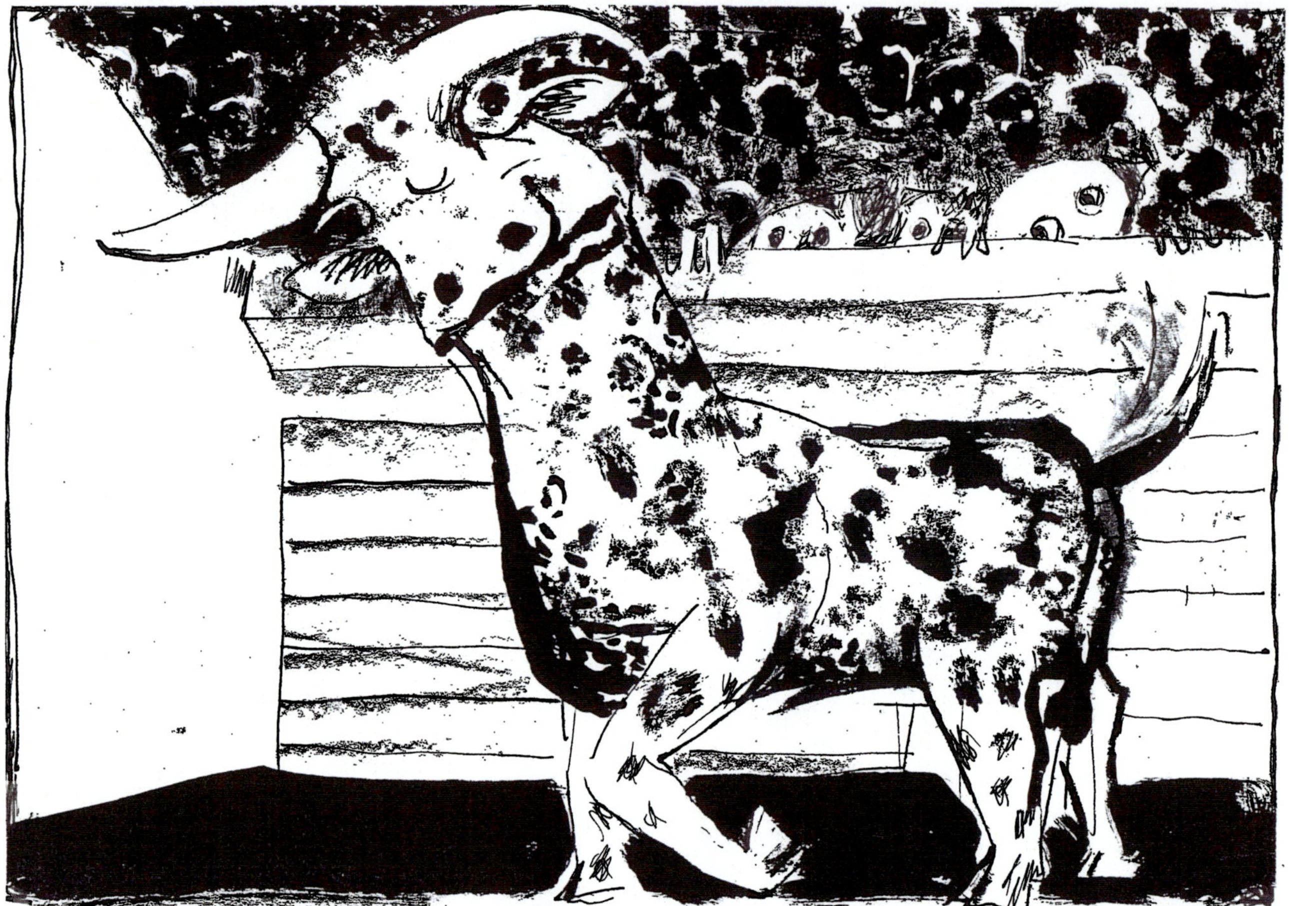

Fig.261 Pantomime Bull   Brush, Pen & Ink

Above: Fig.261 'Pantomime Bull'
The crowd beyond the stockade look on nervously at this aberration of a bull. There's the possibility of conflict between the two voices under the skin, and the worrying unpredictability of this idiot 'Pantomime' creature should he decide to 'let go' — and break out of the compound (bullring).

Right: Fig.262 'Pipe Player'
The horned creature sits on his mythical island, playing and comforting himself. He visualises Aphrodite in the distance, floating inland on a shell.

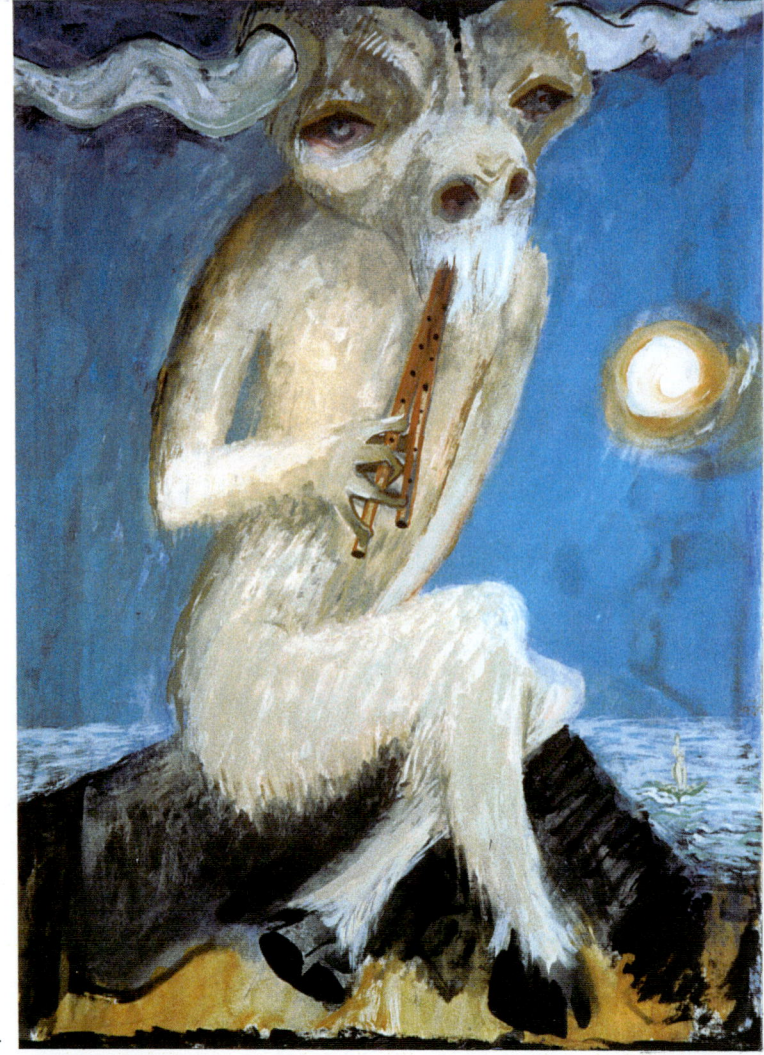

Fig.262 Pipe Player   Gouache

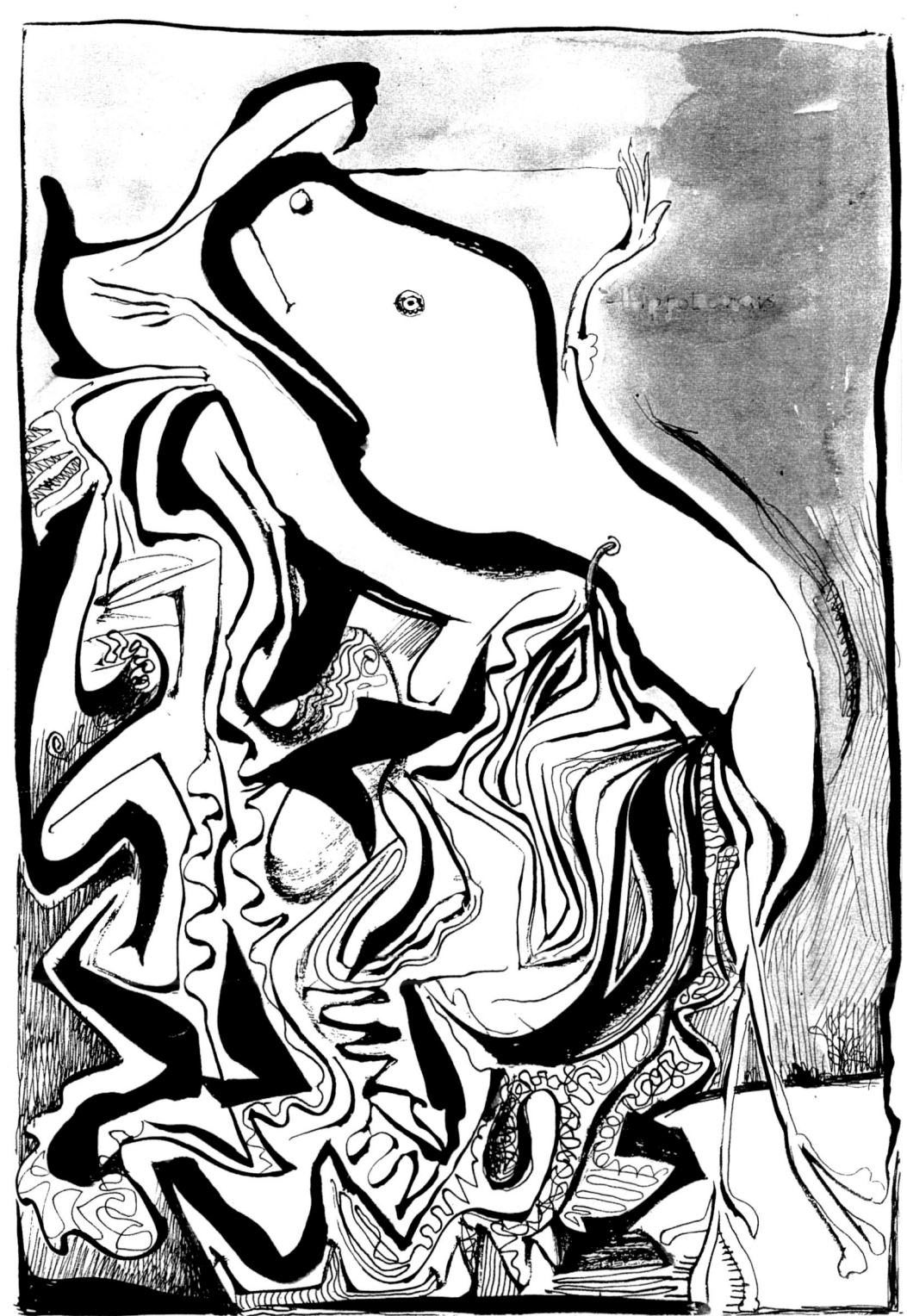

Fig. 263 Old Man with a Quiff   Calligraphic Brush, Pen & Wash

Above: Fig. 263 Old Man with a Quiff
As the ancient flesh sags and wrinkles, the old man's ideas and curiosity regenerate: his spirit — brings into existence through the force of his imagination a newly-formed creature.

Overleaf: Top. Fig. 264 The Guardian.
This neckless monster stands four square, guarding what? The way to the River Styx? Could he be the ferryman, Charon?

Overleaf: Bottom. Fig. 265 A Sea Rescue.
A many-rayed creature rescues a figure overwhelmed by waves of chaotic emotion.

143

Fig. 264   The Guardian   Mixed Media

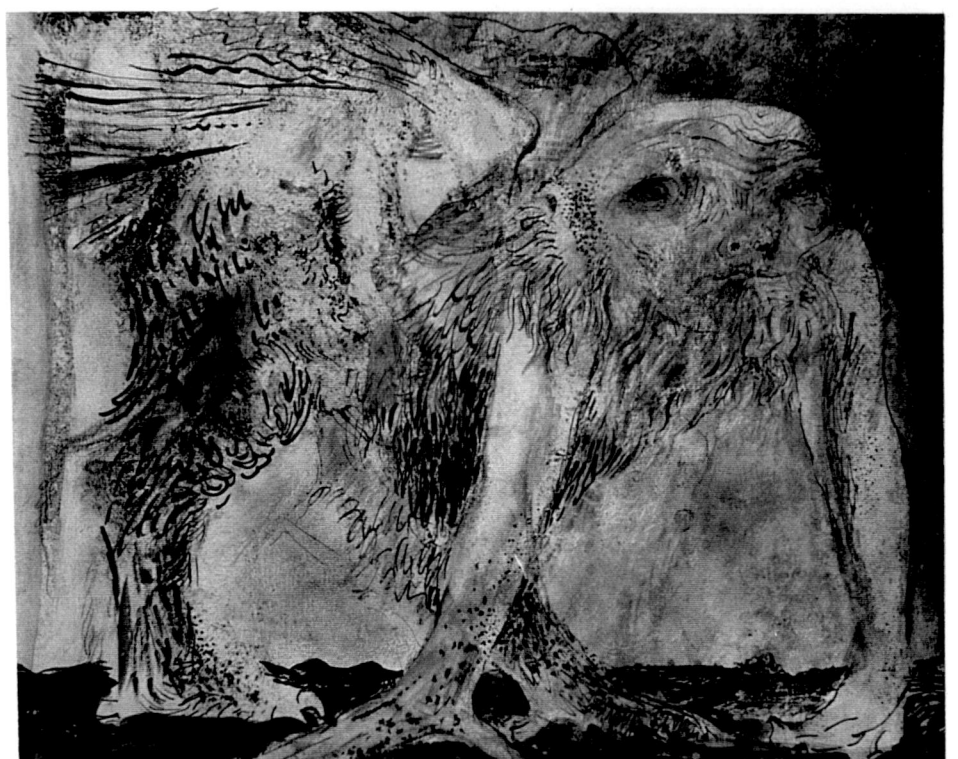

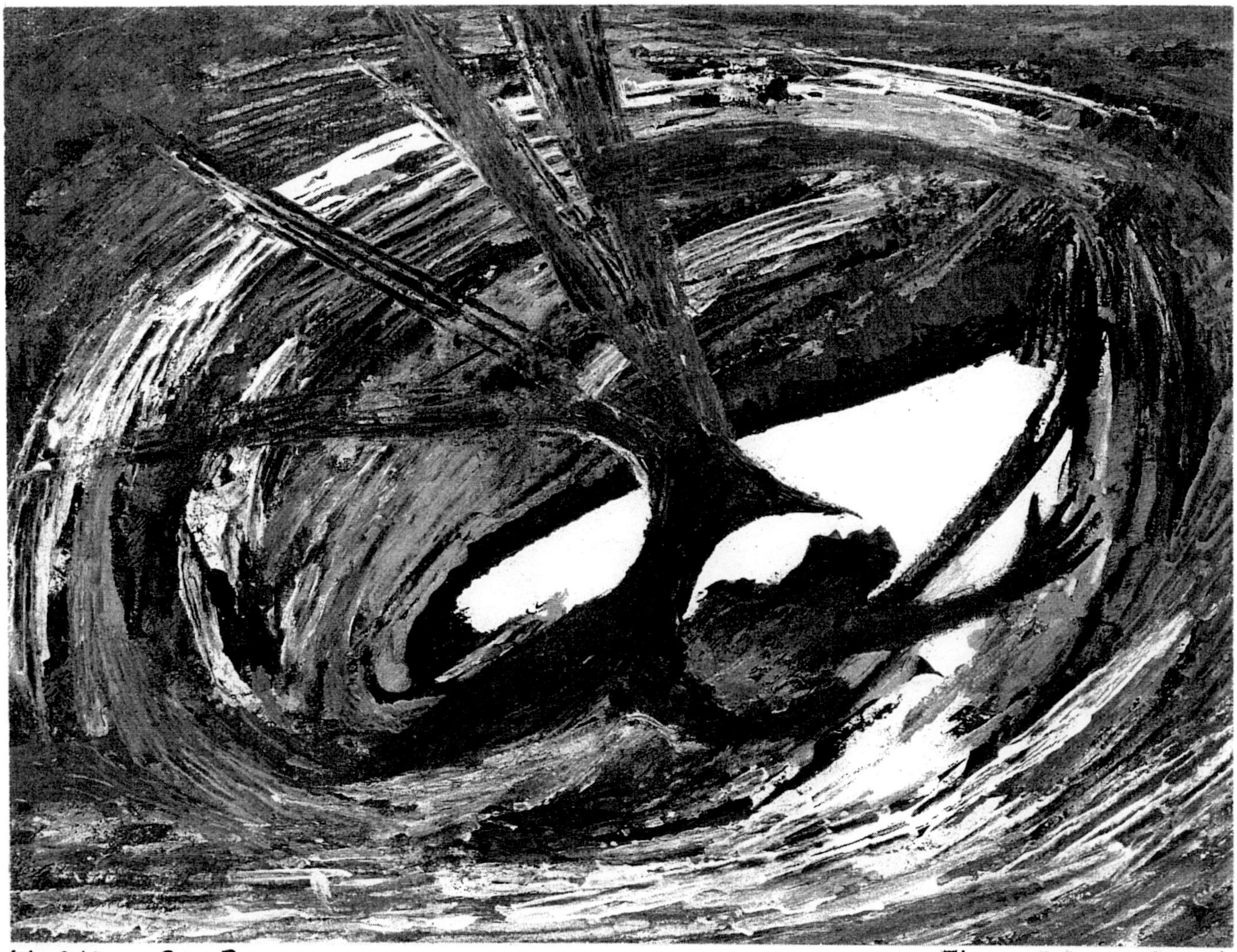

Fig. 265   Sea Rescue   Finger Paint & Brush

6 AN ABSENCE OF LIGHT

Dreams 38, 161   The Shadow Side

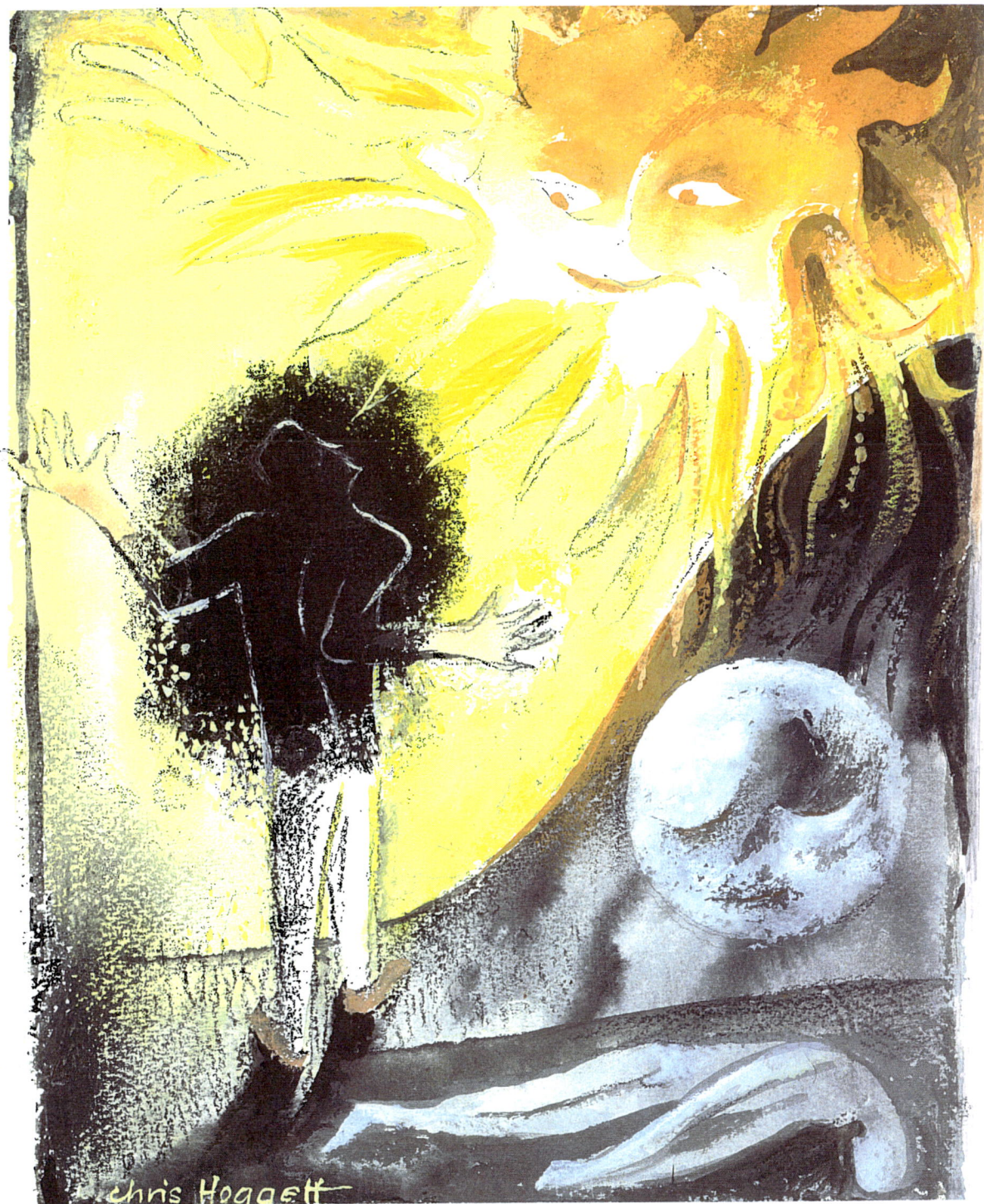

Fig. 266   Darkness at Noon   Chalk & Gouache

Darkness at Noon (fig. 266) touches on the overbearing weight of black depression, even during the brightest and sunniest of days – as well as moonlit nights.

Dream 38   The Black Swimming Pool. & **Dream 161** – The Dark Pit (overleaf)
These two dreams reflect some of the anxiety felt during the breakdown in 1980. This section also includes freestyle artwork which extends the material of the dreams, of attempting to reach out to some partial understanding of the personal fears of the shadow side. The figure clawing his way out of the abyss (overleaf, fig. 267) is the starting place. The Healing Place for Birdman an attempted resolution (fig. 278).

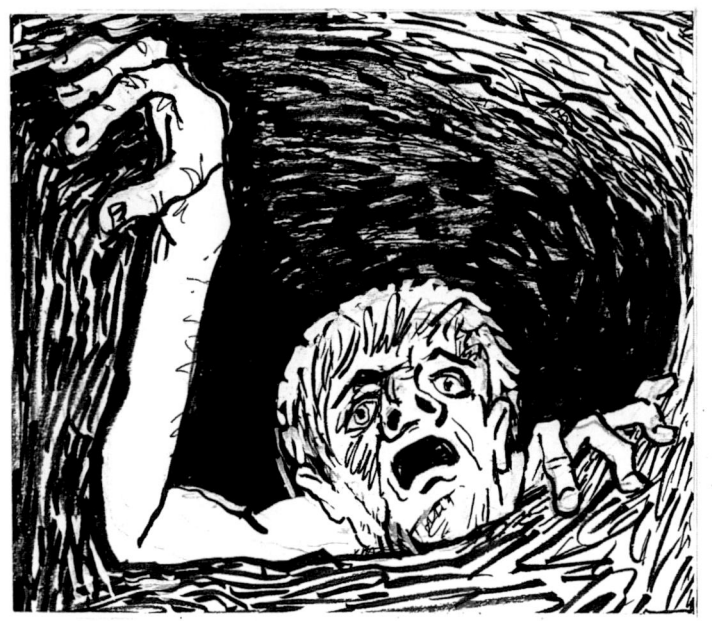

Fig. 267   The Abyss   Pen, Brush & Ink

Left: Fig. 267 'The Abyss'

Crawling out of the abyss — an interpretation of the fear of falling into an inner darkness. The first time this was experienced was on the day of the breakdown in 1980 (see fig. 26, page 16).

From this precursor, dreams like 'The Black Swimming Pool' (below) and 'The Dark Pit' (top right) evolved. Similar dream images seemed to occur at intervals, but these two were the only ones retained and recorded.

It seemed that from this point attempts were made to engage with the fear of the shadow side by using freestyle drawing and painting — some of which are illustrated in this section, e.g. 'The Dark Pool' (bottom right).

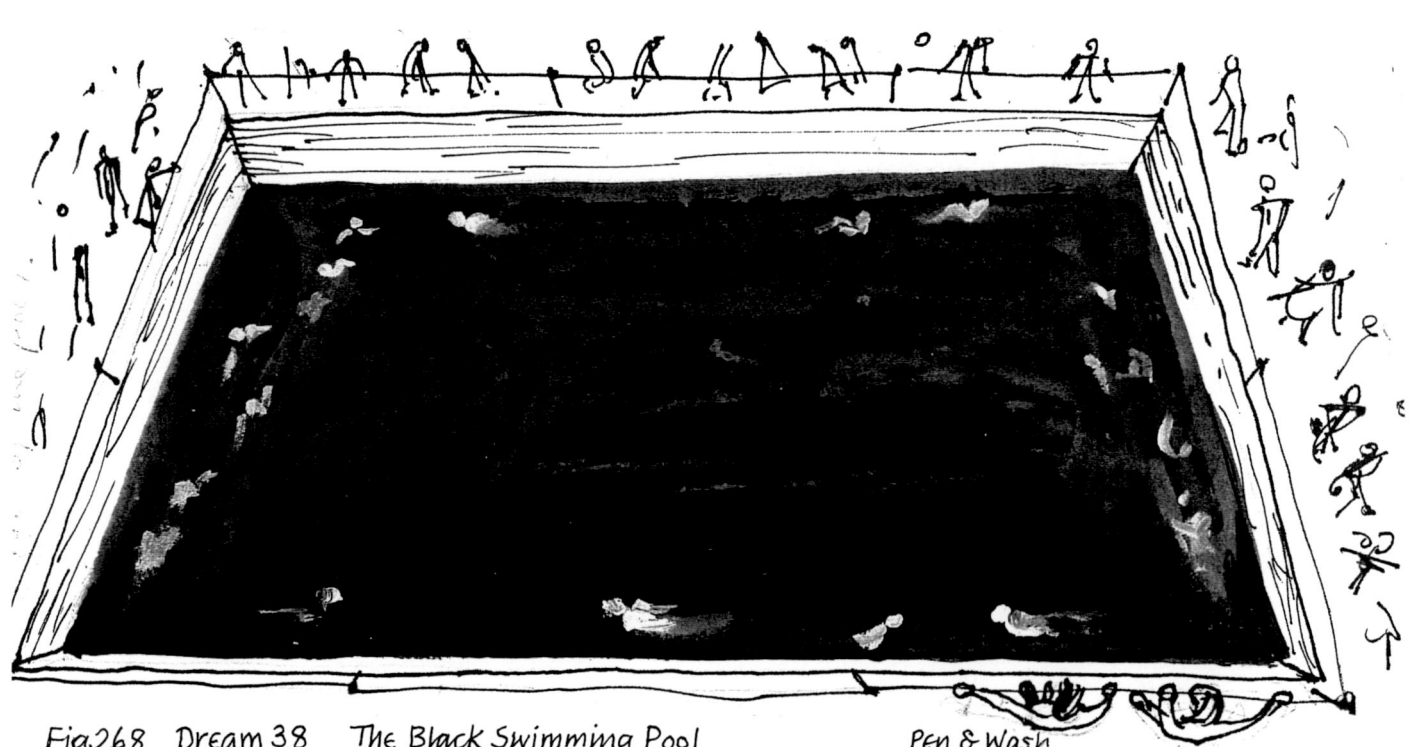

Fig. 268   Dream 38   The Black Swimming Pool   Pen & Wash

Dream 38   23 Sept 1990

Dream Text: A large rectangular black hole with white ceramic walls and a handrail along the edge. A number of intrepid swimmers cause me to turn to the director (from an earlier dream) as we lean against the rail. He tells me it is perfectly clean but for city dust at the bottom. I tell him I can't swim in such darkness. Lacking the courage to take a dip I'm reminded of other dark places, lakes, holes, especially in the Lake District which I find terrifying. Just contemplating swimming there is bad enough. I reflect on my own 'black hole'.

Comment: Reflects the most haunting of the fears which assailed me during the 'breakout' of emotions in 1980s. Looking at one's own dark place was intolerable and terrifying. Perhaps the dream imagery was offering up a challenge to take a leap — this was to be partially resolved in a later painting (Fig. 276 'Antipodian Dive' on page 151).

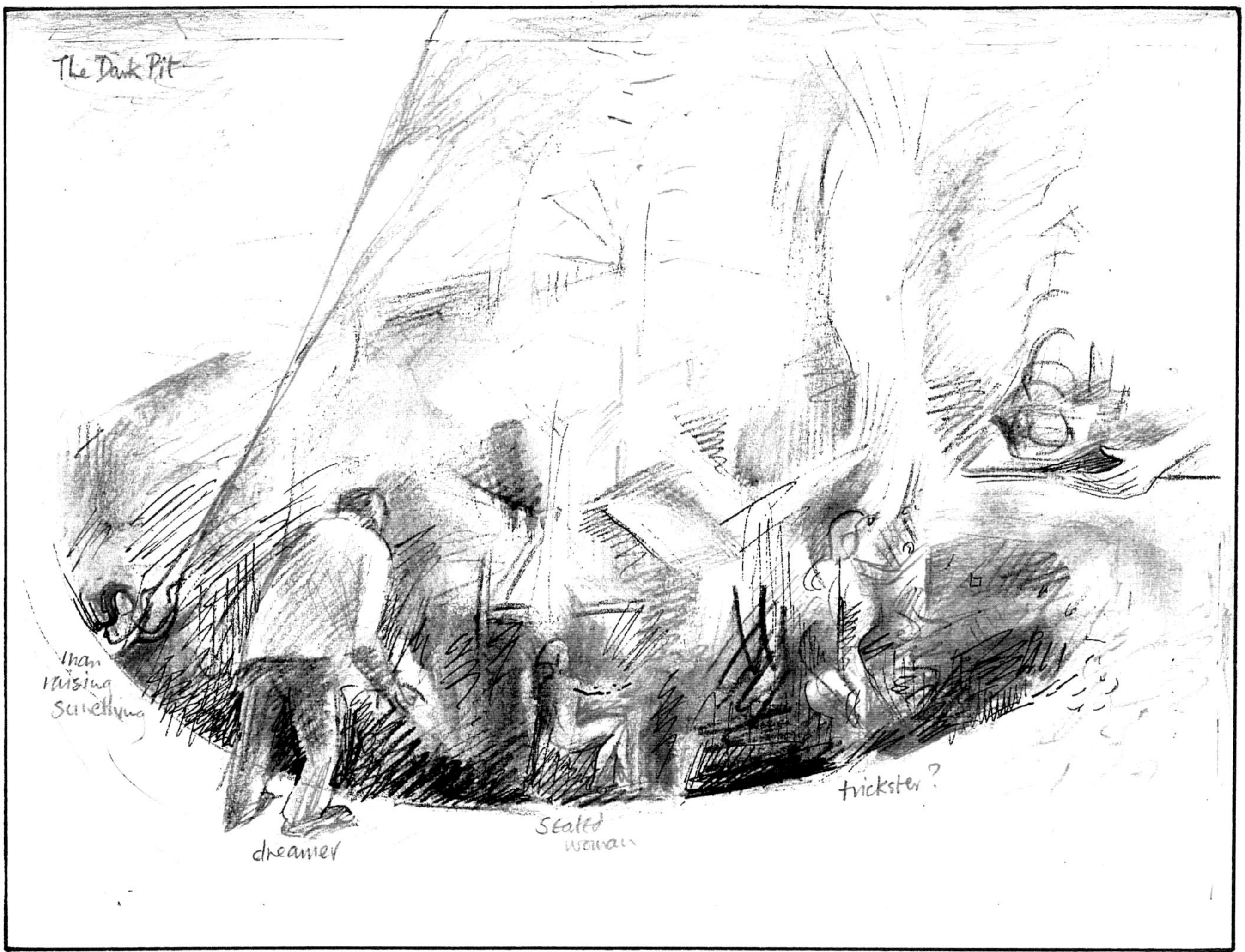

Fig. 269 Dream 161 The Dark Pit   Aquarelle Pencil, Pen & Ink

Dream 161 27 May 1992
Standing at the edge of a smouldering dust-laden, dark pit. Two persons below insist work has to be done. The man to the left is shuffling about, raising and lowering apparent 'emptiness'. He says things are lying about which need to be dealt with.

The seated woman in the central area is working at something, but it remains vague. A more shadowy presence operates within the right side – perhaps a 'trickster'. Later a black object is put on a window ledge above the pit by a (female?) hand. It contains information but, as the observer looks, it starts to levitate and move off, out of reach.

Comment: Looking more closely into the hole than Dream 38, yet I feel anxious about stepping down or leaping into this dark place – but I may soon follow those already 'working' there

'The Dark Pool' - No 1 (Fig. 270. right)
The reclining figure becomes his own black pool, yet looks aside, as if mildly indifferent, as his manikin 'spirit' plunges off into the depths.

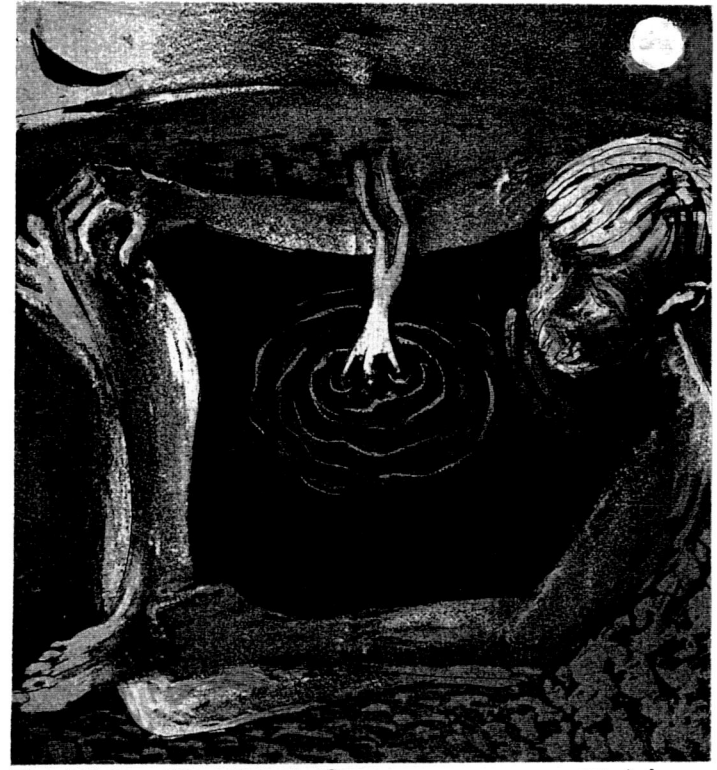

Fig. 270 The Dark Pool   Etching

147

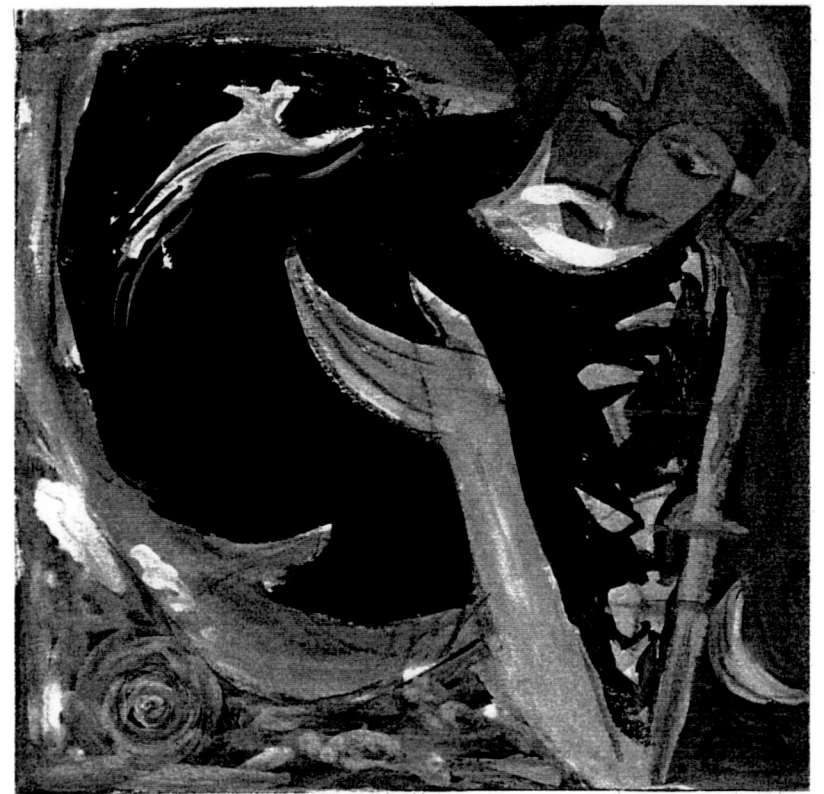

Left: Fig.271 'The Dark Pool N°2'. Again the 'father figure' opens up his blackness and allows the spirit to dive and swim about. But now he offers a concerned and caring gesture, his hand offering assistance into the 'harbour'.

Below: Fig.272 'Floating with the Tide'. Here the dreamer allows himself to be swept away with the tide, crossing from the darkness of the night towards the rays of the morning sun.

Fig.271 The Dark Pool N°2   Gouache

Fig.272 Floating with the Tide   Chalk & Watercolour

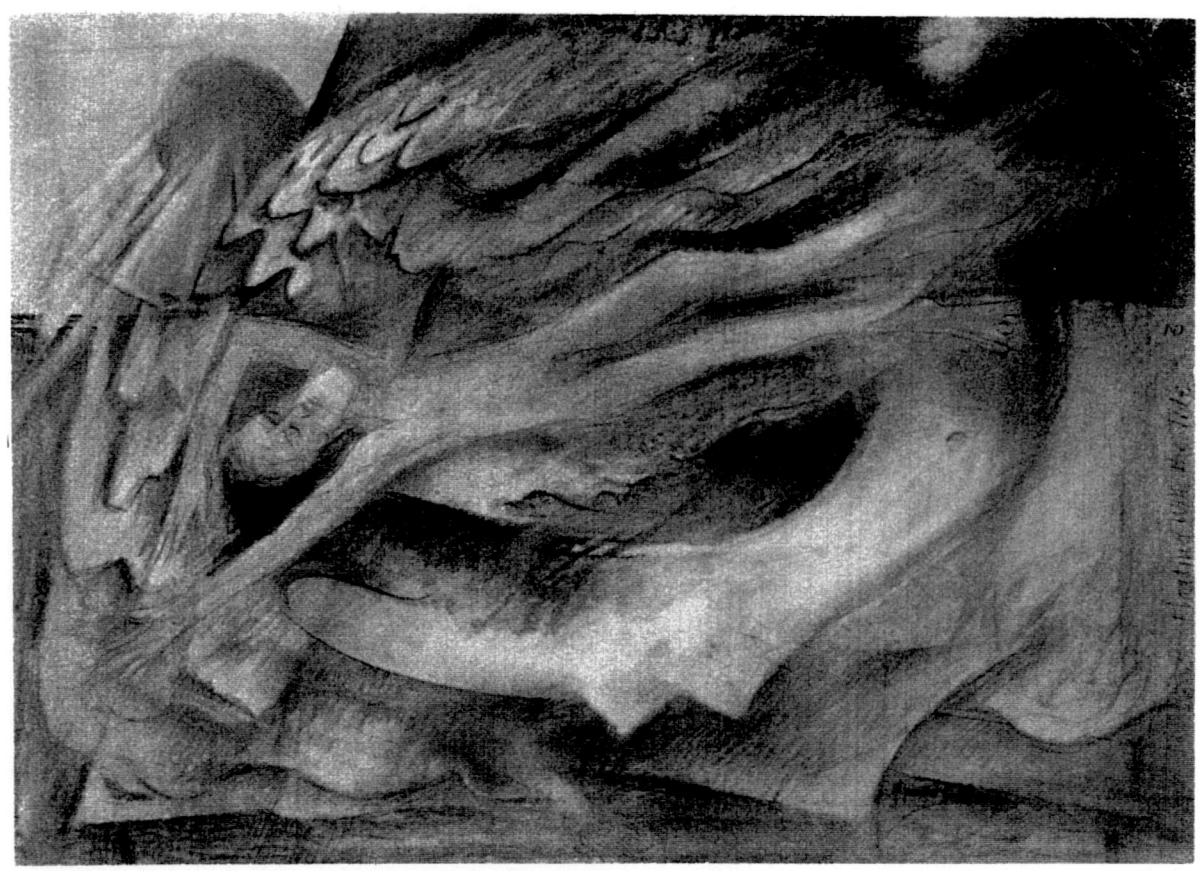

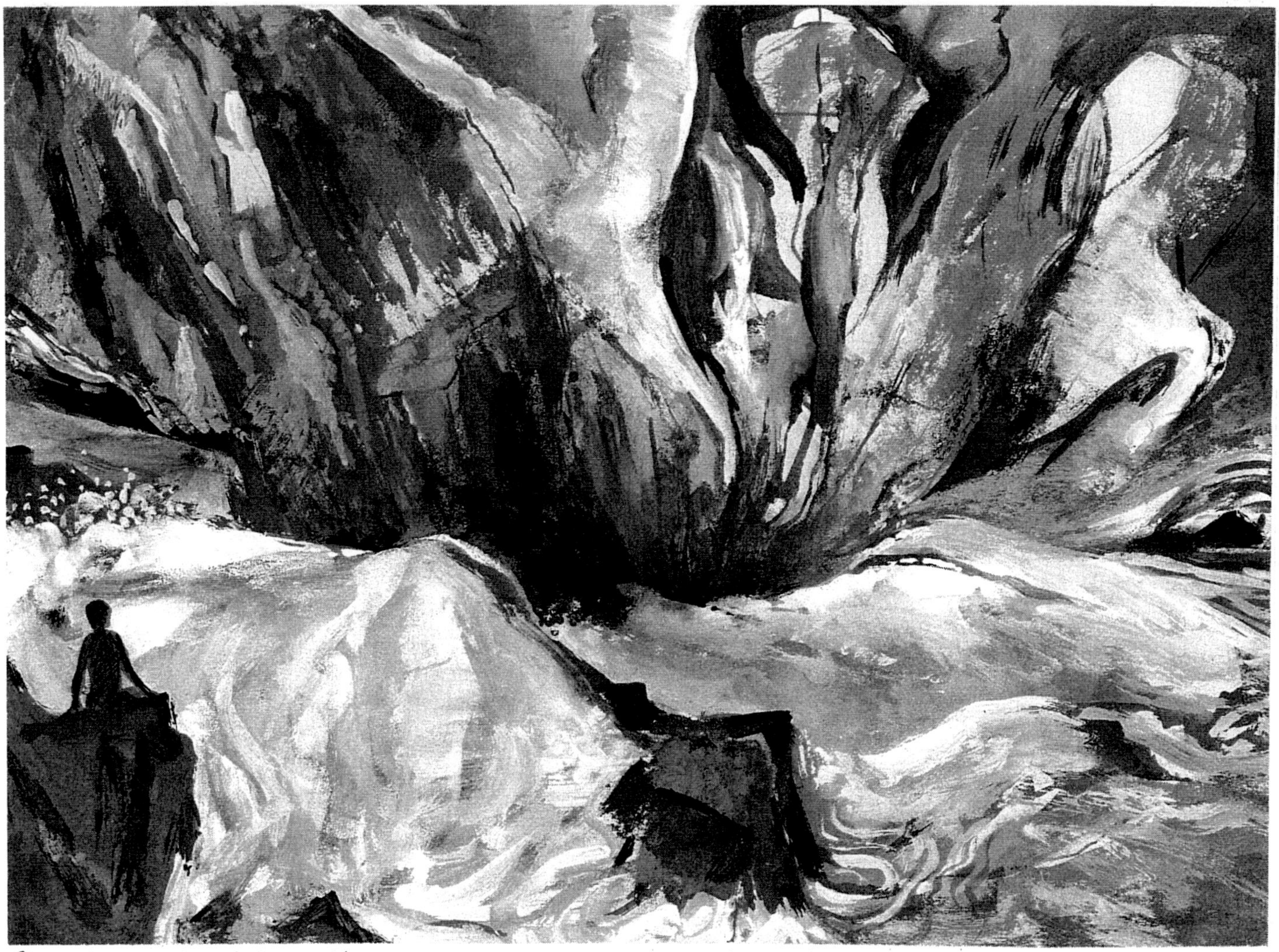

Fig. 273   The Watery Abyss   Gouache

Above: Fig. 273 'The Watery Abyss'
After painting in New Zealand during 1995 and 1996 (see Part Four), various kinds of water formations and movements began to obsess me. Lakes, rivers, estuaries and especially waterfalls. Later, many freestyle drawings based on the latter were developed — similar to the 'Abyss'. Sometimes rocks and water transformed into feminine forms and these led down into 'the deeps' — and I found my 'child' would be watching intensely.

Right: Fig. 274 'Untitled'
Taking the idea further, the waterfall is made up entirely of the female nude; the watching boy becomes an elderly man standing in pit (daring himself to leap?)

Looking back a number of years it is possible now to see how the actual attempts at drawing these images, turned them into the chimeras they now can be seen to have been.

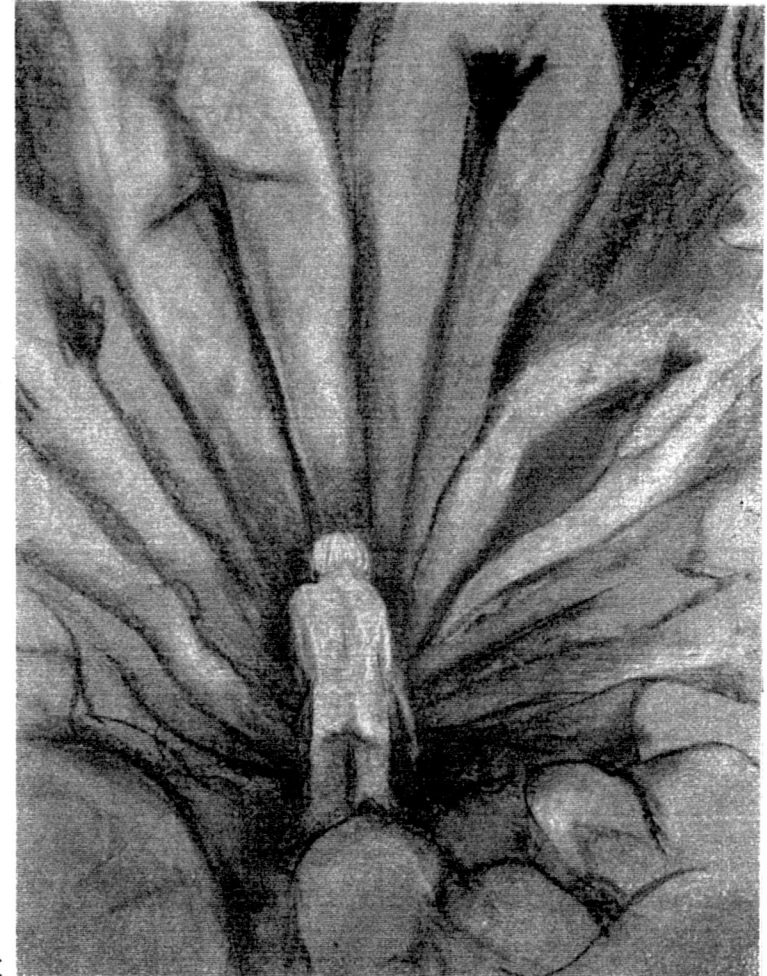

Fig. 274 Untitled   Coloured Chalk

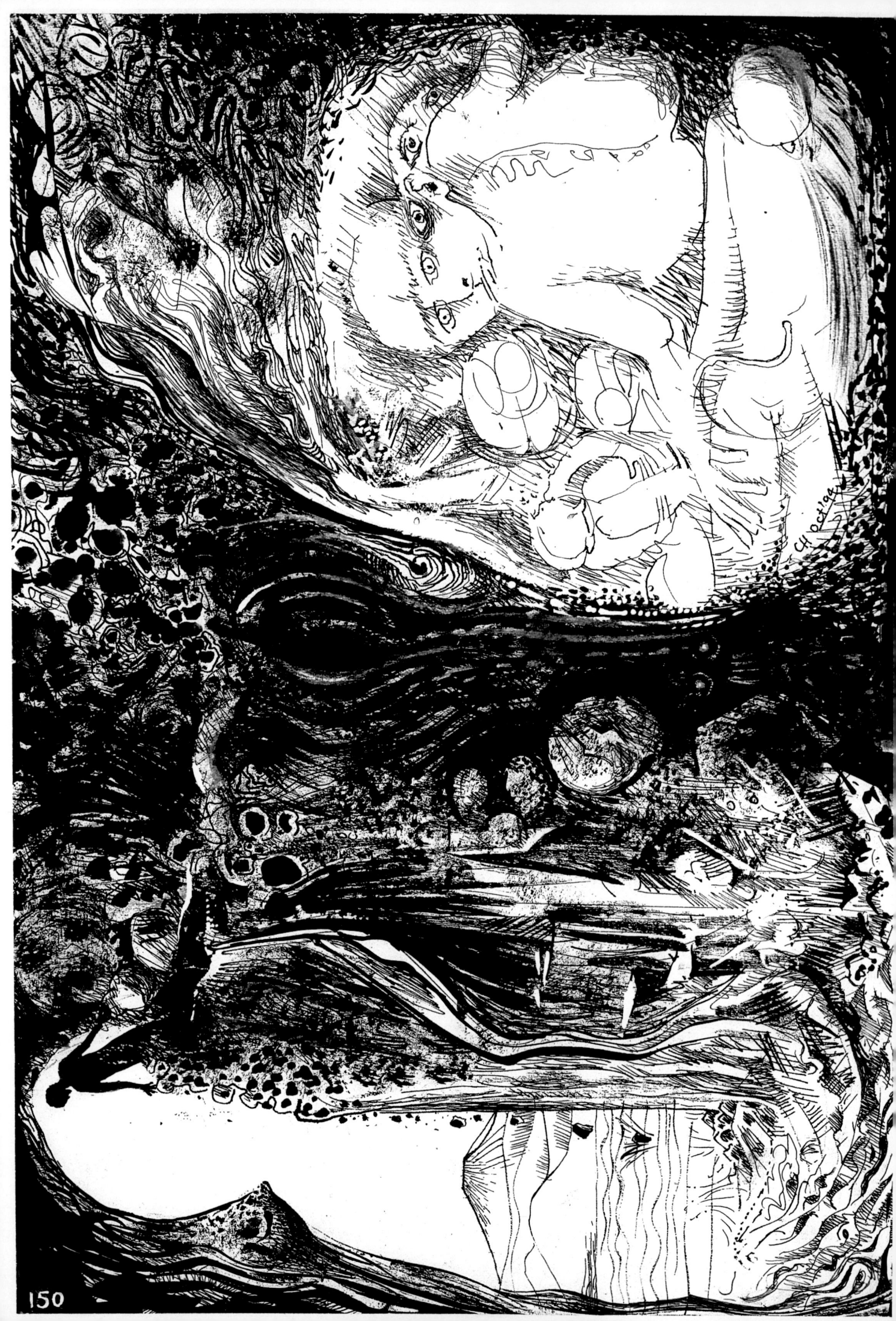

Above: Fig.275 'The Cavern'. Some months before setting off for New Zealand I'd worked on freestyle artwork anticipating the adventure. Contemplating the possibility of change whilst on the tour I saw myself exploring the dark – the unknown – and in this drawing show the birthing place for new ideas if I'm prepared to venture enough.

Below Left: Poem – The Black Pool. Going on a poetry weekend for the first time I decide to continue on the darkness theme. Feeling daunted by many experienced participants, the 'elders' are included in the poem.

Below Right: Fig.276 'Antipodean Dive'. Following the poetry weekend this oil painting attempted to convey the unknown beyond that 'slither of black' – the writing in the painting reads – "Dive up to the far side, an Antipodean Viewpoint".

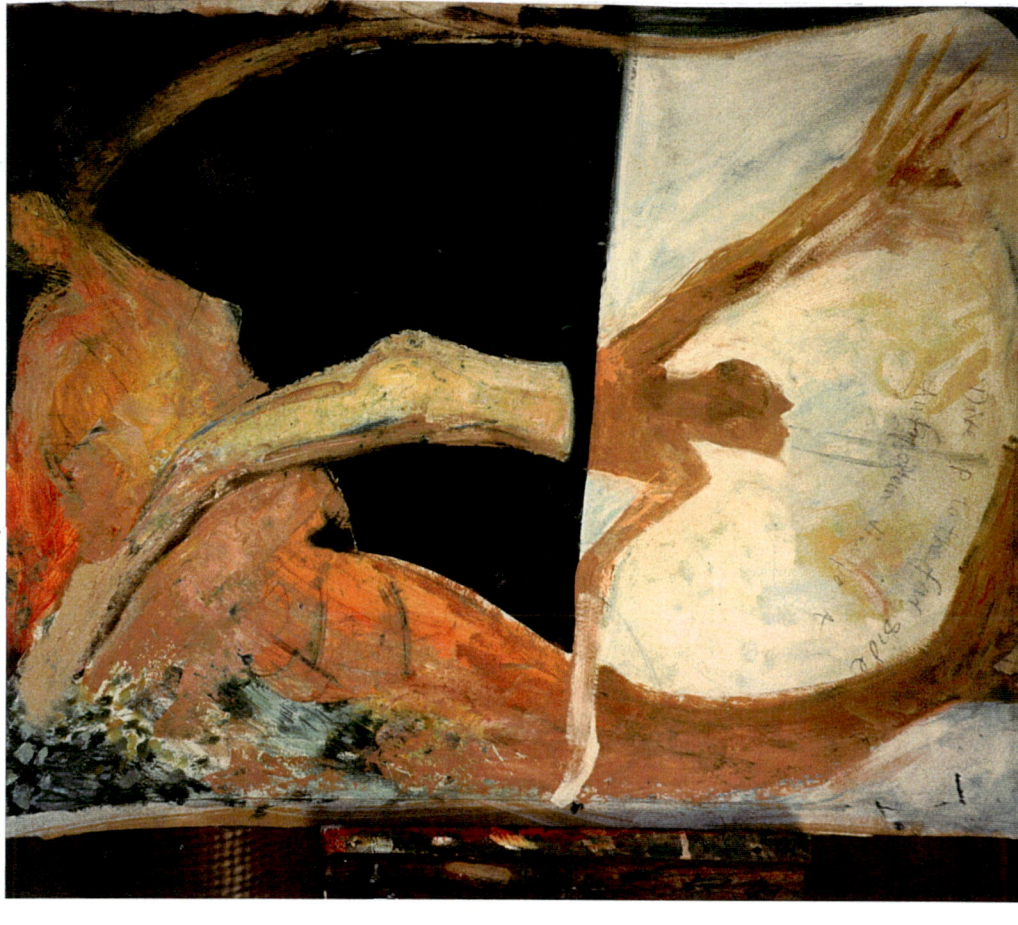

Fig.276   Antipodean Dive   Acrylic

The Black Pool
A Baptism

He knew this was the time.
Just three days, flick, flick, flick.
Old movie style.

In the dreamtime it came in many guises.
Lying just beneath the carpet, antipodean depths,
Slow dissolve to
An ominous rectangular pitch,
Then giant amoeba-like holes.

Entering the valley, mountain-bound,
A slither of sheer black lay before him.
Meld with lampblack and ultramarine,
Not a ripple to make a liquid of it.

The elders, initiations long past,
Gathered at the rim, heads raised.
Watched him leap from a high place,
Flicker out, in slow motion.

One frame at a time,
White flesh coming to kiss
Surface of blackness, until
Finger-touching point–
The membrane gave.

The diver's wrist, elbows, then head
Slipped through,
Flick, flick, flick, to
Final flash of feet.

No great splash,
Rather an environmental change,
Rite of passage, baptismal moment.

5th June 1994

151

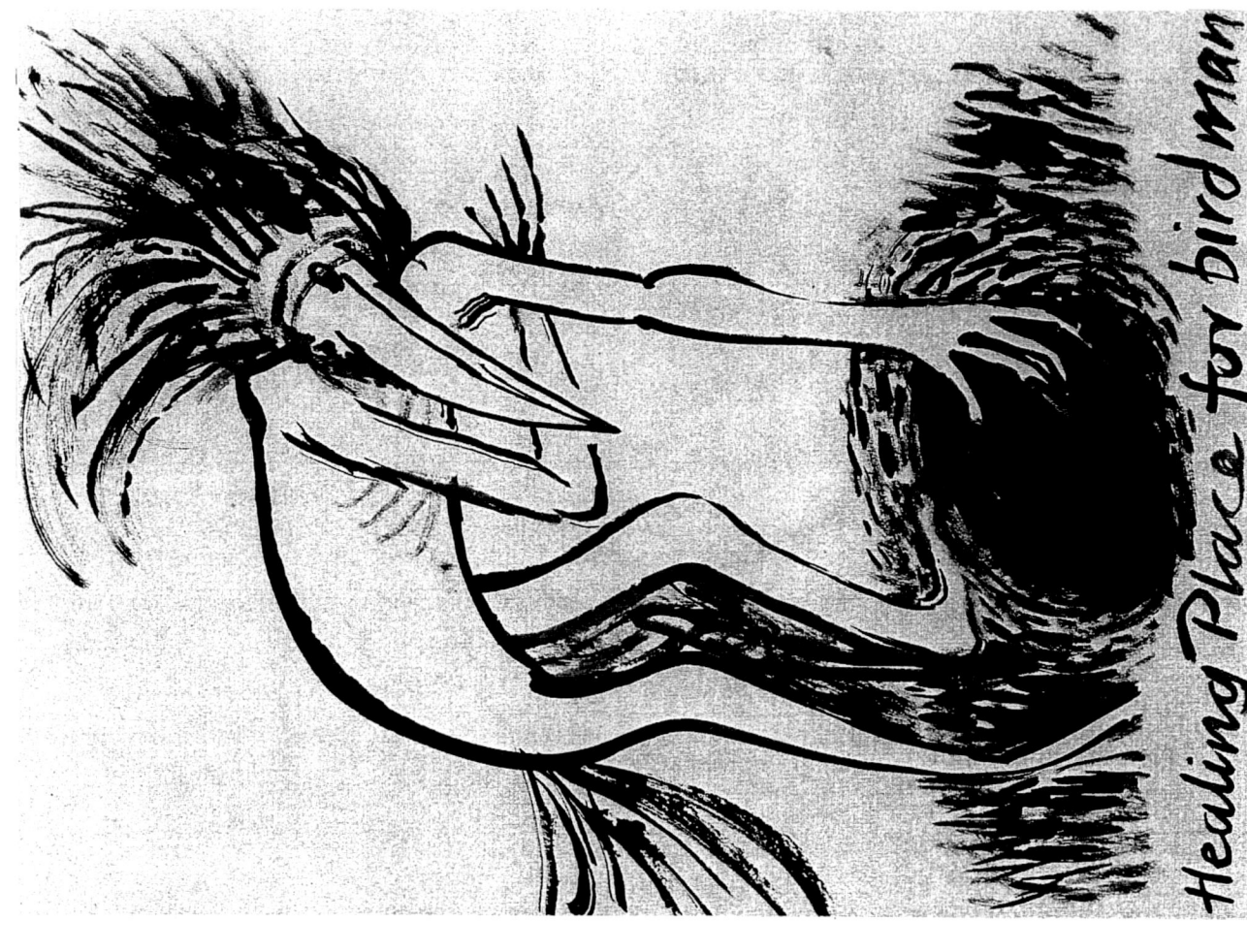

Fig. 278 Healing Place for Birdman   Brush & Black Paint

Fig. 277 Entrance to 'Collins Drive'   Pen & Wash

Above: Fig. 277
The culmination and passing of the 'inner dark' was reached after venturing deep into this old goldmine in New Zealand. It seemed as if Reality was imitating Art in the sense that 'The Cavern' (fig. 275) was the precursor to the actual experience of entering this deep hole. Instead of the 'babes' I discovered a galaxy of glowworms. See the New Zealand interlude in 'Part Four' for a detailed account.

Right: Fig. 278 'Healing Place for Birdman'
The black hole, once the Place of greatest fear is now the centre of attention. That which was most feared becomes a cleansing place, a creative healing place.

7 METAMORPHOSIS

Dreams 64, 67, 83, 134   Growth and Transformation

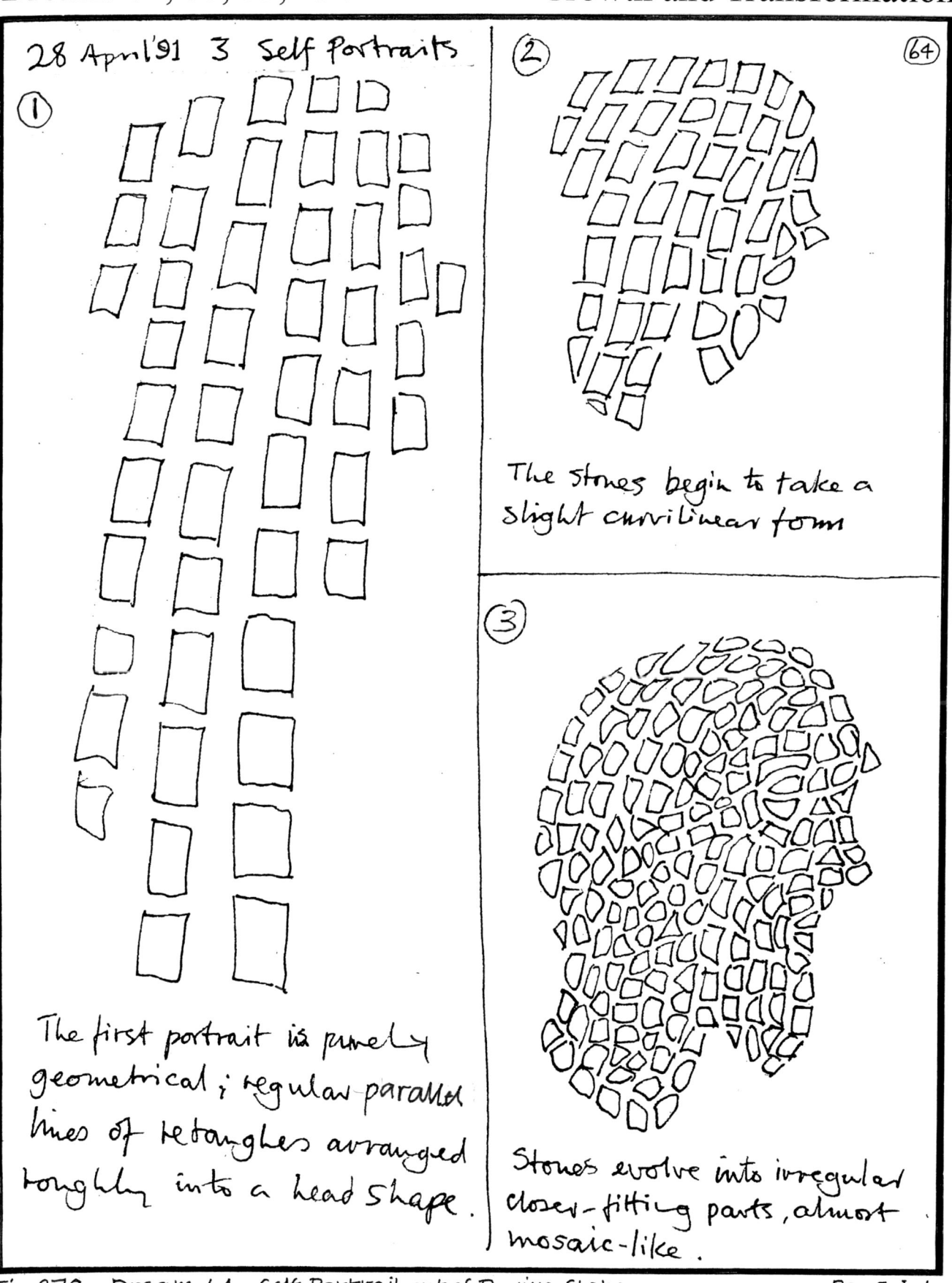

Fig. 279   Dream 64   Self Portrait out of Paving Slabs   Pen & Ink

Dream 64 28 April 1991 & Dream 67 13 May 1991

Dreams 64 and 67 were the first intimations I felt that concentrated on a progressive change of the image. In Fig. 279 - (overleaf) a group of three drawings moved from geometrical/abstract towards a partial realism. Figs 280 and 281 were more figurative and involved the whole body, not just the head. Here, the artist himself makes an appearance as a very angry scribbler with a pencil in hand, 're-working' himself through another group of three images, until he seems to recline along a diagonal line as if content with his efforts.

These dream offerings seemed to open a way towards the conscious, daytime 'freestyle' work which followed. These drawings and paintings pursued the idea of change in portraiture and figure. Initially, having collected these together to accompany the dreams, I'd thought how fragmentary they appeared, that they lacked coherence of any kind - were 'falling apart'. Yet gradually as I started to write

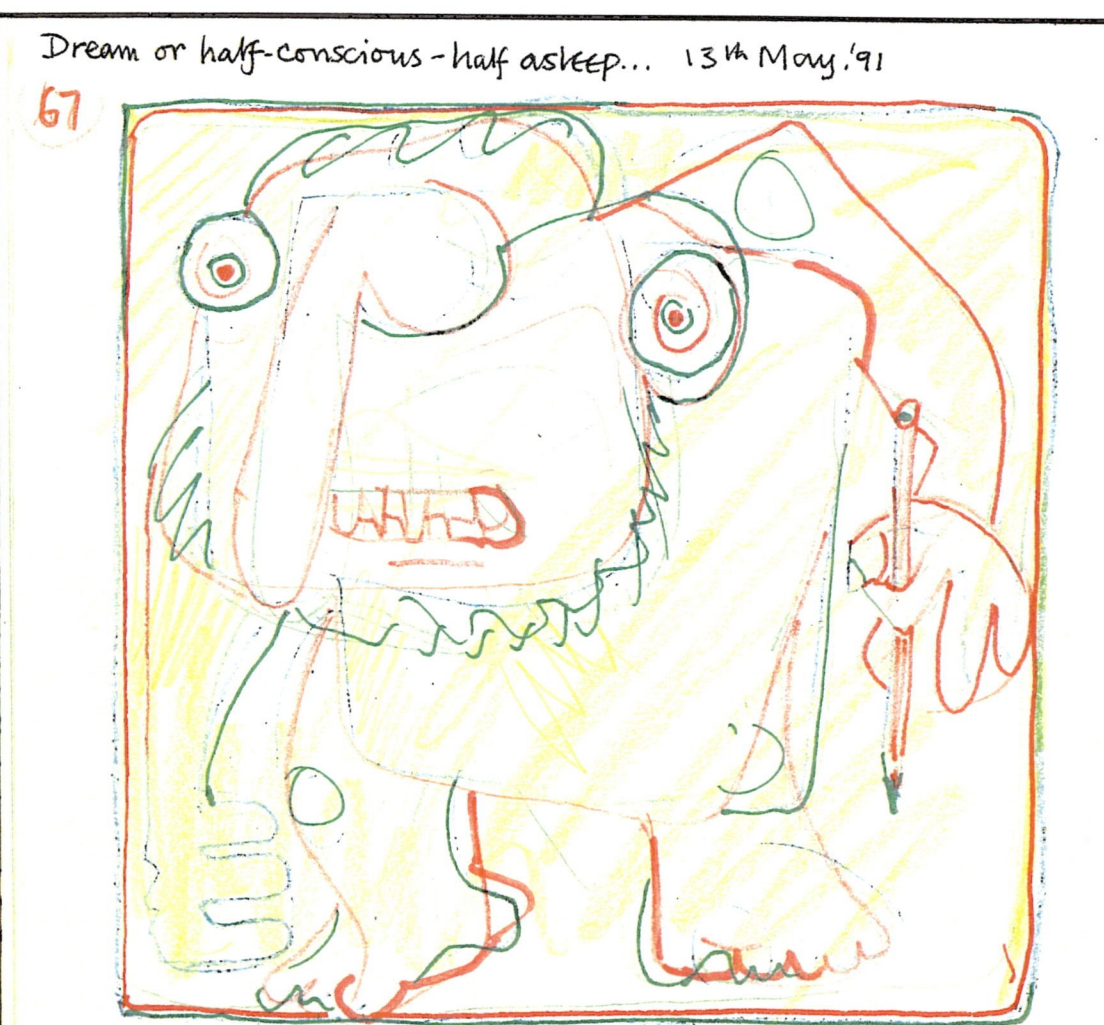

Dream or half-conscious - half asleep... 13th May '91

A loose line drawing as if drawn with coloured crayons. Aware of dissatisfaction with size of head - too large. At same time I've a tummy ache. Holding some kind of drawing tool - brush or pencil. Decide to destroy the image by using a vigorous, angry zig-zag scribble across the shape, noticing that the tool

Fig. 280 Dream 67, part one   Crayons

about them and looked carefully from image to image, the contrary view took hold — perhaps I was looking at a 'coming together' of apparent fragments — a conclusion which implied 'wholeness' as its goal.

stays within the contours, pushing them around without scattering the parts:—
The outline of the head changes shape as each zigzag strikes the edges without breaking the line.

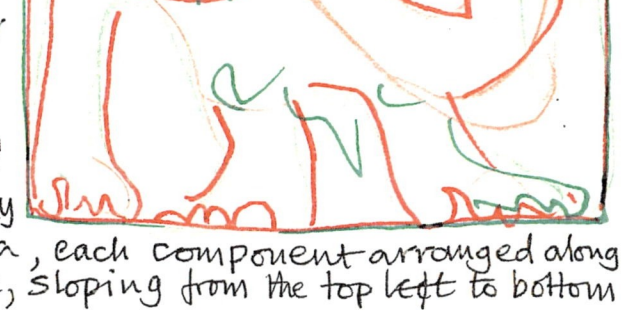

Following on from this angry-frustrated angular scribble I'm aware of the image rearranging itself. It has its own 'logic' — its own creative assembly with a smaller head area, each component arranged along a kind of diagonal line, sloping from the top left to bottom right (dotted line)

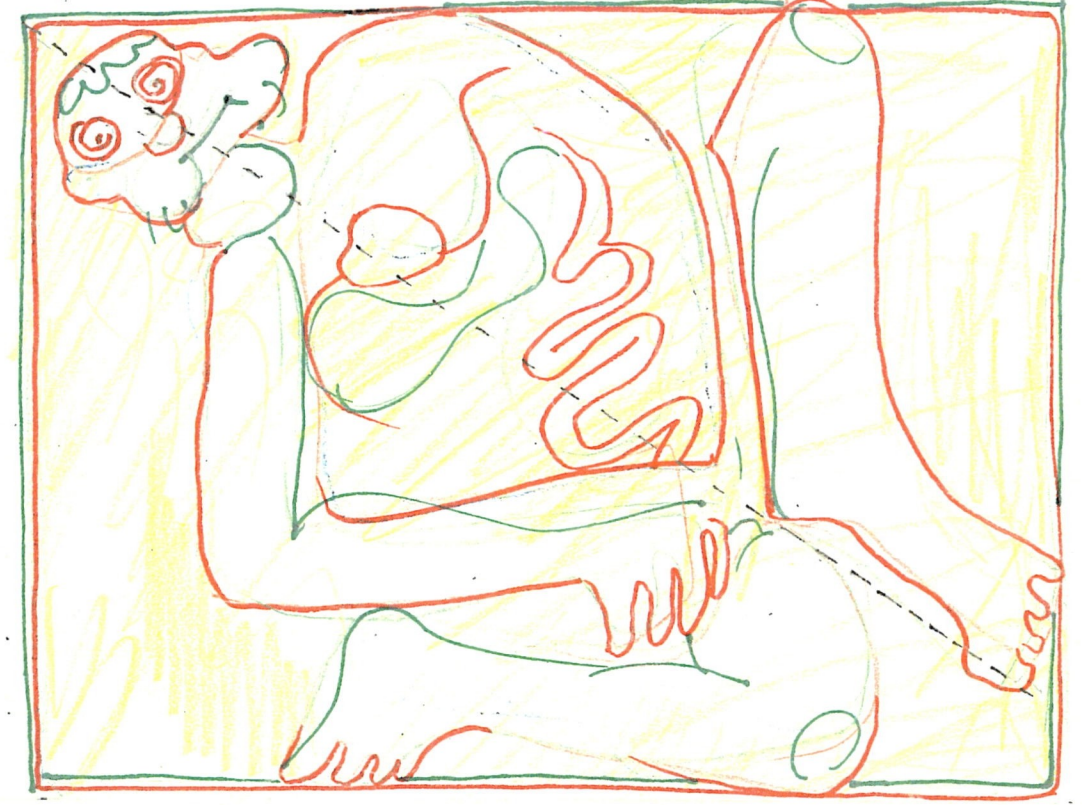

Looking at the image I'm reminded of medical diagrams showing internal organs

Fig. 281   Dream 67, parts two and three   Crayons

Top Right: Fig.283 'Reaching Out'

Structured on a pyramidal shape with the head as its apex, two assertive arms stretch out, dominating the other parts. Head and feet look and move forward, emphasising the search for something. The torso seems absent, unless its presence is hinted at in a plasma-like substance trailing midway to the right side.

Bottom Right: Fig.284 'Woman with a Little Monster'

A standing figure of a woman glances over her shoulder as if disturbed by some unknown presence. A large head, teeth bared, within a TV screen, 'glowers' behind her. In this freestyle drawing there seems, within this random doodling, to be a quest for an understanding of this juxtaposition. A need for the monstrous, balanced by the fear of it perhaps?

Below: Fig.282. 'Fragments before Assembly'

In contrast to 'Reaching Out' (fig.283), all is calmness and order. A neat array of bones and arms, hands, legs and a somewhat inscrutable mask-like face await 'assembly'. Why the body parts should be separated is unknown. Every part seems to be waiting in suspension — a state of expectation, of looking as it were for an instruction manual before the body can be reconstructed.

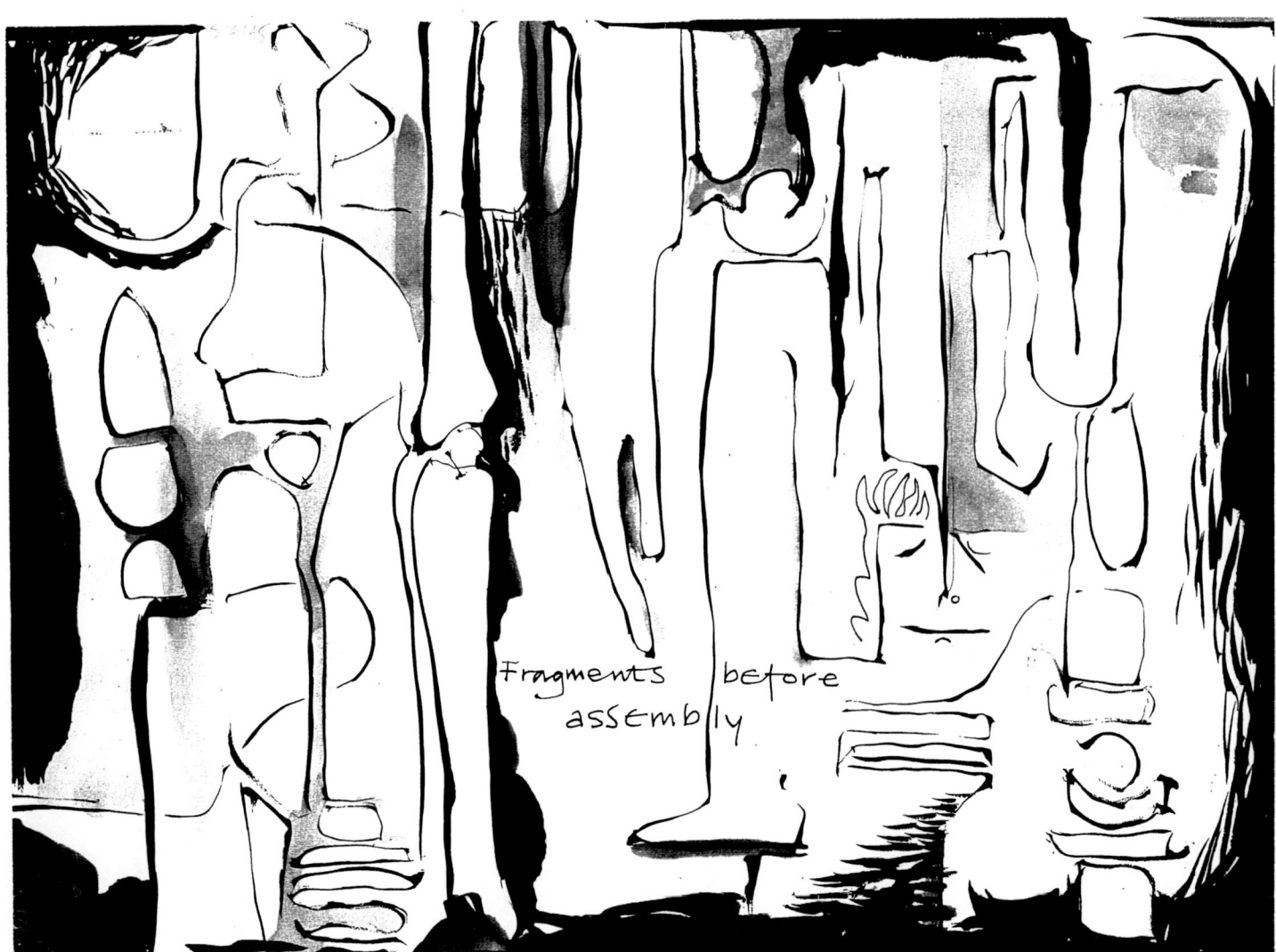

Fig. 282   Fragments before Assembly   Pen, Brush and Ink

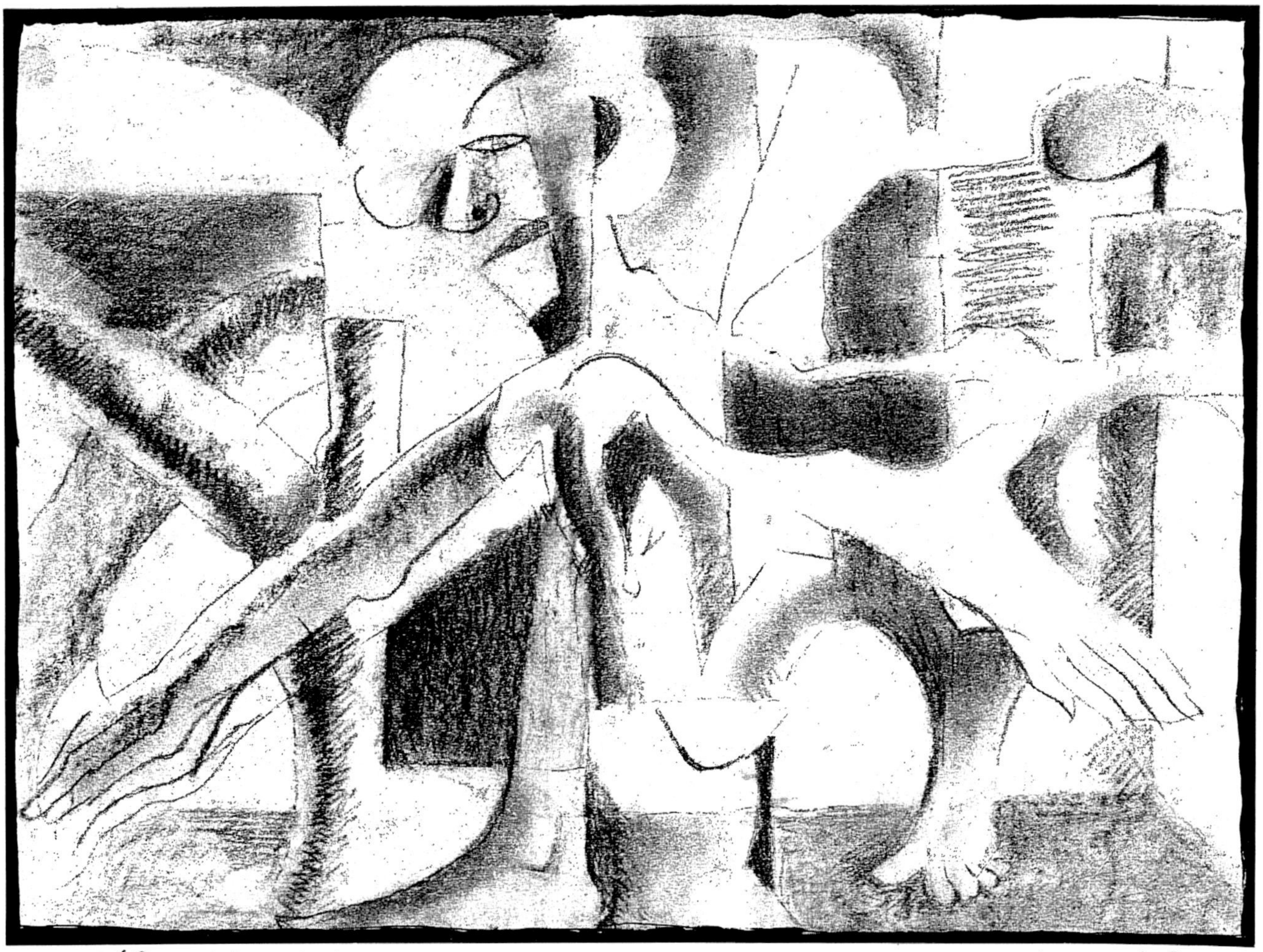

Fig.283 'Reaching Out' — Charcoal Pencil

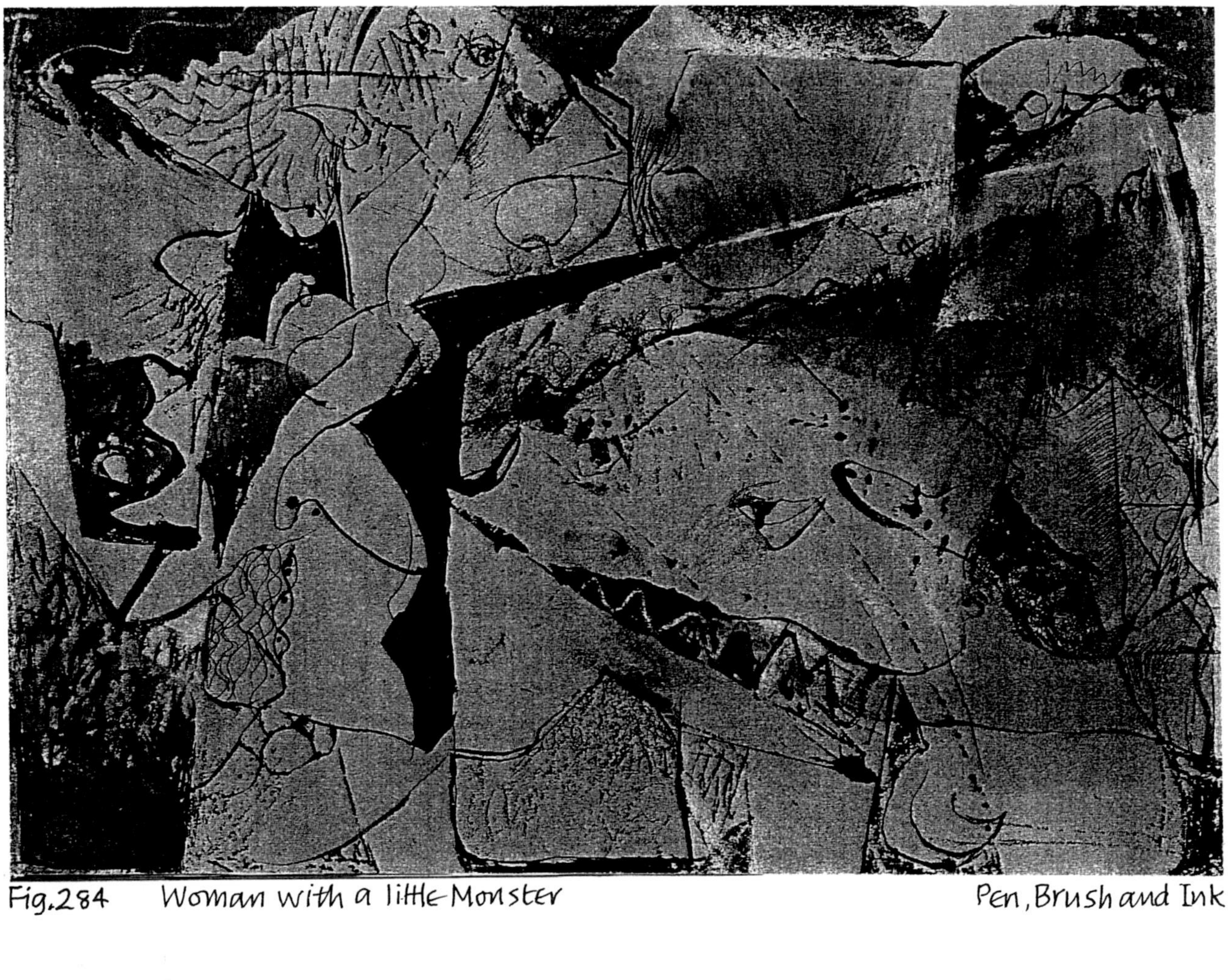

Fig.284 Woman with a little Monster — Pen, Brush and Ink

SELF-PORTRAITS IN VARIOUS GUISES

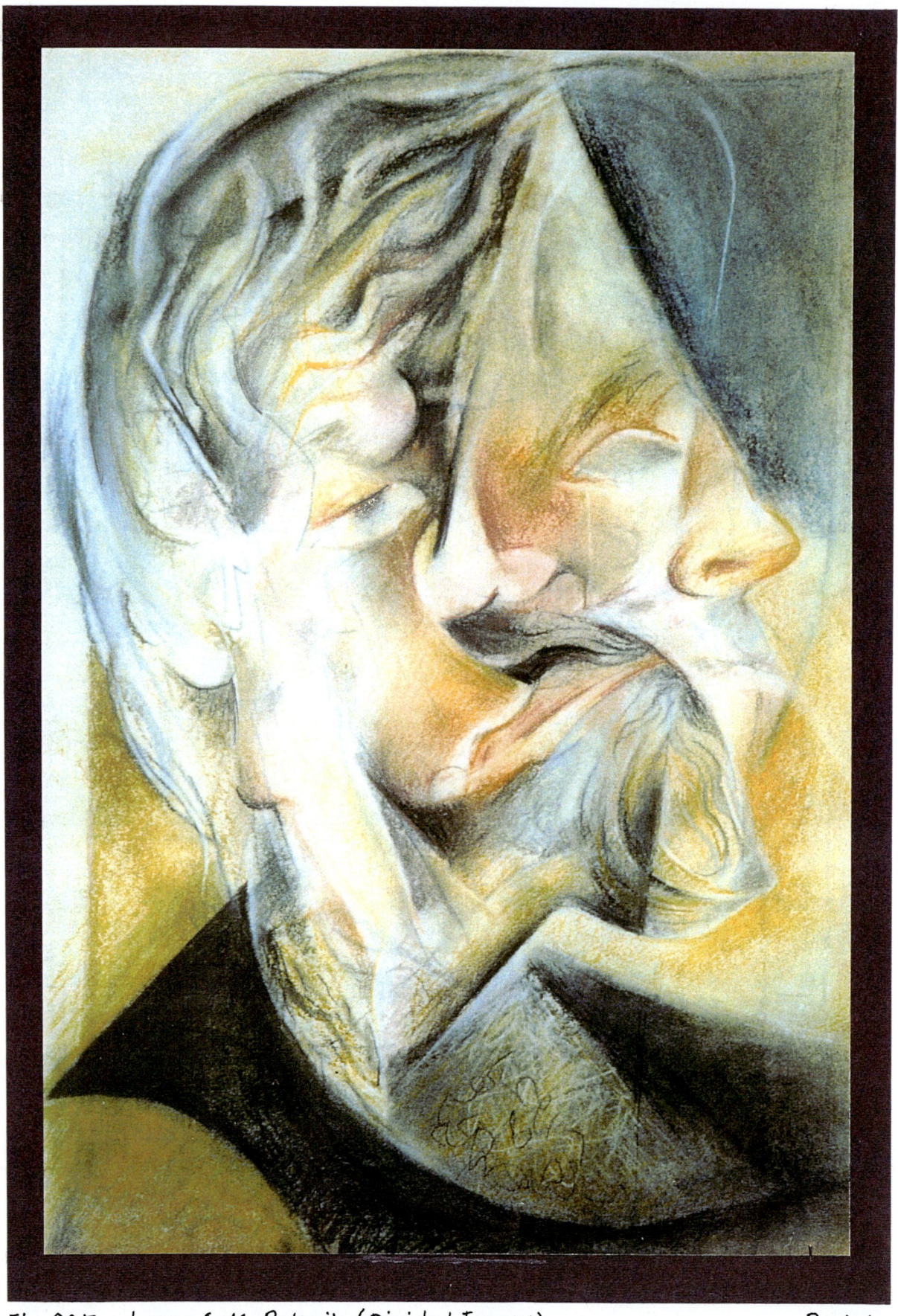

Fig. 285 Large Self-Portrait (Divided Image)　　　　　Pastel

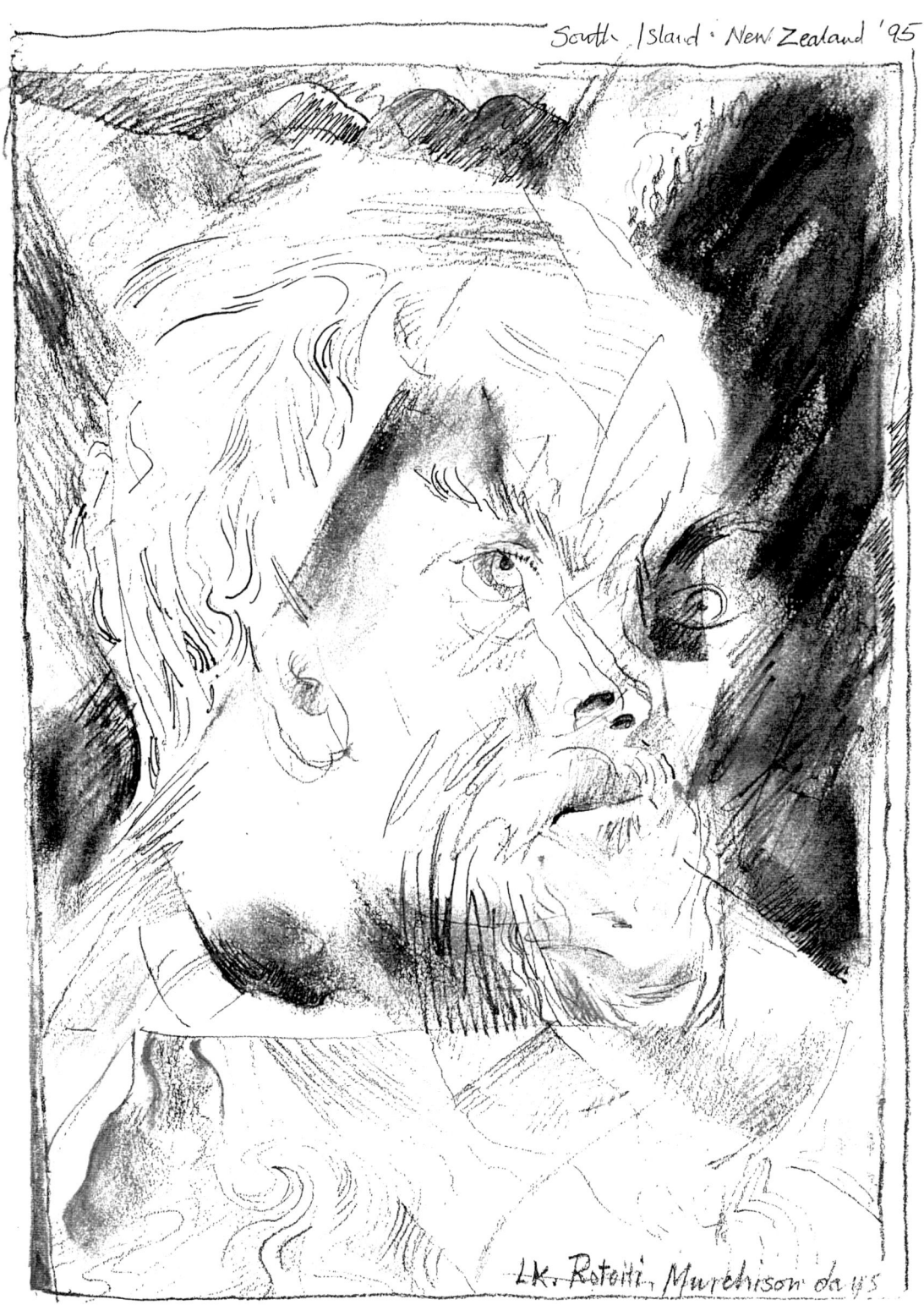

Fig. 286 New Zealand Self-Portrait   Aquarelle Pencil

Above: Fig. 286 'A New Zealand Self Portrait'
A brief visit to the Nelson Lakes in South Island turned into a very bleak day out. The intention to sketch this powerful landscape of lakes and mountains was quickly abandoned as heavy rain and low clouds obscured the view. This drawing epitomises the mood of the day, reflecting loneliness and apprehension. The structure and facial features shift and drift, darkness intrudes.... things begin to fall apart.

Left: Fig. 285 'Large Self Portrait'
Drawn two years after the N.Z. sketch, the head struggles to maintain some kind of structural integrity. The melancholic left side is countered by a more positive right side, whilst a central face presents a more aggressive appearance.

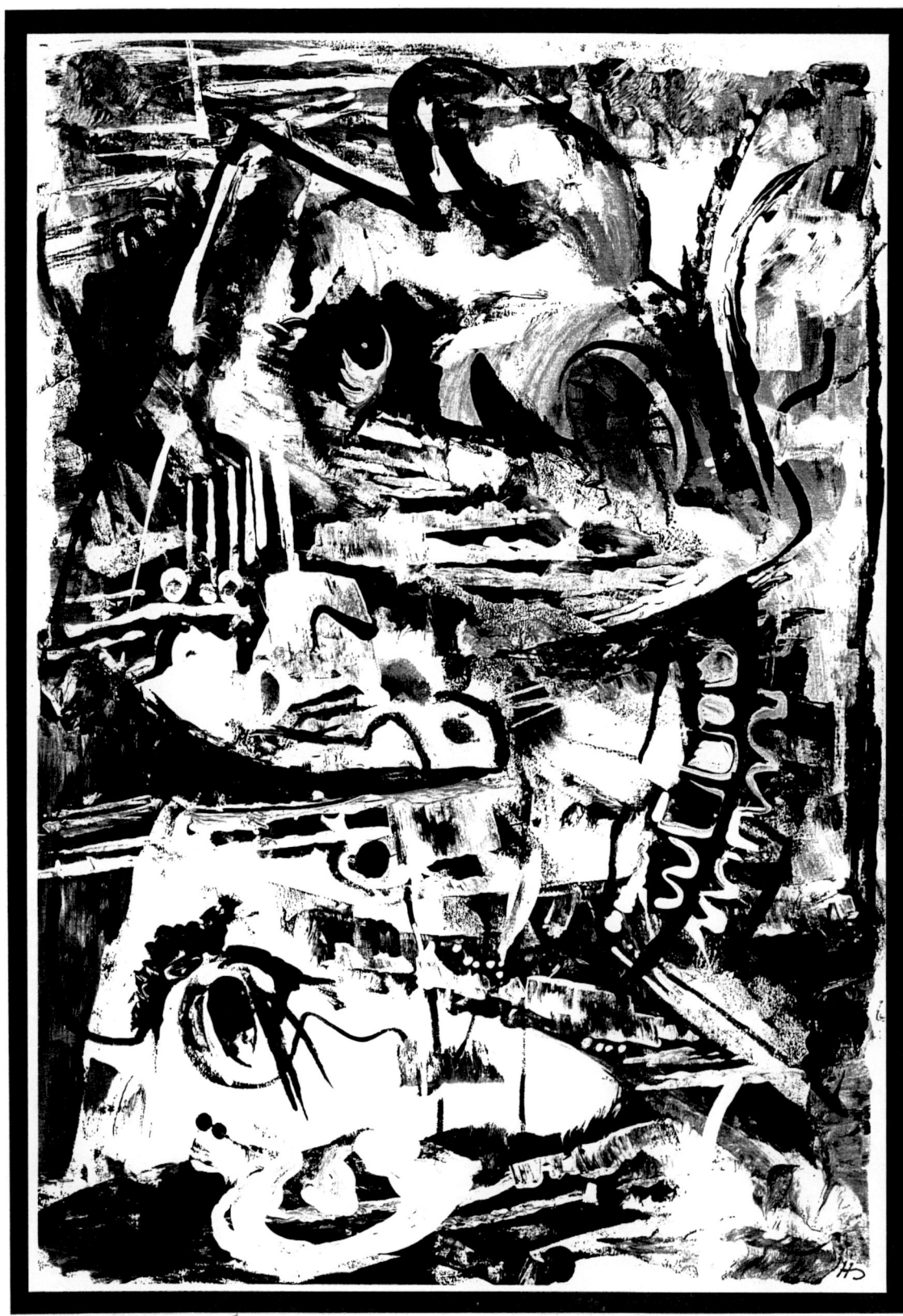

Fig. 287 Mugshot Gouache

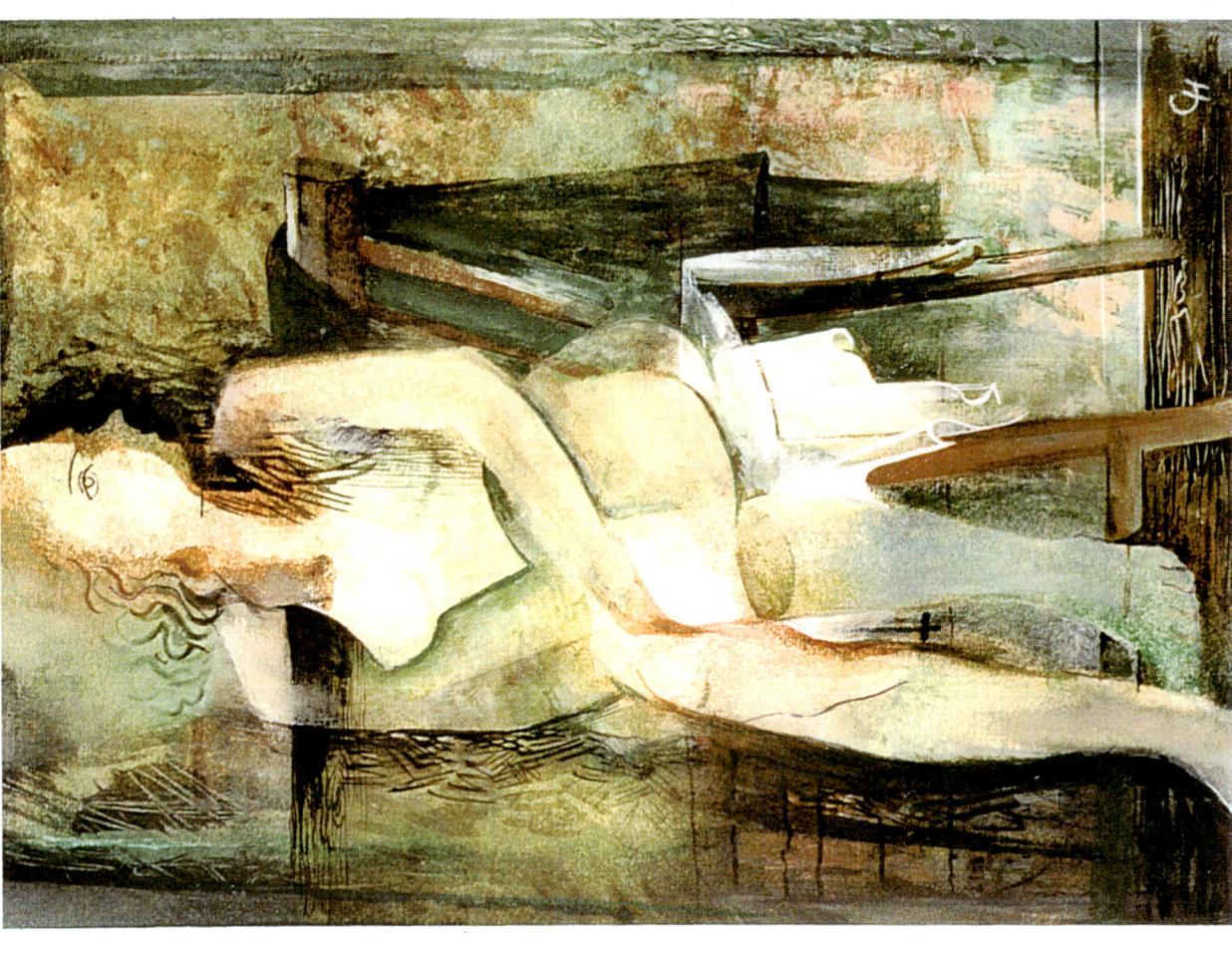

Fig. 288 Nude (Cut-up) Watercolour, Gouache & Ink

Above: Fig. 287 'Mugshot'

'Mugshot' shows a number of disintegrating features. The visual pun of ears as ung-handles (lugs) combined with a flattened top to the head, makes the split face into two villainous 'mugs' wanted by the ego-thought 'police' who demand that this disreputable 'pair' get their act together, become whole again. This temporary fragmentation (regression) disturbs the consciousness; the psychic fantasising disputing the well-balanced 'reasonable' self.

Yet this same-self shows a contrary side, allows the manipulation of a Brush to take over his commonsense and create this troubling 'Identikit' mugshot. At this juncture perseverance is required — the personality is 'at war with itself', trying to find ways to deal with this struggle for change.

Right: Fig. 288 'Nude' (Cut-up)

One of the life drawings worked on during this period, which I thought a dud and was about to scrap, until I reworked it from imagination, surprised how I started to cut up the body into parts whilst still holding the overall contours together. An ambivalent piece showing both fragmentation and coherence at the same time.

Looking for parallels in Cubist work I realised the naturalistic approach excluded that possibility. Perhaps it was yet another example of being at war with oneself — an inability to understand one's own anima.

161

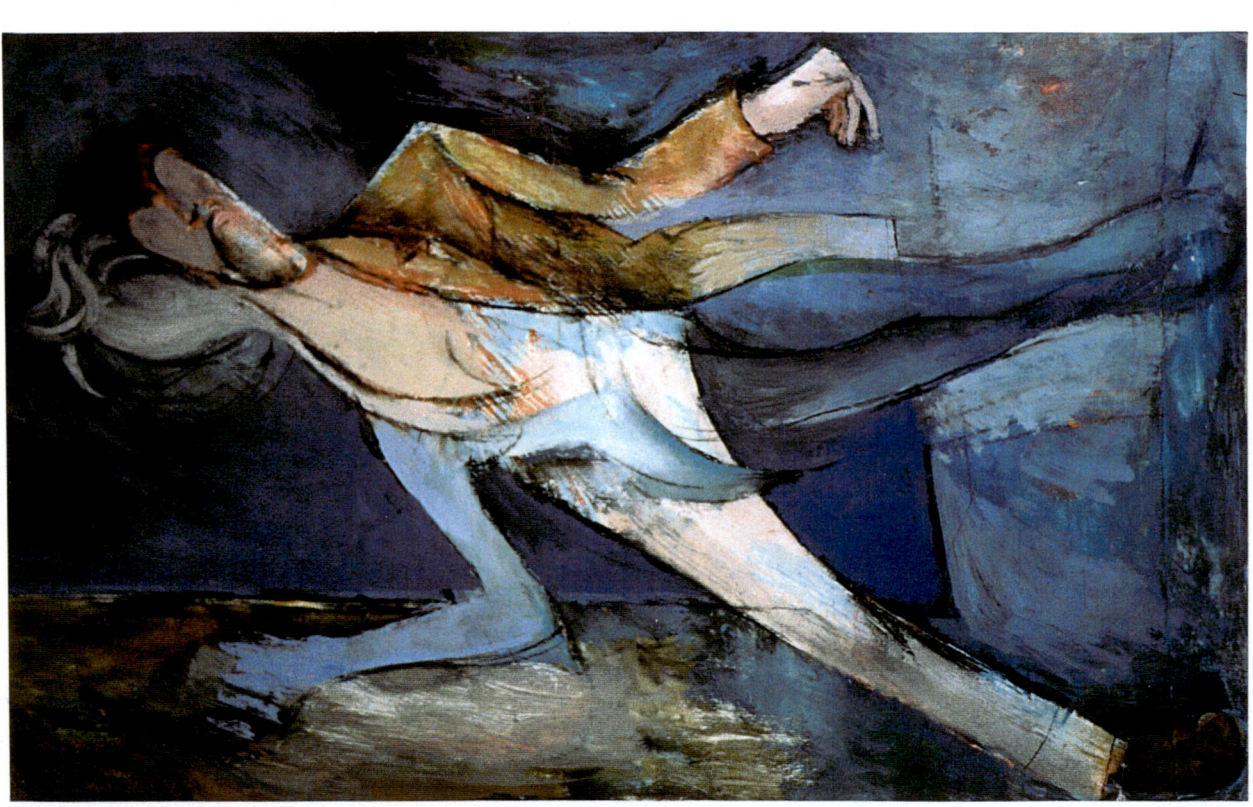

Fig.289   A Question of Gender   Gouache

Right: Fig.290. Tendencies towards Fragmentation – Pen, Watercolour

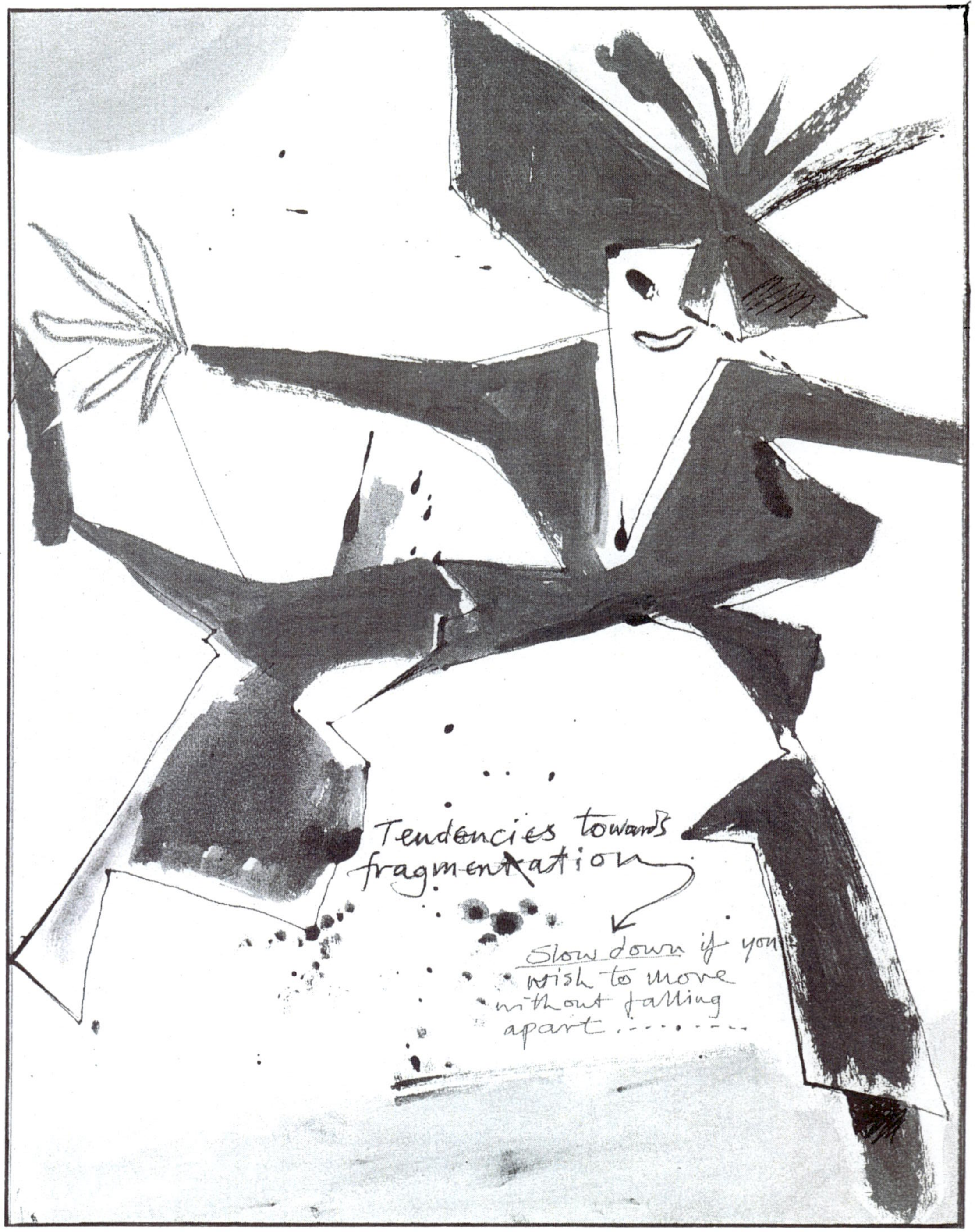

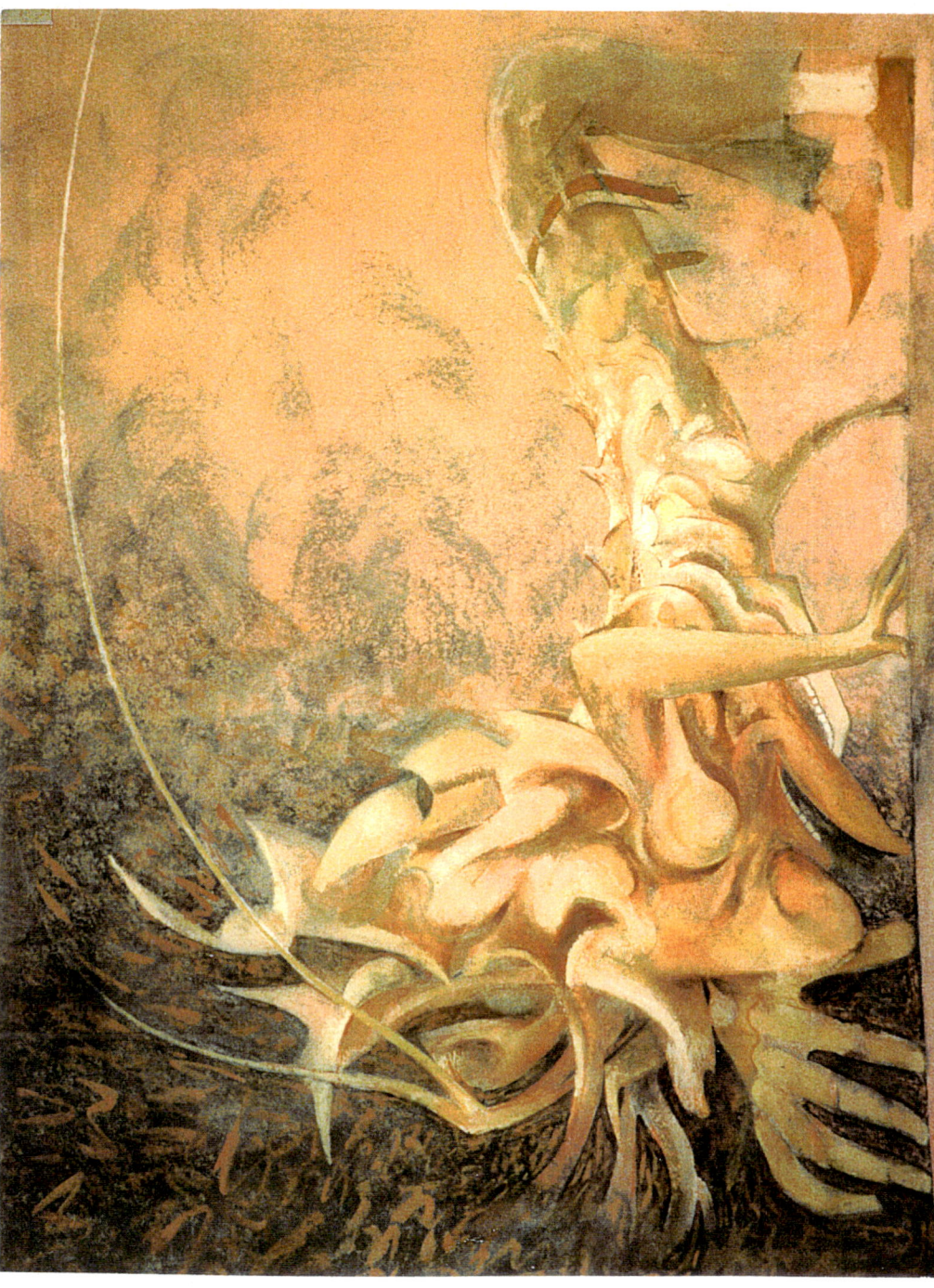

Fig. 291   Metamorphosis   Mixed Media

Above Left: Fig. 289 'A question of Gender'.

Following the cut-up 'Nude', this split identity painting separates in quite a different way. Here a bearded figure sways to and fro with a strange appendage springing off to the left — a blank face with longer feminine hair; an open blouse showing breasts; a suggestion of broader hips. Could this be a hermaphrodite figure, an unconscious merging of male/female identities?

Above Right: Fig. 290 'Tendencies towards Fragmentation'

Handwriting on the drawing reads 'Slow down if you wish to move without falling apart....' I recall writing this spontaneous comment as I finished the sketch, and now feel it echoed the tendency to do too many things at a breakneck pace — of how things were in danger of falling apart.

This Page - Fig. 291   'Metamorphosis'

In retrospect it is impossible to know what compelled eye, hand and brush to form this grotesque fantasy. Although I was reminded of Gregor Samsa's predicament in Kafka's 'Metamorphosis', I'd not read the story for over forty years. There must have been some other explanation as to why this partial change from man to insect appeared. Perhaps it was a quest for the earth and its vibrancy, for both lower jaw and fingertips, together with the 'umbilical' stethoscope seem to feel out the surface of the land. Another possibility occurs — perhaps it's the Joker/trickster in yet another guise. The drawing of the Joker and his Dog ('The Quest of the Joker', page 342) hints at this searching out through touch.

Dreams 83 & 134

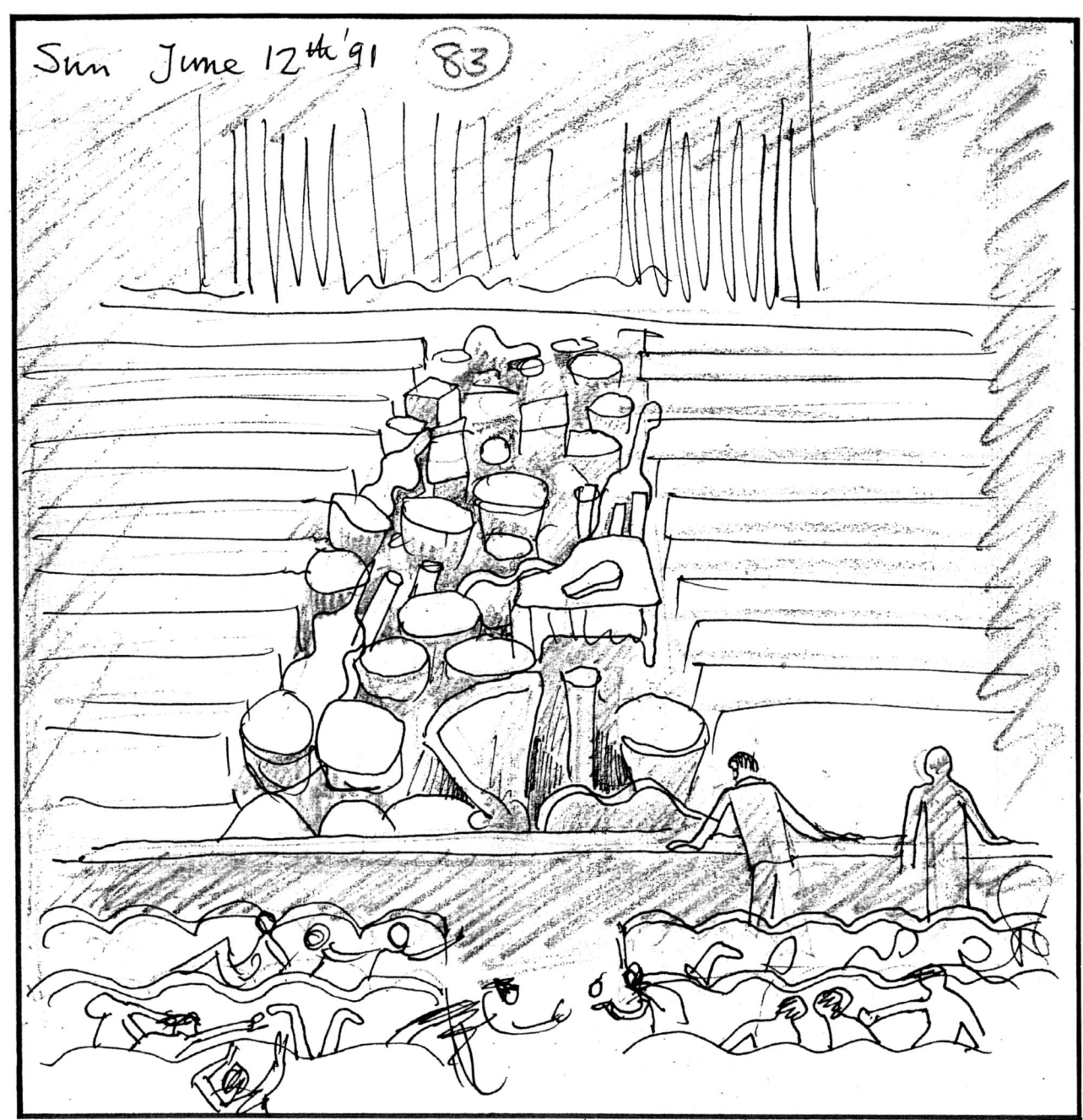

Fig. 292   Dream 83   Untitled   Pen, Ink & Chalk

Dream 83   12 June 1991

A short text in the Dream Journal described the dream image above: "A vast empty hall with a stage at one end and a balcony at the other. The central aisle of the auditorium is exceptionally wide and is crammed with covered musical instruments.

I view the scene from the balcony with a companion as an unruly group of youngsters makes a commotion behind."

With hindsight I see that the text was factual enough but could have said much more about the mood of the dream. Just as the instruments were covered, so also was the stage, reinforcing a feeling of total stillness, the covering suggestive of a pall, symbolising the death of music-making. Behind me an entirely different mood; chaos reigned, the unruly elements (children) showing an excess of life.

Denied access to creating music, they are now out of control — some kind of resolution is needed to redress this imbalance.

Dream 134   6 October 1991

The text accompanying the illustration to dream 134 (part one) describes what is too difficult to convey in drawing — or so it seemed until a second drawing (overleaf) perhaps made the dream story a little 'clearer'. The unruly elements from dream 83 have transformed themselves through a kind of amalgamation (or osmosis?) into various instrumental members of the orchestra. As can be seen in part two some have barely succeeded, showing parts of their former selves.

It now appears that dream 83 was but the precursor for dream 134, the dreamer's psyche perhaps having found a way to bring the orchestra back to

---

Sun 6th/91   The Escalator.   [Note. Find myself needing to give titles to recent dreams — I'm trying to fix the <u>main</u> feeling or vision which often becomes obscured within other imagery.

One of the most difficult dreams to illustrate or describe in words. The sketch I drew a day later after trying to sort out or feel the imagery

So: The underside of an escalator, yet too precise a description — perhaps a downward slope on the move. From its under surface dangle or hang or are suspended an array of pipes/tubes/rounded forms having connotations with something human. (page 183 Fig. 314. The connection seems related to music, the forms are a kind of orchestra and also my 'family' as if I were the conductor/father/mother taking care of them.

'We' were travelling downward on the escalator (on the underside) when something dropped through, possibly hitting parts of my 'orchestra'. The rest of the dream is spent nursing or mothering the supposed injuries. So; supporting, stroking, propping-up, re-assuring and more stroking and caressing of the members of my musical family. I feel we later gave a concert — perhaps!

Fig. 293   Dream 134. The Escalator - Part One   Pencil & Watercolour

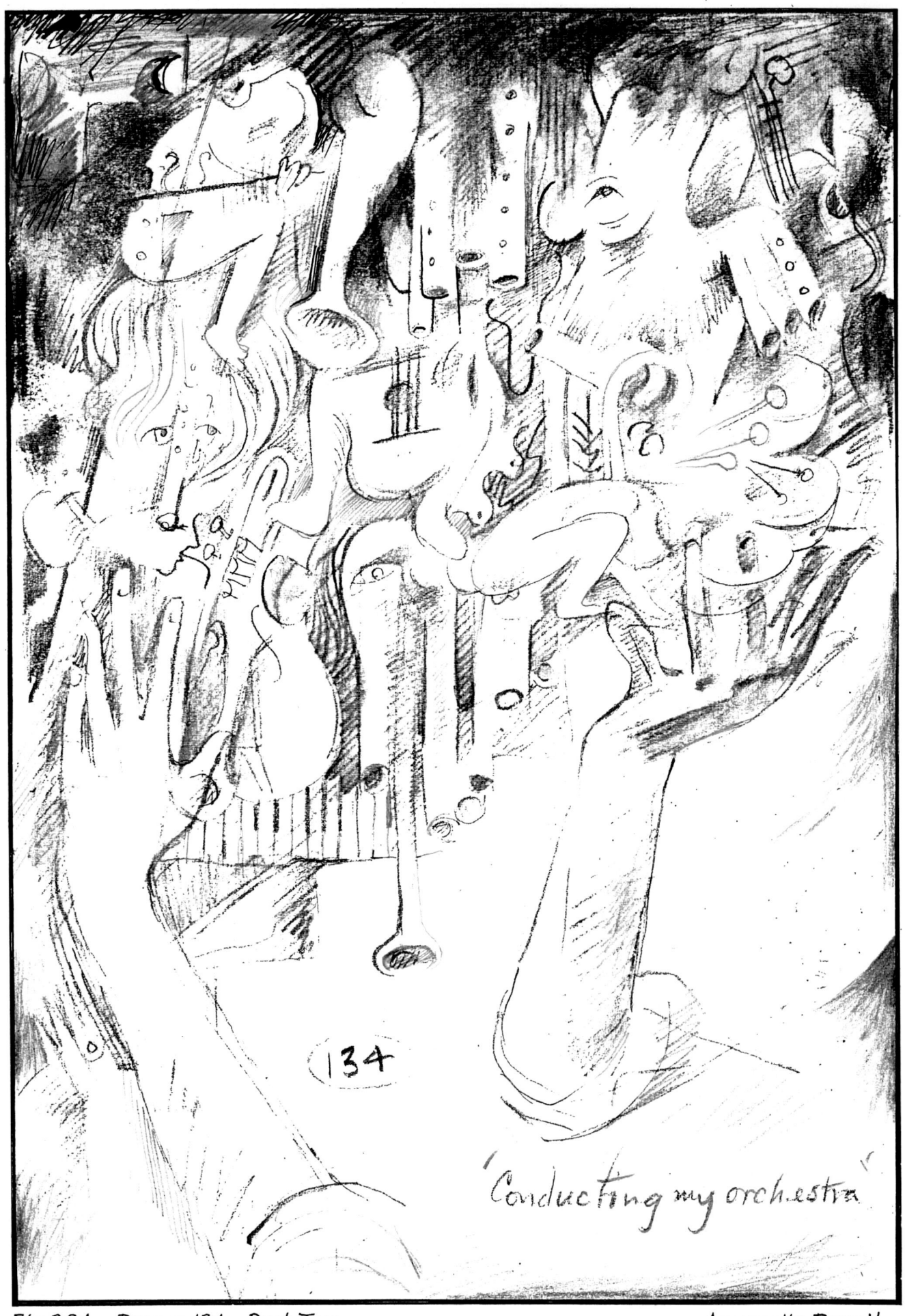

Fig. 294 Dream 134, Part Two   Aquarelle Pencil

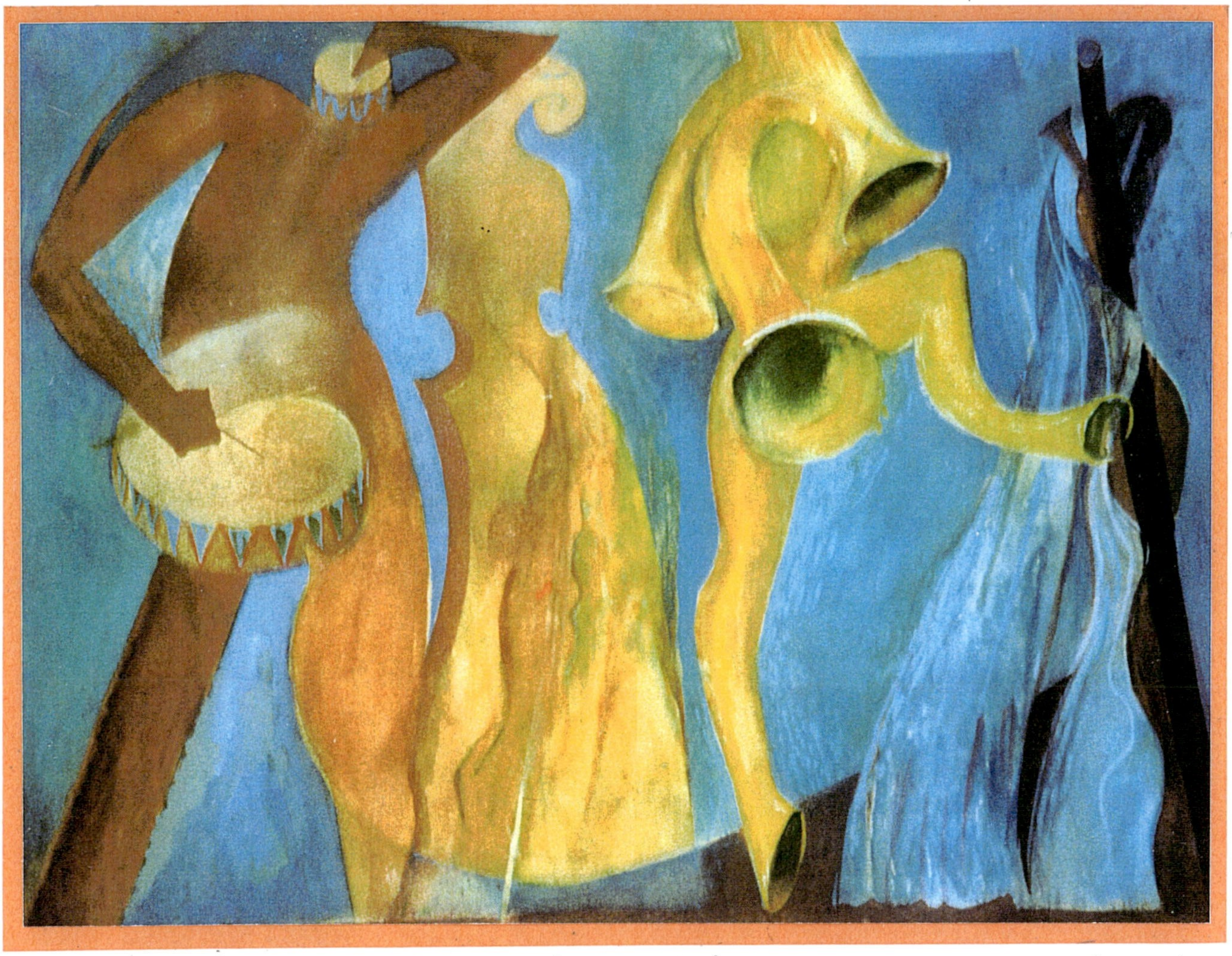

Fig. 295 Percussion, Strings, Brass and Woodwind   Gouache

life — to make music again — whilst at the same time bringing a semblance of order to apparently uncontrollable children. There did seem to be a need to bring disparate elements together to achieve a balance. The 'conductor' by stroking, brings harmony through a fusion of opposites within the dream.

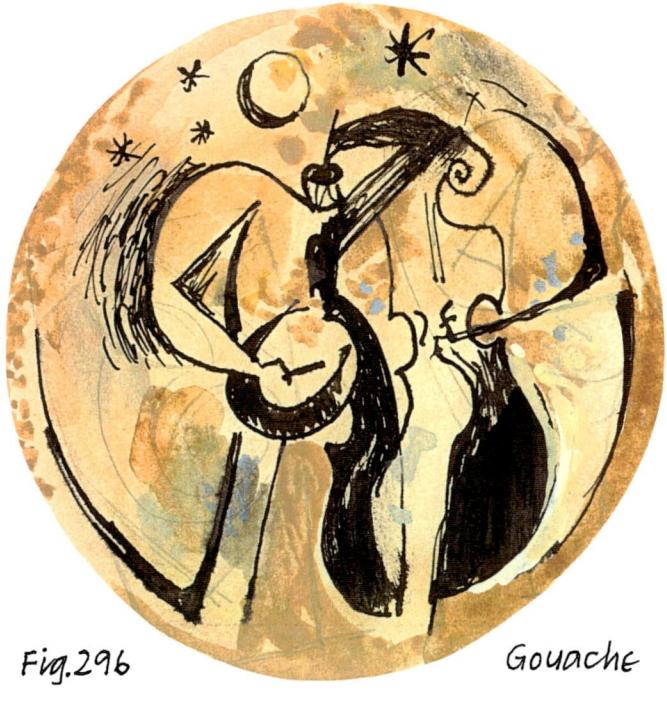

Fig. 296   Gouache

Top: Fig. 295 'Percussion, Strings, Brass and Woodwind'

Influenced by dream 134, this painting of the four 'families' of the orchestra soon followed. It was a more 'conscious' kind of work compared to the more usual 'freestyle' method. — another aspect of control perhaps.

The sharp, aggressive rat-a-tat-tat; the sensuousness of strings; the raucous blast of brass — and the mellow sound of a bassoon — this 'band' of malcontents were incorporated into an 'organised' work.

Left: Fig. 296 Design for a platter in ceramic work. An extension from the painting above — see ceramic section (page 101).

167

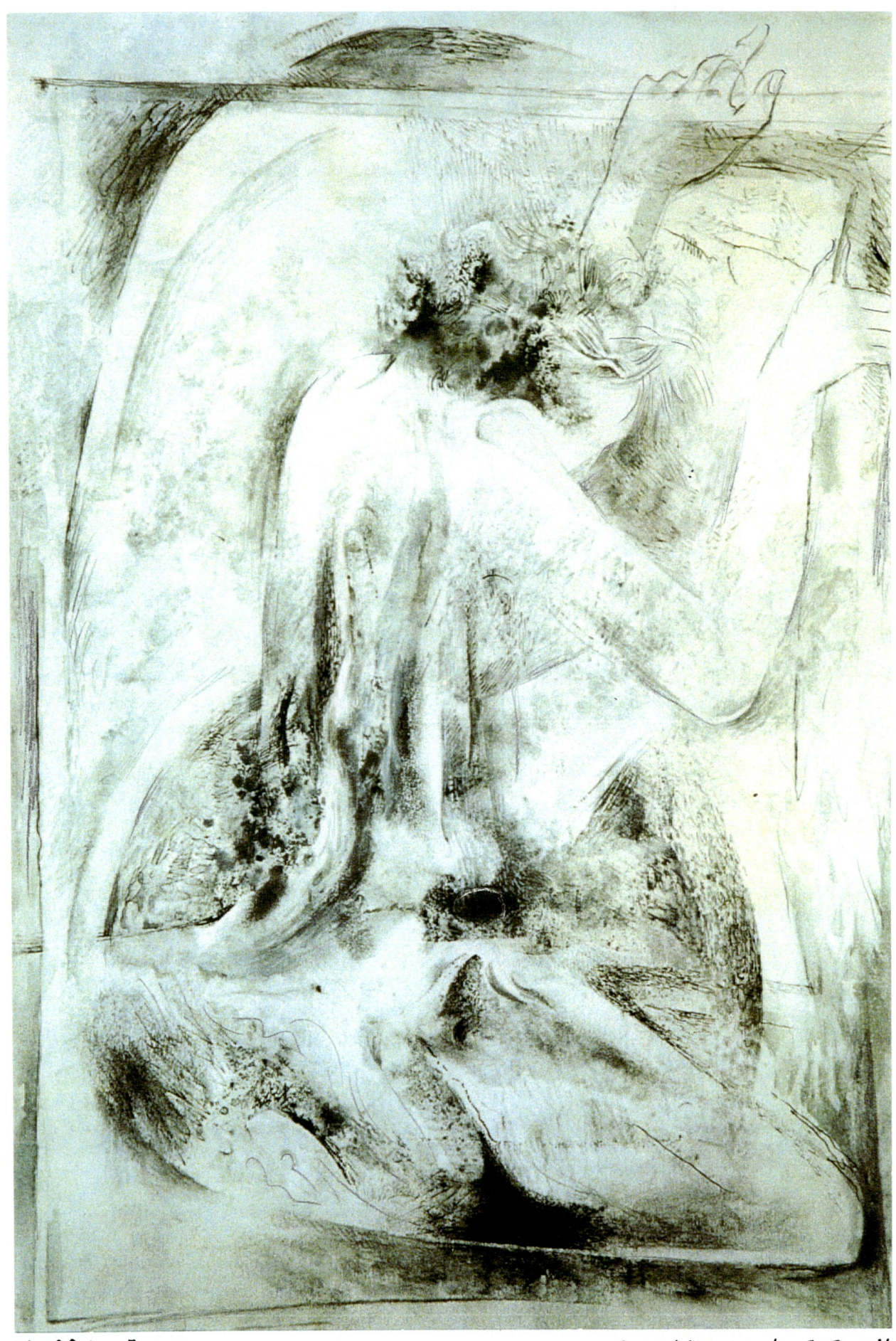

Fig. 297 Impotence Graphite powder & Pencil

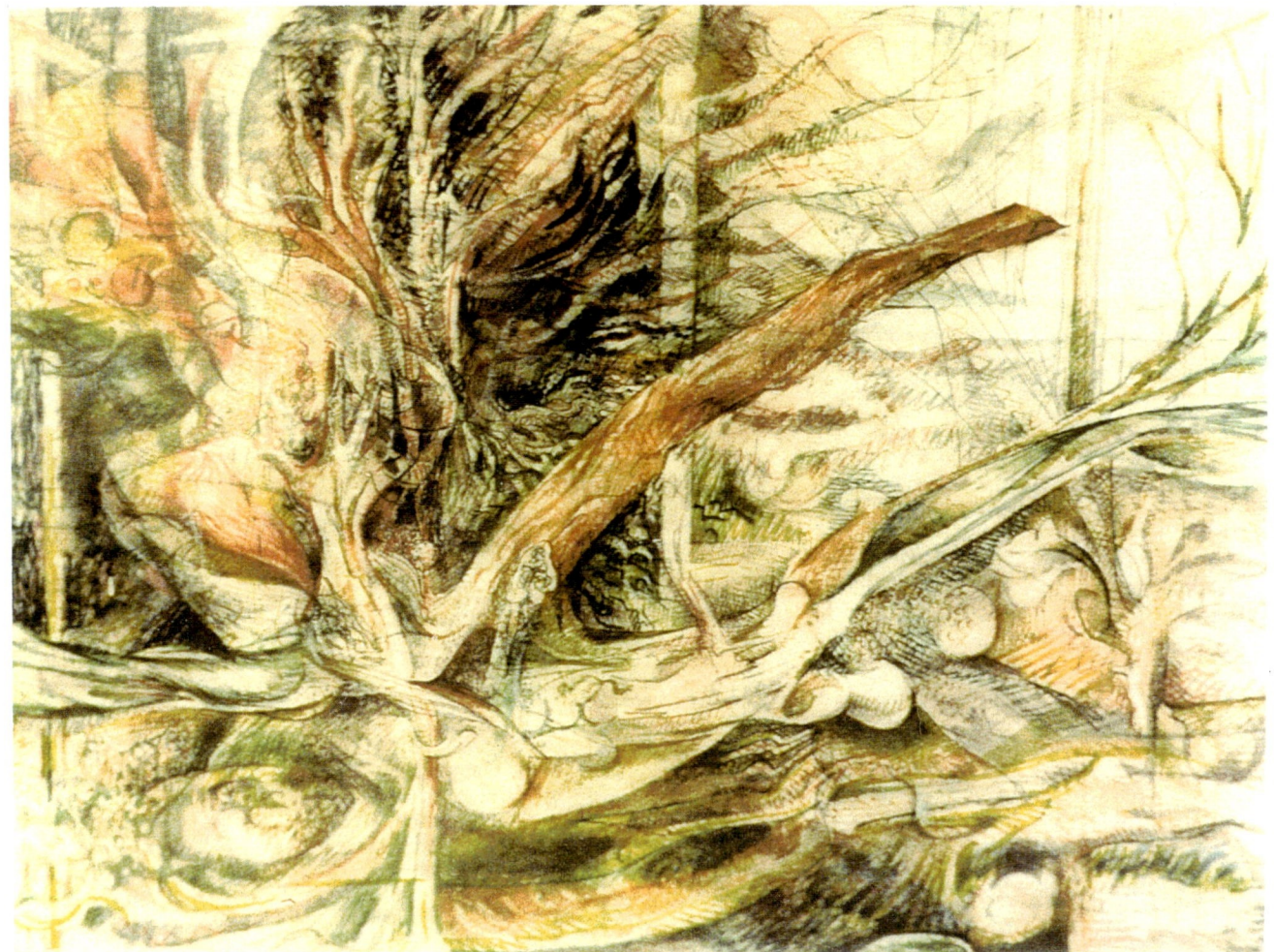

Fig. 298 Woodland Scene   Coloured Felt Tips on Tracing Paper

Above: 'Woodland Scene'

The shadow side dominates — regression, disintegration takes over. In a woodland glade an ancient tree trunk slowly breaks down into its constituent parts with the help of fungi, wet rot, spores, insects, storms and so on... A ghost image is appearing as awareness fuels fears of radical change — in sexual drive, in mortality, in metamorphosis.....

Left: Fig. 297 'Impotence'

An image of disintegration, a dissolving into a slime of nothingness. The head of the figure looks down to see a plughole where his genitals should be — perhaps the consequence of some terrible inertia working away like an acid bath, reducing him to impotence, unable to create a new life for himself. Influenced by the 'fluidity' of the escalator orchestra (see Fig. 294, Part Two) this freestyle drawing picked up some inner darkness. It now reads like a caution or a warning about not dwelling on the past — the self needs to lift itself out of these sluggish waters.....

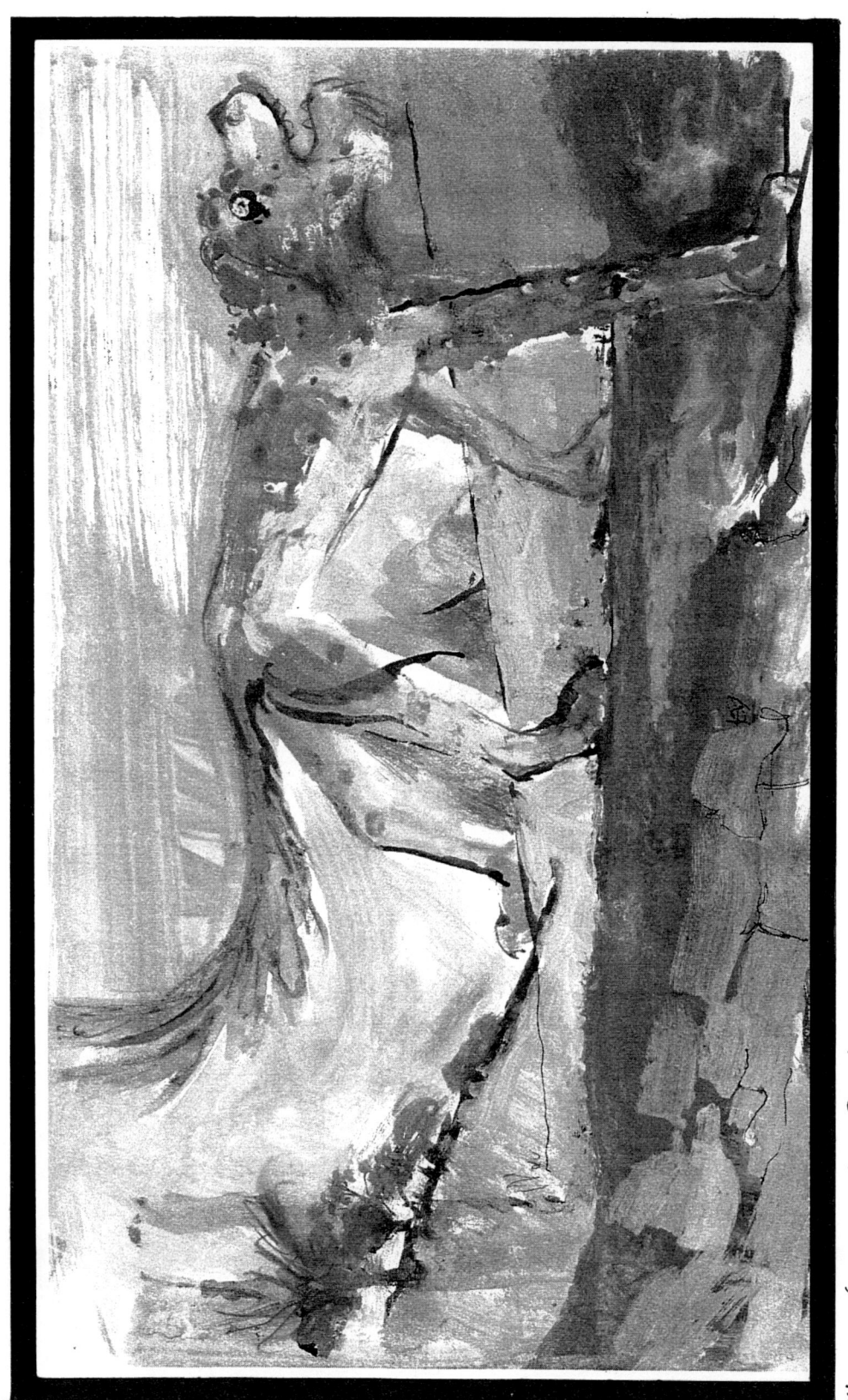

Fig. 299 'Millennium Dog' Gouache

A miraculous creature, capable of straddling several eras at once, Pausing in Past Time, Resting (on two legs) in Present Time and searching forward into Future Time, contemplating new moves whilst resting largely in the Now.. A rather more positive end to this section on change........

8 CONFRONTATION
Dream 65　　　　　　　　　　　　　Conflict and Resolution

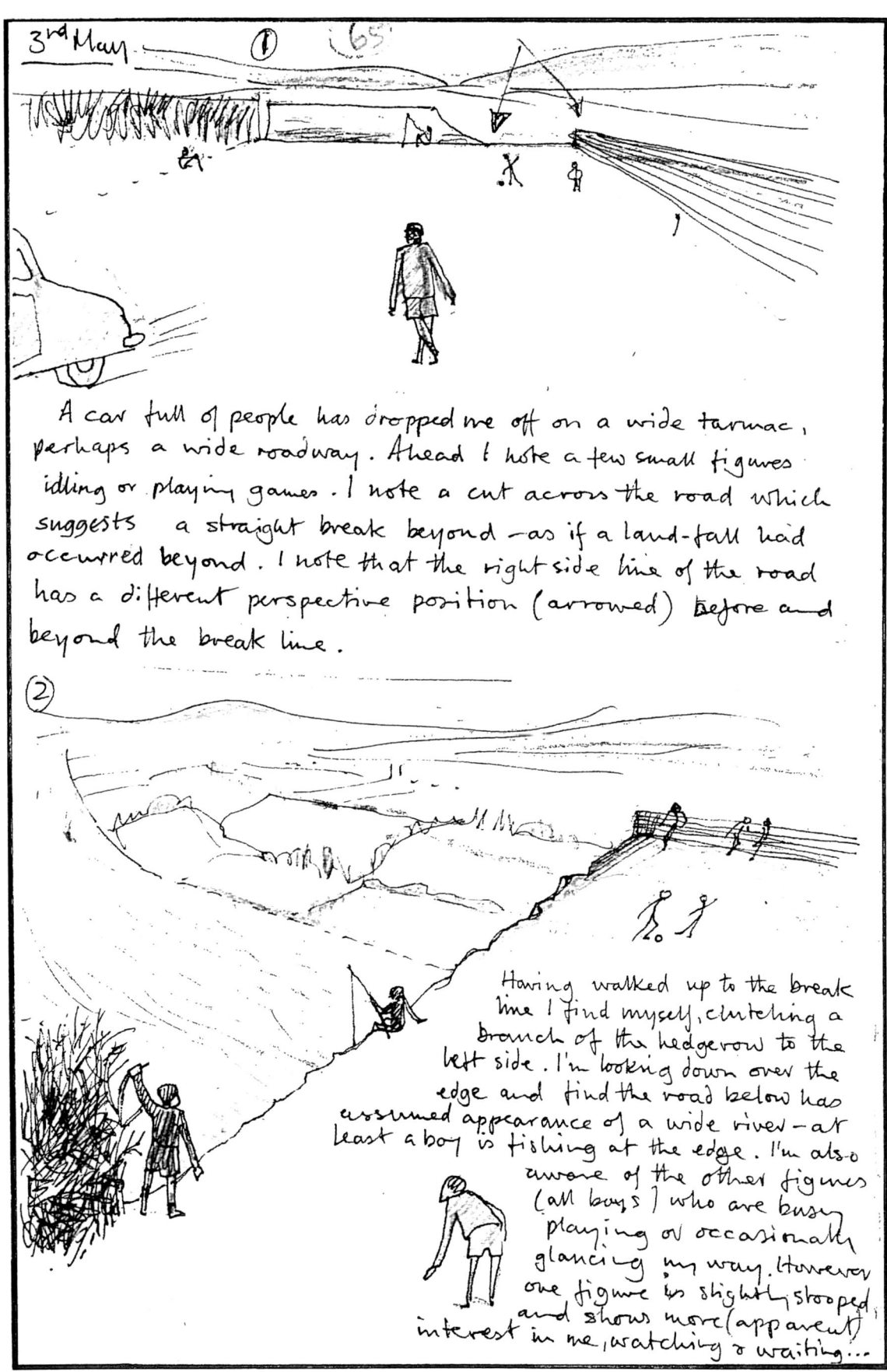

Fig. 300　Dream 65, Parts One & Two　　　　　　　　　Pen & Ink

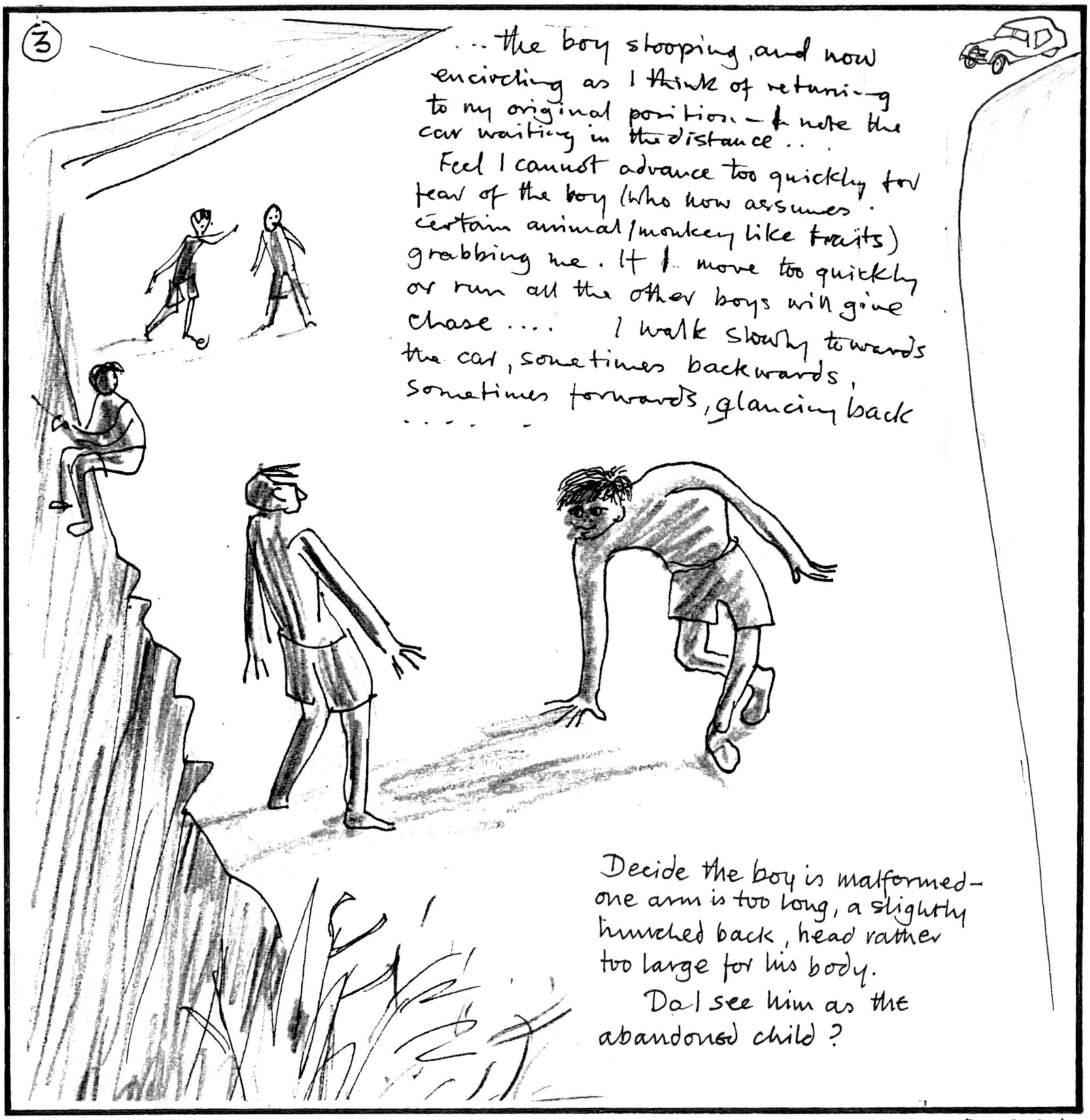

③ ...the boy stooping, and now encircling as I think of returning to my original position — I note the car waiting in the distance...

Feel I cannot advance too quickly for fear of the boy (who now assumes certain animal/monkey like traits) grabbing me. If I move too quickly or run all the other boys will give chase .... I walk slowly towards the car, sometimes backwards, sometimes forwards, glancing back ....

Decide the boy is malformed — one arm is too long, a slightly hunched back, head rather too large for his body.

Do I see him as the abandoned child?

Fig. 301   Dream 65   Part Three   Pen & Ink

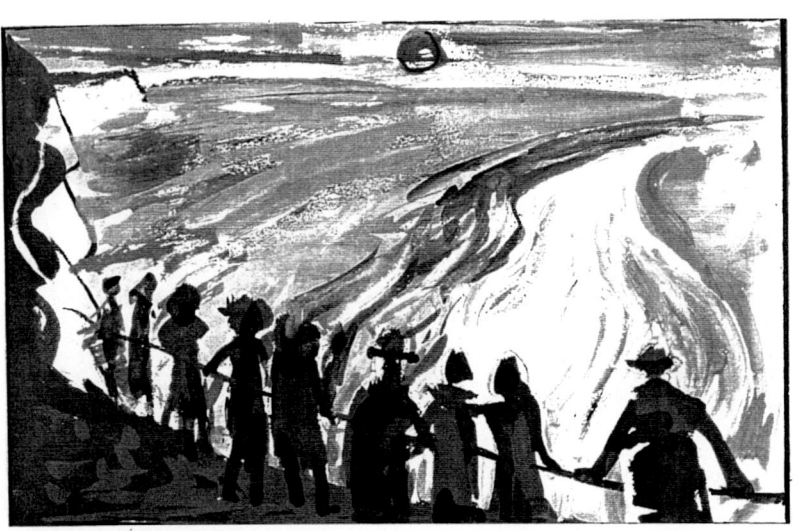

Previous page: Fig. 300. Parts one and two of Dream 65.

Above: Fig. 301 Part three of Dream 65. 'The Hunchback Youth'.

Left: Fig. 302 Dream No. 1A from the Dream Journal. 'Viewing a Great Plain at Sunset'.

Fig. 302 The Great Plain   Gouache

DREAM 65   3 May 1991

Long before being affected by the imagery of this dream, I'd had a premonition centred around the landscape of a much earlier dream. Sometime during '89 an image of a great plain, bathed in evening light, with a broad river flowing towards a high 'cliff-like' roadway, was recorded in a quick colour sketch at the time. Along the high precipitous edge a handrail supported a crowd of spectators looking inwards across the plain towards the setting sun. I recalled how I felt unable to participate, keeping well away from the edge (fig.302, bottom left.).

About a year later, deciding to record dreams in a journal form, I felt impelled to place this dream as number one. It was only then, with hindsight, that I could make a connection between the two dreams, with the geological layout, the curious displacement of a high, sharp-edged road above a great river flowing directly beneath it. The similarities heightened the sense of drama which now occurred in Dream 65.

The spatial displacement of the high, dry roadway with the lush, fertile valley below seemed appropriate contrasts for my anxieties above with the subconscious flow below.

The dreamer, away from the protective shell of the car, walked up carefully to the abrupt edge of the cut-off roadway and watched the boy fishing and others playing tag, etc. Holding on to the hedge at the road's edge a peripheral movement caught his eye — a lurching, shadowy movement quickly clarified into a youth, bent over, one arm swinging close to the ground, swaying gently forwards until pausing to watch me.

The youth seemed hostile. Fearful of the drop behind and of this daunting image of confrontation, I knew instantly this hunchback could not be ignored; he encapsulated in his very posture a symbol of certain encounters I'd experienced on other pathways from my past in the 'real' world — encounters I'd inwardly turned away from and rejected or banished from consciousness — until now.

I have a childhood memory of an old woman in black Victorian clothes approaching me along a pavement. As we draw level I'm appalled by a face which has no nose, only a

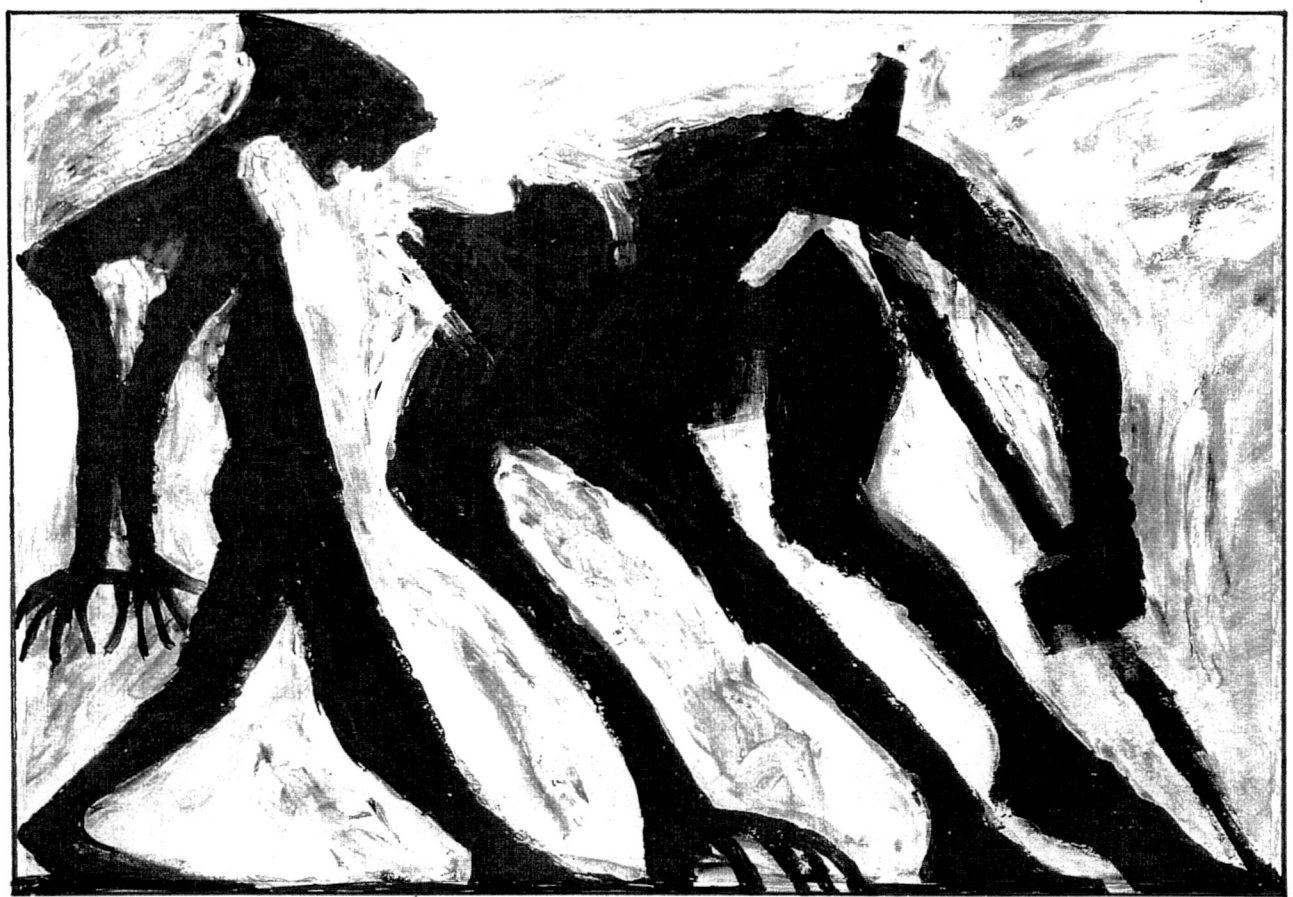

Fig. 303 'Encounter with the Ape-Boy Cripple   Gouache.

gaping hole. Later as a teenager, reaching a road junction I have another encounter, this time with a smart RAF officer with a livid, patched-up flame of a face, the probable result of a plane crash. I attempt to calm my nerves by fantasising a 'dog-fight' and a diving Spitfire from which this stoic hero walks away..... Years later, on a quiet London street I attempt to avoid a lurching shambles of a drunk, hailing me for a light, and, as I side-step, shouting 'What you scared of, Sonny!' Feeling a momentary shame, I offer a light but the swaying figure repeats his words and I walk on ashamed.

In some way these accidental meetings were regenerated through this 'hunchback' image. I wondered also whether the aggressive stance was one certain way of getting a response, and thought it highly probable — confrontation was producing an effect, was claiming my full attention.

It was as if years of emotional chaos, inward fantasising and withdrawal from all disturbing events were now being challenged by this unnerving creature. I felt he had arrived from the depths below, knowing that my self-consciousness was at last receptive enough to listen and able now to look at this mirror image of the neglected child within. This would seem to be the nature of the dream's fear — that of seeing oneself as the emotional hunchback — after years of neglect.

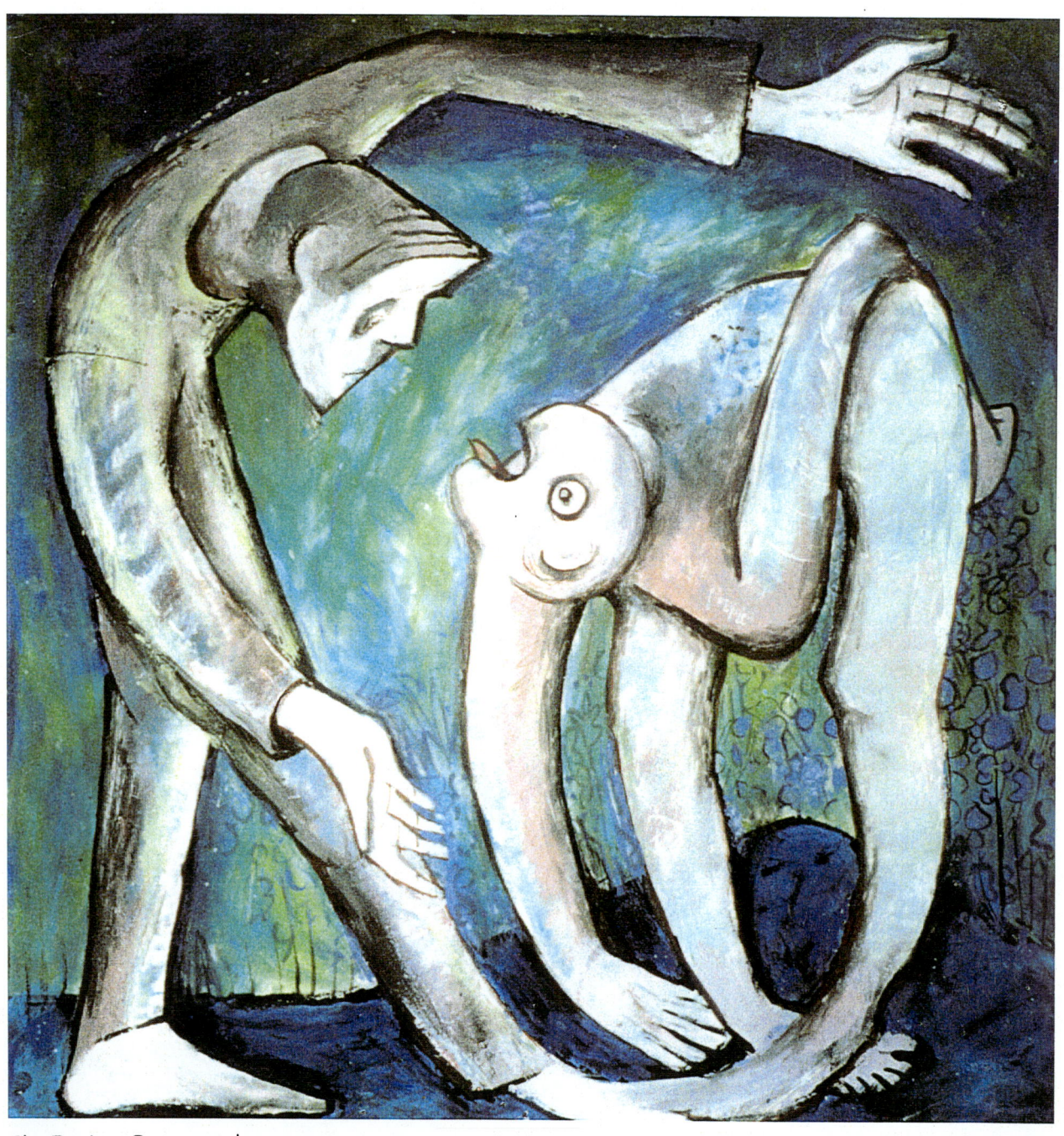

Fig. 304   Rapprochement   Gouache.

Left: Fig. 304 Rapprochement

The boy, now a young man begins to take an interest in the hunchback, his curiosity now awakened, he extends his arms, as if to contain his former anxiety. The 'cripple' looks up quizzically.

Right: Fig. 305 — Gouache. 'An Ambiguous Moment'

A momentary retreat towards the defensive position. The hunchback is capable of delivering a knockout blow at a more cautious youth.

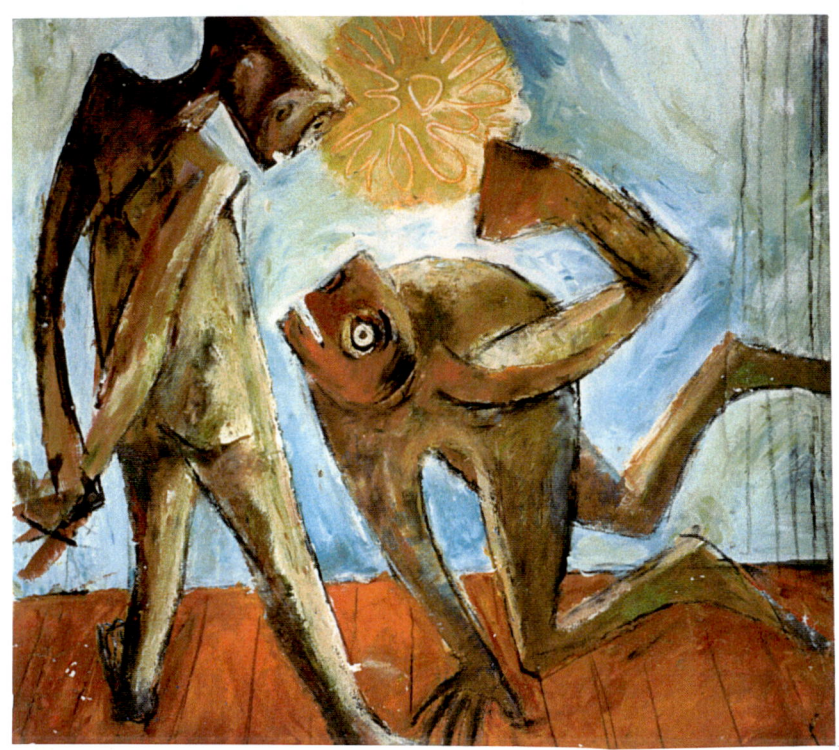

As the effects of the Hunchback dream settled into consciousness it became an obsession to 'revisualise' the original confrontation, and a sequence of variations developed out of this theme. The first attempts emphasised the lop-sided threat of the image by adding a crutch, making him into a cripple. Then he was relegated to an ape as if something still further below the conscious level — (fig. 303, page 173) This painting stressed the intensity and fear of the encounter, the ape youth lurching forward towards the boy who is trapped into a defensive posture, only the thrust of his head hinting at a positive response. Over a period of time the changing relationship between the two protagonists is explored in some ten drawings and paintings.

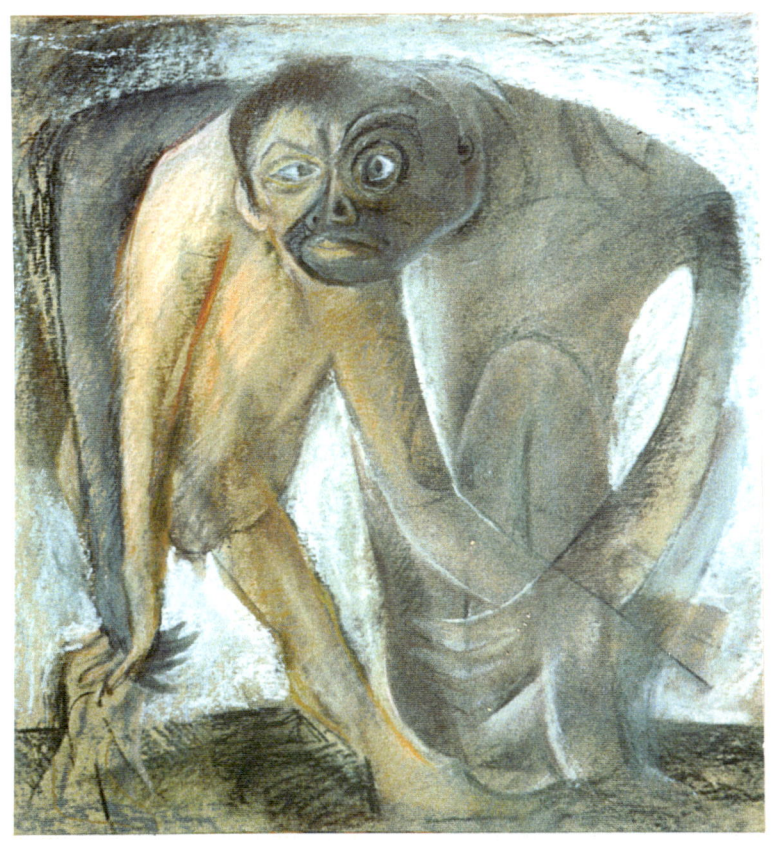

Left: 'Reconciliation'

From a group which attempted to create a 'merger', a kind of Siamese-Twin image, hands closely entwined and the head a symbol of reconciliation as if some kind of equivocal balance had been achieved.

Fig. 306 Reconciliation   Gouache

PSYCHIC INVASION

As if in a totalitarian state the house is invaded by a mob of mercenaries, intent on taking away the dissident.

The idea for the sketch had grown originally from an earlier 'action' painting of a man ascending a staircase (see page 89, fig.173) which now incorporated the confrontational aspects taken from the dream.

I felt later that the invading force was made up of assorted psychic elements who were 'challenging' the ego who was seeking more freedom of expression and was attempting to escape his inner repression.

Of course the inner protective powers wanted none of it! They were determined to return him to the safety of 'prison', away from his risk-taking life of change. Alternatively, if he wasn't willing to comply there was castration or, as a last resort, crucifixion.

Below: Fig.307 Psychic Invasion-1.

The curiosity is the naked ape-like overseer squatting on a window ledge above the stairwell – I feel he's another aspect of my joker or trickster who manipulates the self towards independence. It also turns it into a drama, with an audience of one. Curiously again the 'Hero' throws loaves and fishes to the mob – can he be hoping to assuage their hunger for his downfall?

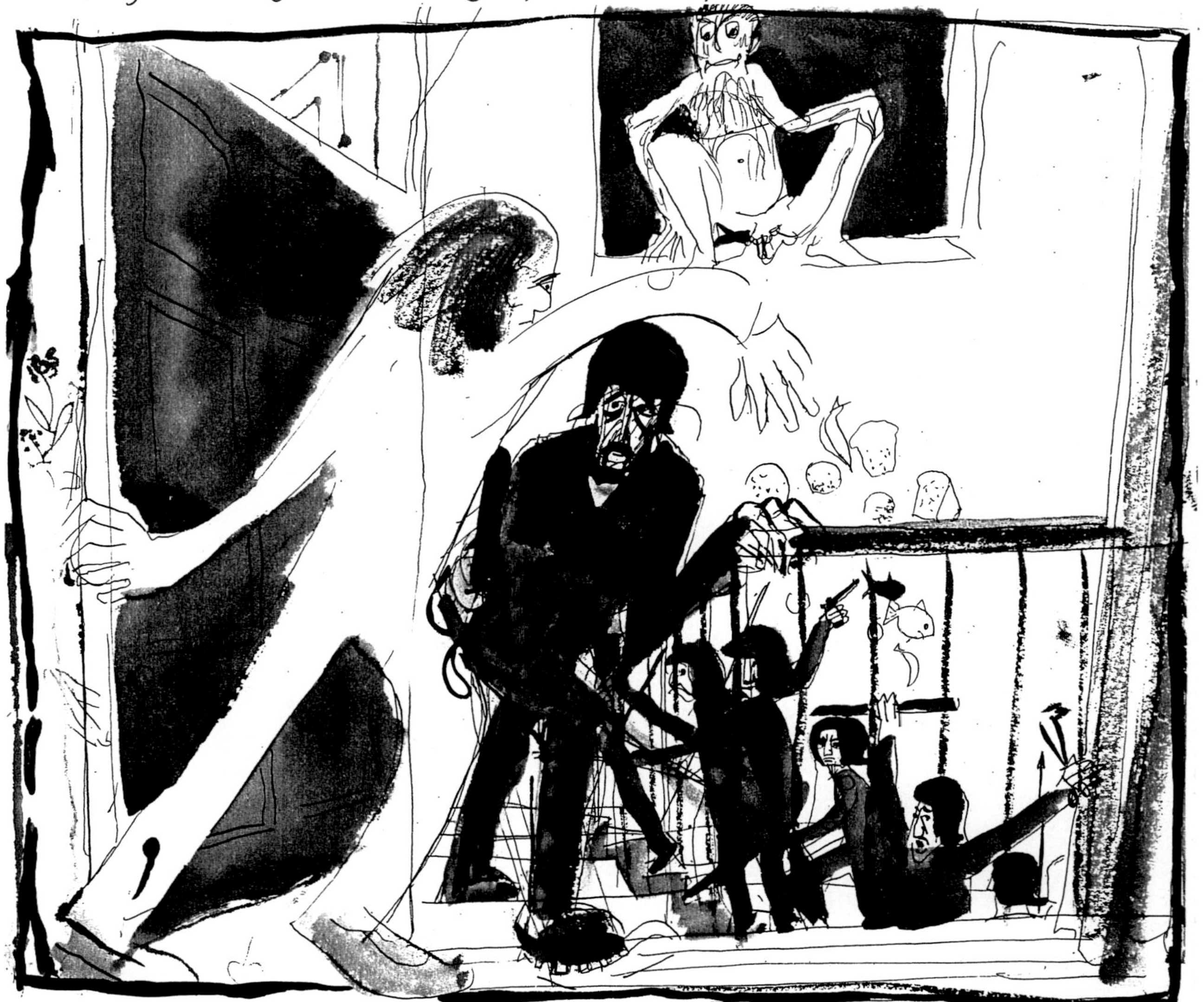

Fig 307 Psychic Invasion – 1   Pen & Wash

Below: Fig.308 Psychic Invasion-2

This version shows obvious biblical references with the long gown, Roman helmets and the cross.

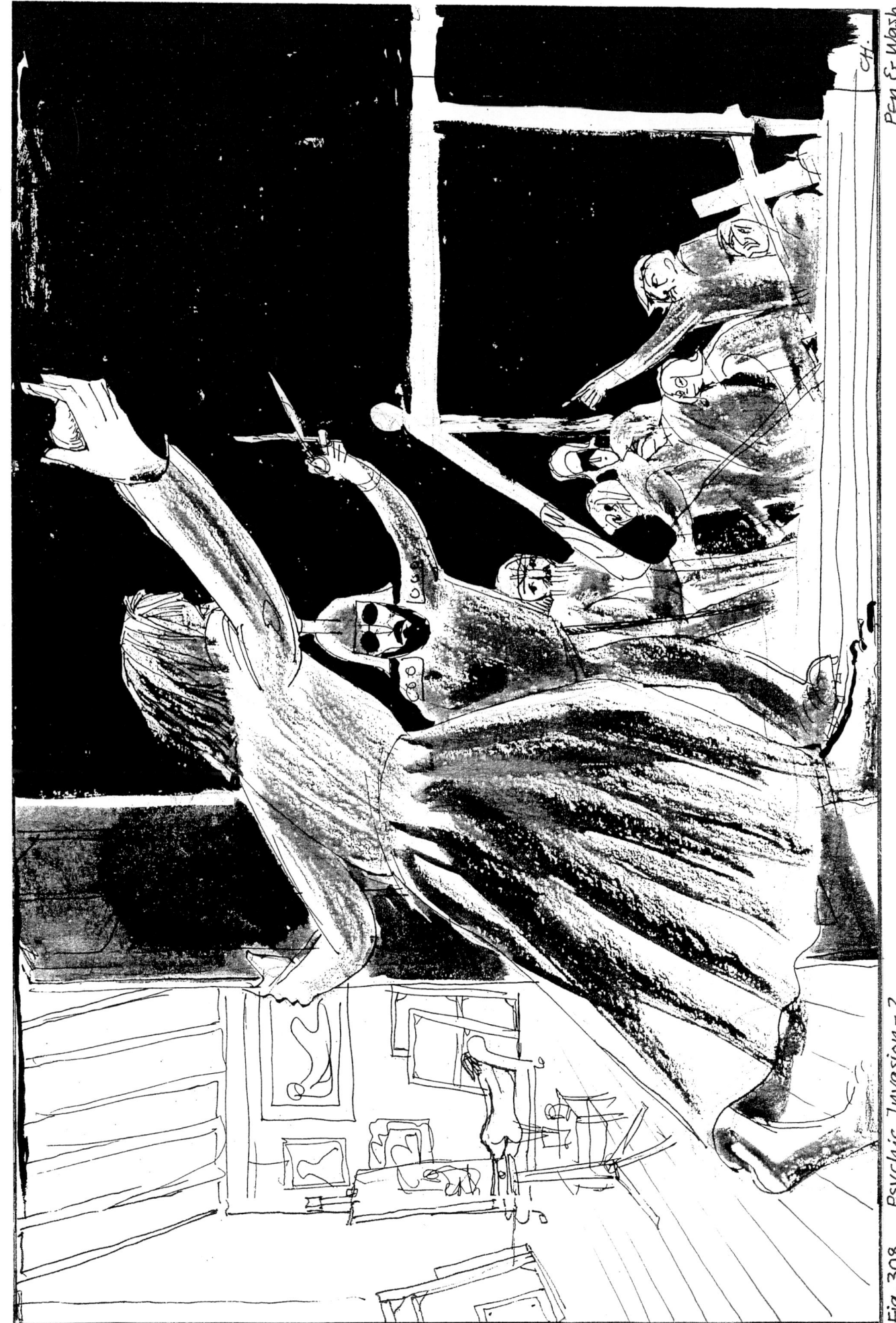

Fig. 308   Psychic Invasion—2   Pen & Wash

MASCULINE-FEMININE ENCOUNTERS

Right: Fig. 310 'Boxed-In'

A drawing showing resistance to any kind of commitment with the woman. Although this could be seen as one large head (eyes, nose and mouth could be visualised as 'shared'), the split through the centre is pronounced and final.

His hair 'standing on end' conveys his terror of commitment with her, his arms negatively turn away and his hands, pushing the sides of the box emphasise his anxiety.

She, as a bird, is ready to take wing from such indecision.

This brush, pen and wash sketch is the study for the painting on page 322

Below: Fig. 309 'The Watery Cavern'

Could this represent the unconscious world — a place of archetypal memory, of retained trauma? A large head glances suspiciously into the watery place where a feminine form guards the entrance. Beyond, water cascades over a dam, making a great waterfall.

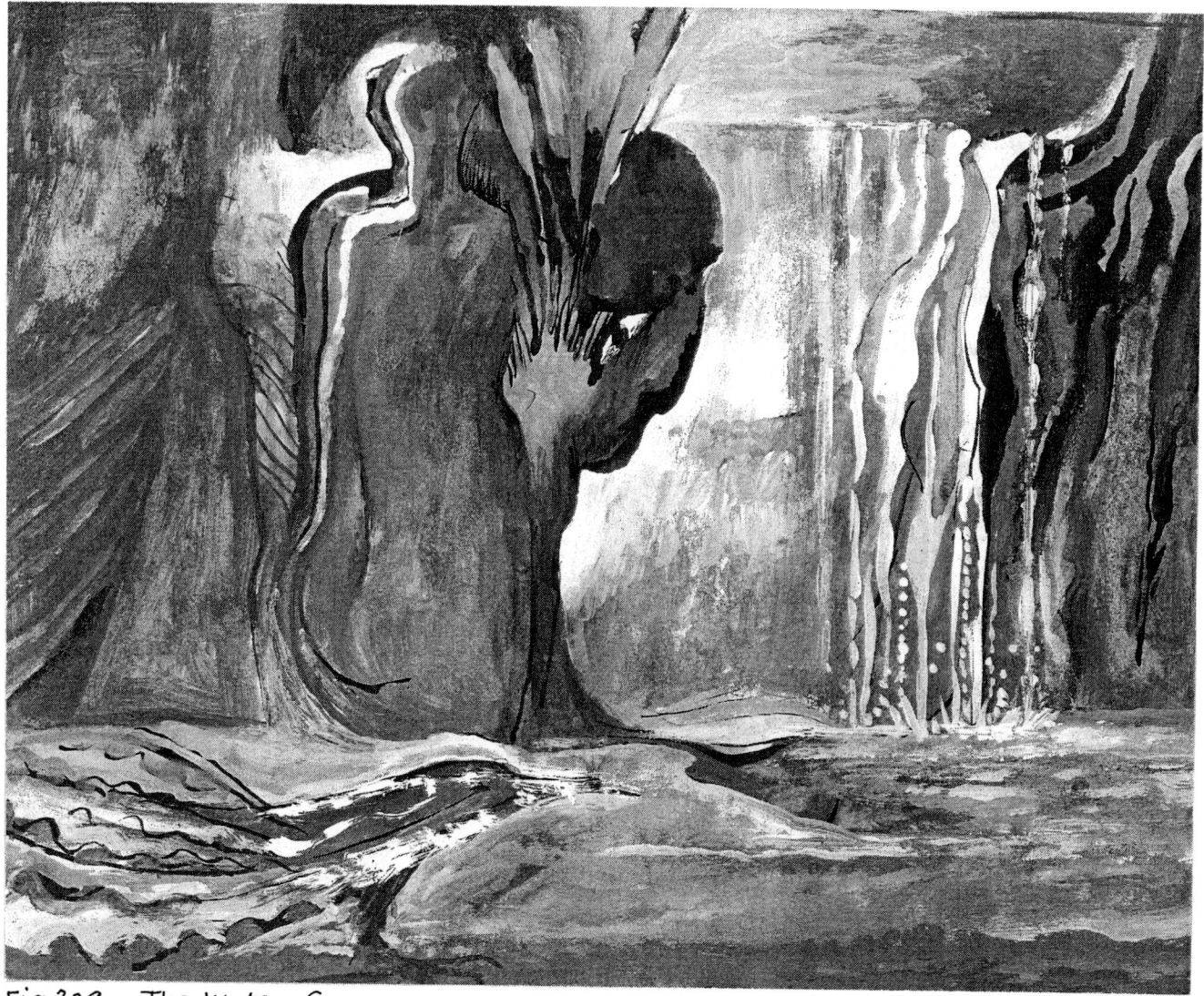

Fig. 309 The Watery Cavern   Mixed Media

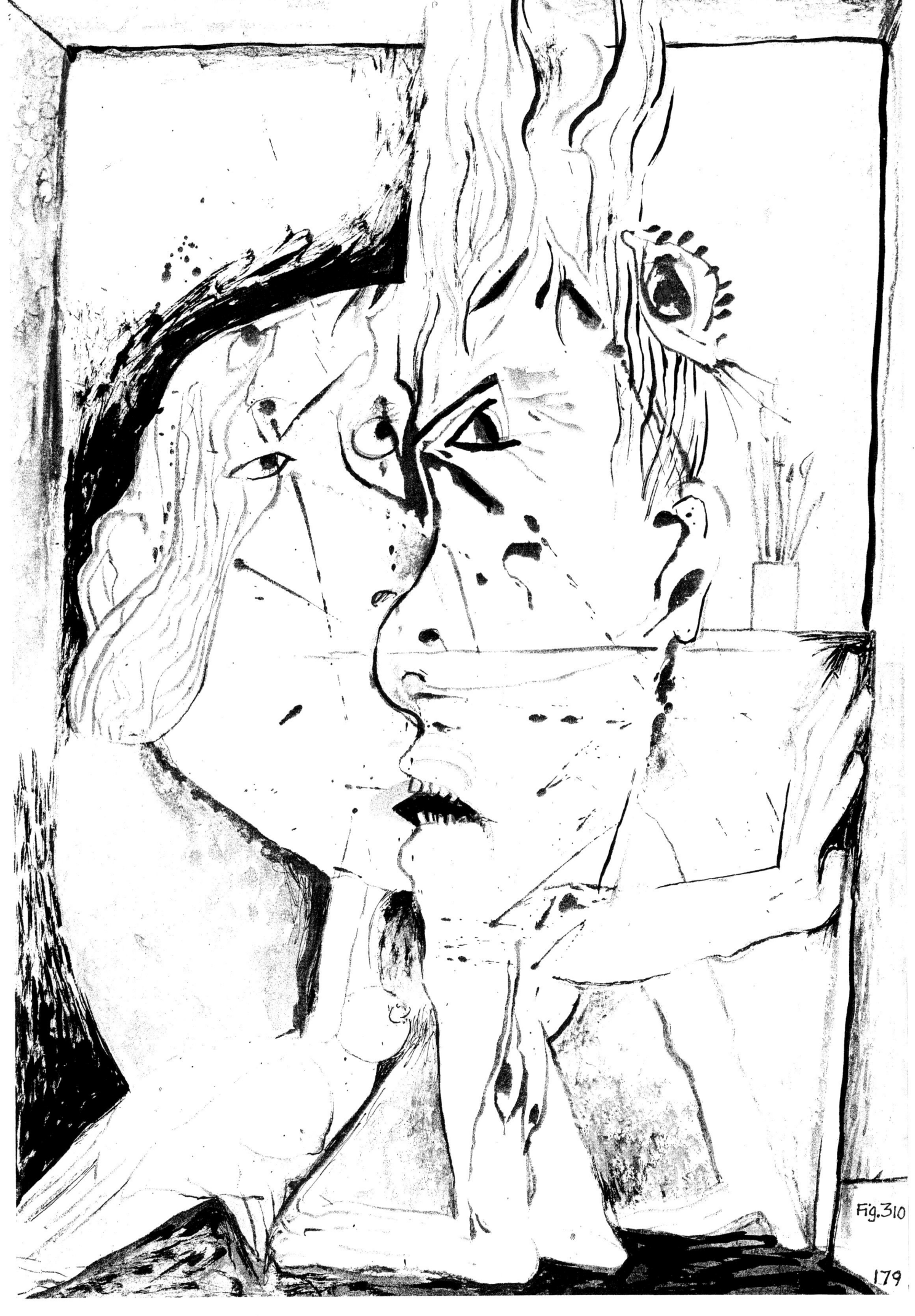
Fig. 310

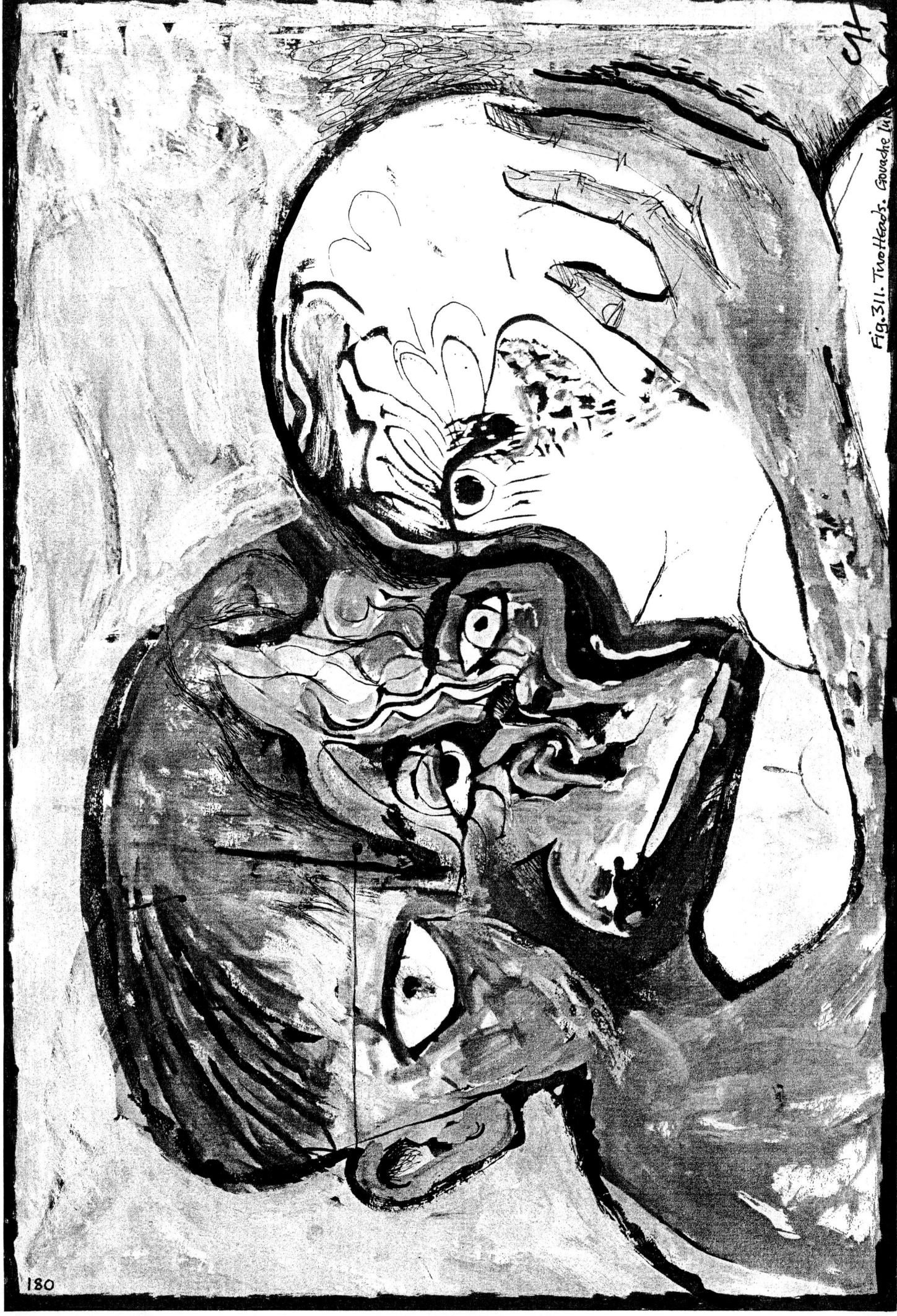

Fig. 311. Two Heads. Gouache (1969)

180

OTHER CONFRONTATIONS

Above: Fig. 311 'Two Heads'

A double portrait of contrasts — the forceful shadow head leans over to embrace the white anxious head whose worried brow suggests that only patience might open out into trust between them.
The shadow's face carries past fears of dream and 'real' deformities which are difficult to accept.

Right: Fig. 312 'Animal Fight'

An animated fight between six creatures — four dogs, a snake and a winged monster.
It's as if face-to-face confrontation is a delight — is something to be welcomed by all the participants.
The small dog (bottom right) is especially enjoying himself. Could it be that the freestyle work was offering encouragement?

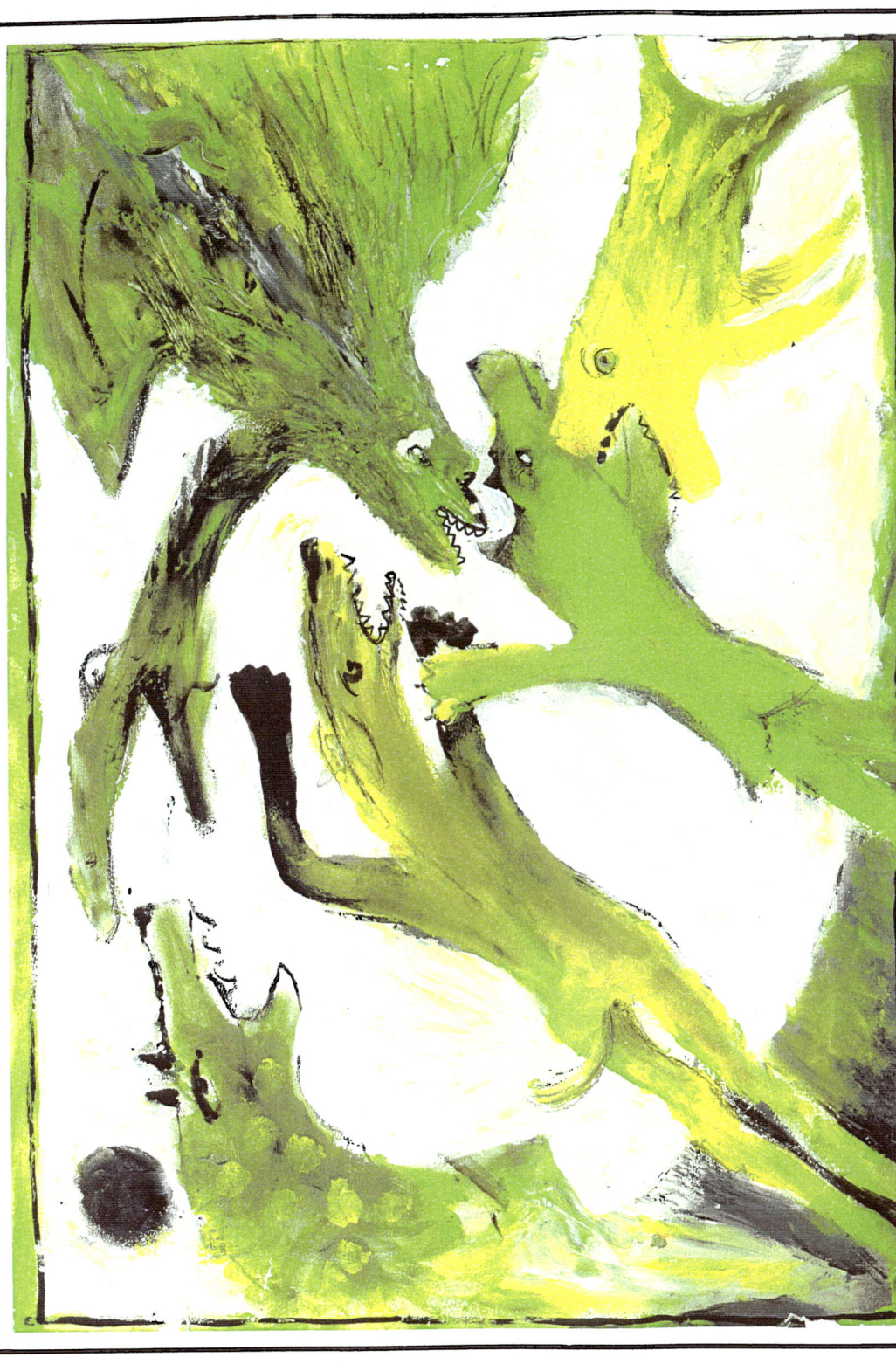

Fig. 312 Animal Fight   Gouache & Pencil

Overleaf: Fig. 313 'The Combatants' Gouache. Following the 'dog-fight' above, this painting shows a more amorphous combat between two warriors. Its ambiguous shapes allow different interpretations whether viewed as shown or upside down.

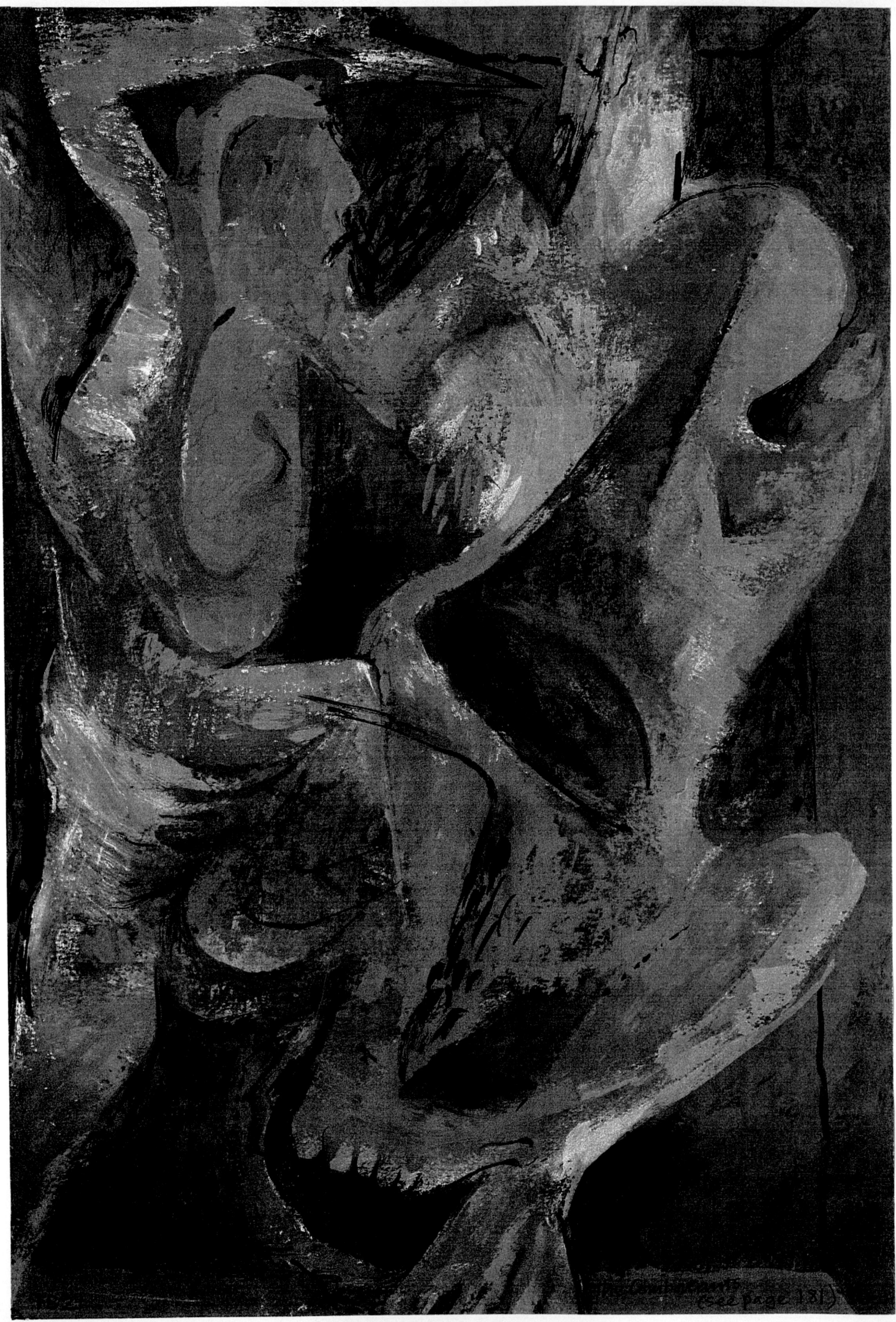

9 MASQUERADING

Dreams 88, 157, 168, 170   Hiding and Seeking

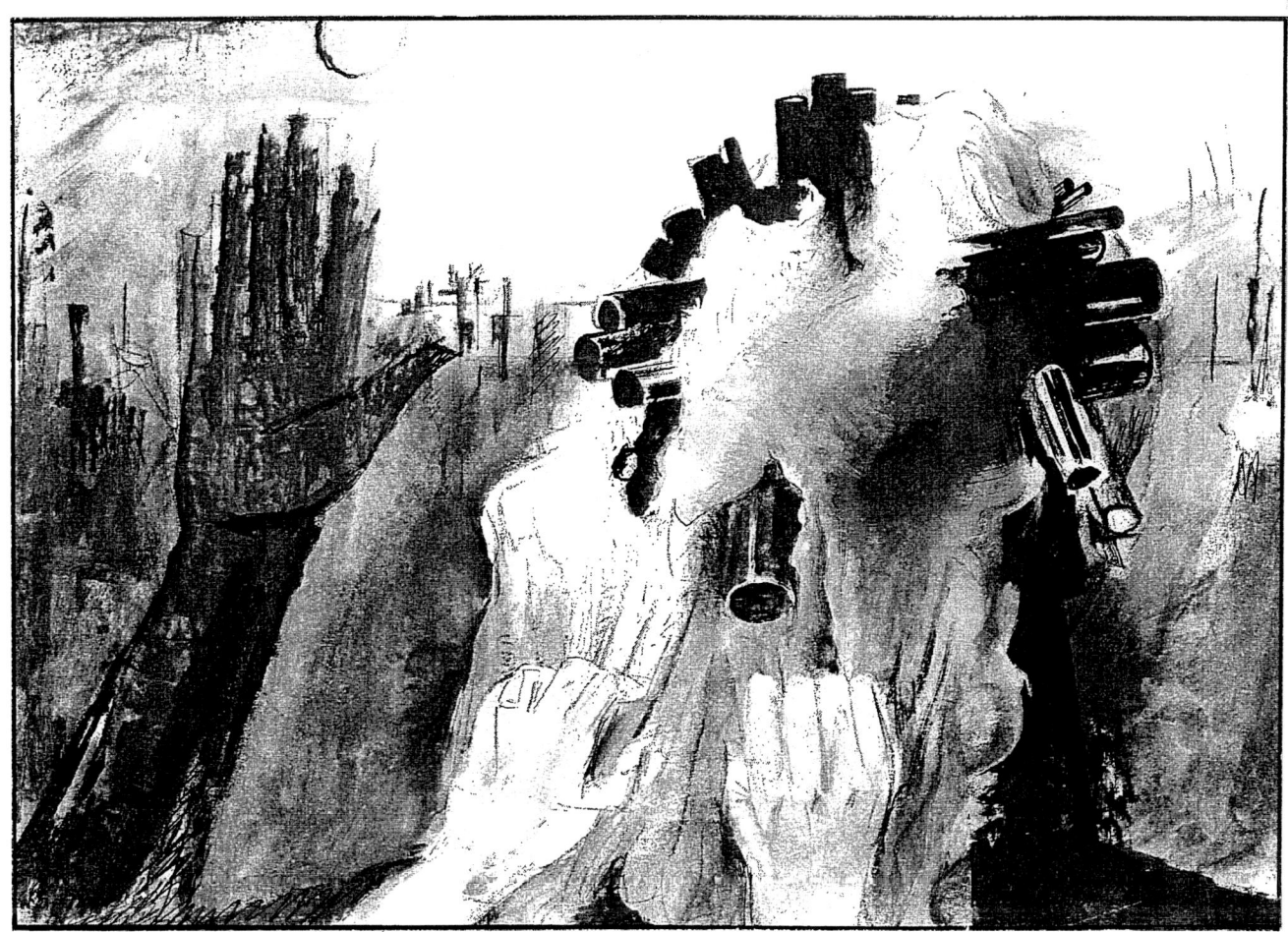

Fig. 314   Dream 88   Removing the Mask   Gouache

Dream 88   30 June 1991

Dream 88 was recorded in June '91. The illustration above had a short text which read: "Pulling a fleece and flesh off a head. Surprised to find black metallic tubes beneath, bound tightly together. Obviously not human yet possessing a presence."

In retrospect, after a sustained viewing of the dream illustration, I felt it represented a figure of power, perhaps a warrior, permitting his vulnerabilities to be revealed. Maybe he is prepared to show his wounds ("pulling... flesh off a head). Many steel tubes seem to have penetrated his head, which are seen as the fleece is pulled away.

The incongruity of black, smooth steel together with the pale yielding softness of wool is startling. Could this odd mix of opposing qualities symbolise the extremities of mood swings I was aware of at this time?

The meaning behind the raised hand is ambiguous. Does the hand advise caution in the removal of the mask, or is it raised in an act of salutation, welcoming the the hands of one wishing to reveal the man beneath the mask? Could the pale hands represent the conscious self searching for subconscious elements? The scene is set on some kind of roof level, suggesting a higher (conscious) desire to understand the underlying structure.

It now seems possible that this dream offers a flashback about a manic/depressive experience caused by unforeseen circumstances during a rehearsal of a drama project some twelve years previously.

MASKING THE ALIENS

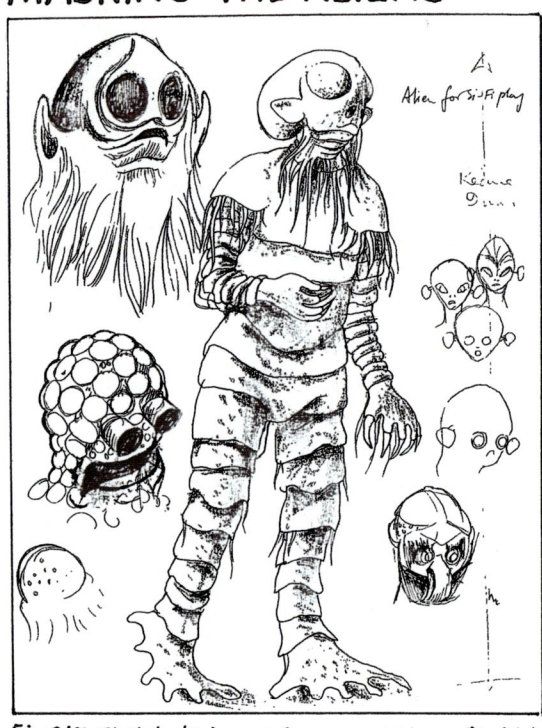

Fig.315 Sketch designs: Swamp creature. Pen & Ink

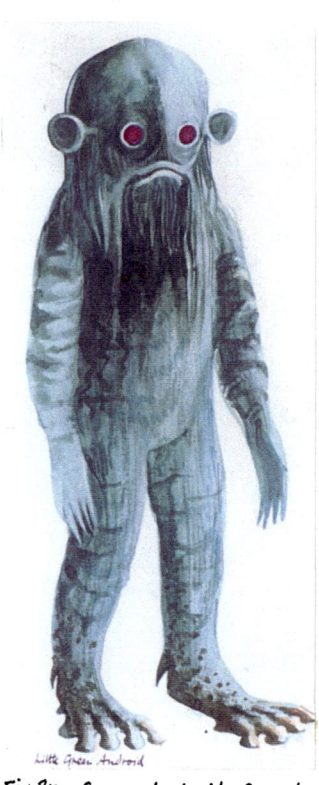

Fig.316 Green Android. Gouache

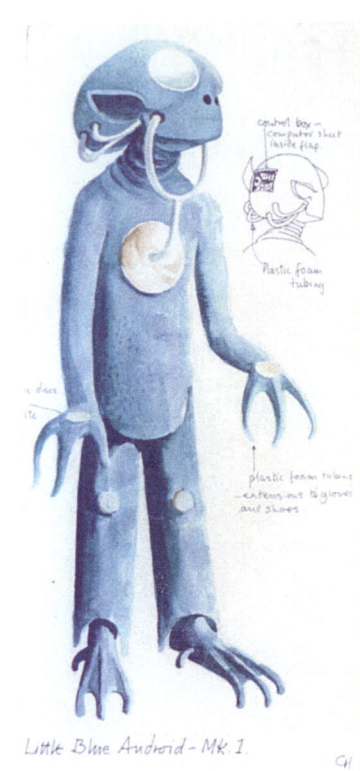

Fig.317 Blue Android. Gouache

Following years of work on traditional school plays, it was a refreshing change in 1977 to be invited to sketch out ideas for masked costumes for a Sci-Fi production. Having not made masks before, the design and construction of alien creatures presented plenty of challenges. Exploring the technical problems of using new materials (latex, etc.,) could stimulate the imagination to 'find new 'alien' forms. Alternatively, these might come from reflection, forms growing out of some inner response.

From the time of this production onwards, I was fascinated by 'masking' - its ability to conceal and disguise interior happenings and, at the deepest psychological level, protect the vulnerable self.

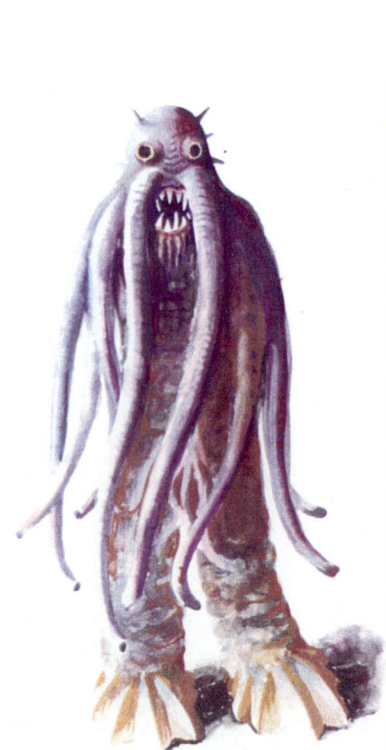

Fig.318 'Elephanus' design. Gouache

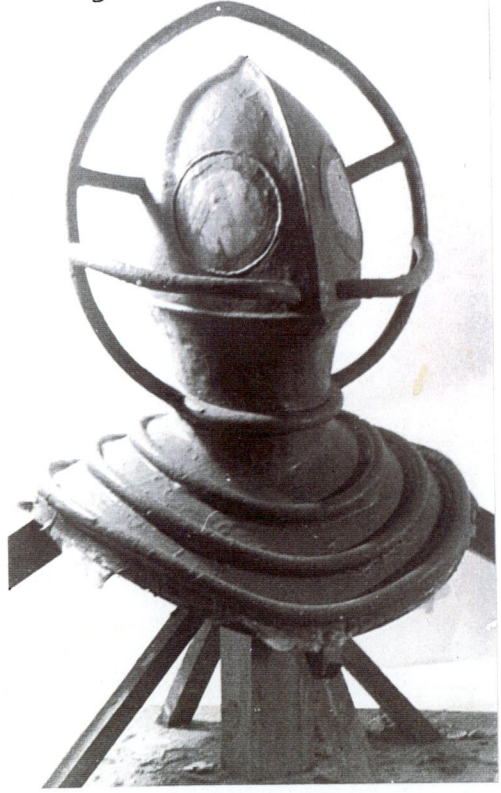

Fig.319. Making an Alien headpiece. Photo

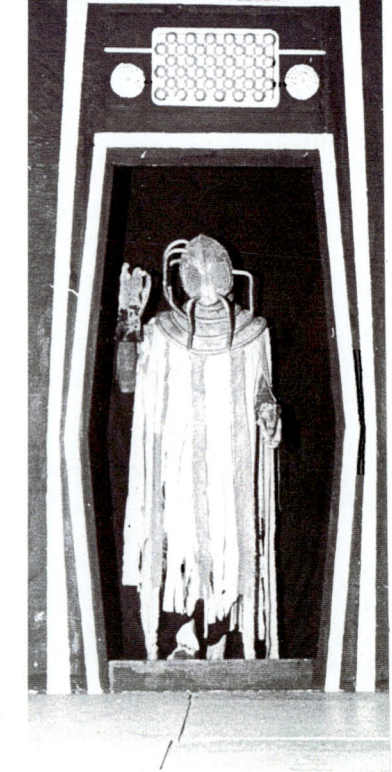

Fig.320 Alien on stage. Photo

COSTUMES FOR A SEA DANCE DRAMA

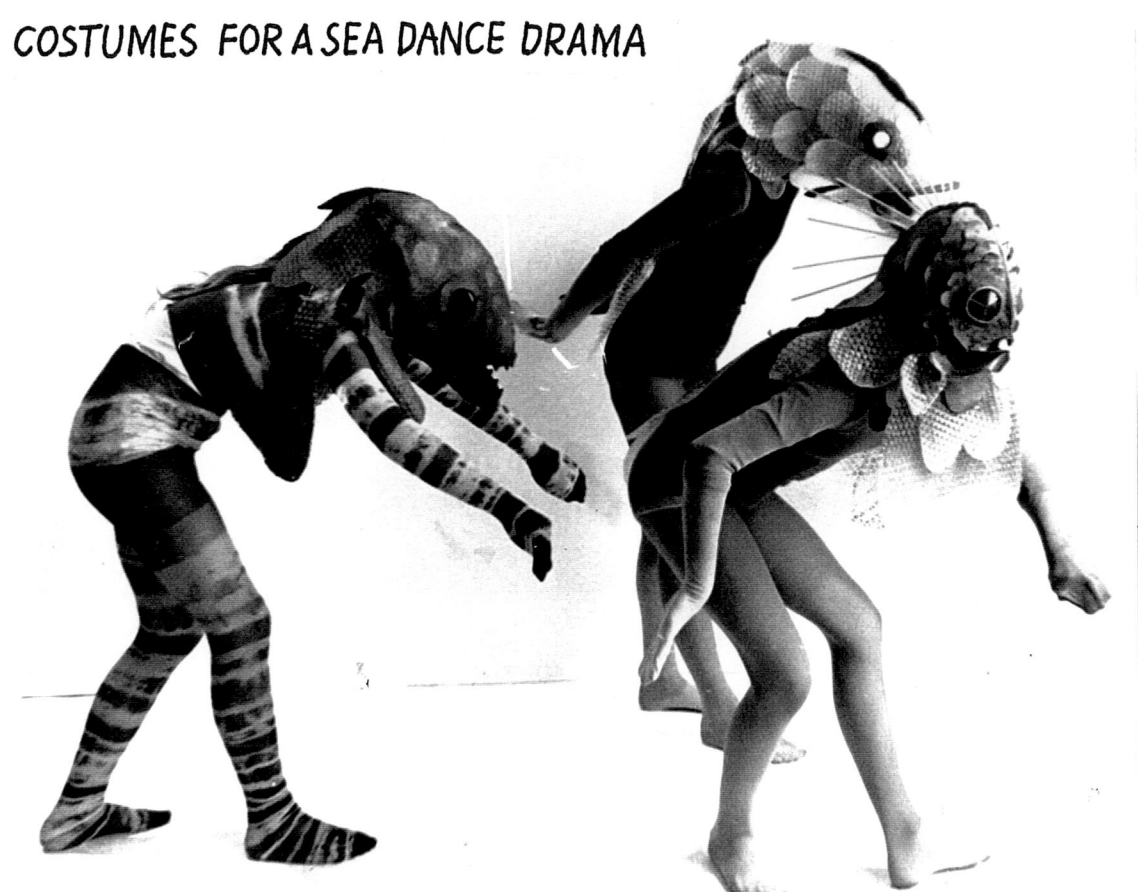

Fig. 321 Fish Masks and Batik-treated tights (left). Photo

The following year I devised a dance drama based on Joan Aiken's story 'The Kingdom under the sea', deciding to participate myself as the 'Lobster Monster' (Bottom right and page 131). Some 40 costumes were made for a travelling show to take to primary schools, where the pupils could dress up, rehearse and dance within one day.
It was a show which encouraged me to attempt a much more ambitious project. The consequences which flowed from this are described overleaf.

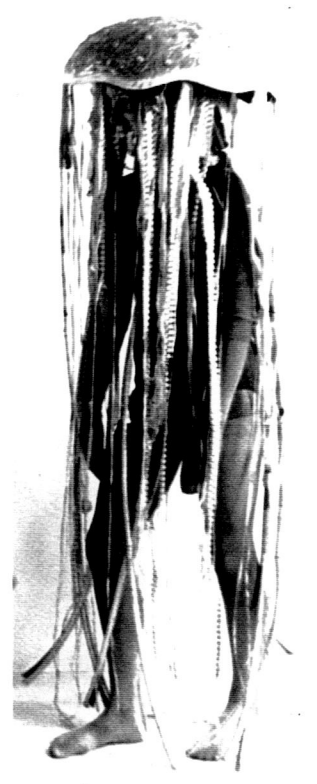

Fig. 322. Portuguese man-of-war. photo

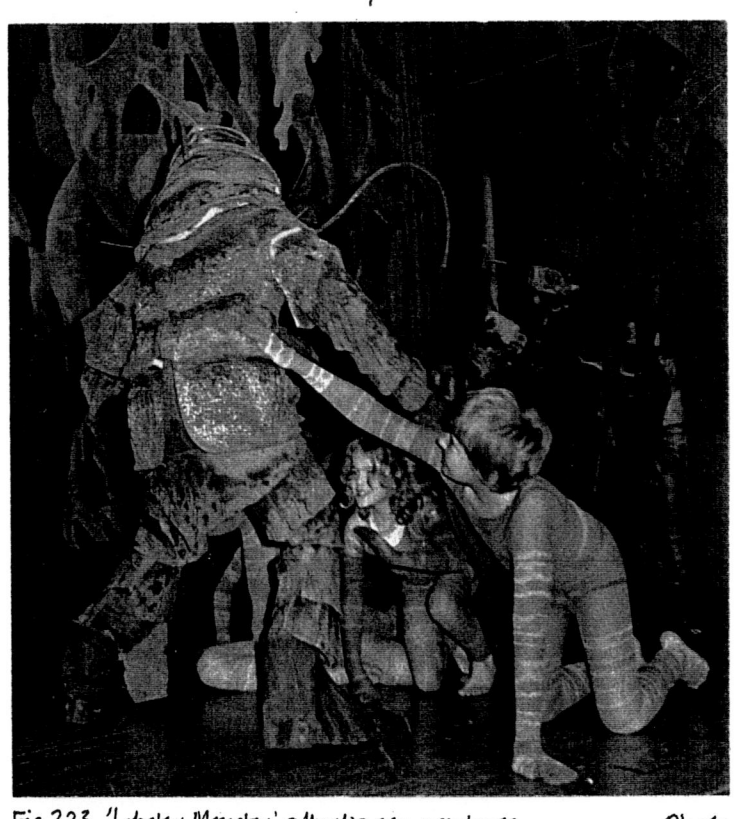

Fig. 323 'Lobster Monster' attacks sea creatures. Photo

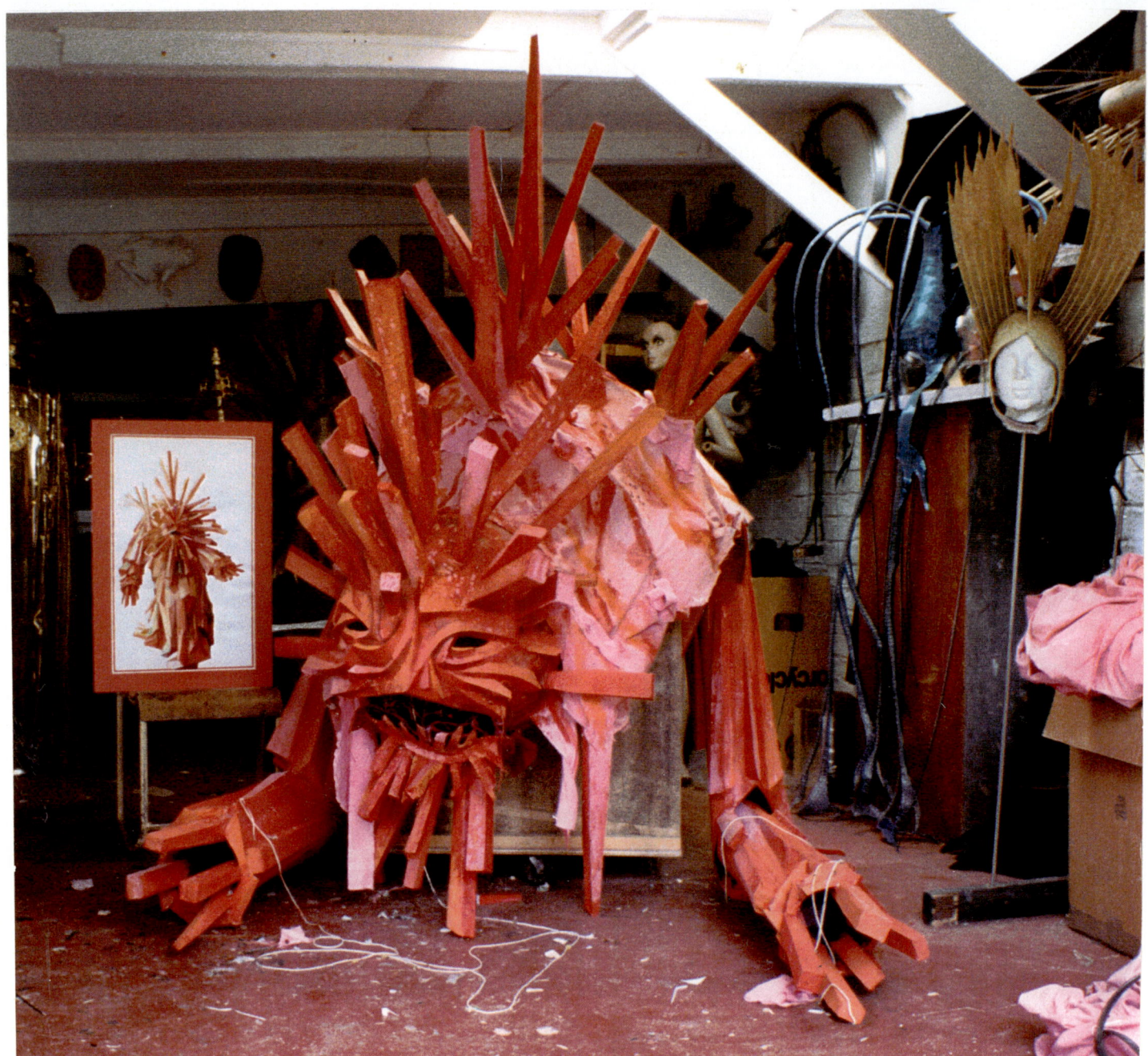

Fig.324. Persephone – Costume for the Titan Briareus, the Demeter headpiece on right   Photo

The composer, an ensemble of musicians and a recording specialist were now at the rehearsal stage. I'd already found a choreographer willing to find and train a group of dance/drama students for the leading roles.

Months earlier I had become obsessed with a vision which, I felt, if translated to the stage, would make an exciting dance drama. The Persephone myth I'd read led me into a state of manic enthusiasm and, within weeks, many costumes were designed with a few nearly completed.

This version of the myth opened with the Titans – Briareus, Enceladus and Typhon. I became fixated on making Briareus and then operating his ten foot tall enormity from within the costume. Shadow play would, hopefully, suggest the two other giants.

With hindsight I now realise that the start of a manic mood accounted for all this activity and would soon transform itself into a darker and more anxious phase. Briareus was now the symbol of manic aspirations and yet was, in real practical terms, only peripheral to the main story. The giant echoed all too well the inflated egomania I was now enduring.

Following the music rehearsal things began to unravel. The recording engineer was not satisfied with the sound quality on the tape and suggested I recall the musicians – yet I'd no financial resources to pay them again. Then the choreographer quite suddenly took ill and the dance students, who should have been training, failed to materialise. The final straw was that the local college stage was no longer available.

This 'production-that-never-was' became a metaphor for the internal transformation then beginning to take effect – a microcosm for the real breakdown which later followed.

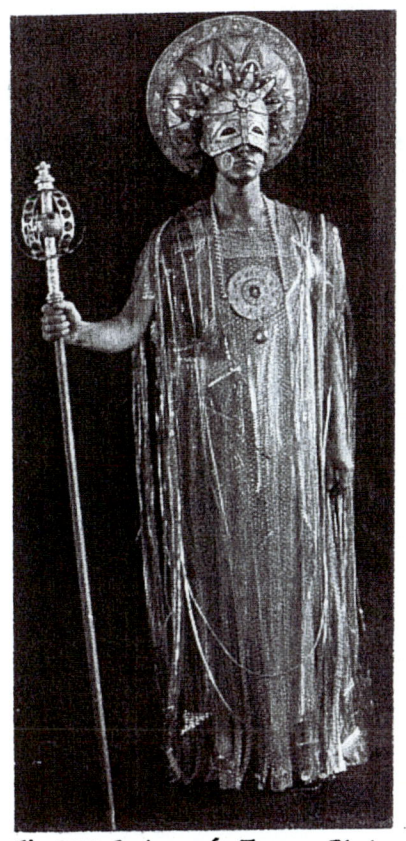

Fig. 325 Costume for Zeus   Photo

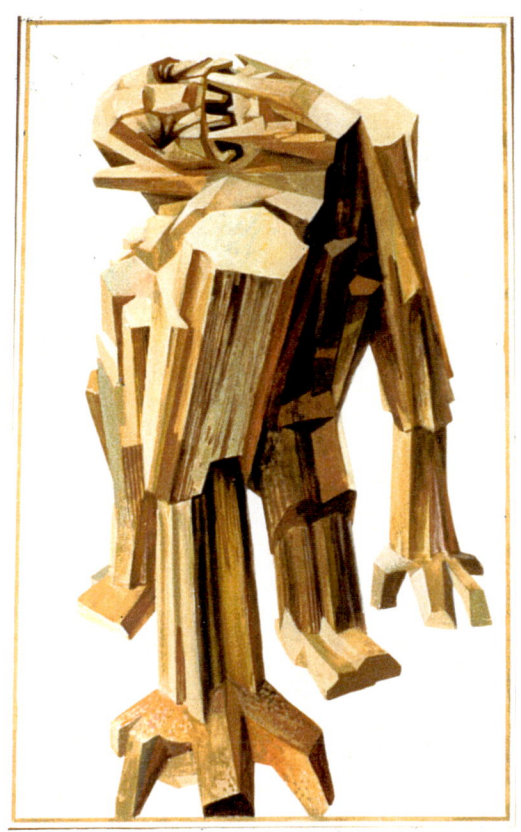

Fig. 326 Design for Enceladus   Gouache

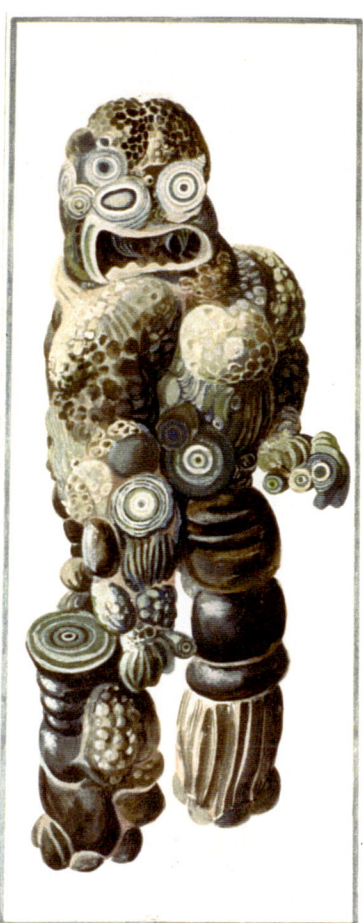

Fig. 327 Design for Typhon – Gouache

DESIGNS AND COSTUMES FOR 'PERSEPHONE'

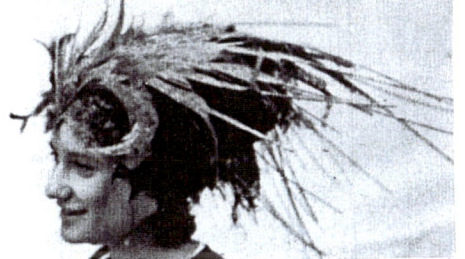

Fig. 328 Headpiece for Persephone – Photo

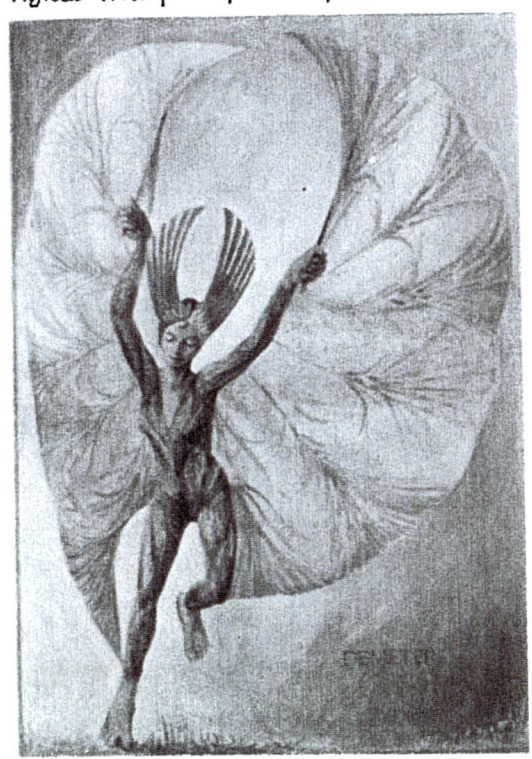

Fig. 329 Design for Demeter   Gouache

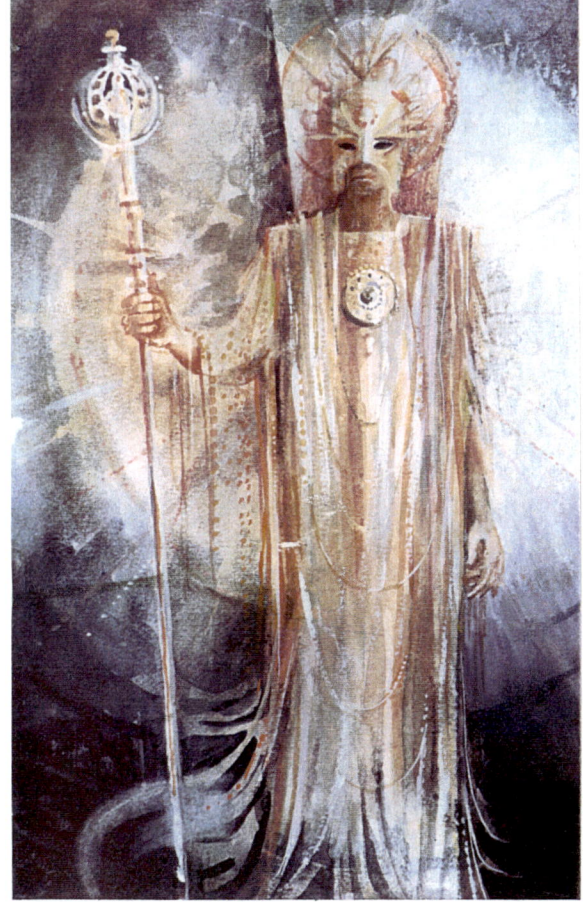

Fig. 330 Design for Zeus   Watercolour & Gouache

Dream 157   23 April 1992 'The Music Examiner'

Entering a vast hall I notice a young woman in the furthermost corner, practising on a flute. The sun's rays streaming through windows behind casts her in shadow and, as I advance, the sun dazzles my eyes. The flautist, and now other performers, welcome me as I approach and I offer to accompany her on the piano.

I look about and now notice a large man hunched over a table writing. I approach him, offering my apologies when I realise he is the music examiner. His head is large and pear-shaped and has 'saucer' eyes. Surprisingly he has no other discernible features. Only the faintest of marks for a nose but no mouth.

He can't respond to me. He expresses no emotion nor can he speak. He can only write down comments about the music.

I now notice another man on a stage with similar mask-like features. I'm told that he is a magician and will perform tricks.

On waking I realised how mesmerised I was by the examiner's and magician's faces. All the surrounding young people seemed unimportant. The dream's message - masking could stifle communication.

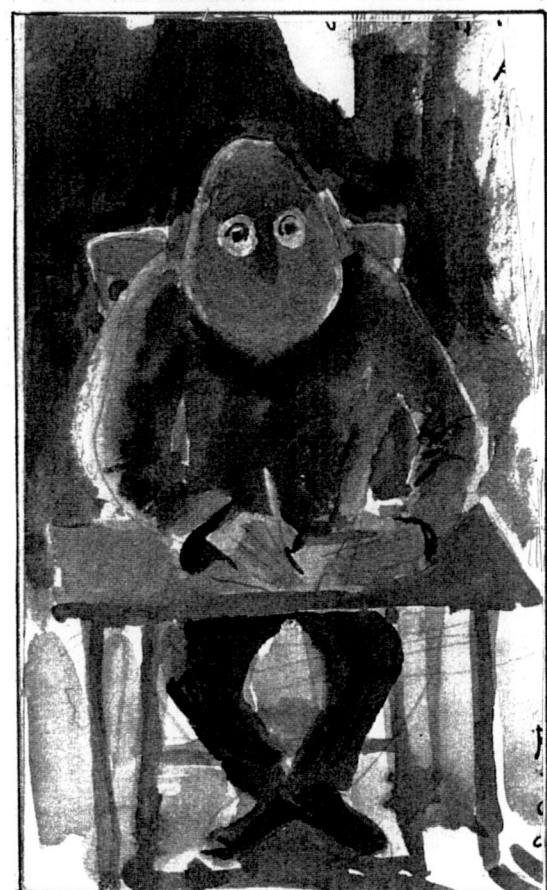

Fig. 331   Dream 157   Gouache

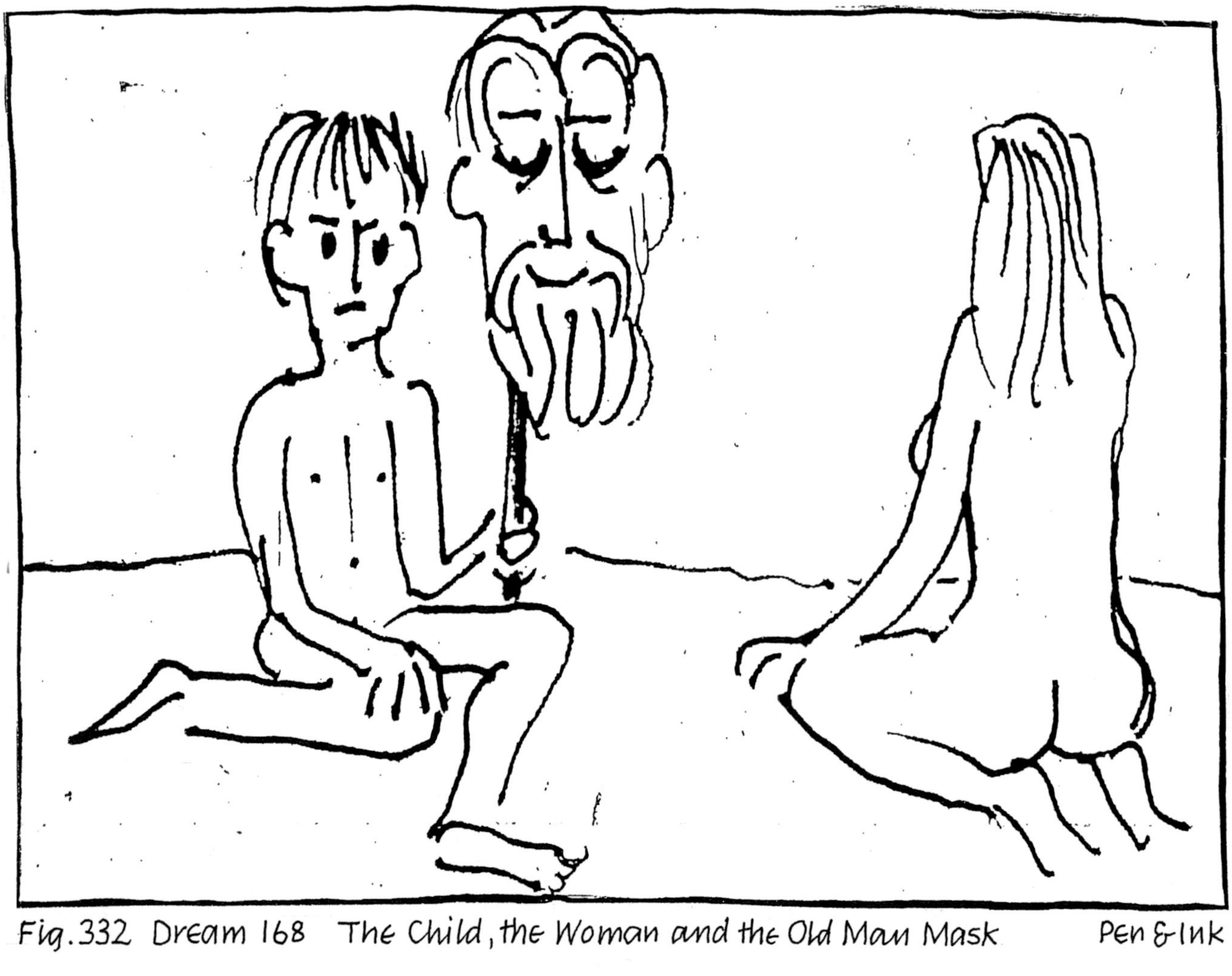

Fig. 332   Dream 168   The Child, the Woman and the Old Man Mask   Pen & Ink

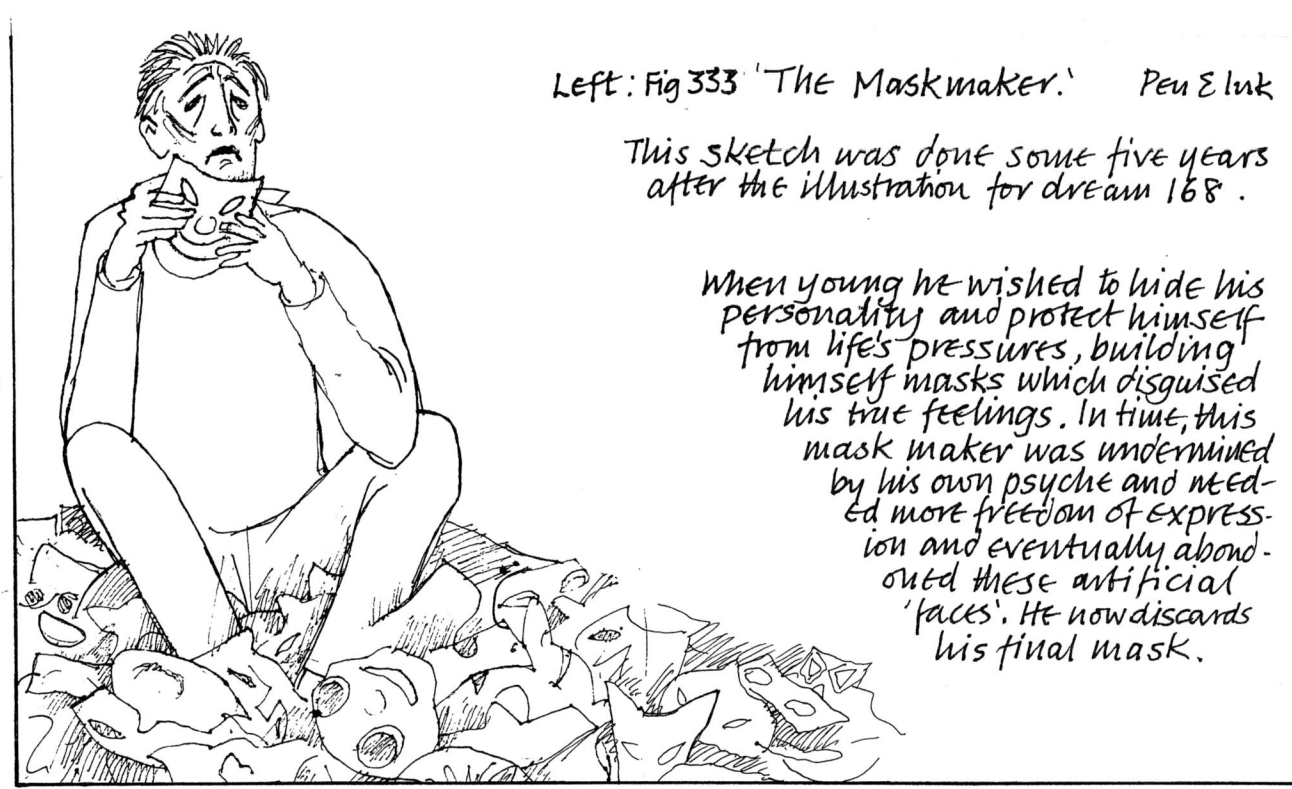

Left: Fig 333 'The Maskmaker.'   Pen & Ink

This sketch was done some five years after the illustration for dream 168.

When young he wished to hide his personality and protect himself from life's pressures, building himself masks which disguised his true feelings. In time, this mask maker was undermined by his own psyche and needed more freedom of expression and eventually abandoned these artificial 'faces'. He now discards his final mask.

Bottom Left: **Dream 168**   7 August 1992

"A frightened child fears being consumed within a relationship and is busy making masks to avoid a confrontation. But it is too late, the young woman has arrived. The seductress confronts him but he is just in time to raise his most protective mask — that of an experienced older man."

This quote, written alongside the dream illustration above (fig.333) had much to say about my past apprehensions about women. Youth and age together face the mature woman, showing my vulnerability when confronting the child-mother relationship — the macho 'old man' mask heightens this show of self defence.

In retrospect I'm now aware that half-way through the therapeutic process my therapist had stressed the necessity of forming a relationship between us. The dream image was hinting that this would come about when I could trust her — that the anxious look of the child would vanish when he realised this and abandoned his 'old man' mask.

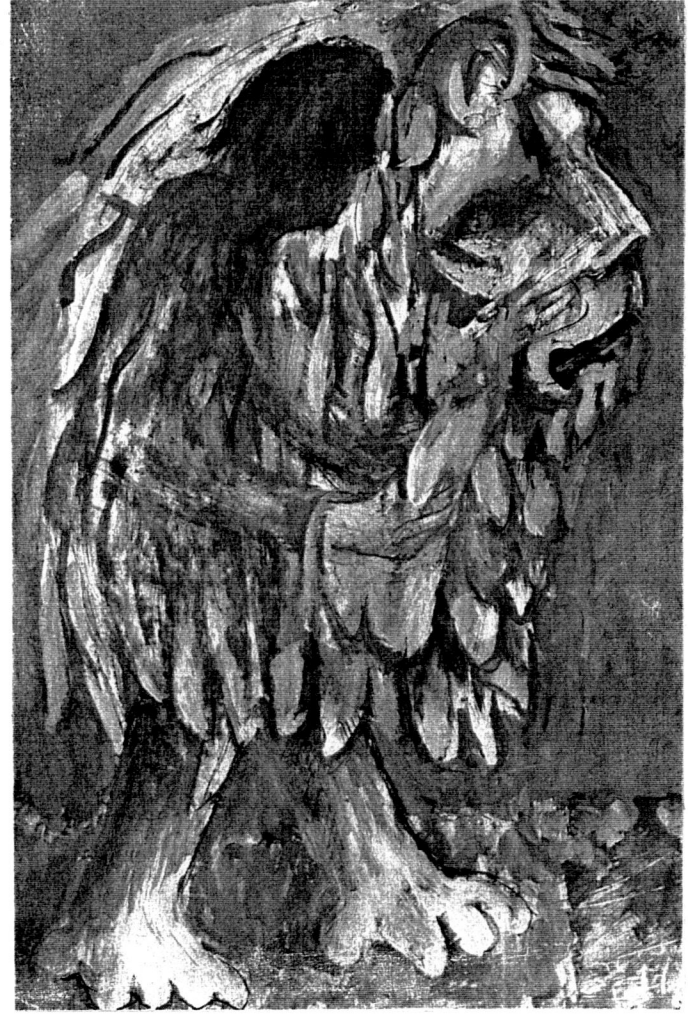

Right: Fig.334 Pantomine Lion   Gouache

This later painting shows parallels with the dream above. The theatre costume replaces the mask, the timidity of the adult performer echoes that of nervous child in dream 168.

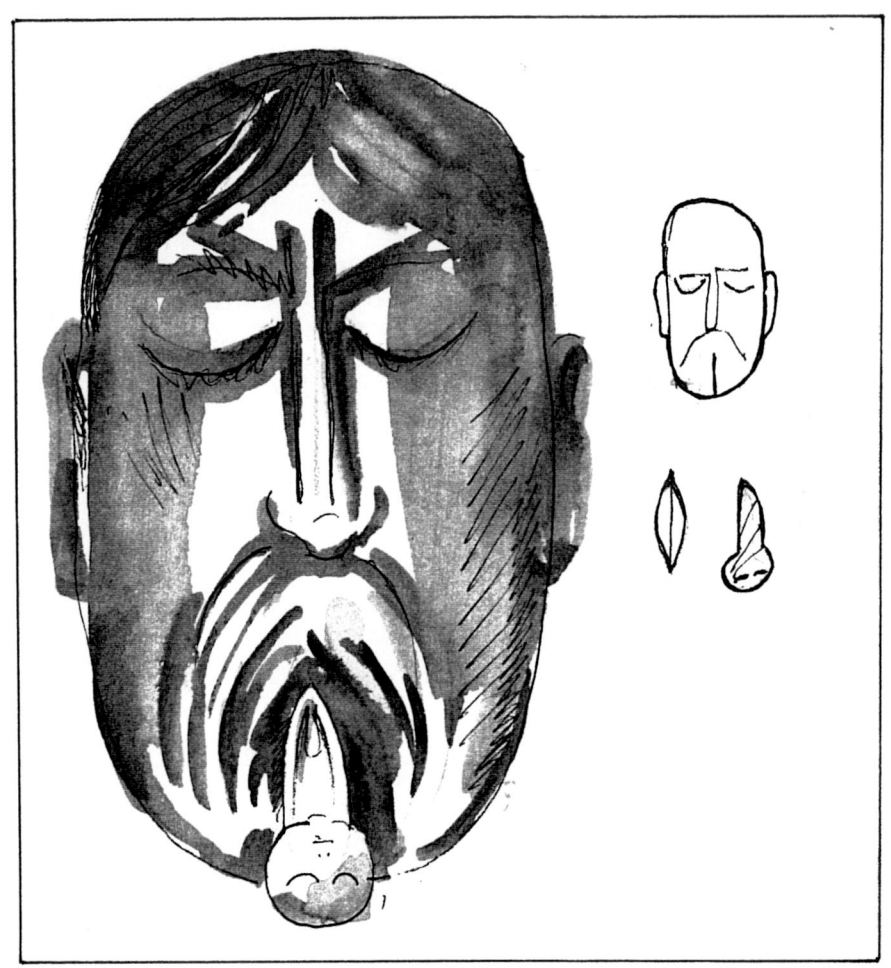

Fig. 335   Dream 170   The Birth   Pen & Wash

Dream 170   1 September 1992

"A craftsman/maskmaker is carving a large head. At the mouth a baby's head appears. There is a certain embarrassment that the mouth/vagina ambiguity might cause offence, so the sculptor is thinking about making separate parts - a head, a mouth/vagina and a baby/phallus which might be fitted separately."

Initially, for me, dreams are invariably obscure, only becoming revelatory with hindsight, sometimes years later.
Dream experiences are essentially free in expressiveness, showing darker and 'outrageous' aspects of our hidden fears and desires. Imagine my curiosity when I discover an internal, puritanical censor laying a dead hand on the contents of the dream. A 'certain embarrassment' causes the sculptor to rearrange the offending parts so that they are detachable and could be fitted 'later' - if 'suitable'.
Perhaps this is a dream 'coding' - a way of highlighting the genital hermaphrodite aspects within the head where both the vagina (mouth) and phallus (swaddled babe) are suggested. Could this be the dream's way of offering an insight into the need to find the anima/spirit - to seek out the feminine aspects of creativity within?

10 DECAPITATION

Dream 94 — Death and Regeneration

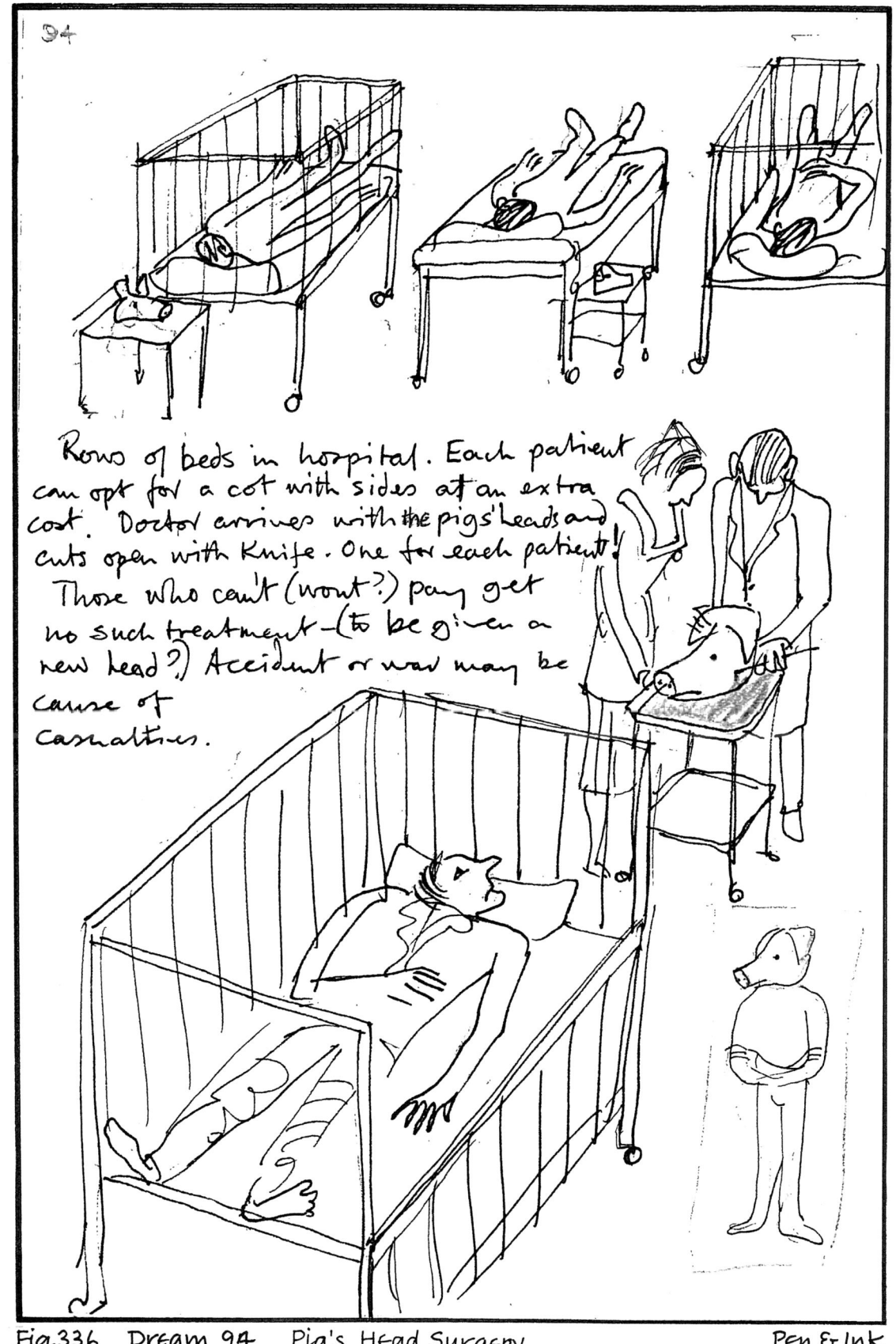

Fig. 336   Dream 94   Pig's Head Surgery   Pen & Ink

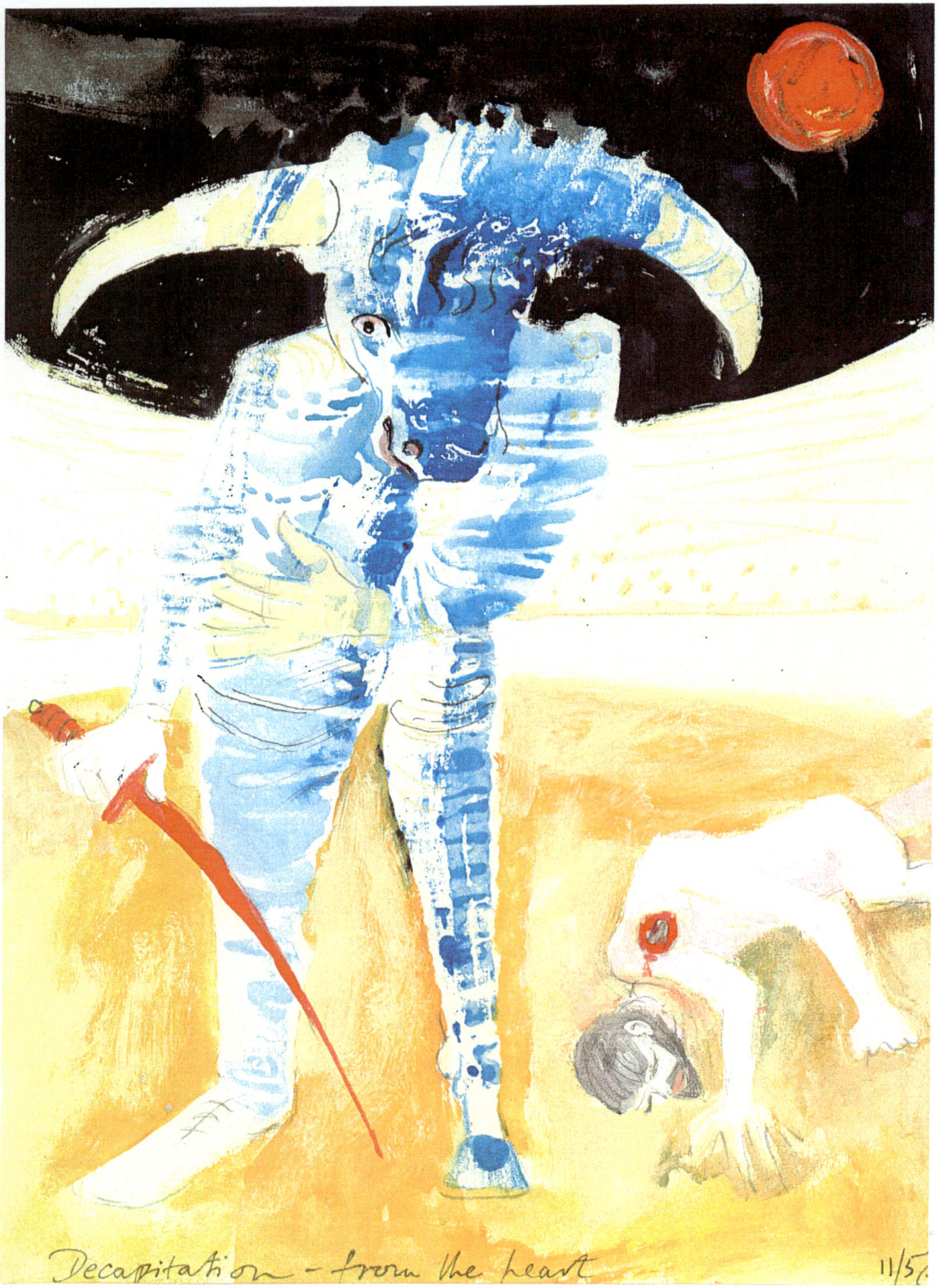

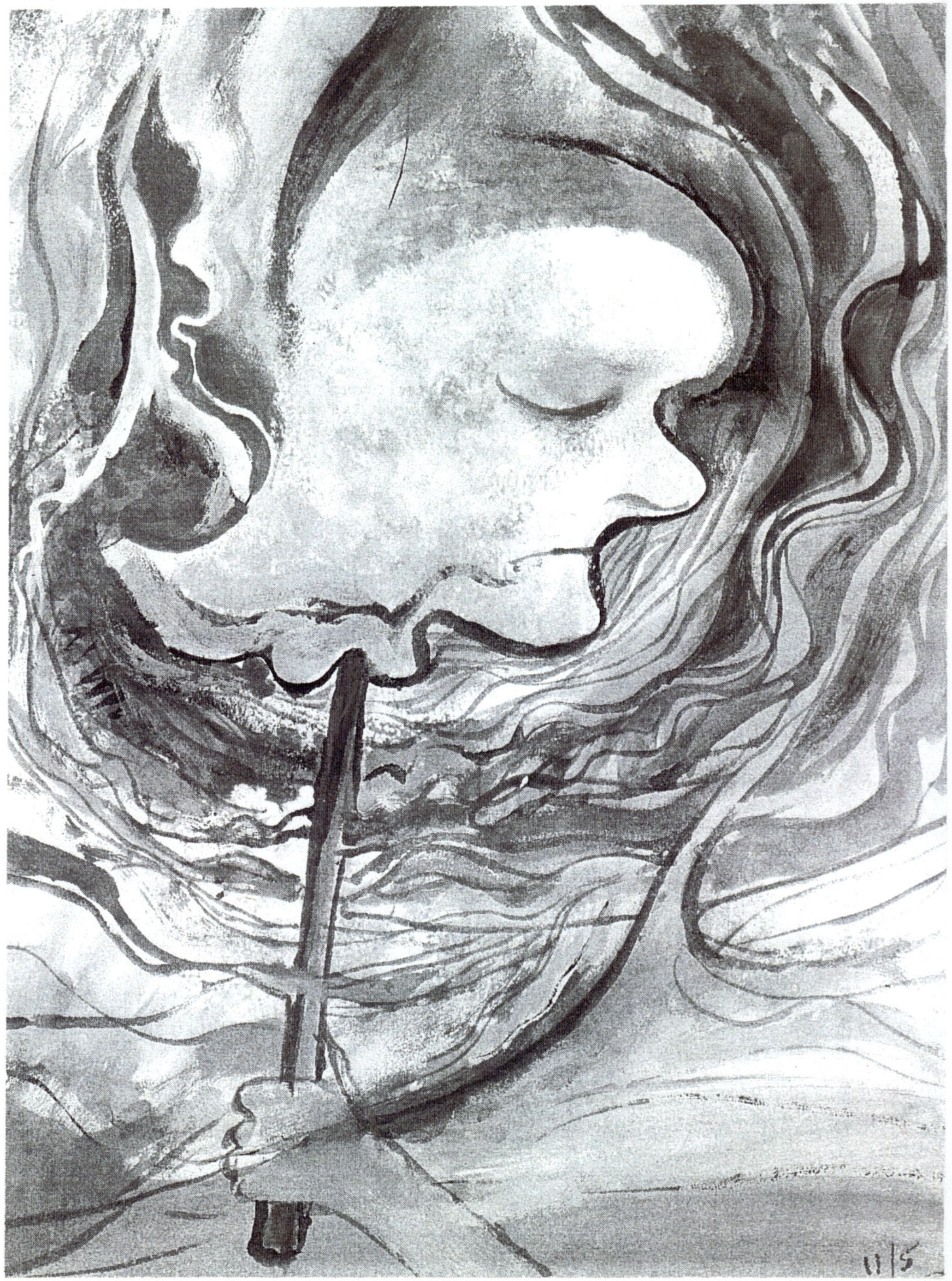

Fig. 338 Revolution! Gouache
Left: Fig. 337 Decapitation - from the heart. Pen & Gouache

192

Dream 94 (page 191) The curious content of this dream pin-points the vulnerability of the neck. In the past frequent neck-ache had troubled me enough to seek medical advice, without any conclusive outcome. It made me reflect on some explanation. I recalled a sense of loathing on occasion, of not being quite in touch with my body (without any substance abuse!). To receive a pig's head seemed like a semi-comic entry into a child's magic storybook of changing identity — I would have preferred a head, say, of some-one like Jung who could have helped me analyse the dream! The 'central' idea of a cut neck seems to stress the idea of a psychosomatic malfunctioning and this was where one should concentrate the mind.

Above Left: Fig. 337 'Decapitation from the Heart' Pen & Gouache

The subconscious draws the Matador slaying the 'bull-self' — the heart pays back the rational self for its neglect.

Above Right: Fig. 338 'Revolution' Gouache

Shows the guillotined head of the King, raised in triumph by the emotive masses.

Left: Fig. 339 'Warrior Head'

The warrior, a daydreamer, is lost in thought - enough to lose both his horse and his body

Overleaf: Fig 340 'Black Tuesday' Oil Transfer & Pen

A painting resulting from a particular Tuesday in 1994 — a day of deep depression. Three heads oblivious of each other stare out into space. The reverse viewpoint shows a lighter mood, a sea creature enjoys a meal — a whale's head rises......

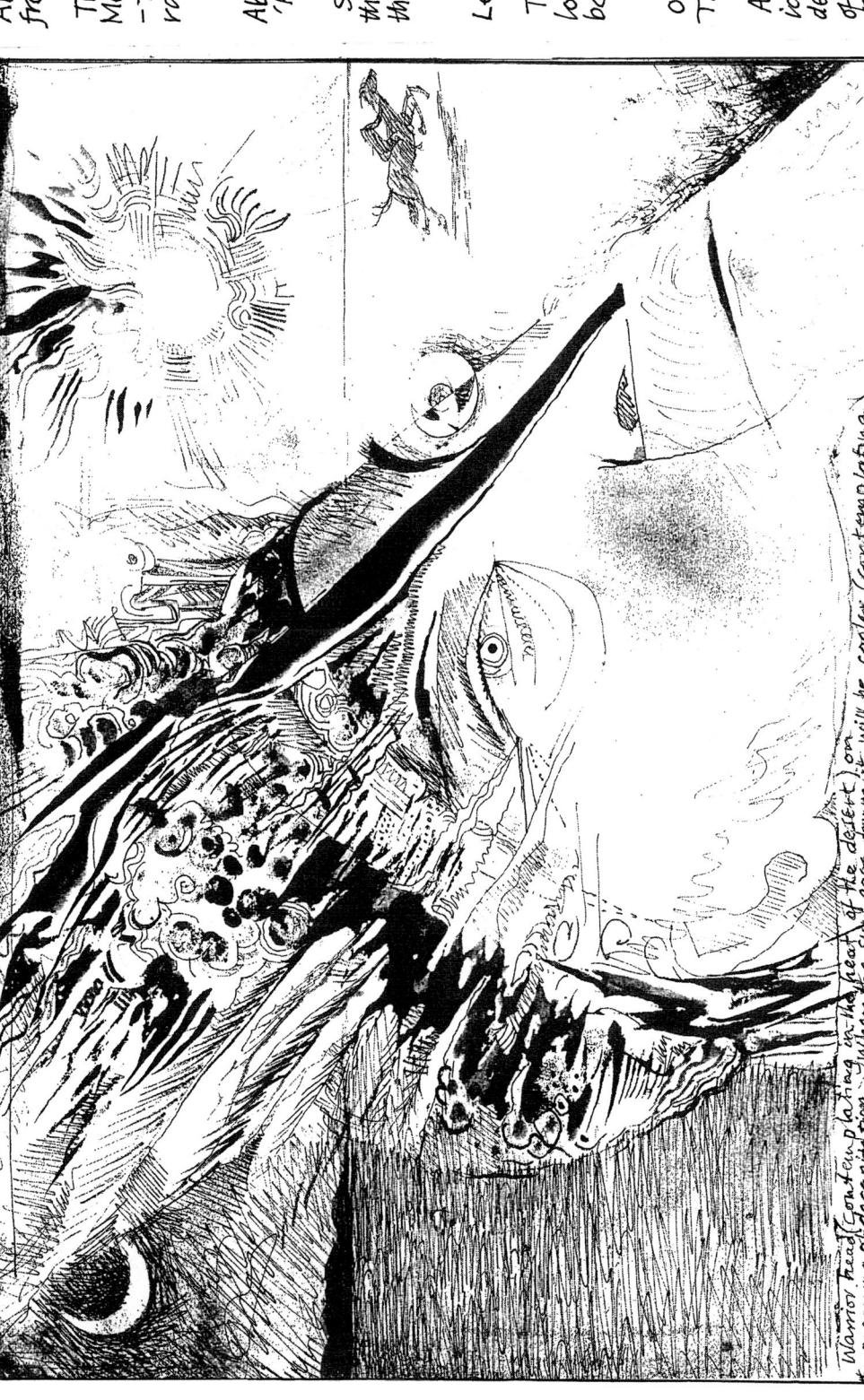

Warrior Head (contemplating in the heat of the desert) on the morning of decapitation. (When the sun goes down it will be cooler (contemplating on the coldness of the desert at night). Staying with change, movement, transformation.. ⚔ FRIDAY 13th MAY '94

Fig. 339 Warrior Head Pen, Brush & Ink

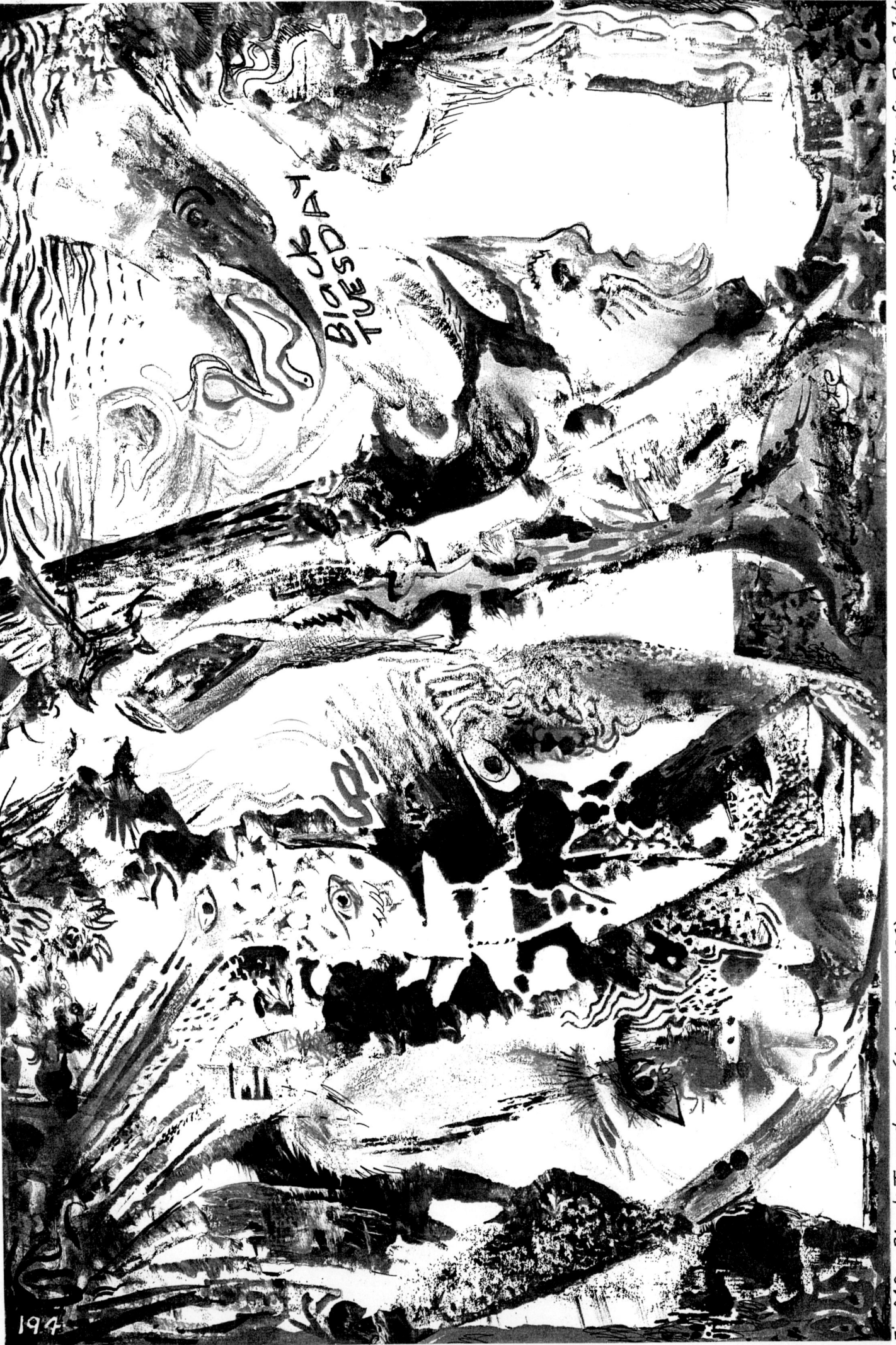

Fig. 340 Black Tuesday (text-page 193) Oil Transfer, Pen & Ink

11 VICTIMS AND SACRIFICES

Dream 96   Acceptance

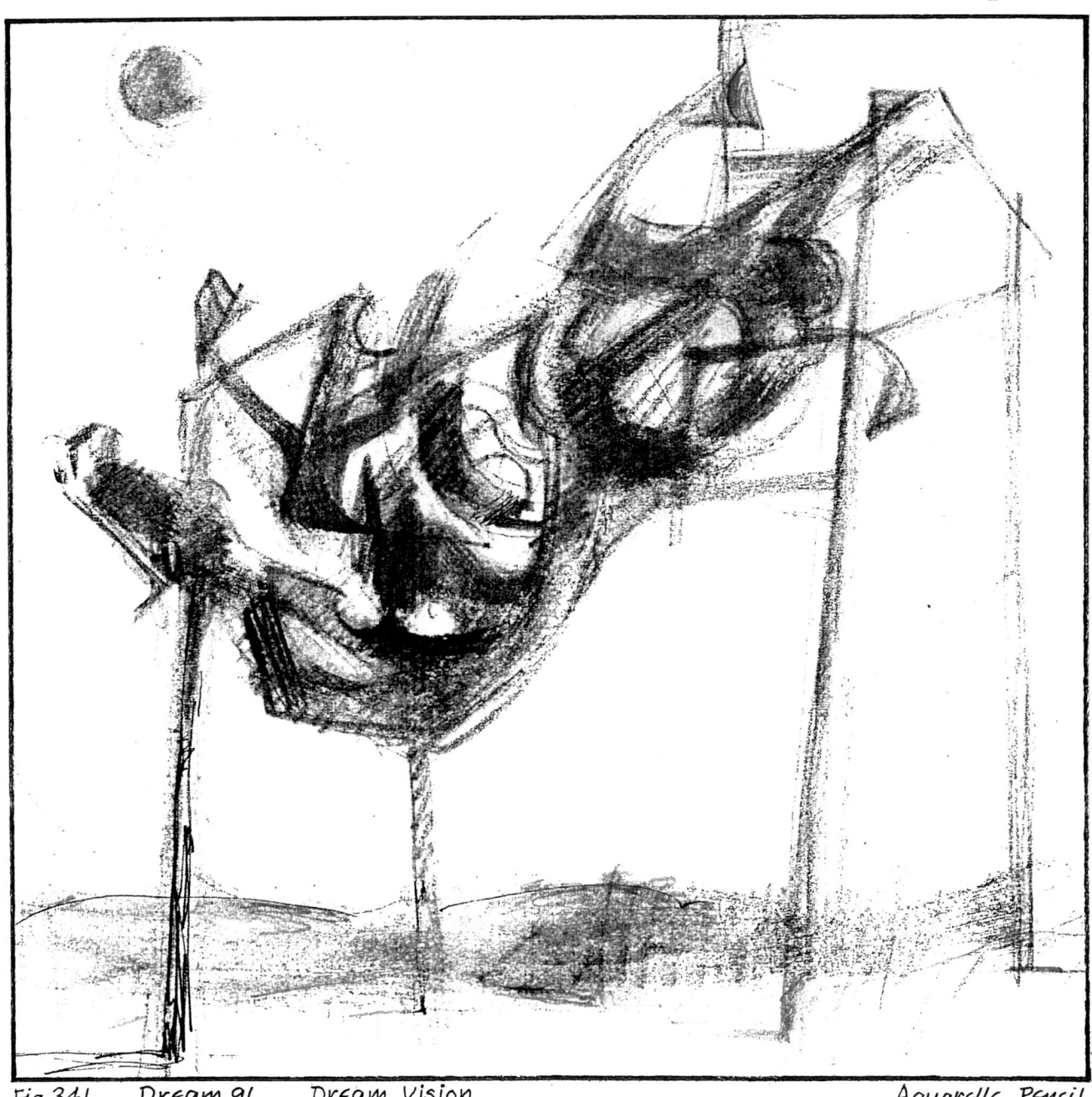

Fig. 341   Dream 96   Dream Vision   Aquarelle Pencil

Dream 96   26 July 1991

'Until this moment the walk over the hills had been without incident. Someone earlier had remarked how lonely the landscape was — or had I misheard, had the voice said 'lovely'? But by then other voices had intruded, we're witnessing something quite other, something unnerving and terrible. They talked in hushed tones about the nature of the apparition which had confronted our small party of art students out for a day's sketching.

The four poles held a strange trussed-up form. Some voices argued that it was horse-like, others that it was 'humanoid', whilst I felt that both creature and supporting frame together made a complete object.

Now, eight years on, I'm looking again at this dream image and a short sequence of pen sketches I made soon afterwards (fig. 342 overleaf). There is still the jolt of surprise

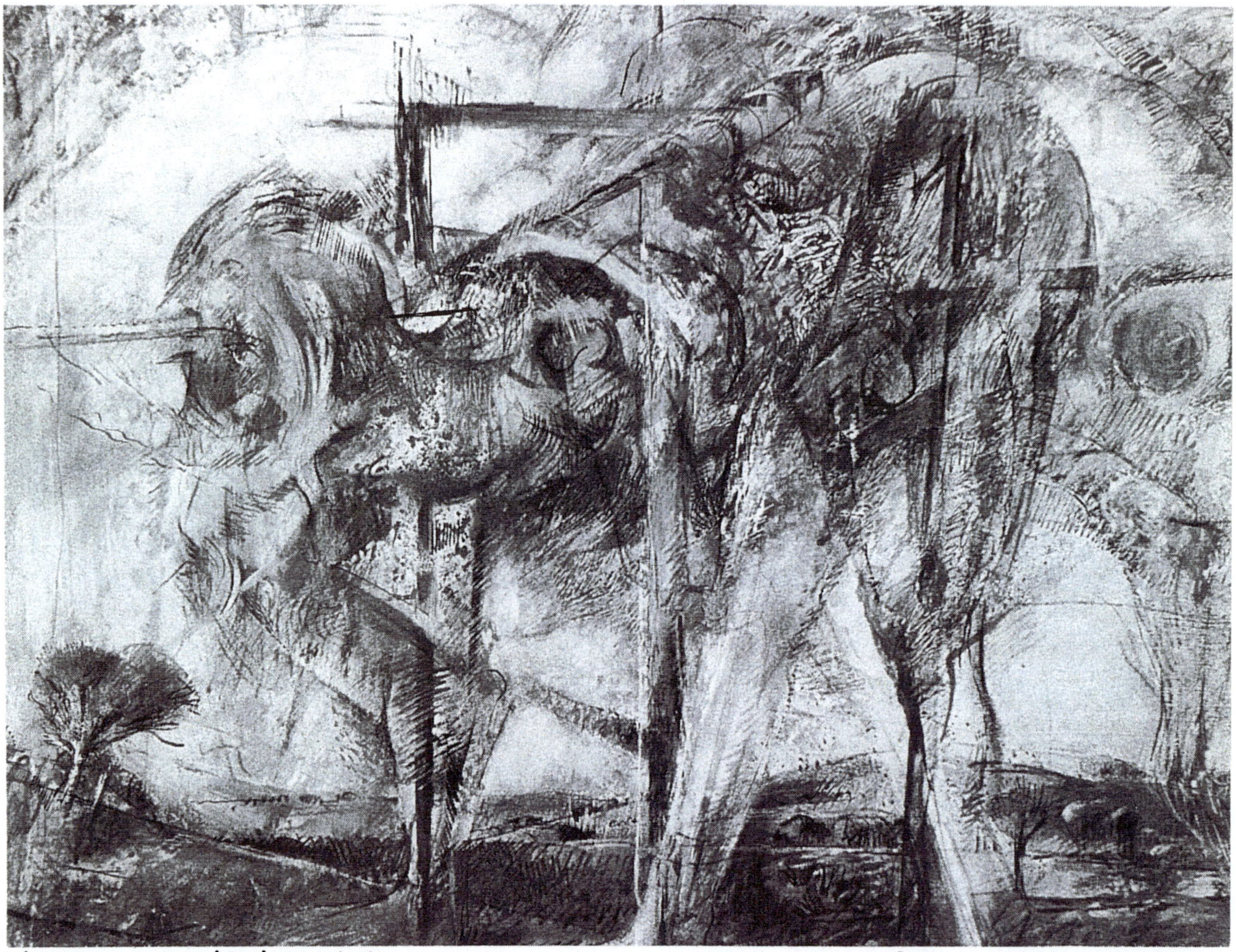

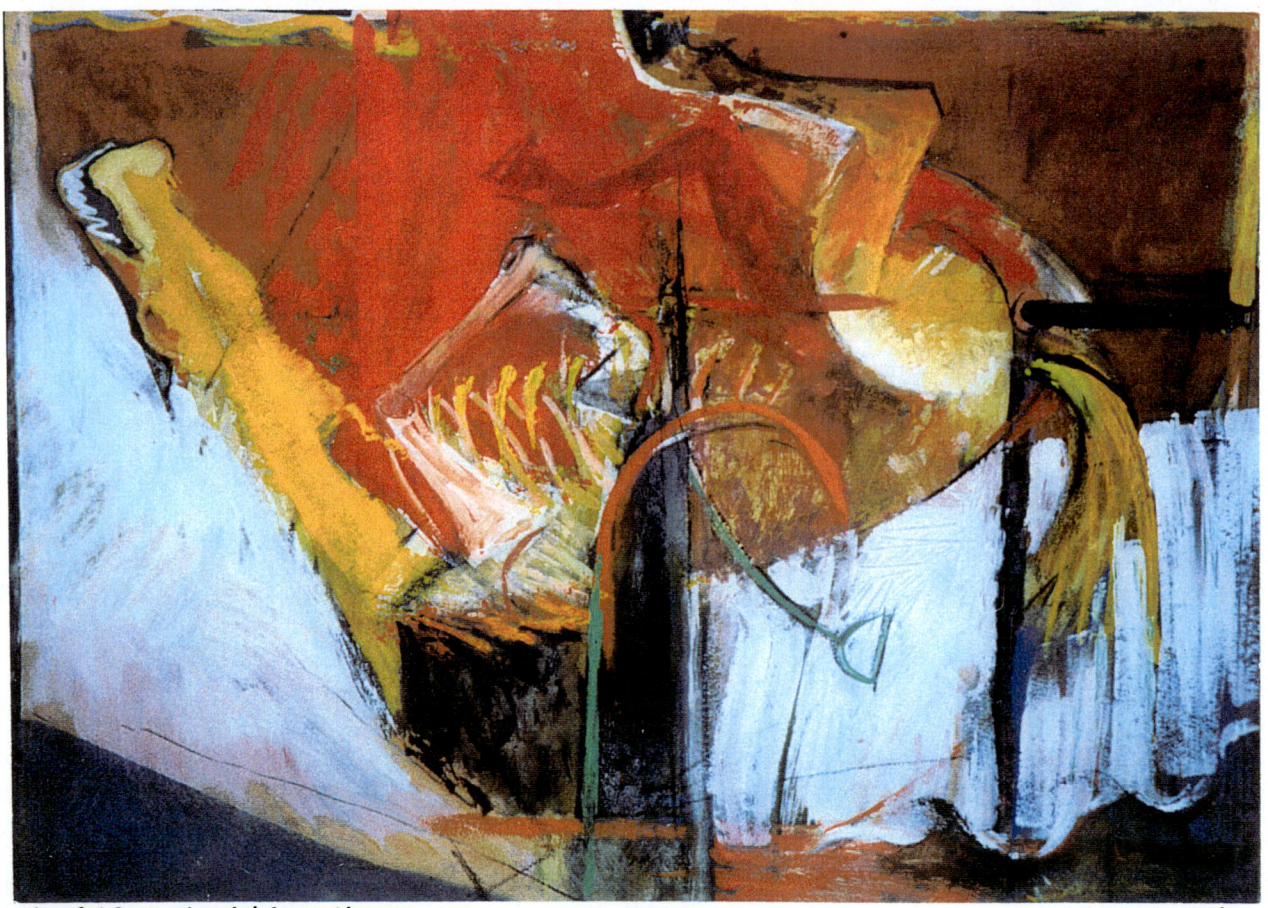

Fig. 342 Sacrificial Victim   Aquarelle Pencil & Paint

Fig. 343 Writhing Horse   Gouache

and a momentary shudder as I contemplate the amalgamation of soft flesh with the rigid wooden framework. The mix is brutal, the suspended figure of a trussed-up victim now like a cruxifixion. It seems a symbol of some profound agony, the anguish of frustration, of indecision, of being 'knotted-up'.

The 'Sacrificial Victim' (top left) painted in 1996 was a recent reflection on the original dream inasmuch as both were about trussed up victims. In the recent drawing however it is a human bent up into an awkward posture. It is as if the content is one of self-immolation rather than a sacrifice on behalf of others. Perhaps this 'man-in-a-grid' was a self-portrait expressing my own 'self-inflicted victim' situation

The other picture 'Writhing Horse' (fig. 343 Bottom left) is more problematic and I have difficulty acknowledging it as my own work, which somehow makes it the most intriguing painting in this small group of works. It started off in my now well practised freestyle or 'automatic' technique without any conscious direction on my part.

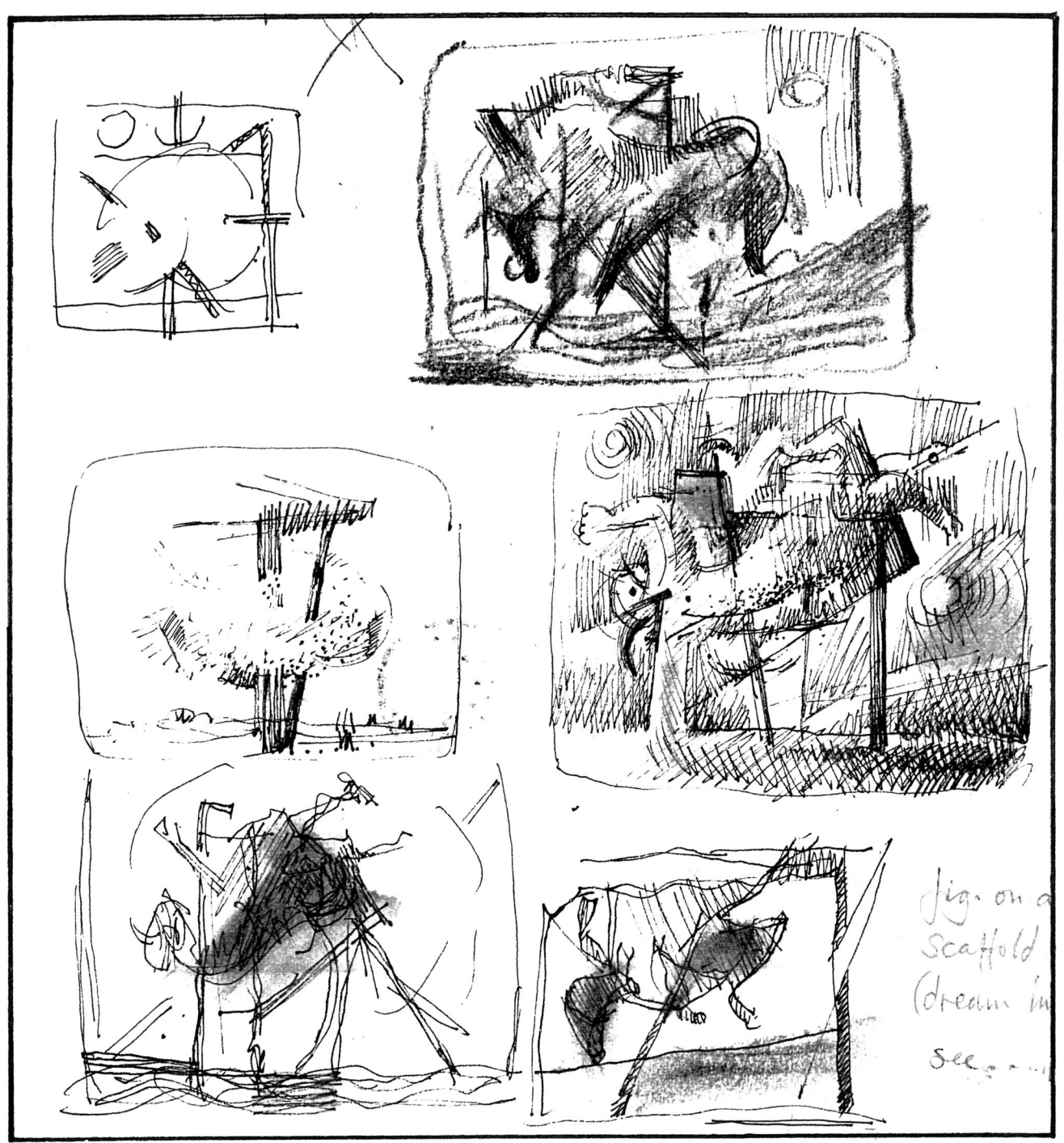

Fig. 344 'Six sketches based on Dream 96'   Pen & Ink, Crayon

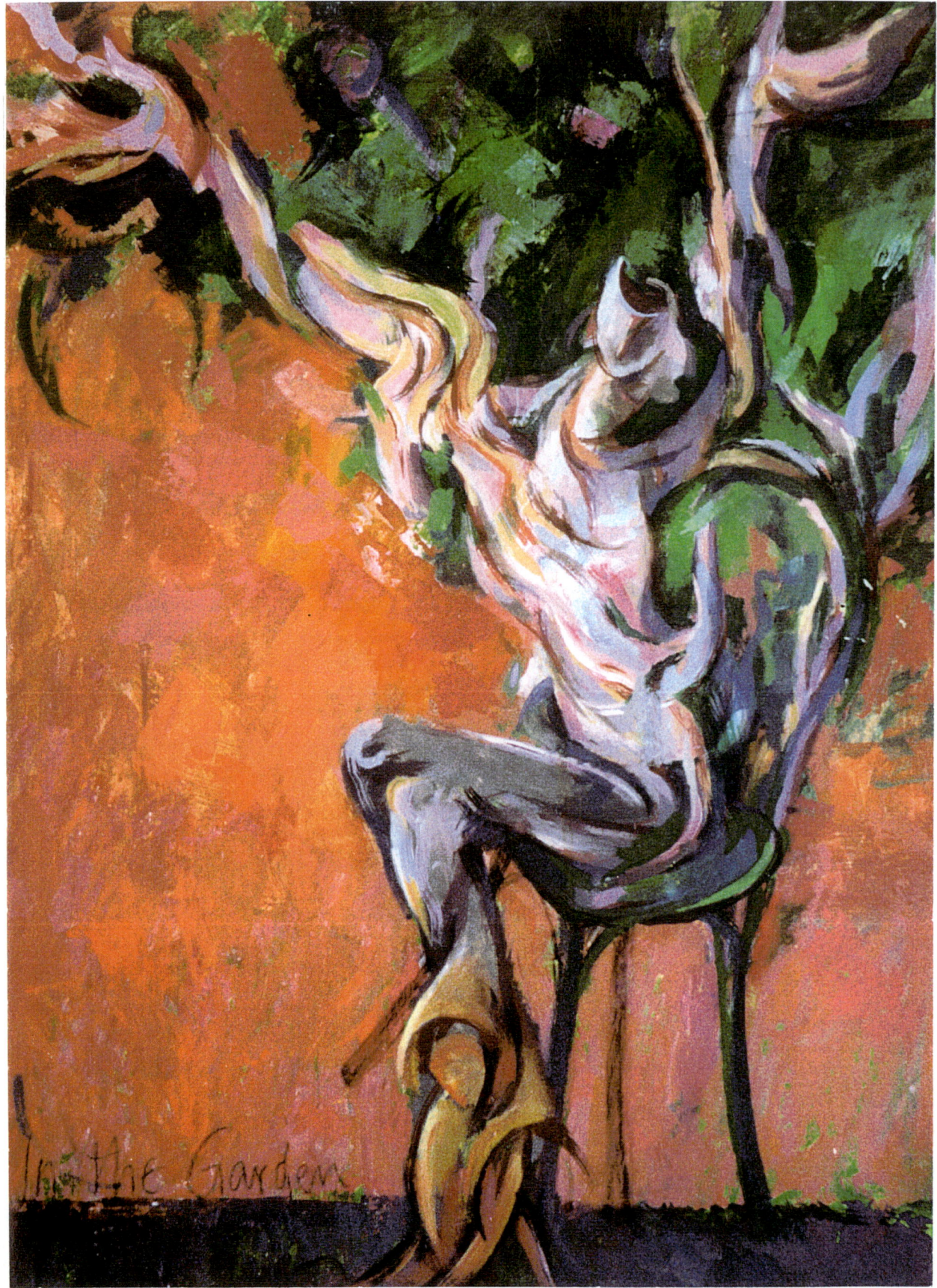

Fig. 345   In the Garden   Oil on Board

A development of the drawing on page 23, this painting is closely related to the breakdown of 1980. Here, in the interlocked lower limbs and twisted torso and arms, with the hands arranged for an imaginary nailing to a cross, was a personal 'Agony in the Garden'. It seemed to emphasise the sense of 'knotted-upness' experienced in the later dream.

PART THREE

The Volcanic Zone: Breaking out, Bursting forth

'. . . running just under the surface of anything you and I think we understand. '

From *The Man who had singing fits*   A Zolynas

THE VOLCANIC ZONE   200

1 THINKING THE UNTHINKABLE   201
    The release of anger, rage and repressions –
    a more aggressive approach to life

2 STRETCHING THE WINGS   215
    Birds and winged creatures as symbols of independence –
    of letting go and moving on

THE VOLCANIC ZONE

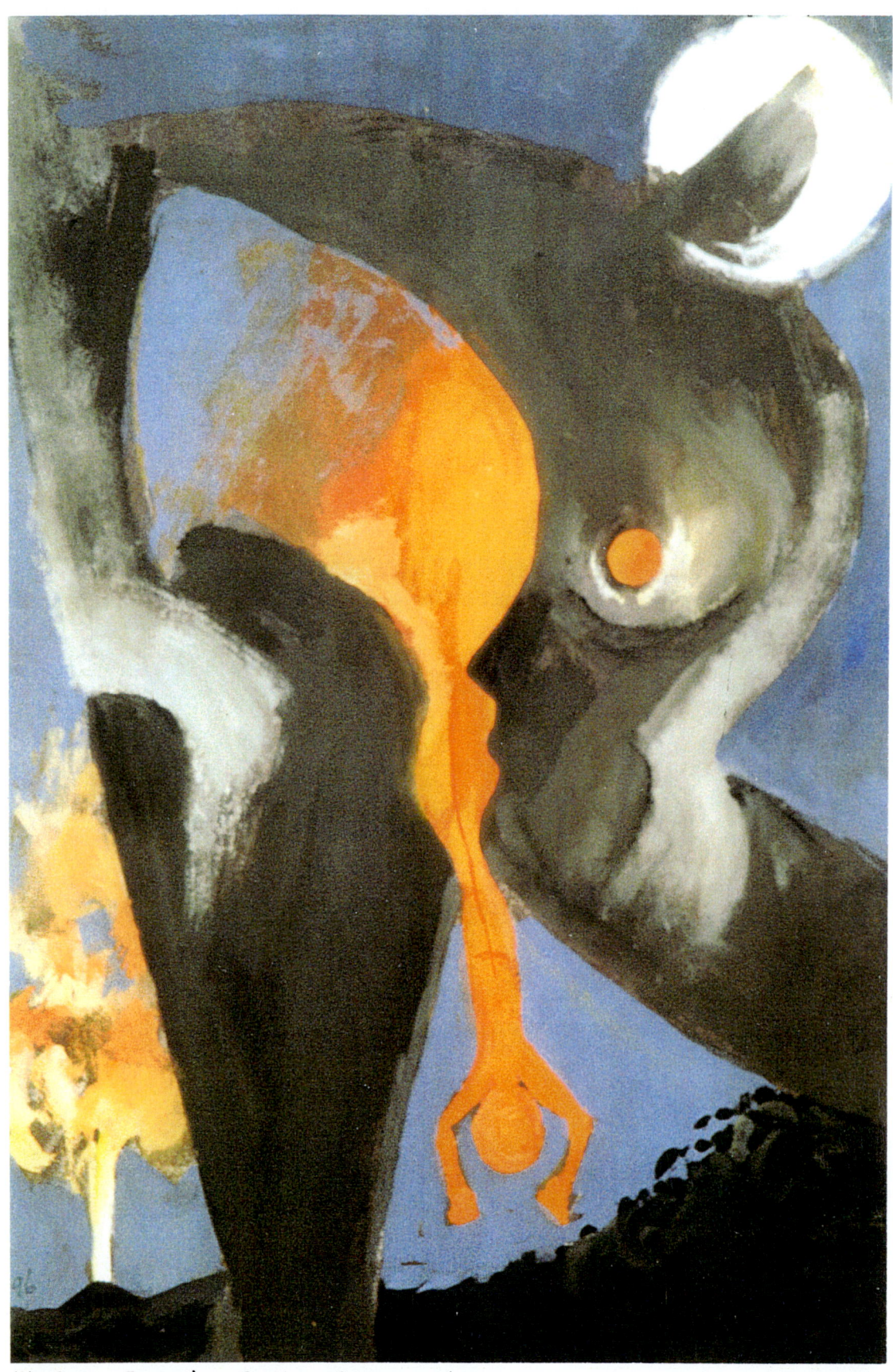

Fig. 346   Bursting Forth – Regeneration   Gouache

1 THINKING THE UNTHINKABLE
Breaking out - Letting go

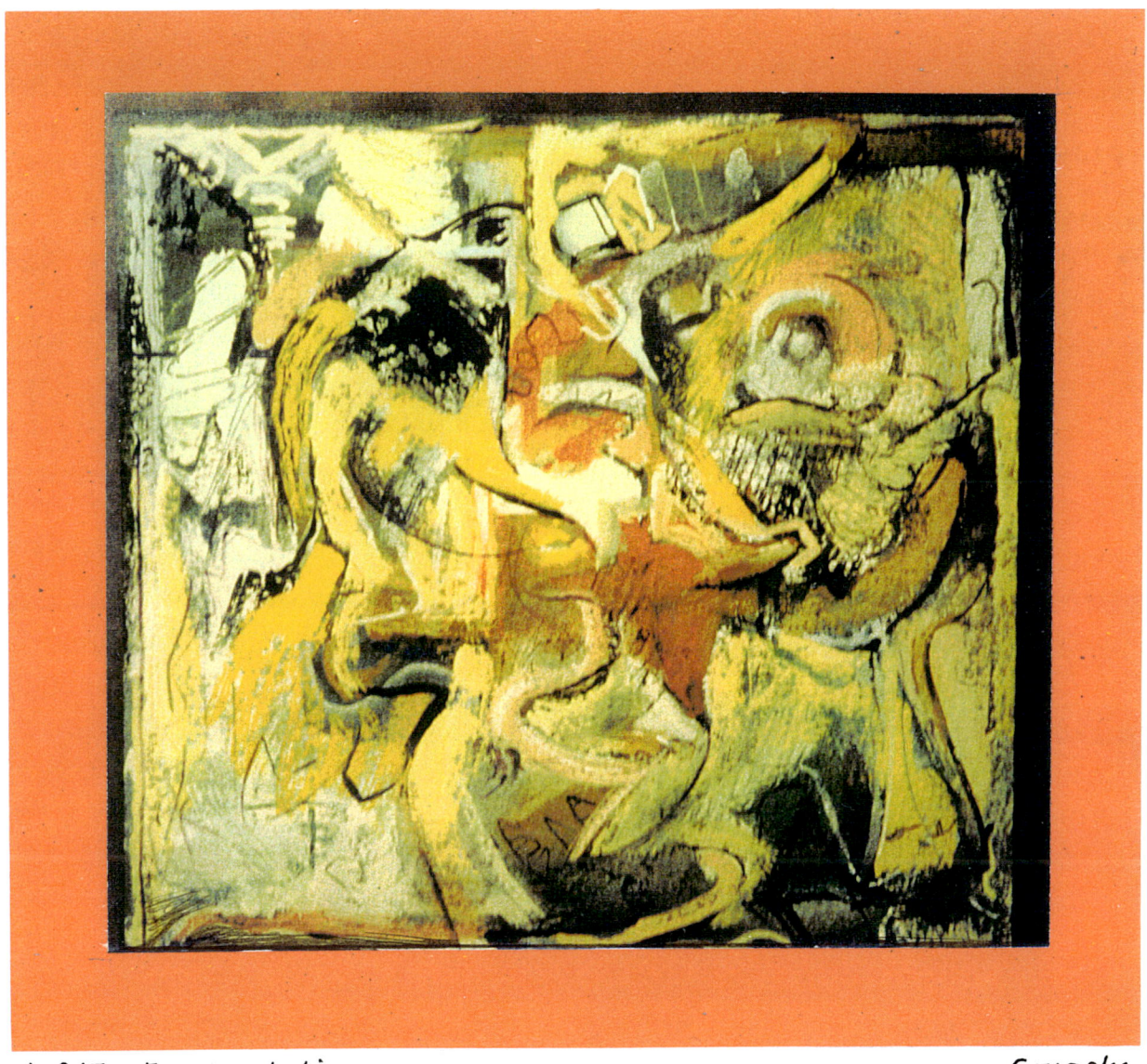

Fig.347   Fragmentation   Gouache

Thinking the unthinkable was the equivalent of doing the impossible. It was beyond reason for me to contemplate expressing anger without a corresponding fear of some form of retribution, usually in the form of rejection. To avoid this feeling of exclusion from the family (thus also, society, friends or whatever) the tendency was to keep quiet, play my cards close to the chest. To 'sit on the fence' was the safest place, otherwise one might step down into a minefield on either side.

Confrontation had had to be avoided at all costs, especially with women (given that I'd been 'boarded out' on frequent occasions) and a strong sense of guilt did nothing to assuage the problem.

It wasn't until after the session with 'C', where I could allow silence to alleviate my anxieties around this subject that a great release of energy allowed surges of anger and rage to operate (pages 202-214). Now I could experience the sense of letting go, of breaking out of this psychological stranglehold on self-expression.

This section illustrates images which grew out of a developing method of 'free-style' drawing, expressing the long suppressed anger.

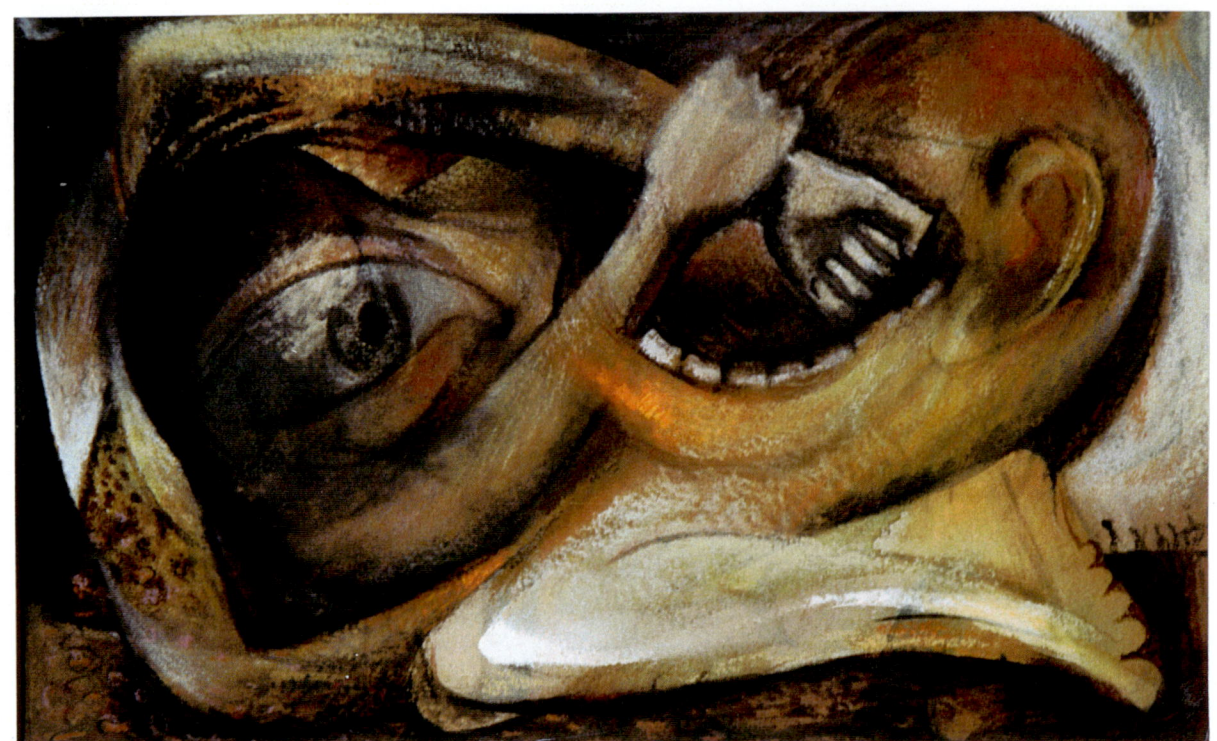

Fig. 348   Self Hate   Gouache

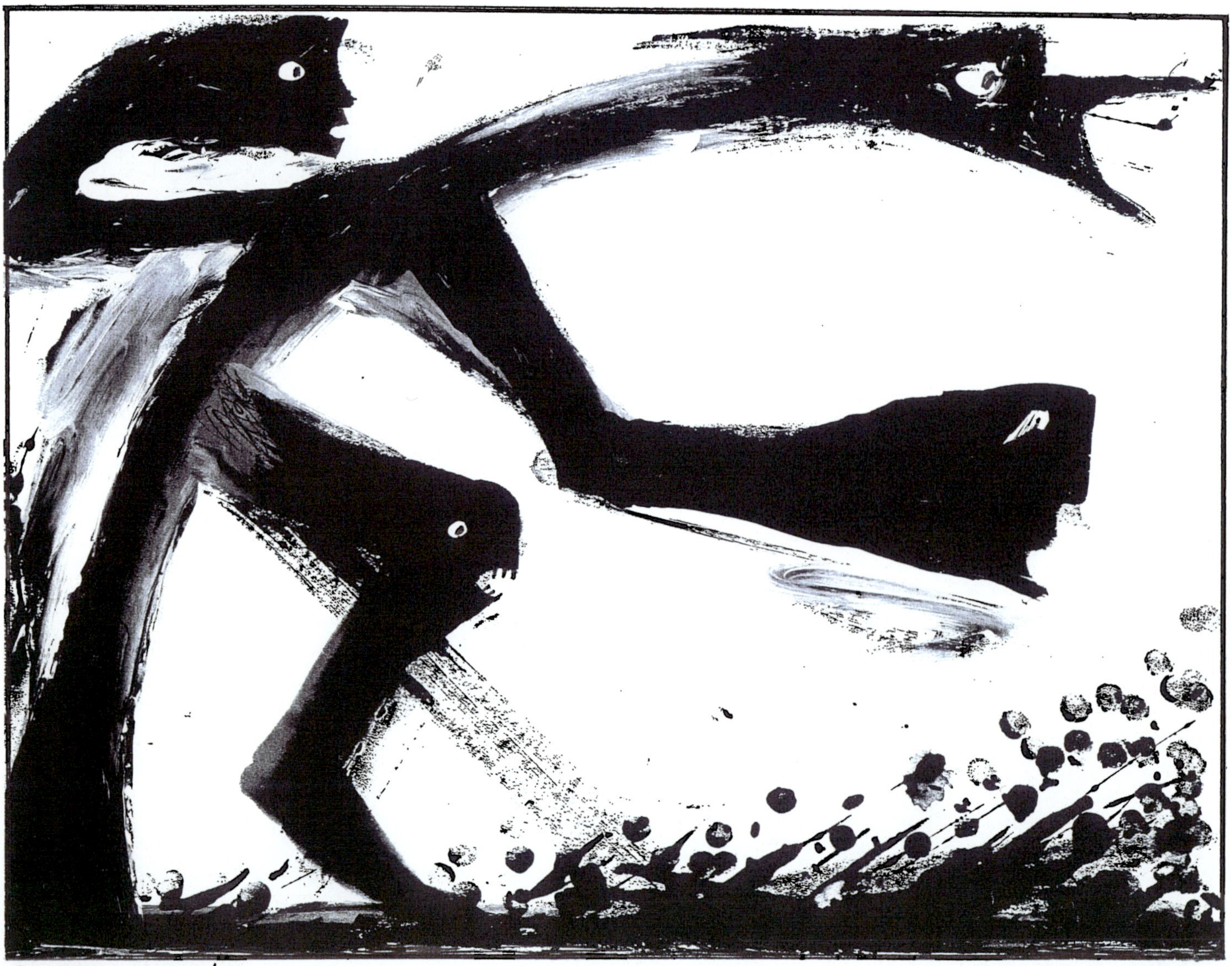

Fig. 349   Untitled   Brush & Black Paint

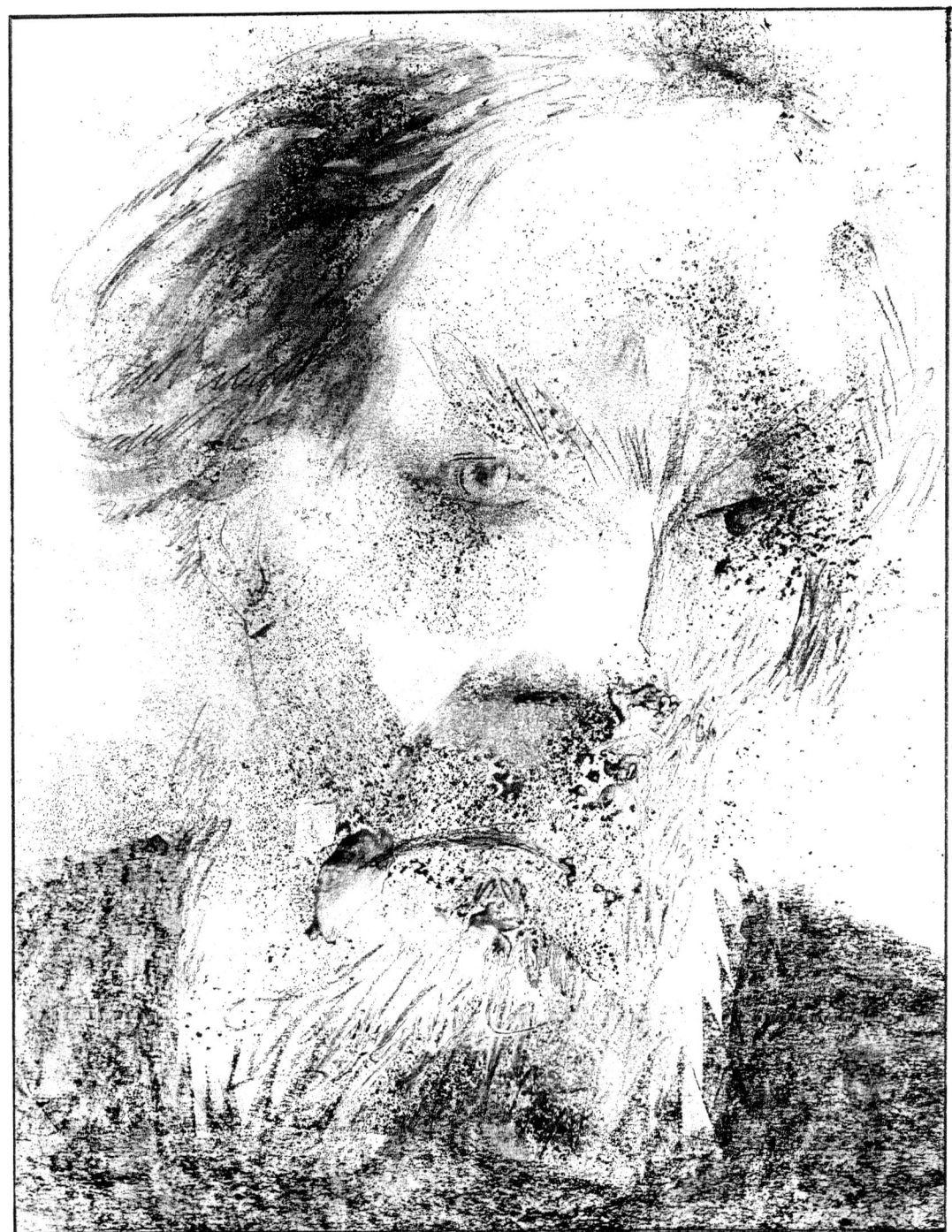

Fig. 350 Alter Ego Graphite powder & Pencil

Above: Fig.350 'Alter Ego'. An unforeseen likeness of my internalised dad created out of a 'free-style' accidental drawing. This father, assimilated into the self, brooding and ready to boil over in rage conveys everything I loathed about my own reticence to speak out freely when questioned on controversial issues. Now the hidden rage is externalised, his repressive power is diminished. Once his 'cover is blown' this internal saboteur is impotent and rendered harmless. It might take a short while for the benefits to filter through, but this particular chimera is laid to rest.

Above Left: Fig.348 'Self Hate'. Vision of a self-made hell, attempting to eat oneself, but even in this apparently negative imagery a restraining hand prevents the other from entering the all-consuming mouth.

Bottom Left: Fig.349 'Untitled'. A vulnerable creature. The trick of convincing the enemy that he is outnumbered — a typical joker's strategy. He only 'kicks up a rumpus' — a wholly defensive attitude.

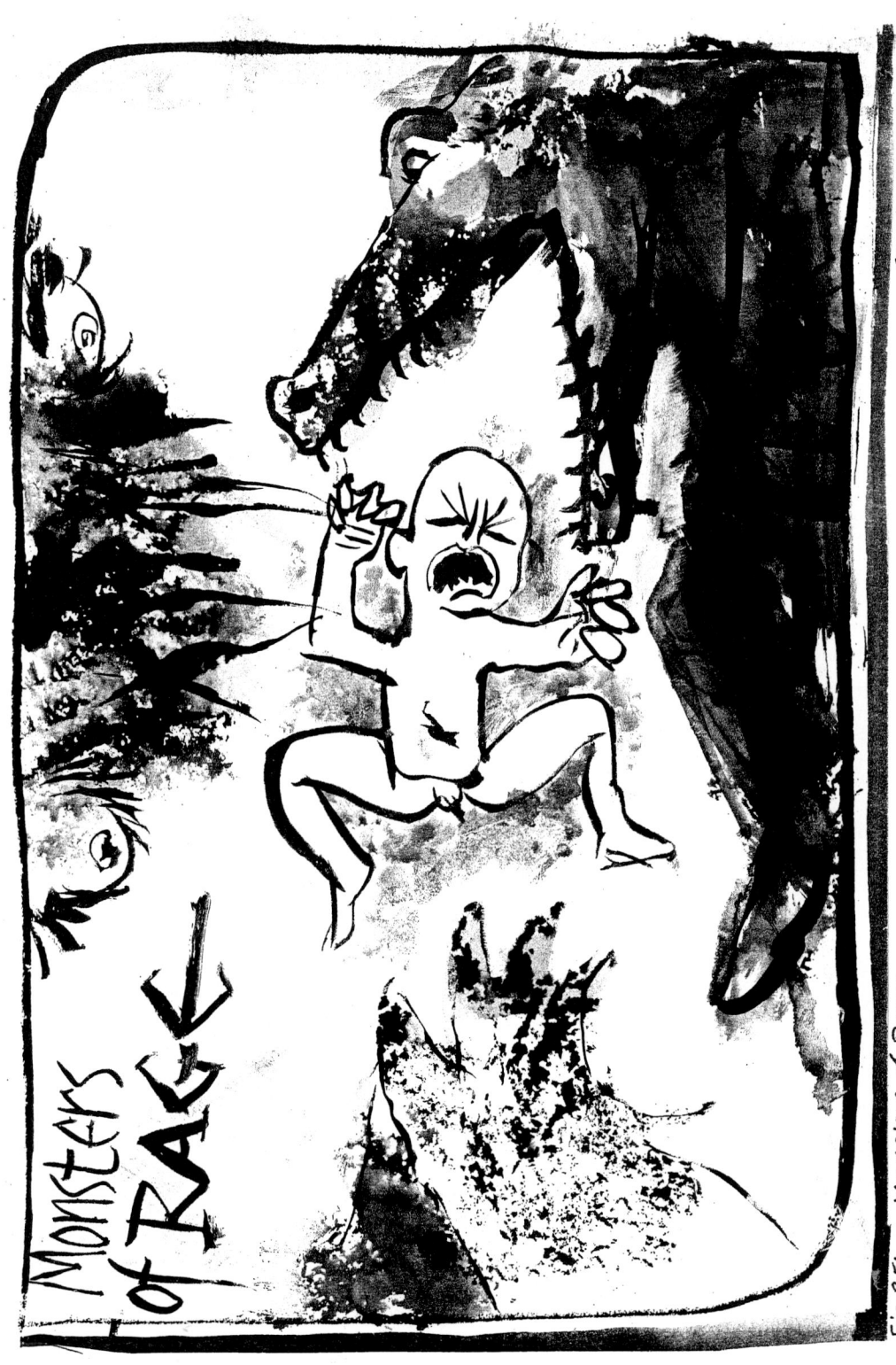

Fig.351 Monsters of Rage   Brush and Ink

THREE IMAGES OF THE INFANT 'LETTING GO'

Above: Fig.351 'Monsters of Rage'. The neglected baby conjures up his monsters of frustration — of not getting what he wants and needs.
Below Left: Fig.352. 'Bile' An outpouring of verbal excrement.
Below Right: Fig.353 'Serpent of Outrage' The baby vividly re-presents his feelings.

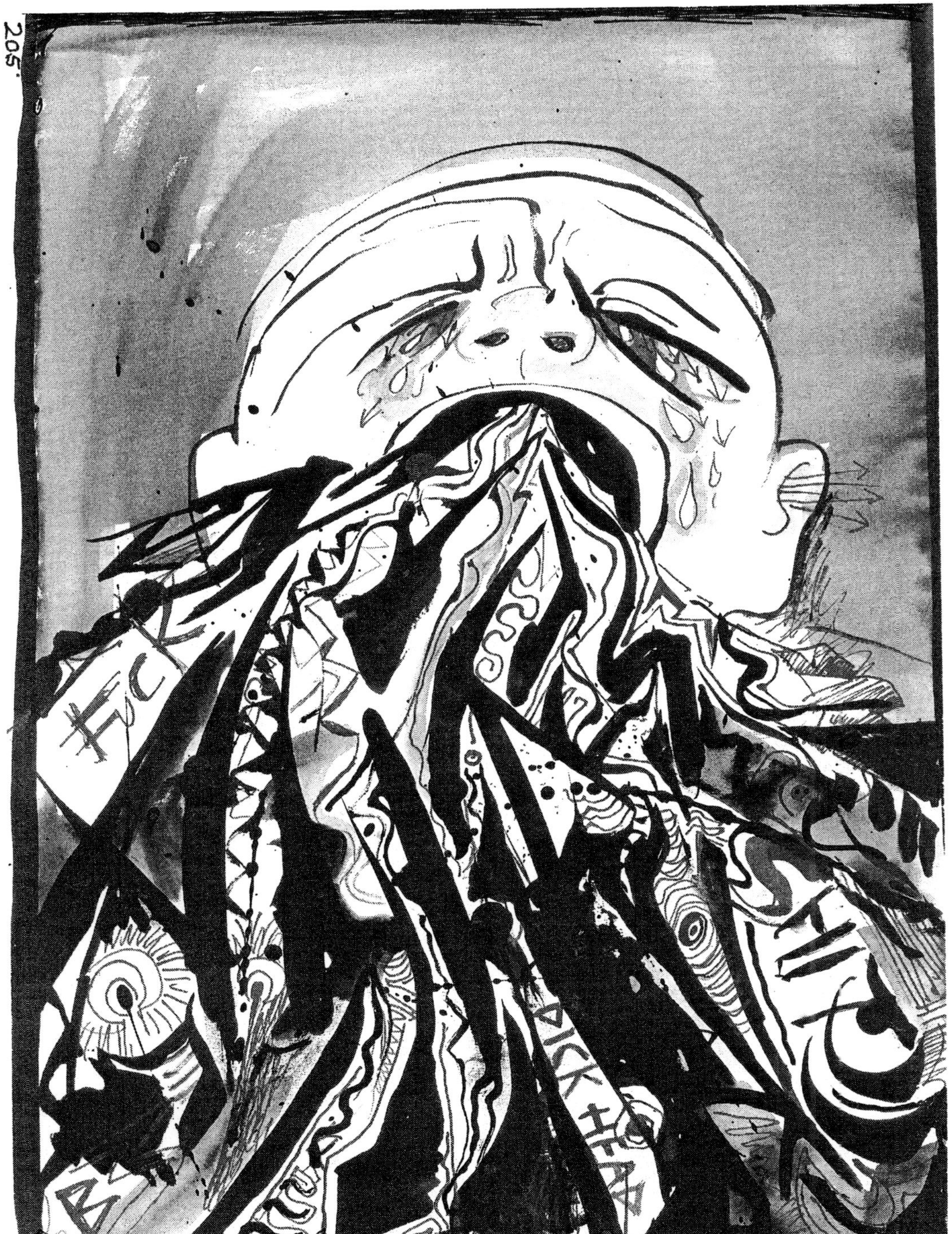

Fig. 352 Bile Brush & Ink

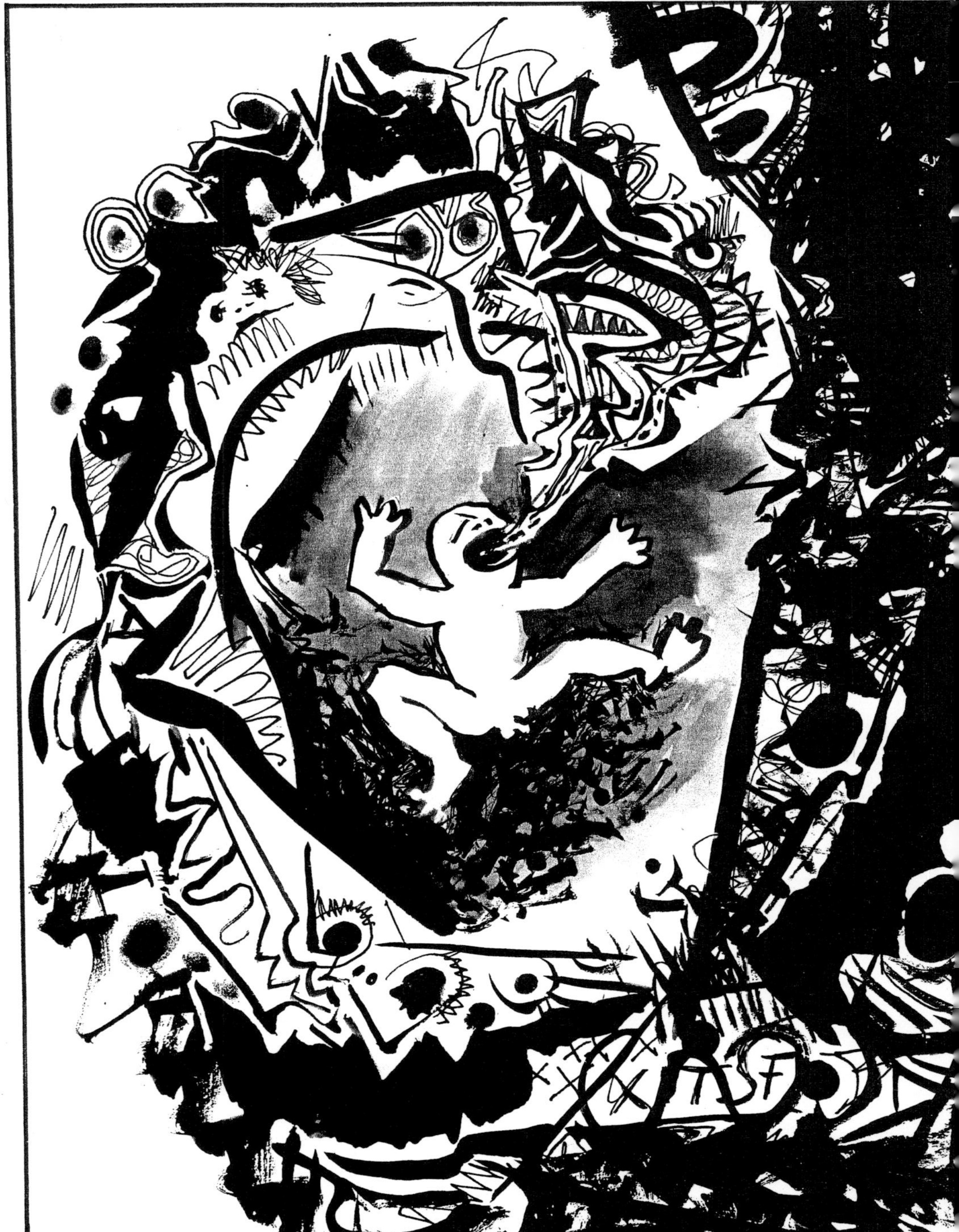

Fig. 353 Serpent of Rage Brush & Ink

205

Right: Fig. 354 'Hospitalisation'.

These sketches stress the hard pull on the arms; the distorted face shows the rigidity and suspicion the child feels.

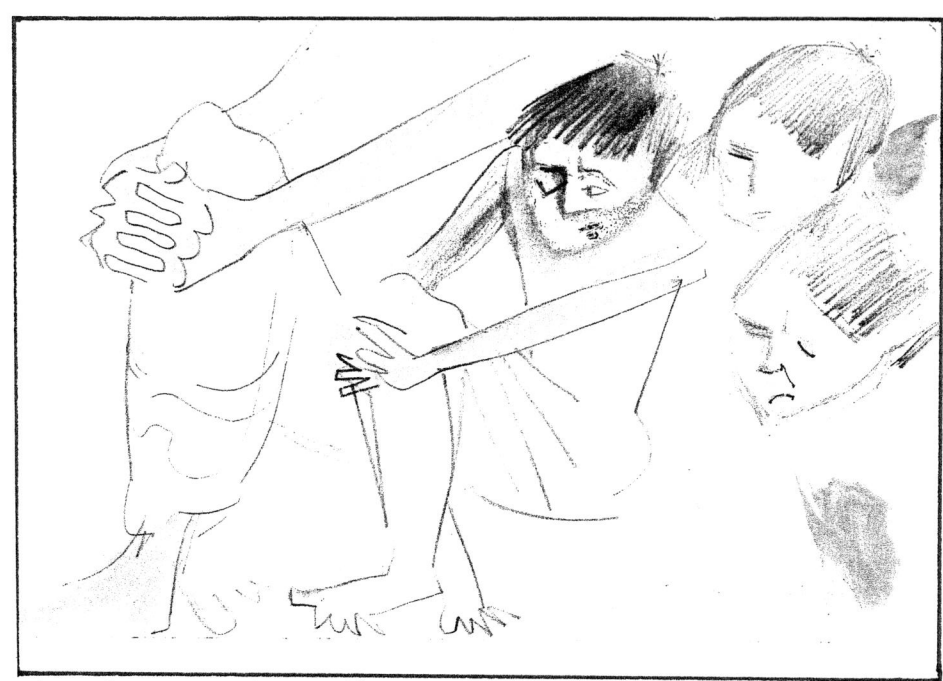

Fig. 354   Hospitalisation – a page of sketches   Pencil

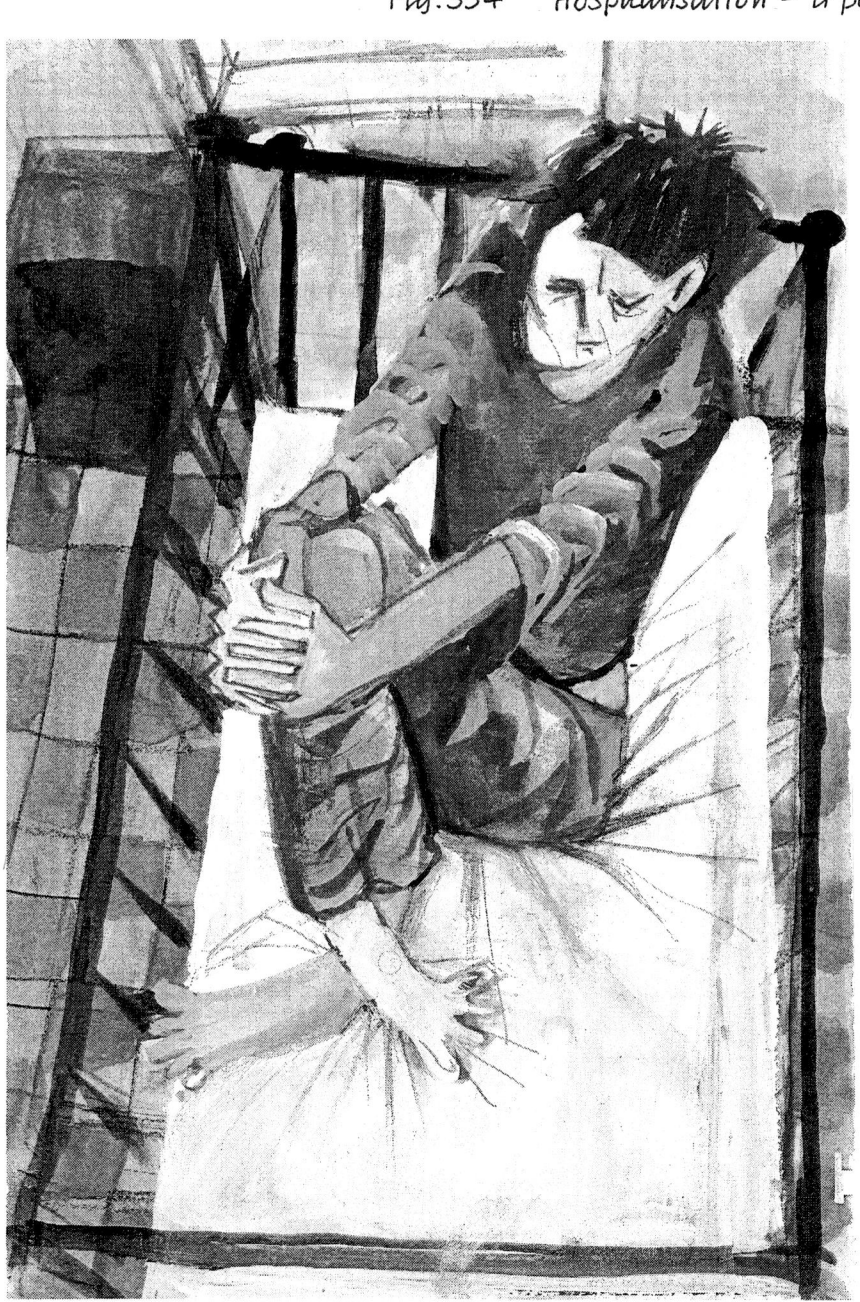

Left: Fig. 355. Hospitalisation.

Based on the sketches above, this gouache painting attempts to convey the repressed anger, the 'locked-in' emotions of the neglected child.
(See also references to paintings as extensions or variations based on dream sketches on page 82).

Left: Fig. 355 Hospitalisation   Gouache

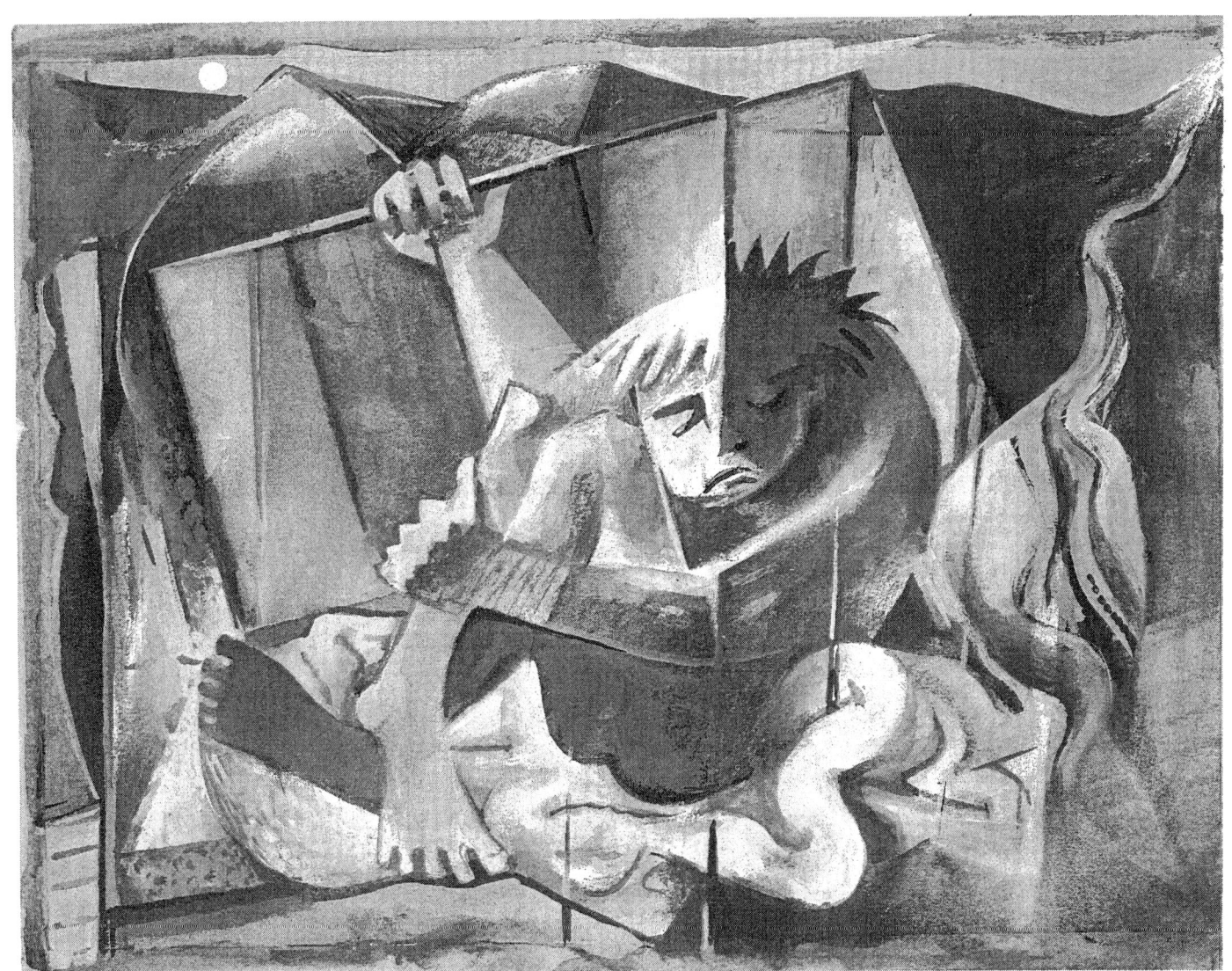

Fig 356   The Prisoner   Gouache

Fig. 356. The Prisoner.   The incarceration in hospital when about ten years old for a period of approximately twelve weeks led to a large amount of time inside a high-railed bed. It was one of those experiences which, in retrospect, had a strong repressive influence on the child. The long hours of boredom and loneliness were increased by very restricted hospital visiting (Sunday afternoons only according to mum) and also the fact that children were confined to the railed cots for long periods. The overall feeling was one of abandonment.
   The cot or bed rails came to represent the iron bars of a prison cell. I feel that in 'The Prisoner' the repressed anger of the child is fully expressed by the body language; the intertwined feet, the clutching of hands to bars and legs; the surly facial features, all express the withdrawal into the self — the loss of freedom beyond the bars.
   A river of life flows down from the mountain top, lightly catching the child's back. The wave movement transfers over to the cot sheet — the child dreams of his freedom......

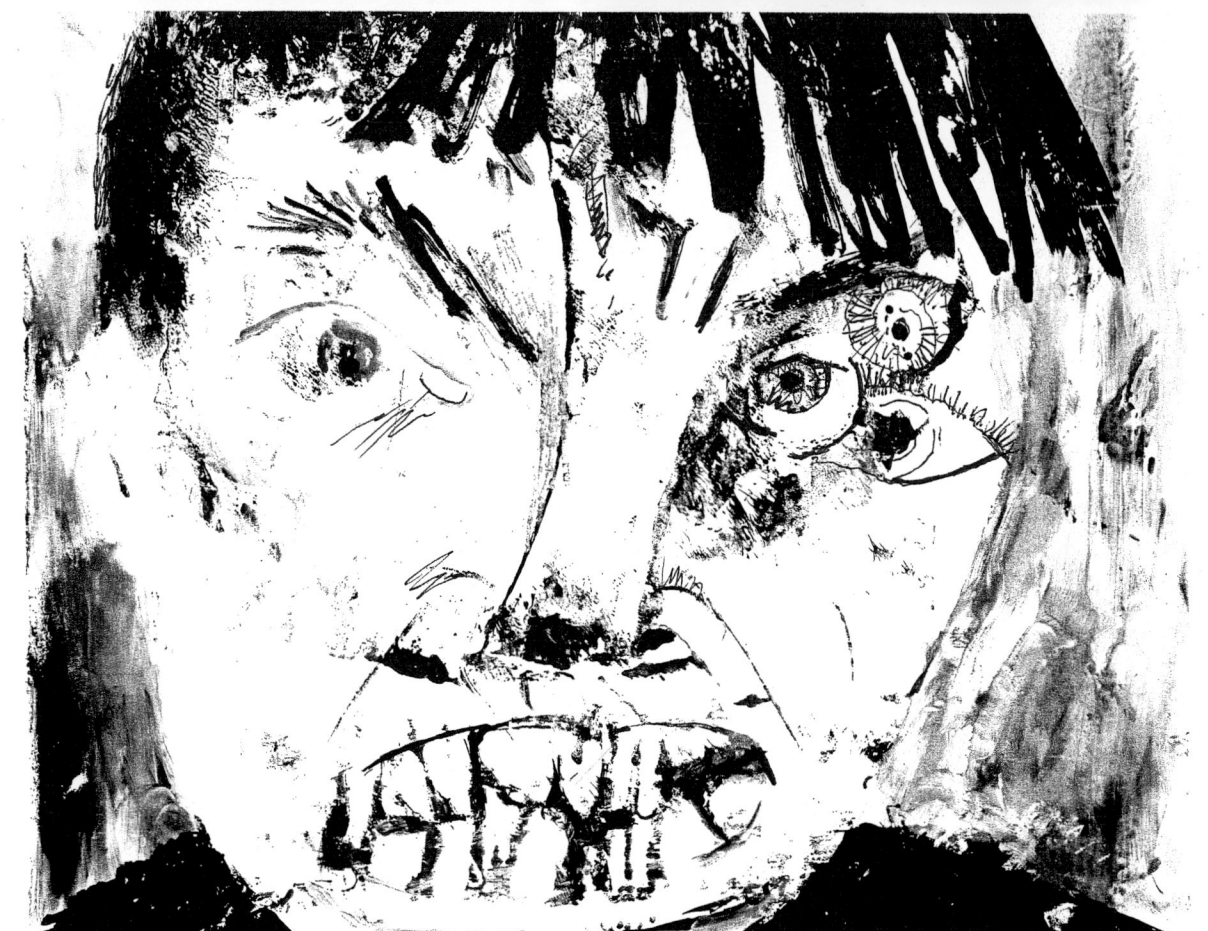

Fig. 357 The Enraged Boy — Gouache & Pen

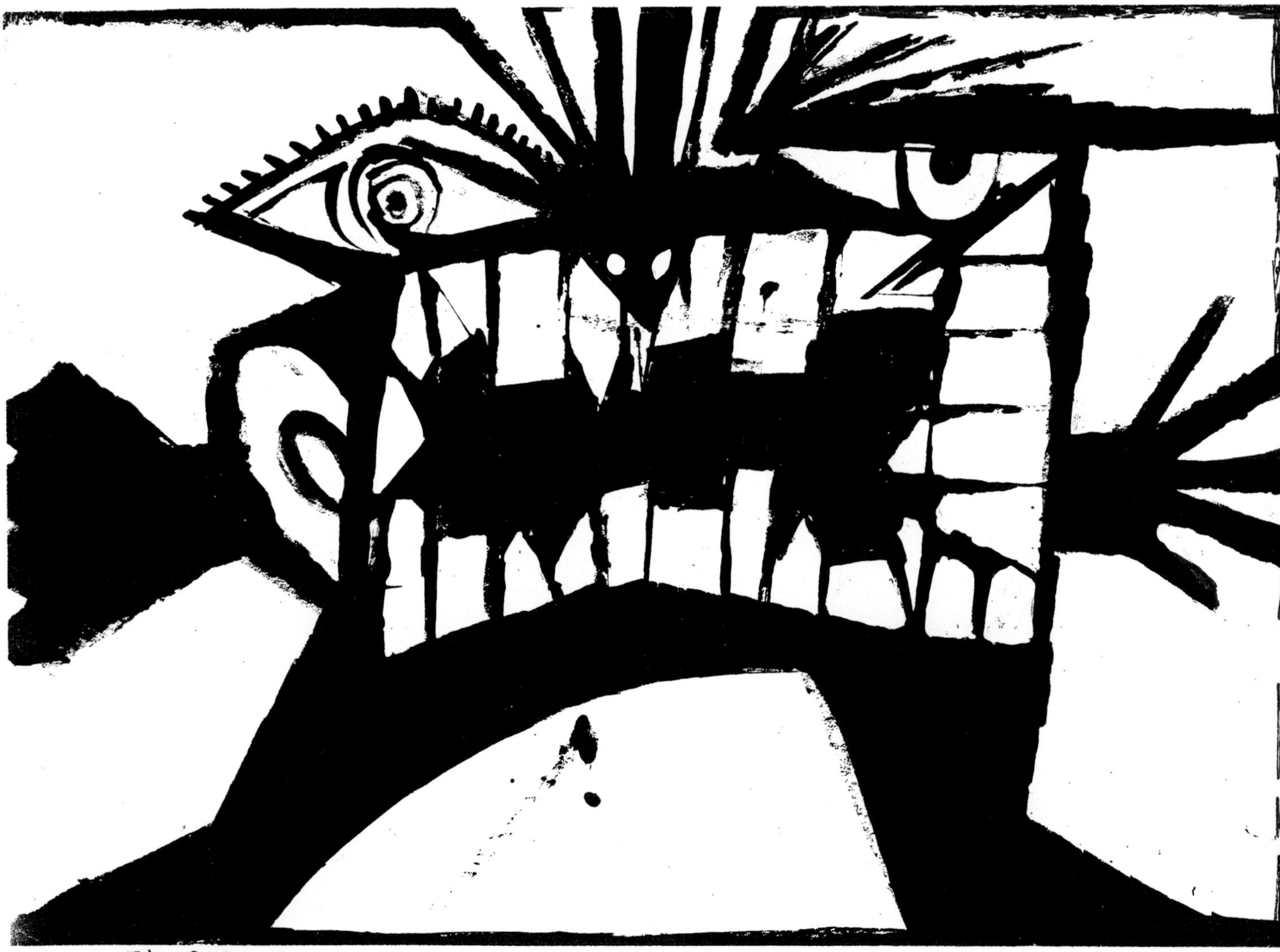

Fig. 358 Rage — Brush & Ink

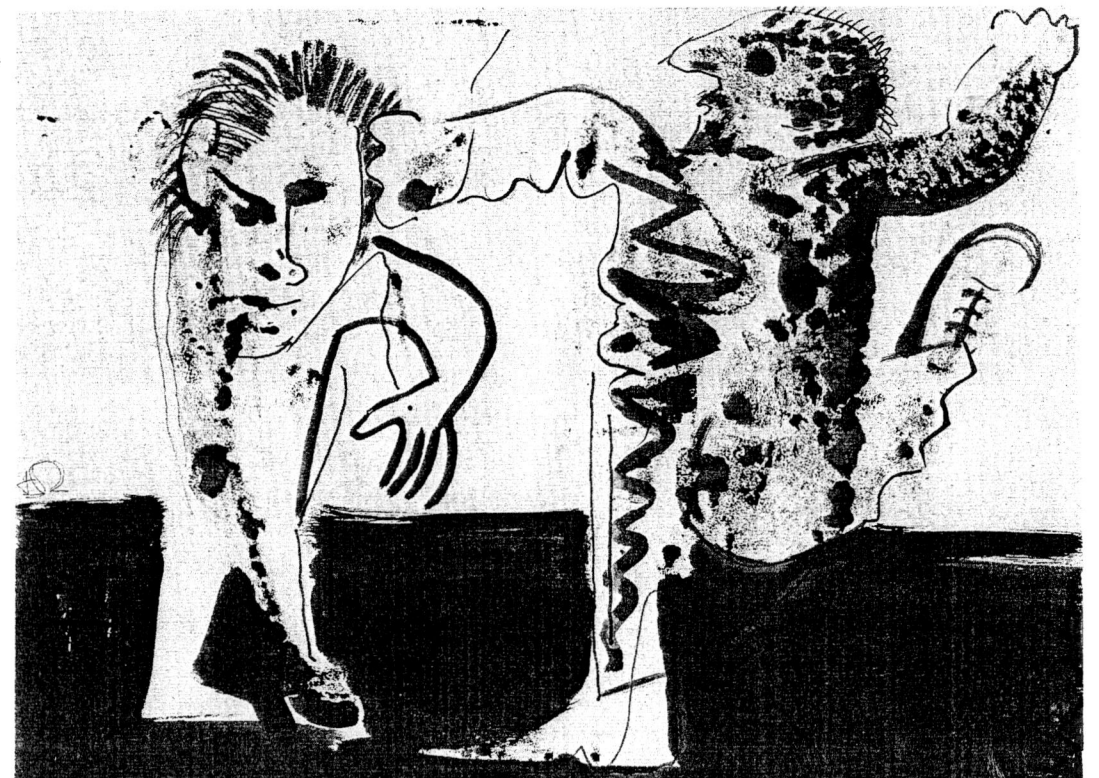

Fig. 359 'I'll knock your head off, you little Sod!'   Print, Pen & Brush

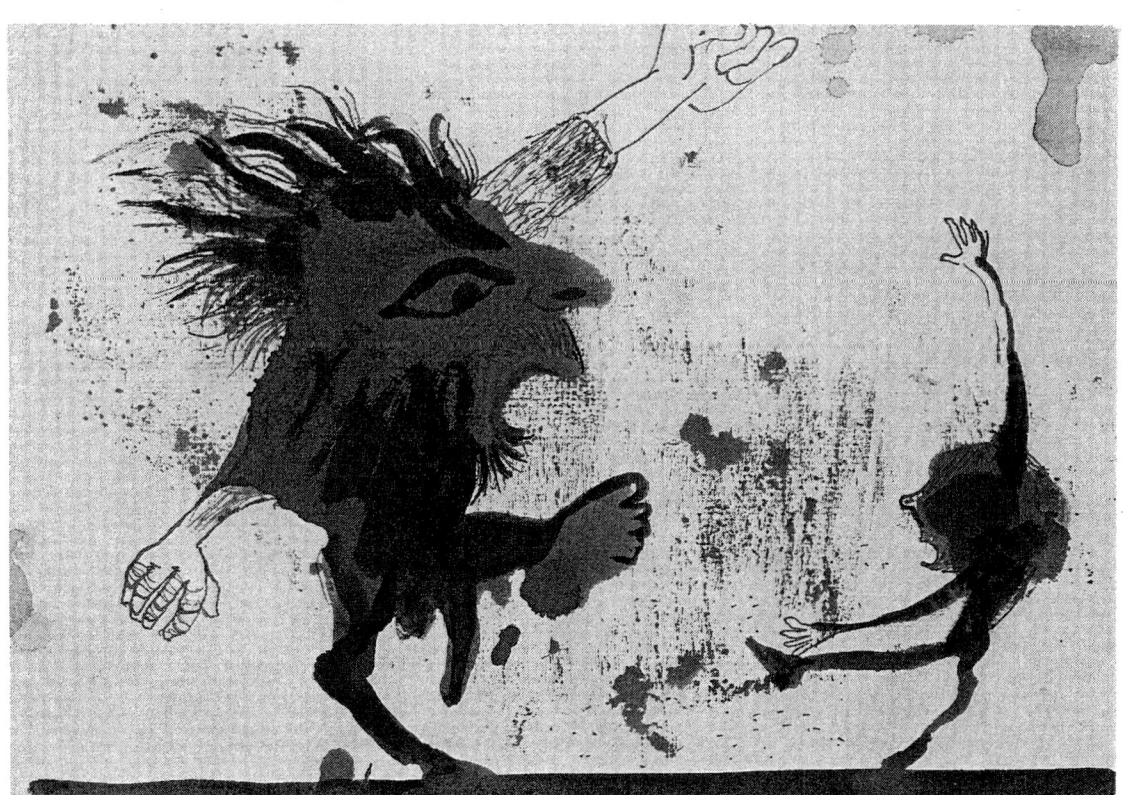

Fig 360   Kick-Boxing   Pen, Brush & Blots

Top Left: Fig. 357 'The Enraged Boy'. Like a suit of armour the angry facial expression protects the boy from external and internal fears.

Bottom Left: Fig. 358 'Rage'. A stylised version of 'The Enraged Boy'. Only the extremities of the body are needed to convey his aggressive stance.

Top: Fig. 359 'I'll knock your block off, you little Sod!' The internalised father acts aggressively towards the child who has taken control of his own life.

Bottom: Fig. 360 'Kick Boxing'. The father is shocked to find his son retaliate if his freedom is curtailed. The confrontation implies independence.

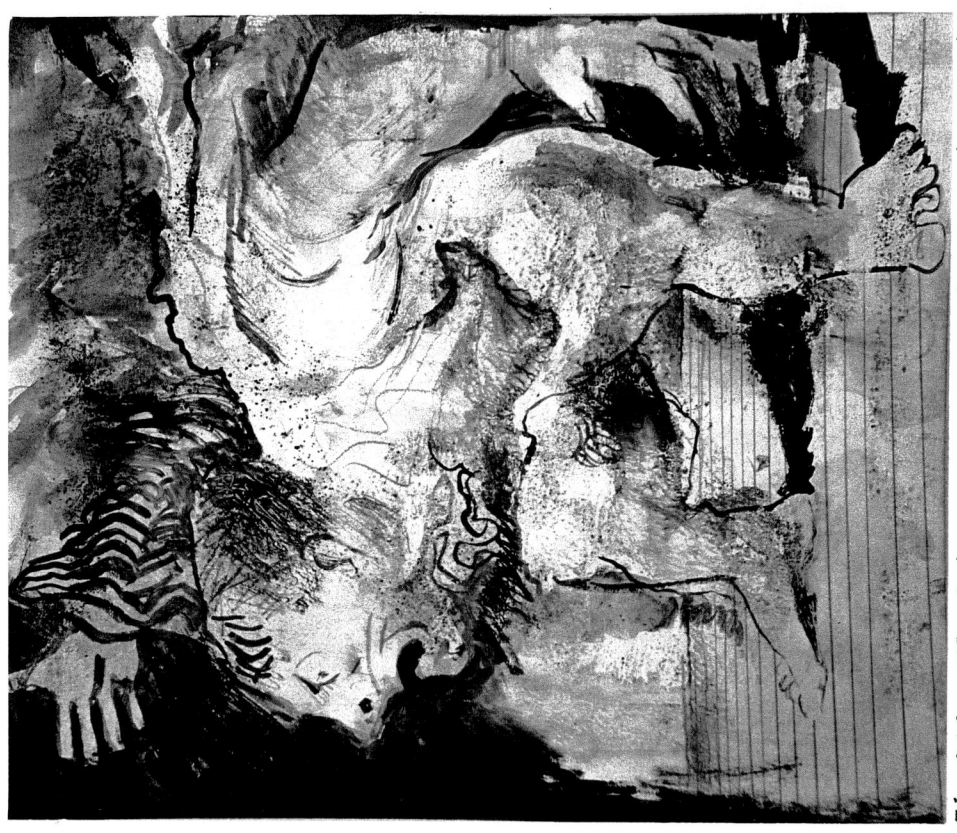

Fig. 362 The Actor Paint & Graphite Powder

Left: Fig. 361 The Mask of Rage Paint, Pen & Ink

The two performers above cast off their costume armour and try wearing masks of rage — or hurl invective at an unseen audience. In both cases the aim is to express anger — not to retain it.

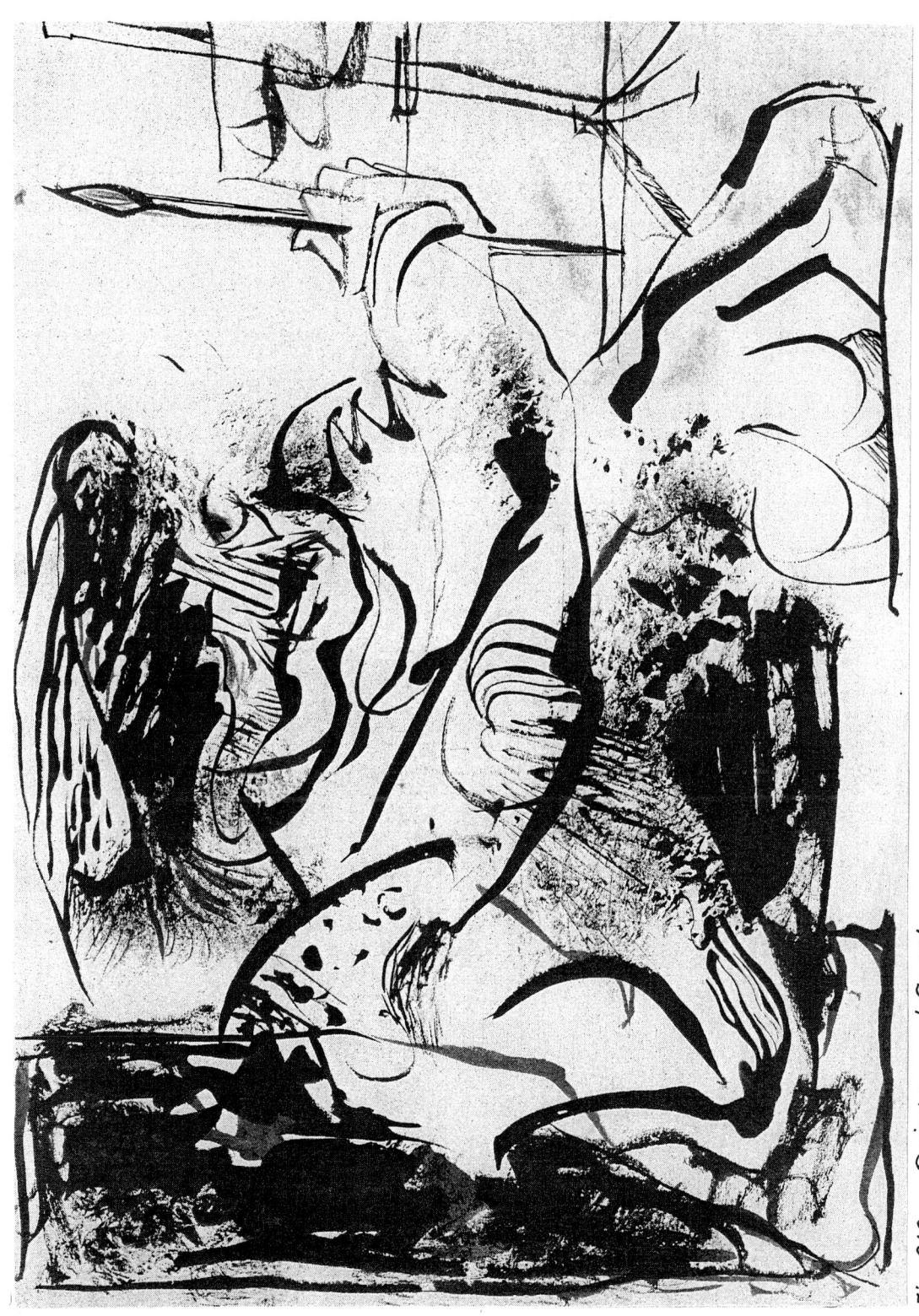

Fig. 363 Painter and Easel

Pen, Ink, Brush & Stippling

Above: Fig 363 'Painter and Easel'. As retentive matter is released, newly discovered energy is directed towards the canvas on the easel. Anger becomes a creative generator. The stance and gesture of the painter show confidence. The large feline paw symbolises the stalking for the hidden imagery.

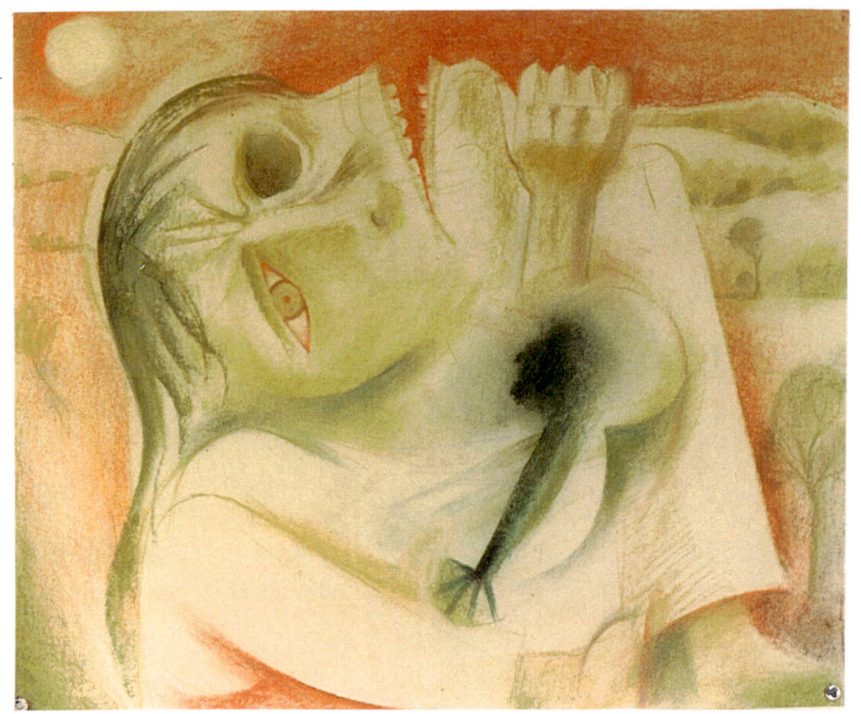

Fig. 364   Mother and Child   Pastel

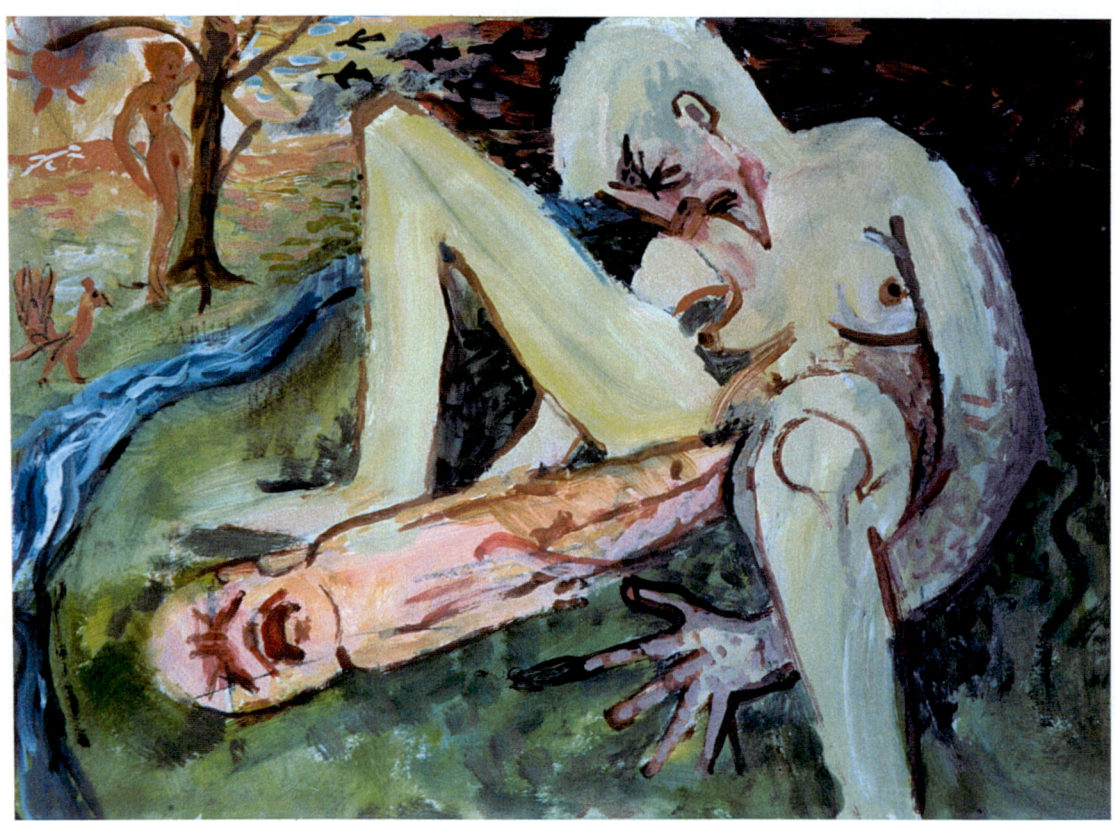

Fig 365   East of Eden   Gouache

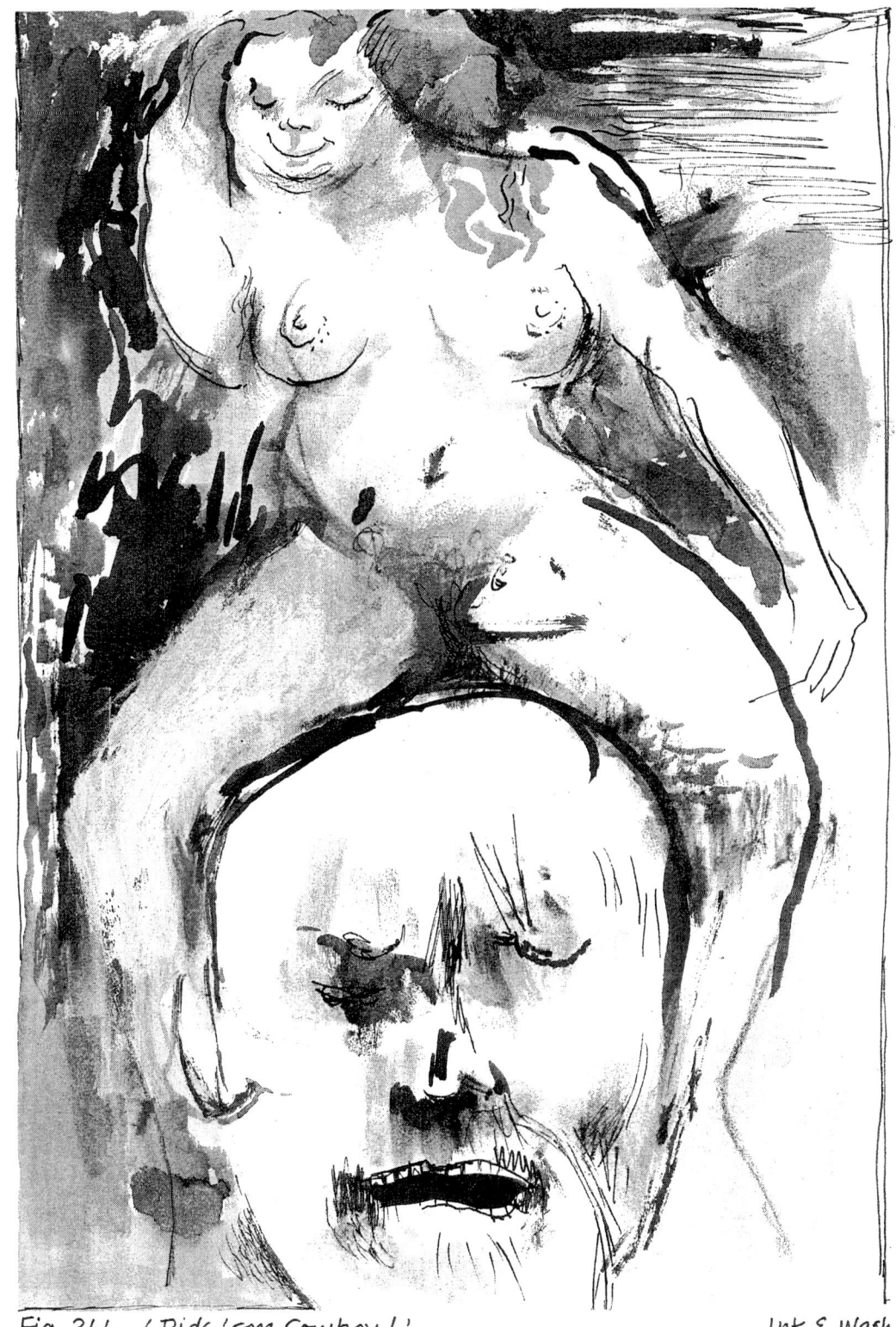

Fig. 366   'Ride 'em Cowboy!'   Ink & Wash

Figs. 364, 365 and 366. Two examples of expressing fears about the woman and of the rage directed at the mother, of creating one's own world without the woman — East of Eden?
   Above: On the fear of being controlled.

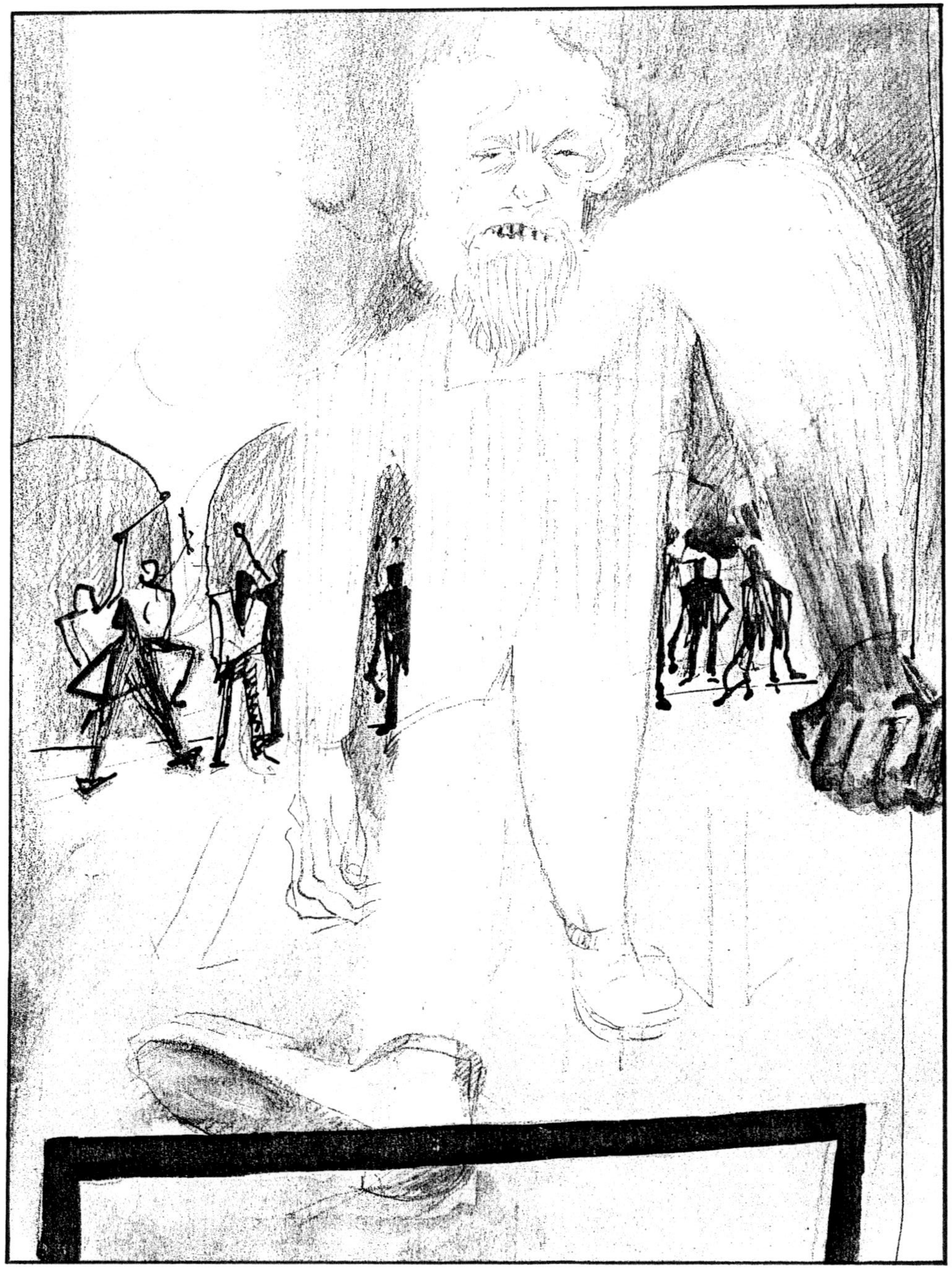

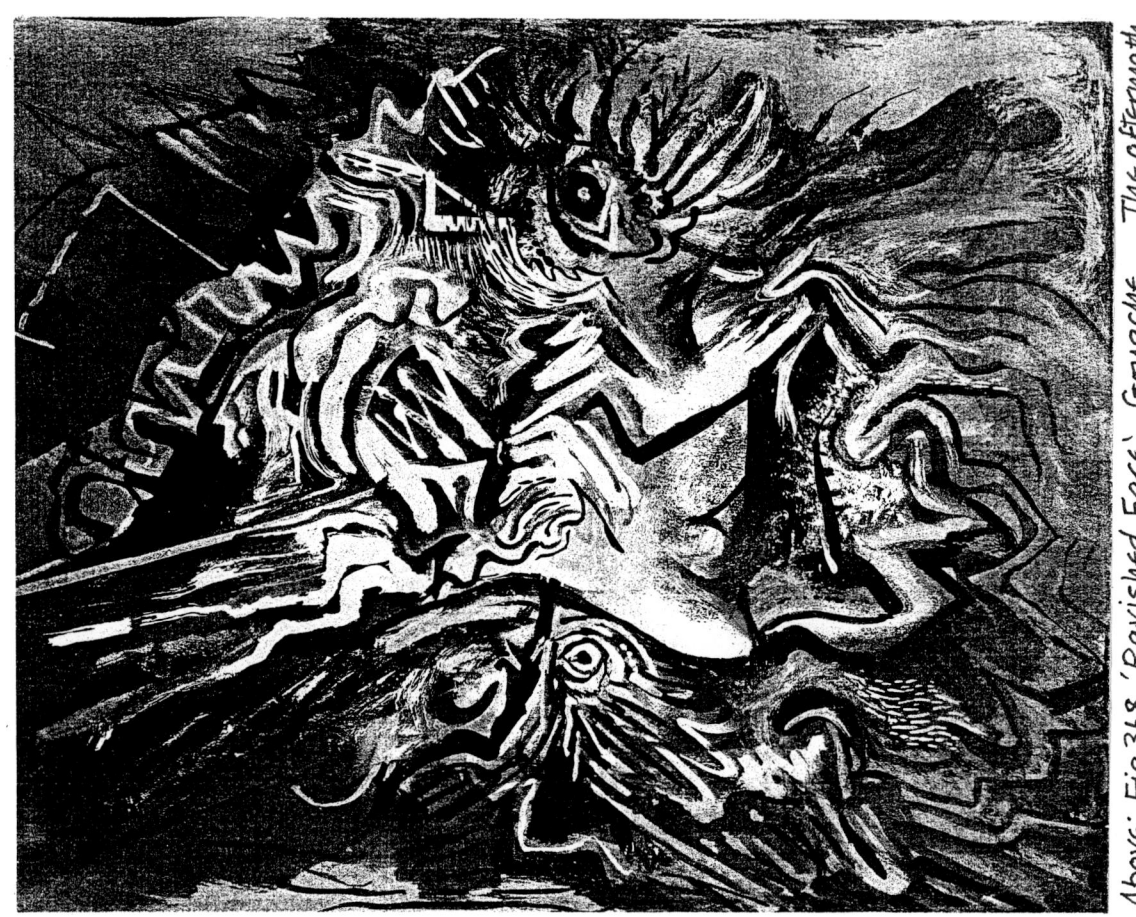

Above: Fig. 368 'Ravished Face'. Gouache. The aftermath of emotional outpouring - the face waits for rejuvenation.

Left: Fig. 367. 'White Hot Frenzy'. Chalk and Ink. My alter ego returns with gang of hoodlums to beat me up - from a 1994 dream, when inner doubts seemed to be overwhelming me. I stood firm and he retreated.

2 STRETCHING THE WINGS
Opening out - Taking off

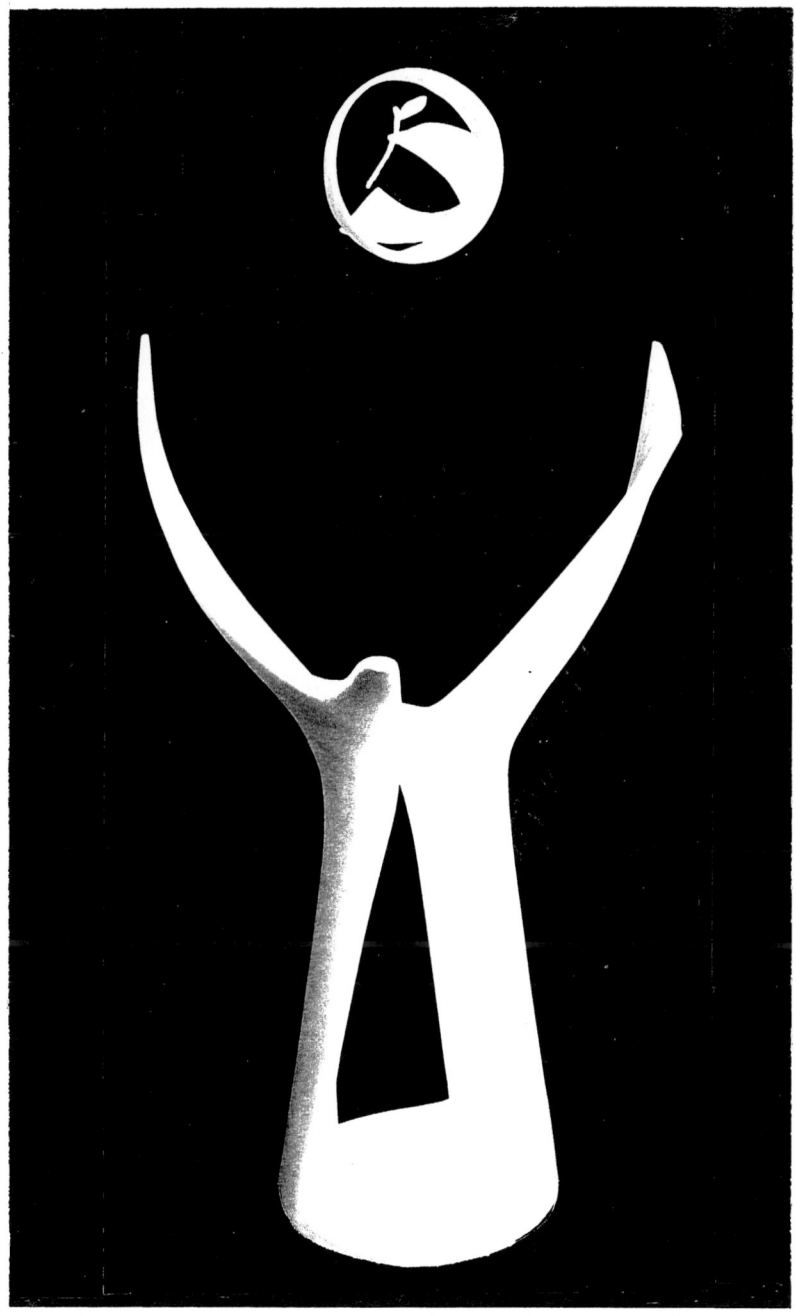

Fig. 369 Peace Sculpture   Glass fibre & Cellulose Spray

This sculpture is the precursor of a sequence of bird images which stress the idea of a nurturing or 'holding' place.
  A pair of hands in an attitude of supplication changes into a bird about to take to the air. Turning very slowly on a turntable the sculpture encircles the suspended upper part, a spherical dove of peace which represents the world. The dove is held just high enough to convey a sense of 'containment'.

STRETCHING ONE'S WINGS

This section is concerned with a variety of winged creatures both 'real' and mythological. Birds, angels, dragons, men attempting to fly with appendages to aid flight (i.e. Icarus), and people performing as birds on stage.
In many of the pictures the emphasis is on an 'opening out' and, by extension, a lifting off, as a fledgling might leave its nest.

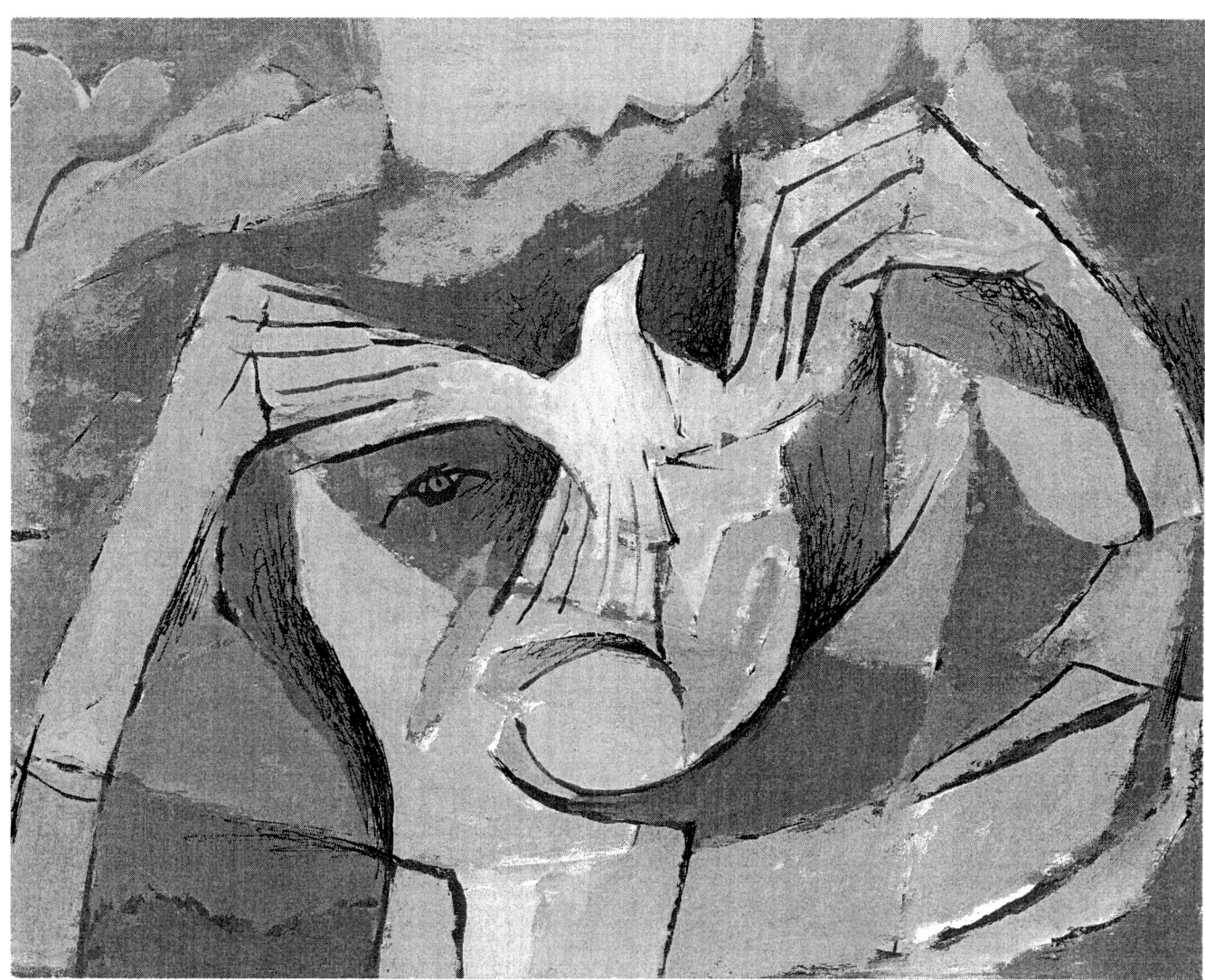

Fig. 370   Stretching One's Wings   Pen & Gouache

This painting has some affinity with the peace sculpture (see previous page and footnote at end of this section, page 240).
Just as a priest elevates the chalice, so the child raises his arms to hold before his gaze a bird cut-out, his fingers helping to form the wings. This symbol of his aspirations carries the hope of a transformation from idea to reality.
The inner child, having sensed an absence of nurture and family relationship during formative years is now attempting to reach out to the internalised father via the bird.
It now seems possible to imagine this bird as a symbol both of stability (during a nesting phase) and of freedom (as a fledgling reaching out to its true environment).

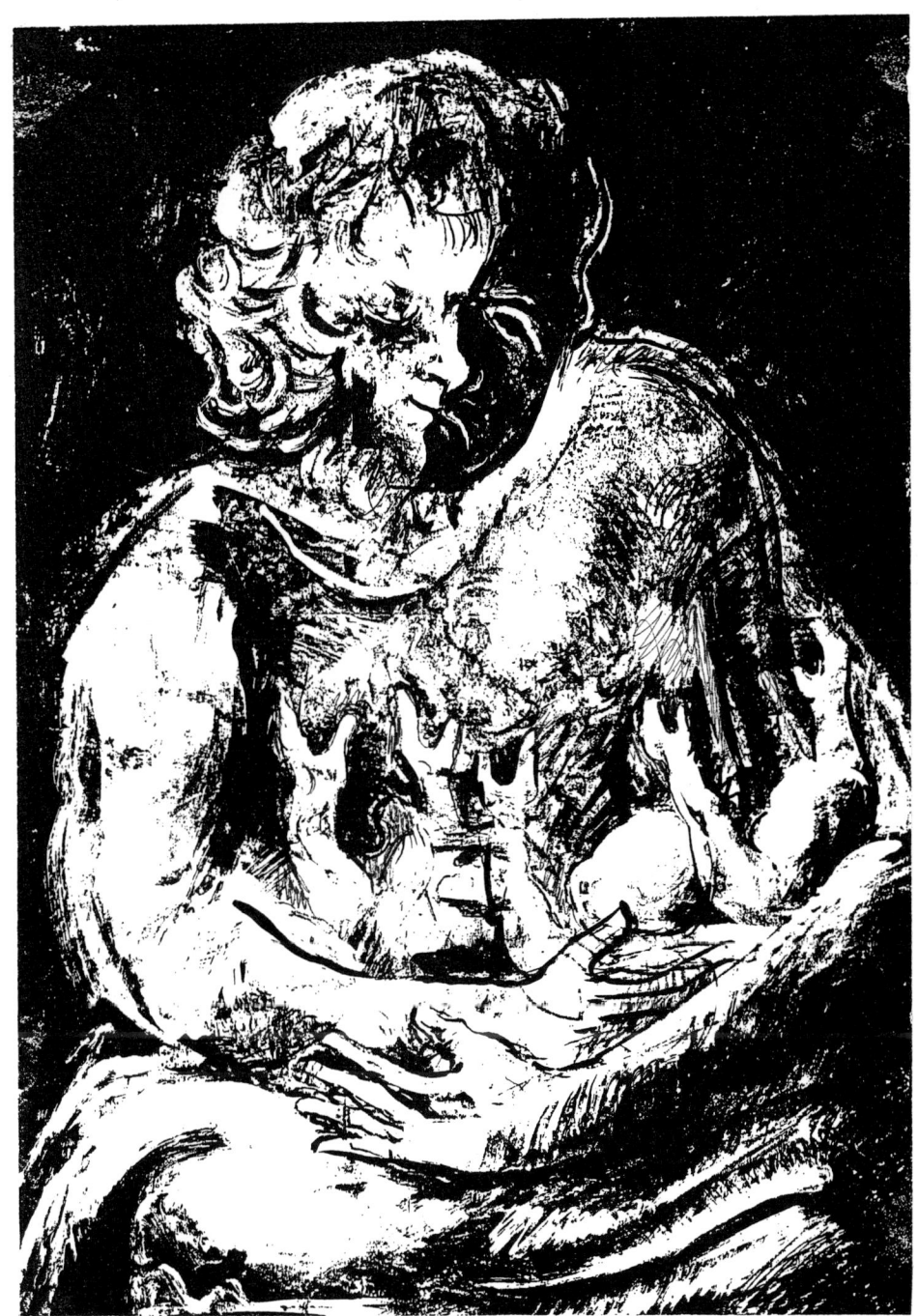

Fig. 371   Mother's Lap – Bird's Nest   Pen, Brush & Ink

'Mother's Lap – Bird's Nest'

Sometimes the content of a picture is ambivalent. Here the babies' hands reach out to the mother and then change into beaks of chicks, mouths wide open for food.

The mother's lap can then be experienced as a nest.

The mother's face is also open to interpretation. A light and smiling aspect is dominant, but a darker hidden side gives a feeling of uncertainty......

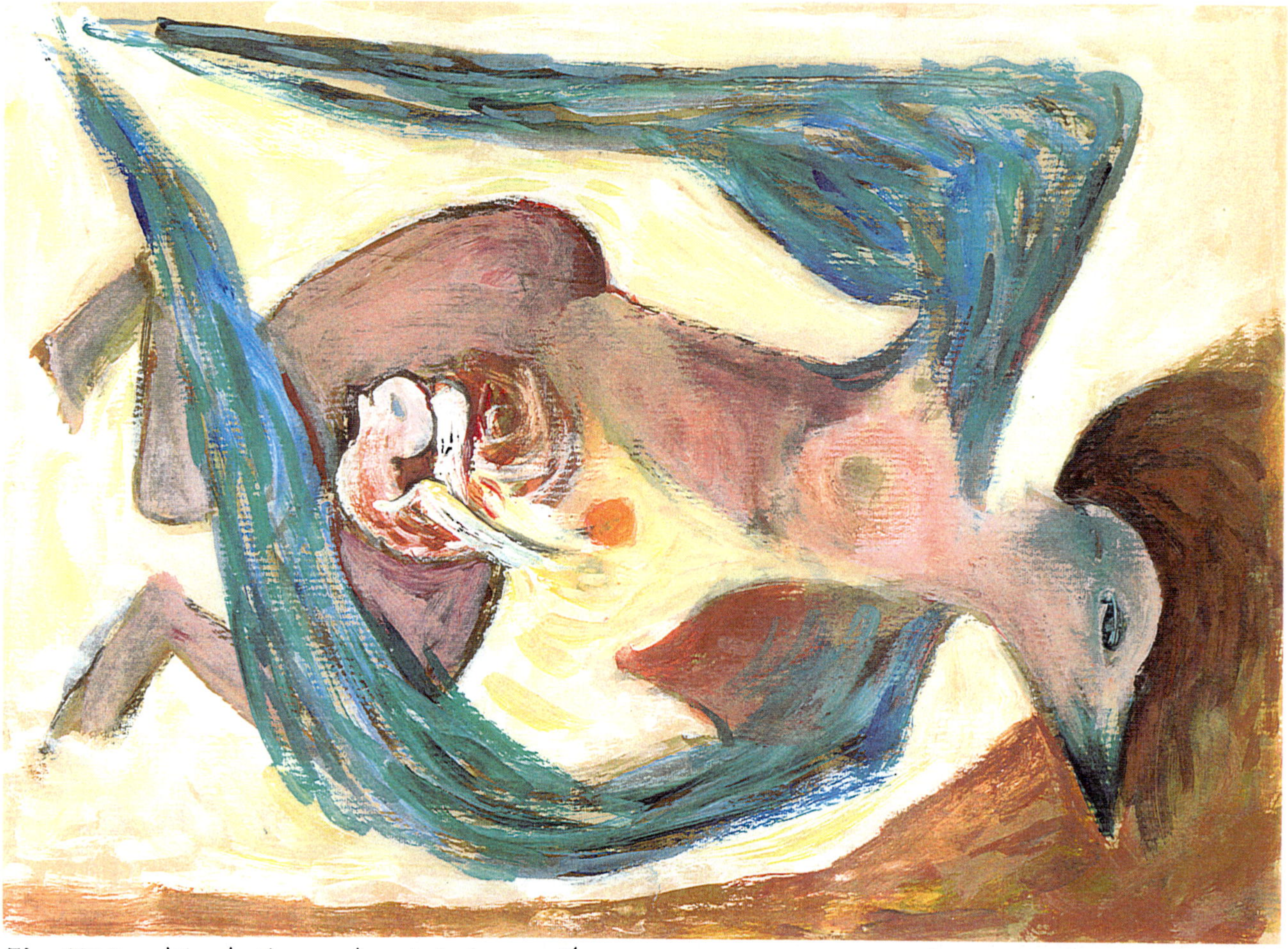

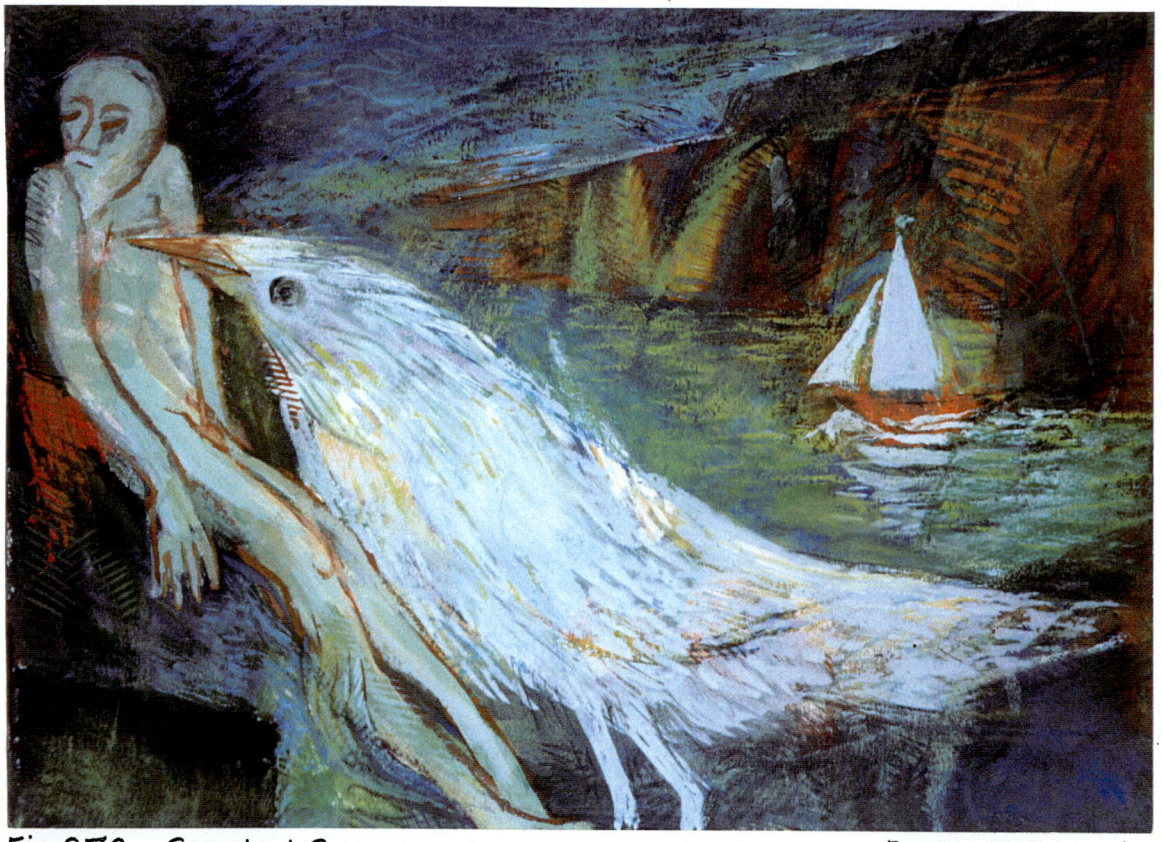

Fig. 372 Fledgling about to leave the nest — Gouache on toned paper

Fig. 373 Coastal Scene — Pastel & Gouache

Birds as 'Carers'

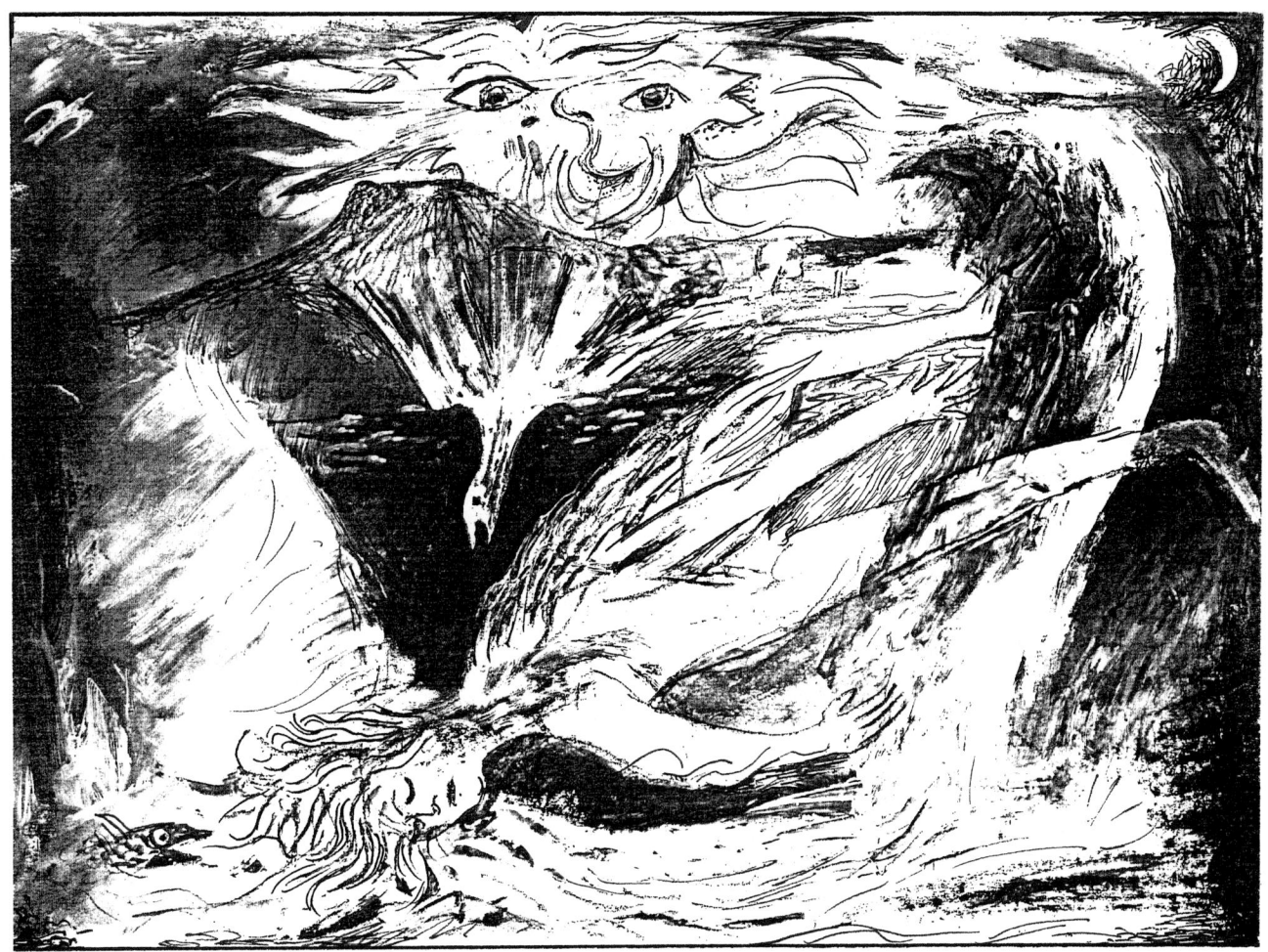

Fig. 374   The Drowning Youth   Pen & Wash

Above: 'Drowning Youth'

Above a dormant volcano the sun is smiling. Below a bird dives towards the sea where a drowning youth floats in a trough between towering waves. The bird is concerned about the youth but the sun appears nonchalant.

Top left: "Fledgling about to leave its nest'

A humanoid bird soars above the land, her blue wings encircle her baby chick who is about to fly from her lap/nest.

Bottom left: 'Coastal Scene'

A sea cliff and a small sailing boat make a backdrop for a sickly looking man who leans back against some rocks. A large white bird attends to him. Showing compassion it leans against the man's legs, its beak gently nudging his chest. A sense of nurturing seems evident.
The boat is toylike, harking back to childhood memories.

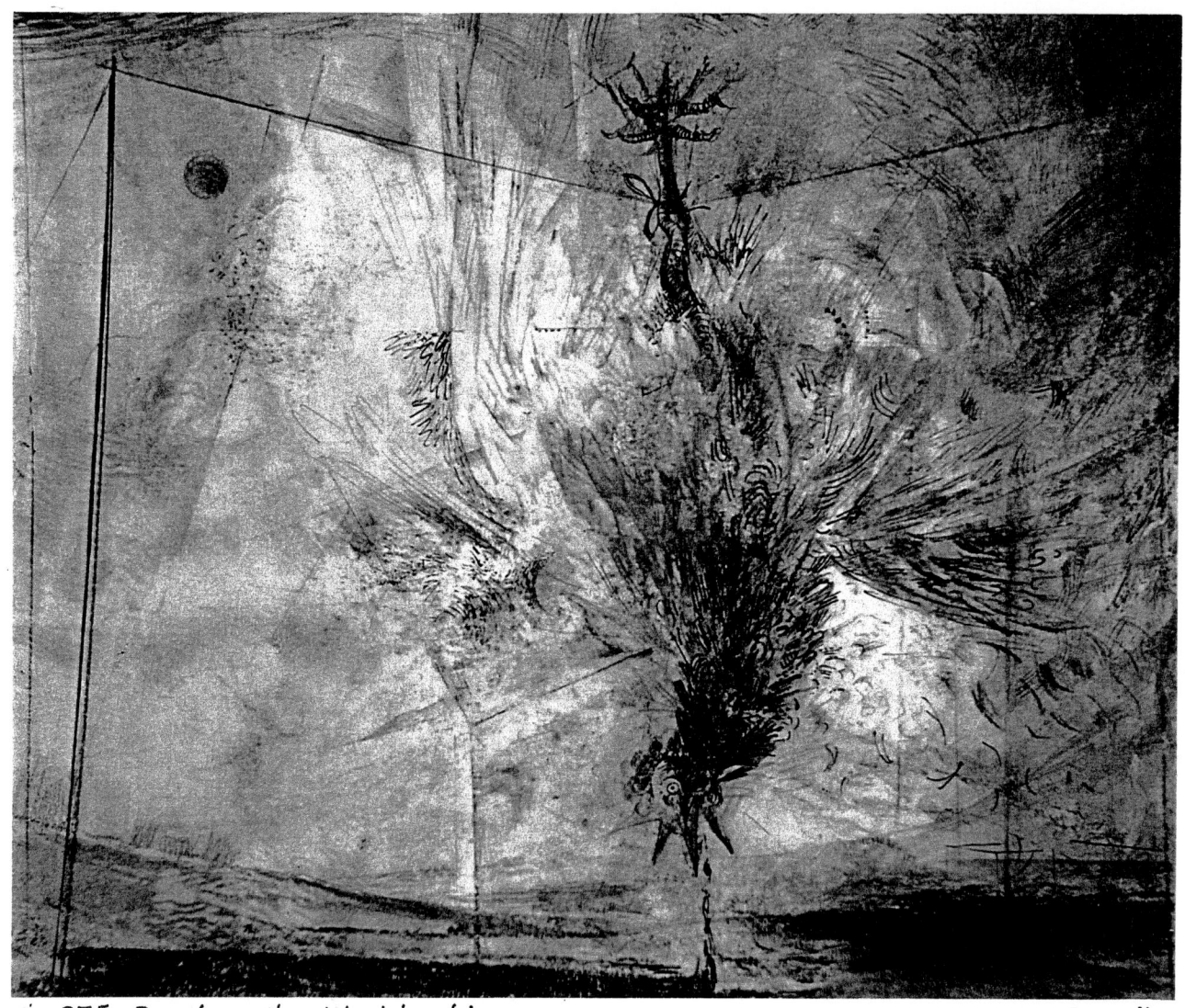

Fig. 375 Death on the Washing Line   Pencil

Birds as Victims

Some of the freestyle bird pictures were far from being aspirational and emphasised a much darker aspect of retained childhood memories.

During the mid to late 1930s, between the ages 7 and 10 yrs, my brother and I were boarded out on a farm during the summer holidays. At market times I recalled a disturbing and vivid memory of the killing of chickens. The farm's washing line was put to a quite different use when Walter, the old farmer, tied up five or more birds by their legs with twine. Then, taking a sharp penknife from his pocket he would move swiftly along a thrashing line of chickens cutting out their tongues. The flapping turned to a frenzy as I stood nearby, both appalled and fascinated by what I was witnessing. "It's alright lad, they don't feel anything, and the meat comes out whiter", said Walter, perhaps seeing my distress.

After some fifteen or more minutes of blood letting I could well believe this latter point but had my doubts about the former.

Now, drawing and painting these memories and feelings, the experience remains as real as the actual event some sixty years ago. The pencil drawing above (fig 375) emphasises the representational aspects: the vigorous wing movements, the claws tied to the washing line, and the blood dripping from a jerking head.

The two freestyle paintings opposite stress the empathy I felt, and are perhaps more challenging responses. Both release old retained anger and feelings of a child's despair.

The bird's body metamorphoses into my head; my body into its head.

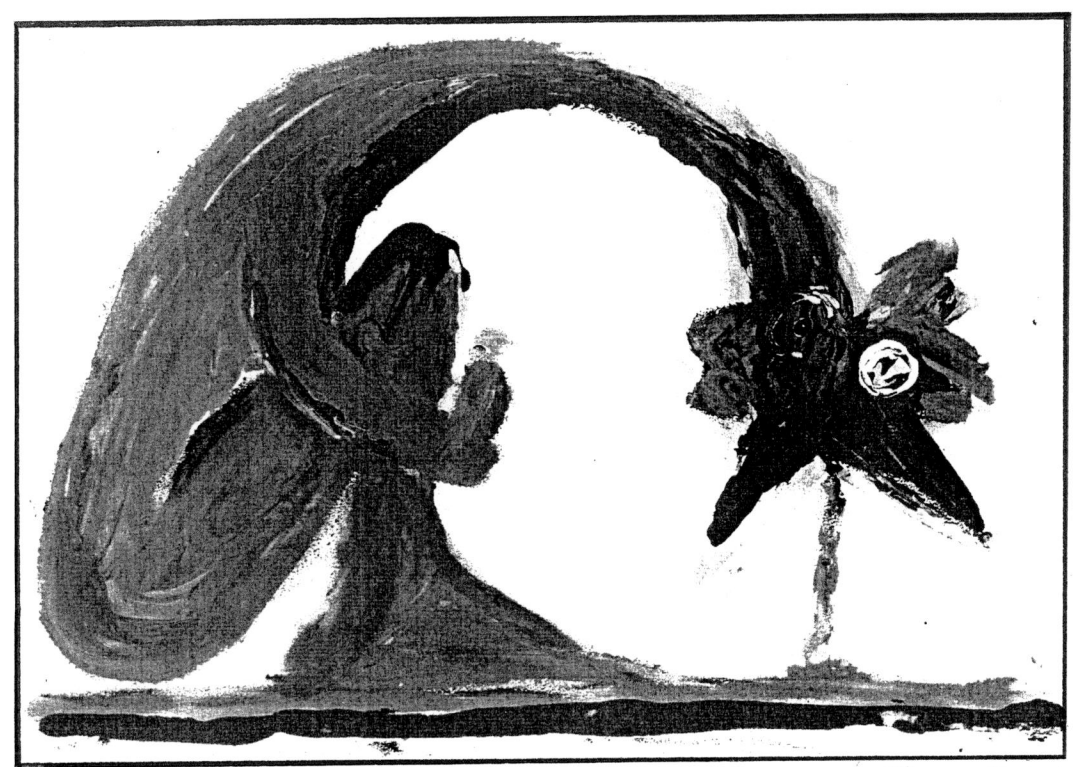

Fig. 376 Metamorphosis Nº 1 Finger Paint

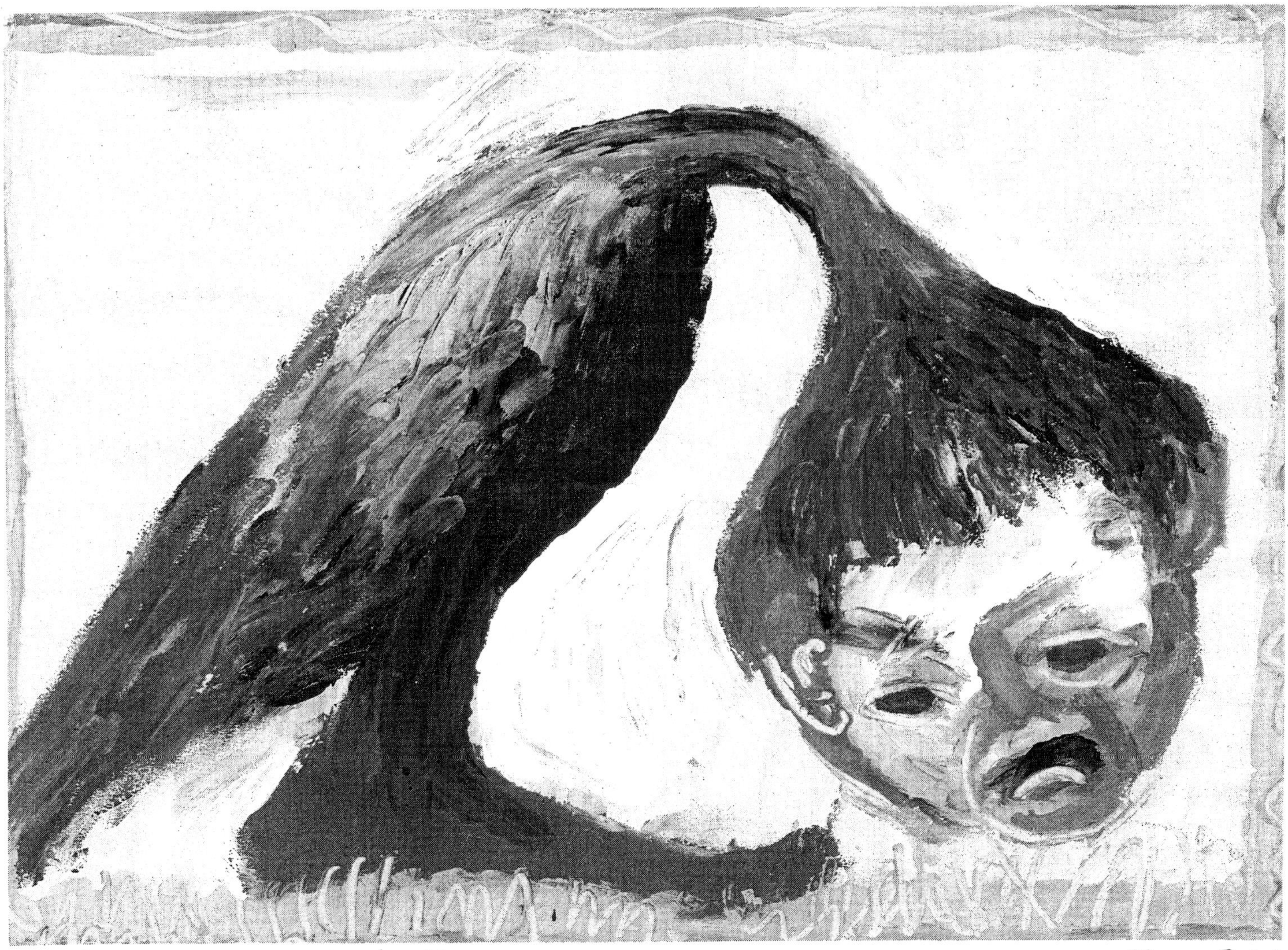

Fig. 377 Metamorphosis Nº 2 Finger Paint

The Company of Birds

Three bird groups showing flocks of migrating birds, of birds masquerading as actors on stage, and people masquerading as birds.

Top right: 'Bird Theatre I'

Preening their wings, puffing out their feathers, 'strutting their stuff', some joining in a chorus, the bird actors look contented and happy. The bright stage lighting and colourful plumage emphasise the 'showing off' of the birds as in a light-hearted comedy.

Bottom right: 'Bird Theatre II'

Sometimes the accidental nature of freestyle artwork leads to quite unnerving imagery. The almost Alice in Wonderland atmosphere in this painting with its crowded spatial unease seems curiously disturbing. The standing figure in the left backstage sets the mood. His suspicious, retentive look (perhaps a psychotic personality) reflects on the figures of his own imaginings, strutting and standing around him. He envisages people dressed up as, or changing into, birds. One has a hydra-headed arm, two wear trousers, perhaps wishing to change back into people. The scene has changed from comedy to tragi-comedy.

Below: 'Migration'

This large flock is either anticipating flight or has already taken to the wing. A feeling of restlessness prevails, migration beckons... a need for change is evident..... seeking another environment.....?

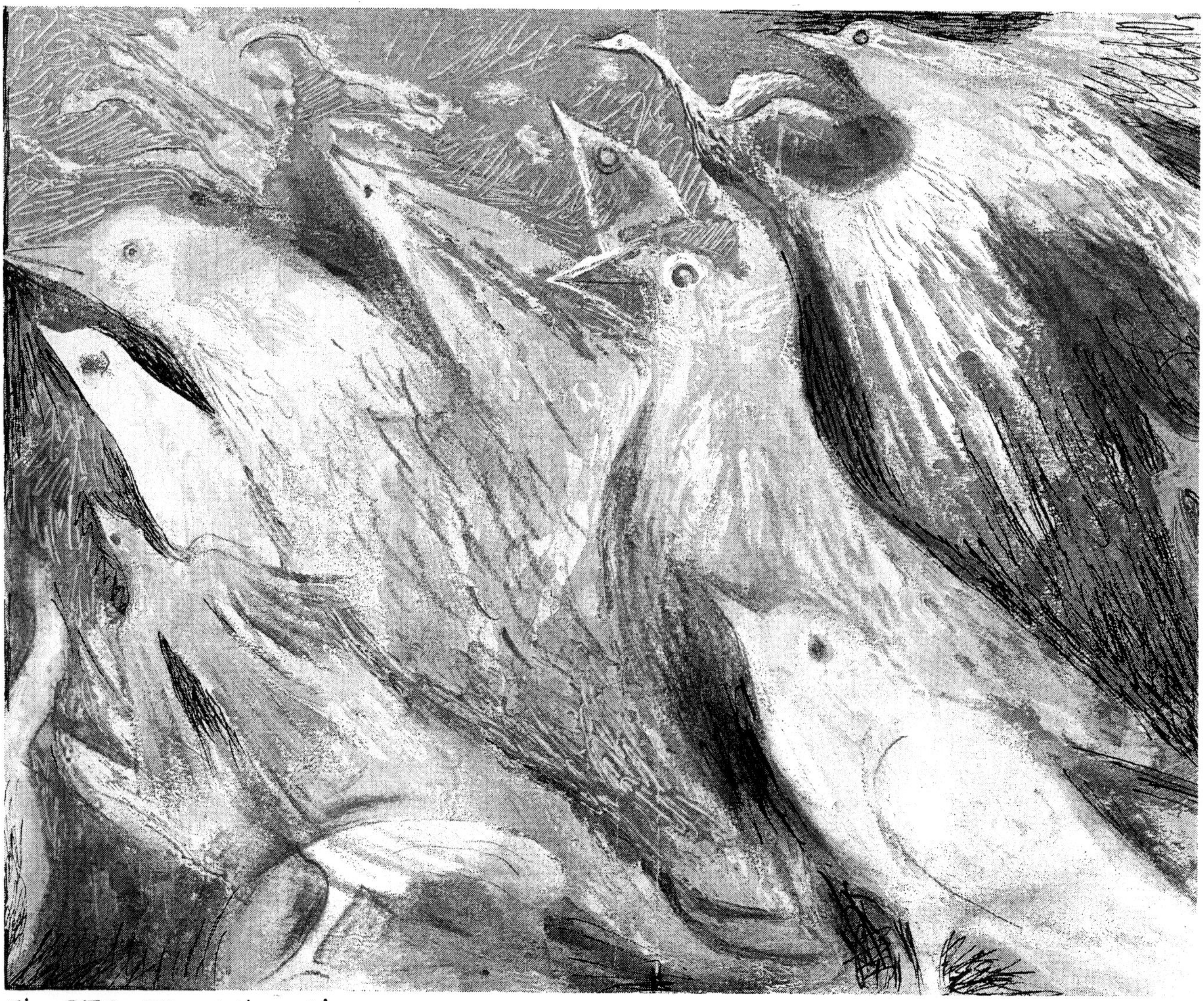

Fig. 378 The Migration   Finger Paint

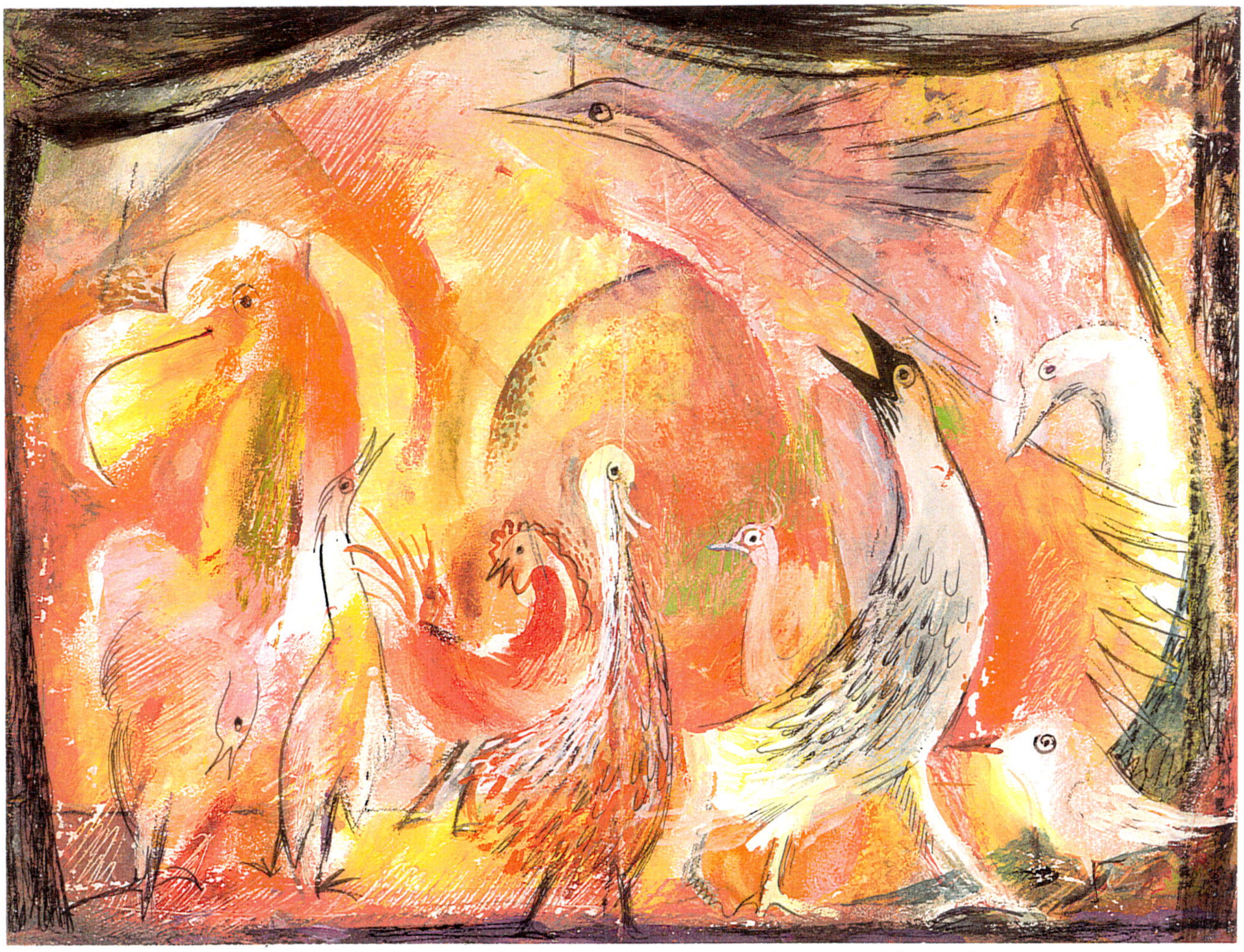

Fig.379 Bird Theatre № 1 — Finger Paint   Below: Fig.380 Bird Theatre № 2 — Pencil

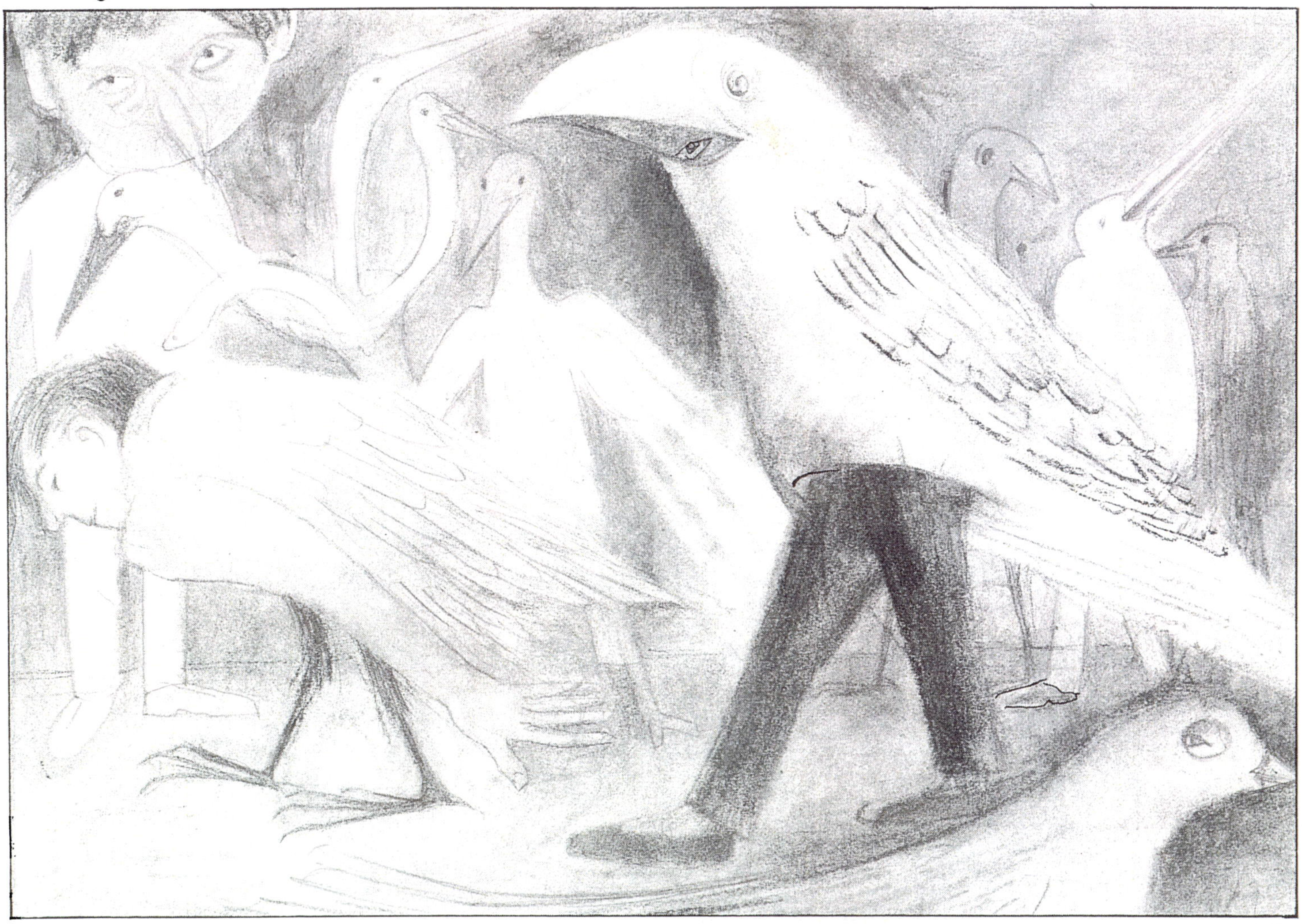

223

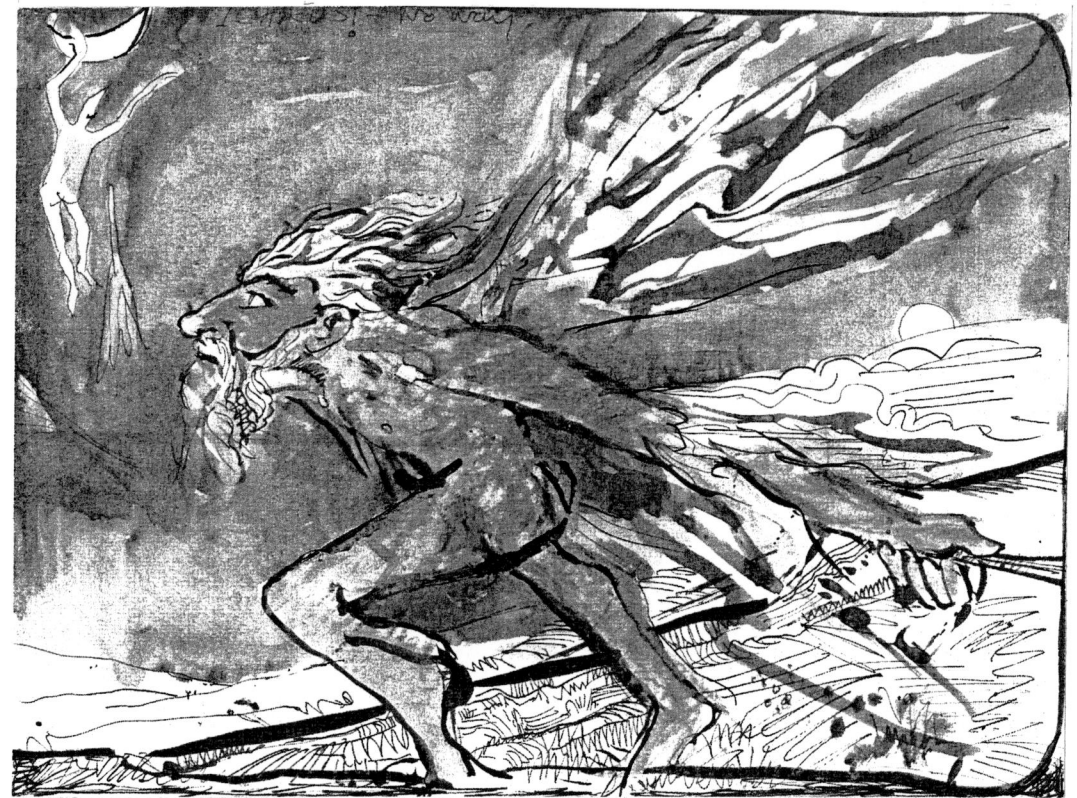

Fig. 381 A Strenuous Effort   Ink & Wash

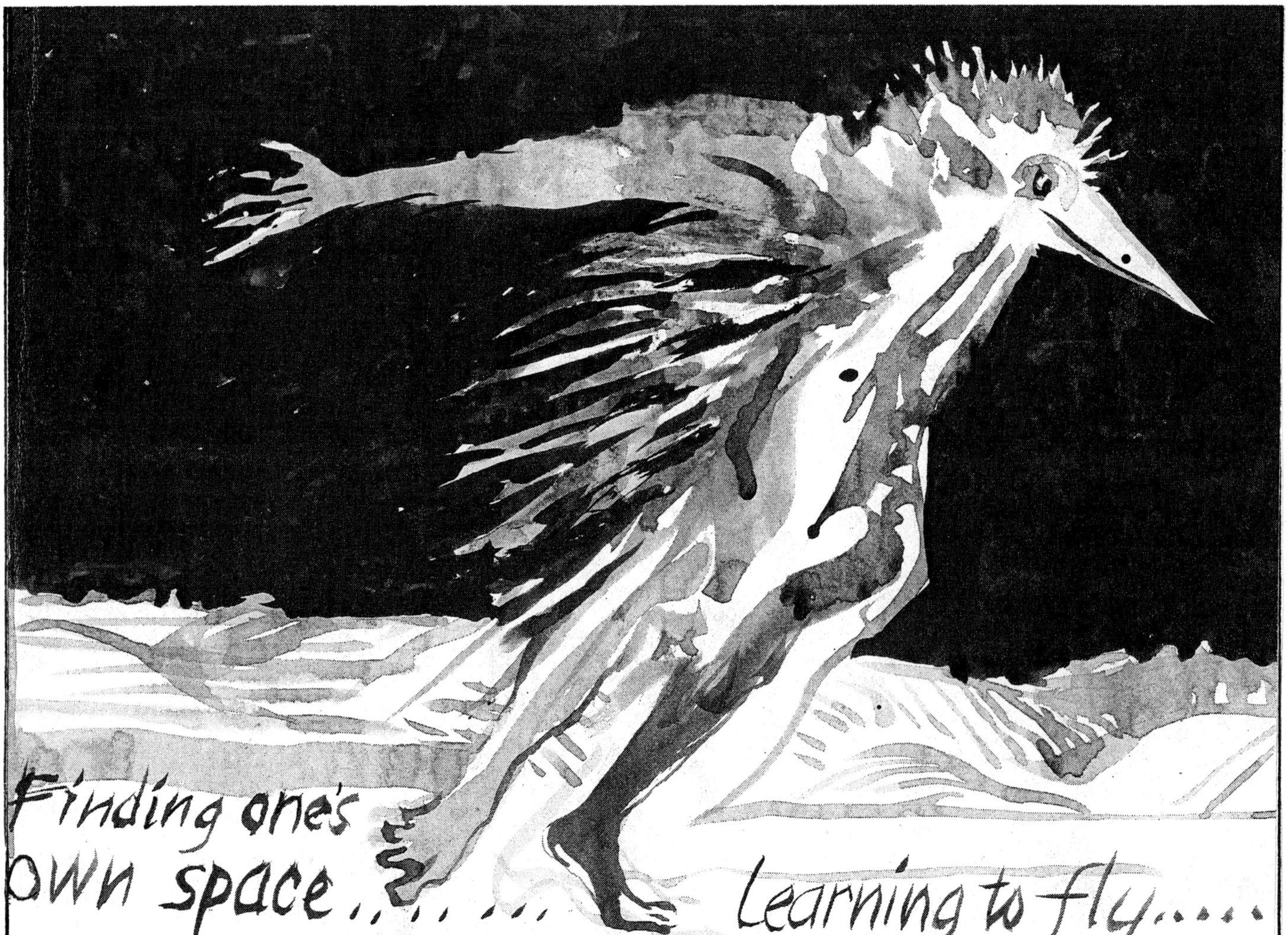

Fig. 382 Learning to Fly   Brush & Wash

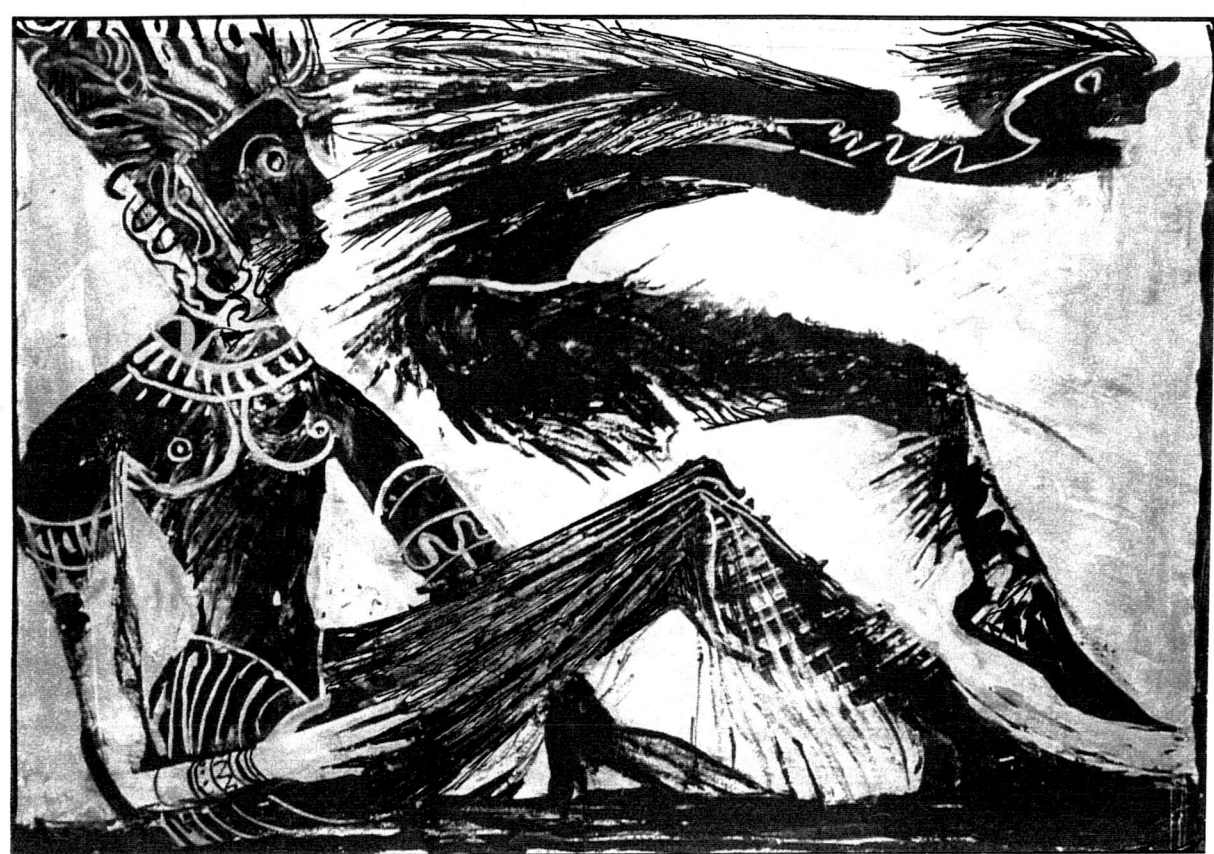

Fig. 383 The Fledgling   Brush, Pen & Ink

Taking Off

Wings, from sheeting attached to shoulders, and hand-held devices become signs for psychological 'lift-off'. The work gives a sense of moving on and up — of lifting the self out of the doldrums.

Top Left: 'A Strenuous Effort'

A Blakean figure, willing himself to take off. He glances up, determined to meet the challenge of the already airborne figure. The impression is one of effort and strain to achieve his desire.

Bottom Left: 'Learning to Fly'

In contrast to Fig. 381 an altogether more light-hearted approach to flight. This Joker character suggests using an easy, uplifting run without effort. Just find your own space, his pose seems to say.....

Above: 'The Fledgling'

An echo from the Joker's run, 'Learning to Fly'. Leaping from his mother's lap this fledgling child acquires feathers and sallies forth in his search for freedom and independence.

Overleaf: 'Lift-Off'

A cartoon-like brush-and-pen version of achieving lift-off. My hopeful flier gathers momentum like a rocket and seems to hit his head on the ceiling of the sun. There is considerable internal fragmentation. Perhaps he pricked himself on the desert cactus — a warning to those who run before they can walk! The cumulative effect, however, is one of exhilaration.

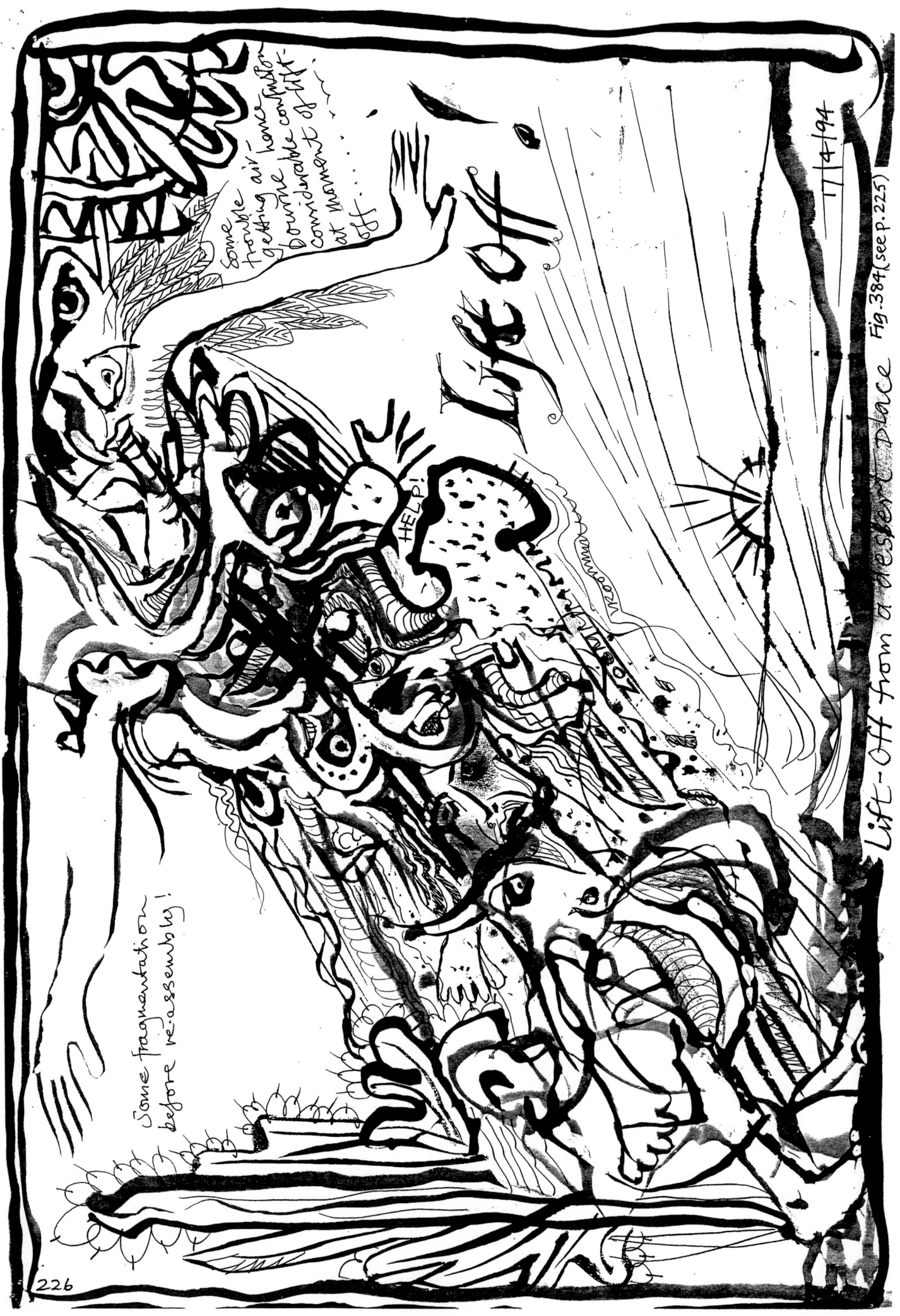
Lift-Off from a desert place Fig. 384 (see p.225)

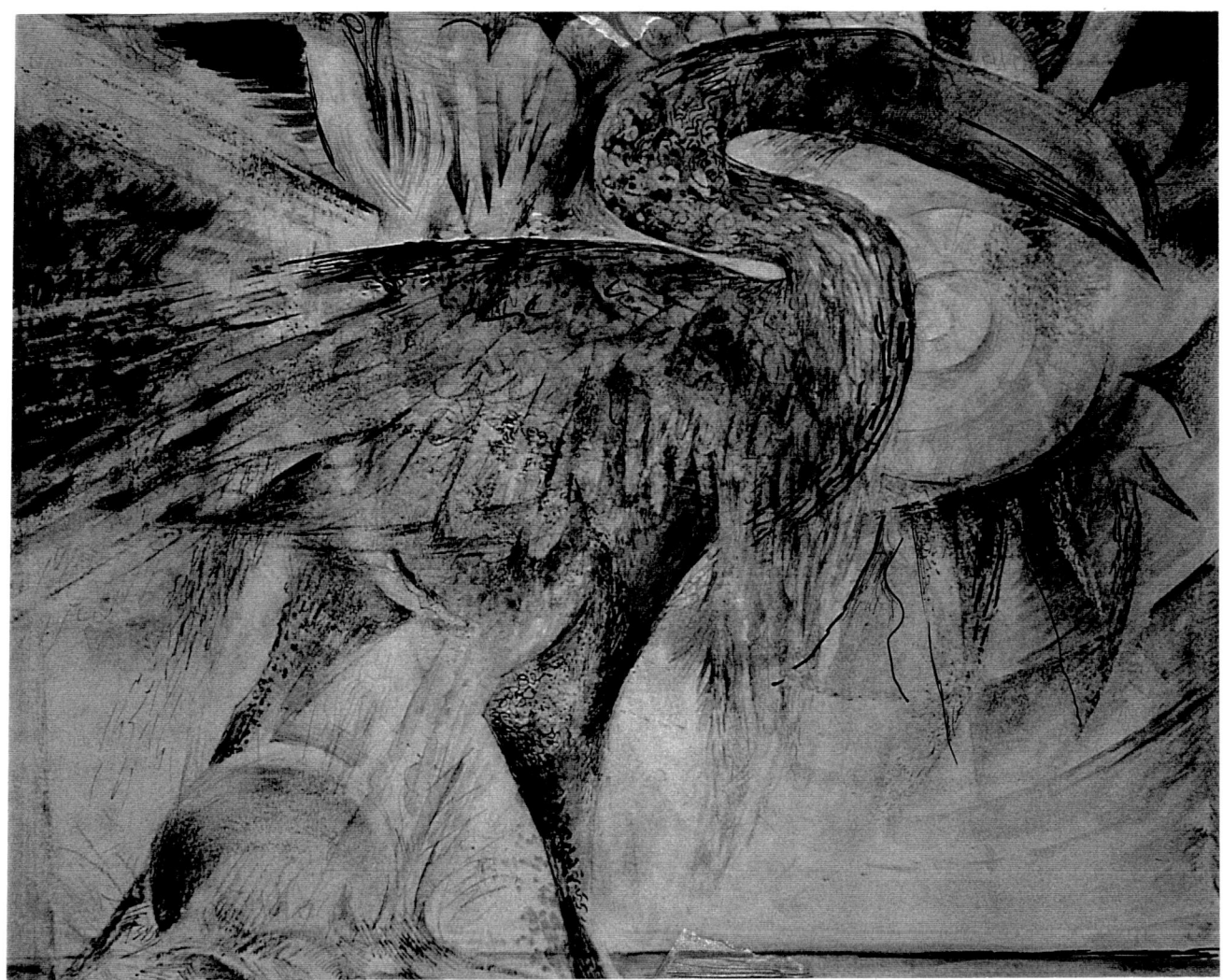

Fig. 385 Origin of the World   Pencil

Origin of the World

Of the many myths centred around the origins of the world, the one which described a giant bird laying a world egg on the waters came to mind as I developed a freestyle drawing. The totally ambivalent textures and lines gradually revealed two strutting legs, a sunburst and a long neck and beak.

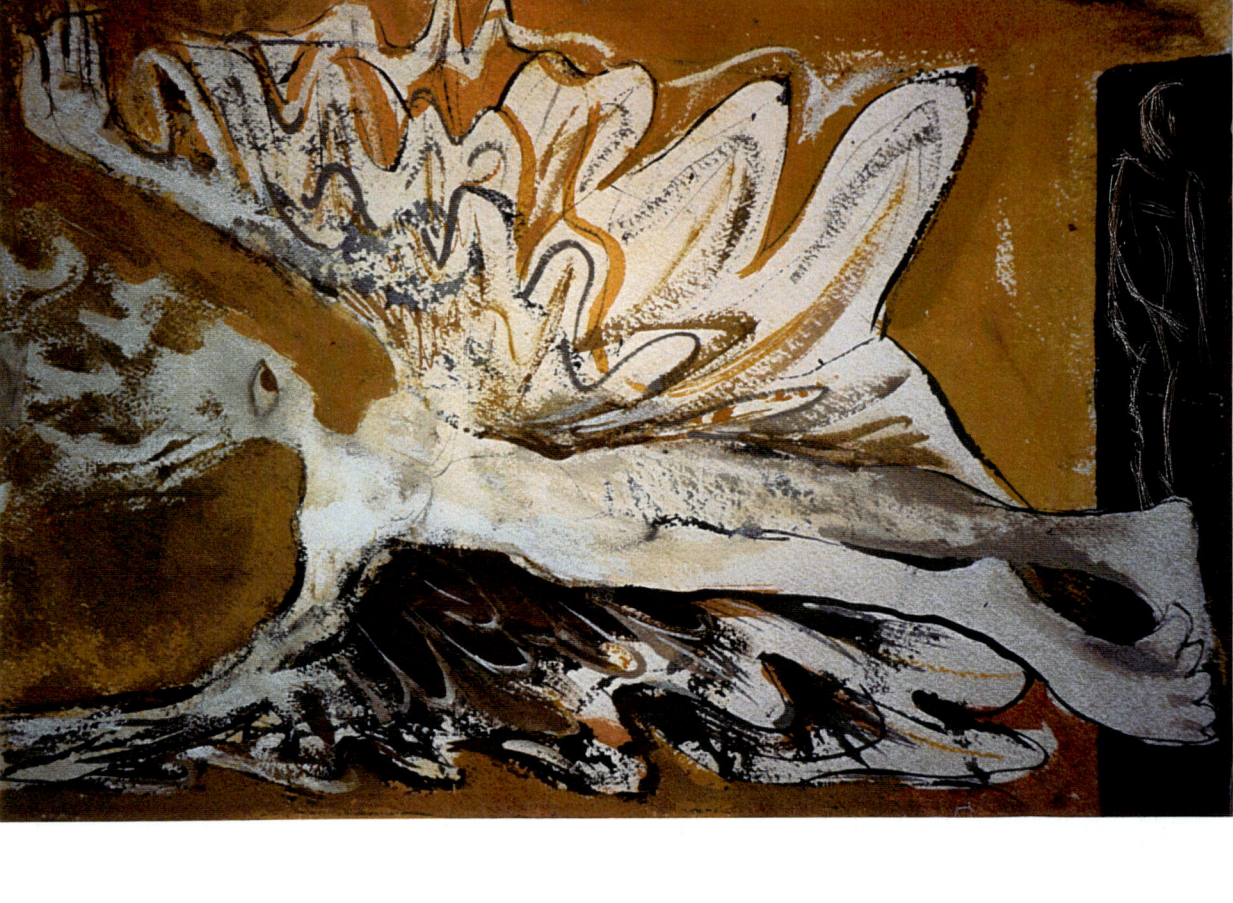

Fig. 387 Surprised Angel — Gouache

Angelic Forms

Below: 'Wings'

There often seems to be a hiatus between dream and reality. Sometimes, when we attempt to express the idea or dream in painting, nothing seems to mirror the expectation. 'Wings' is perhaps a visual interpretation of this mood. Five characters rest in a landscape near a cliff edge watching an apparition form in the sky above. There is no sense of urgency, no rush or agitation to see what winged being might materialise. The self is probably hinting, 'You need to exercise more patience'.

Right: 'Surprised Angel' — A club-footed (guardian?) angel stands on a tomb showing a faint outline of a body.

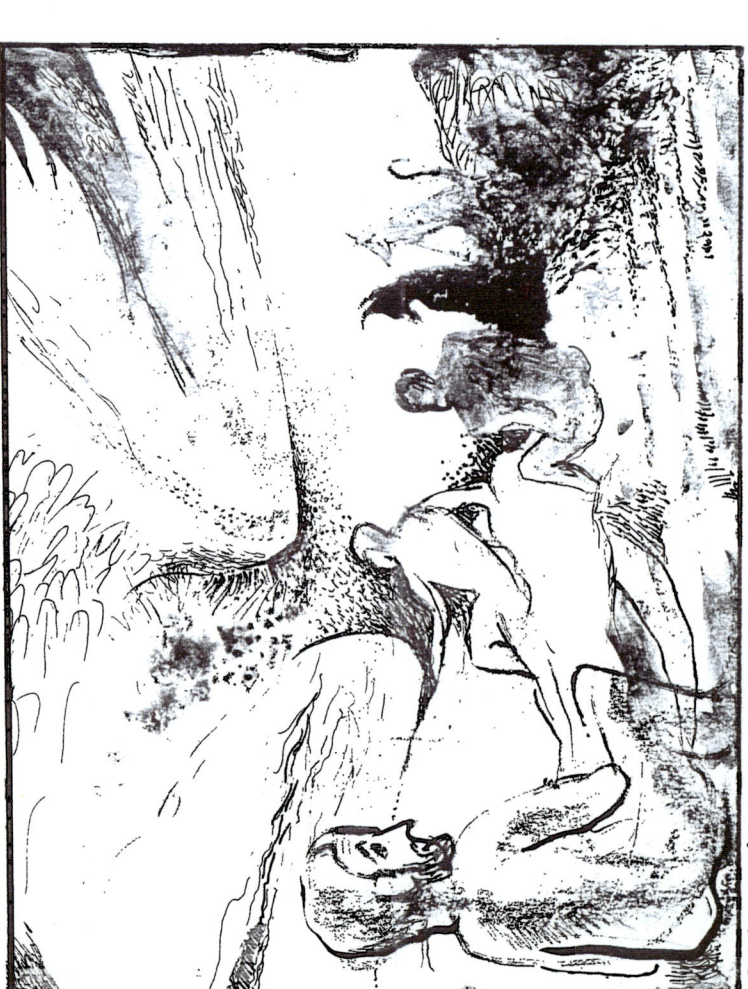

Fig. 386 Wings — Pen, Brush, Ink & Chalk

Below Left: 'Death Wish'

Above, a mosaic reminiscent of a God-the-Father figure in an Orthodox church leans forward exhorting the two struggling angels to rescue someone who prefers to give up the struggle. (This scene may have been triggered off by the memory of an ancient cemetery in disrepair).

Below Right: 'A Desert Gathering'

Perhaps inspired by a car journey along the Desert Road on Southern North Island in New Zealand (see page 251). It was such a bleak piece of landscape I could have peopled it like this. Young angels converse with an elder, others are airborne while a host gathers further away in the desert.

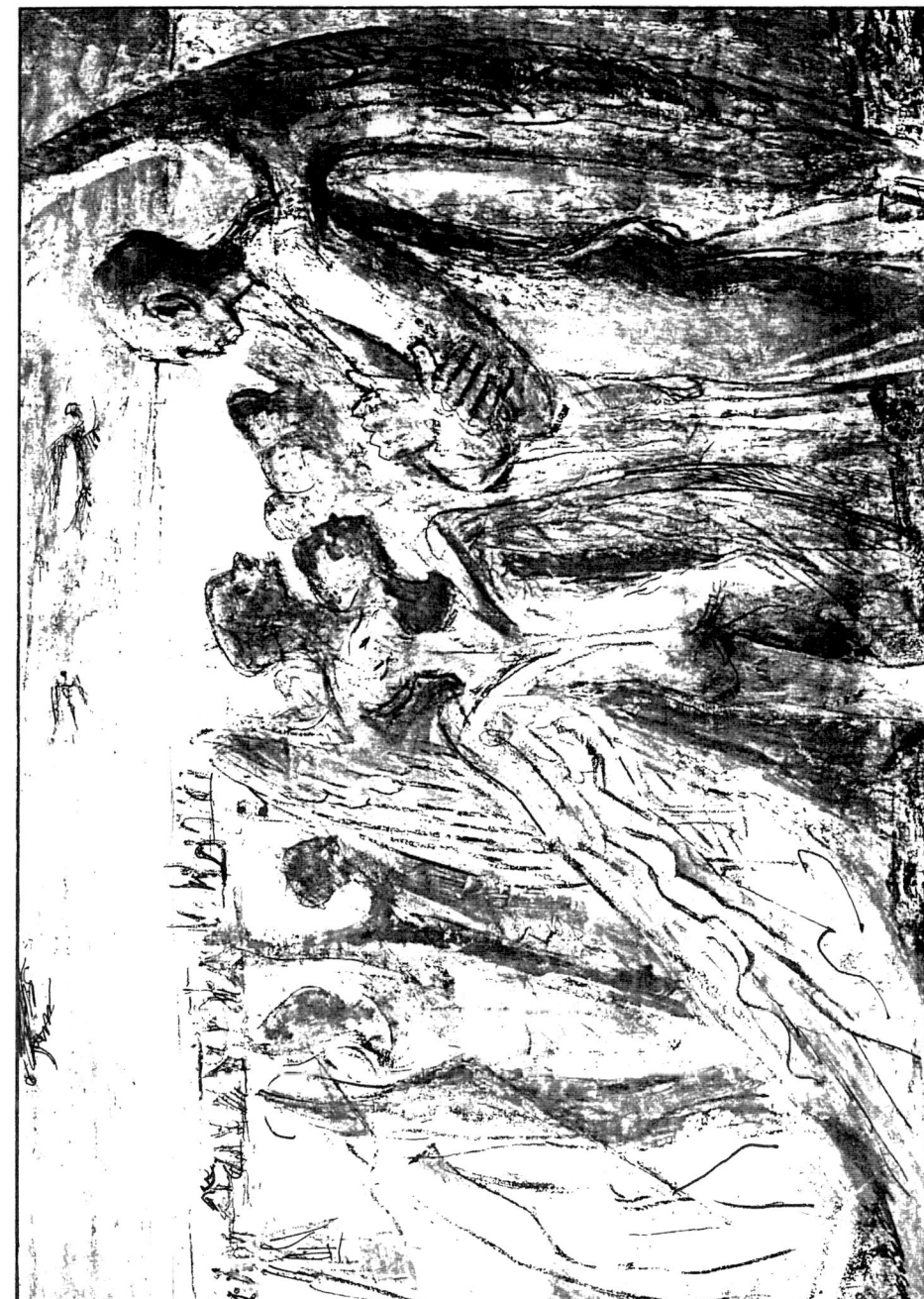

Fig. 388 Death Wish   Ink & Gouache

Fig. 389 A Desert Gathering   Gouache, Pencil & Pen

229

More Mythological Winged Creatures

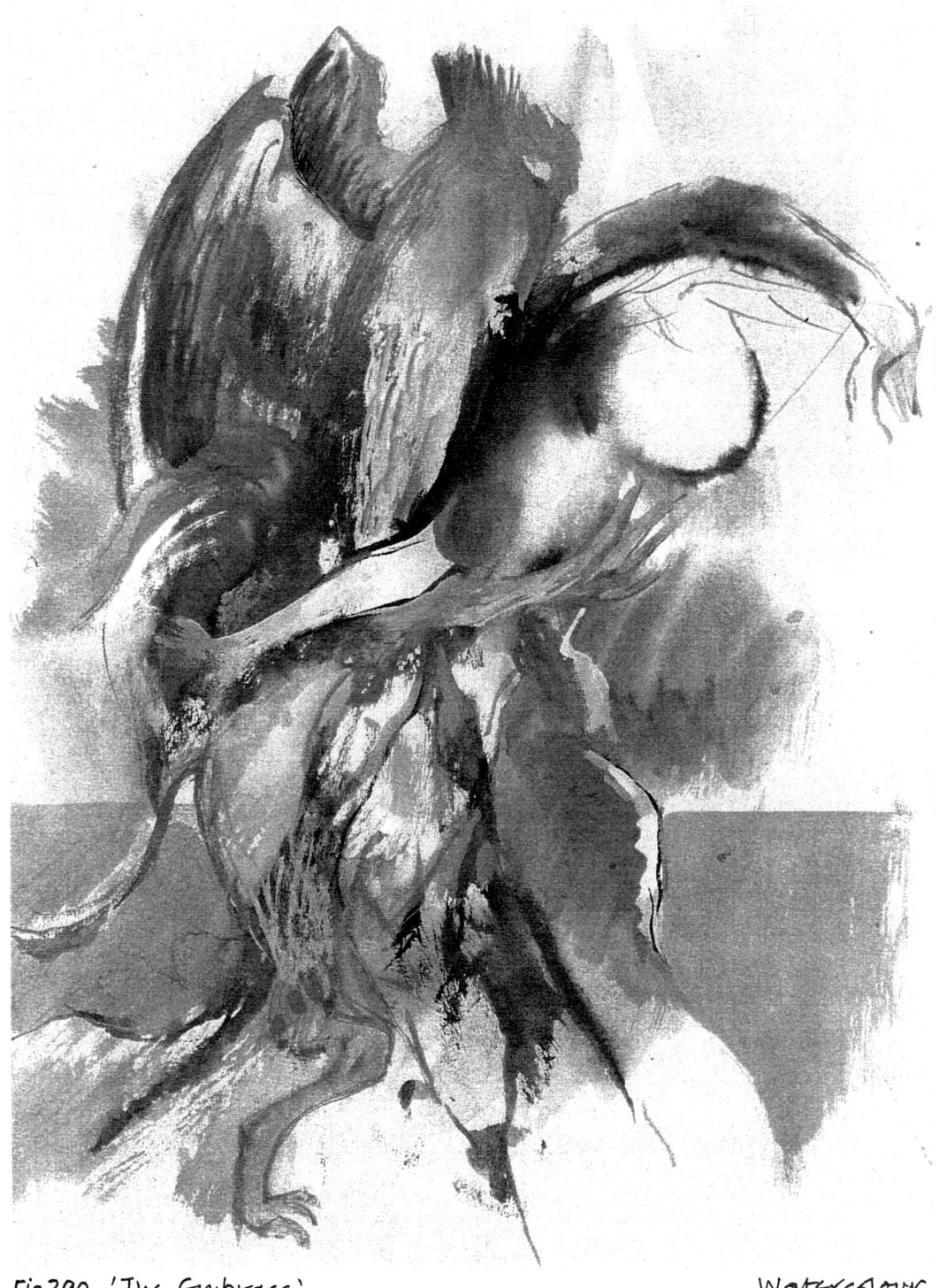

Fig.390 'The Embrace' Watercolour.

Above: 'Mythological scene - The Embrace'

An equivocal confrontation, possibly sexual, clasping a dark angel to one's bosom; perhaps a power struggle, or light seeking a balance with darkness.

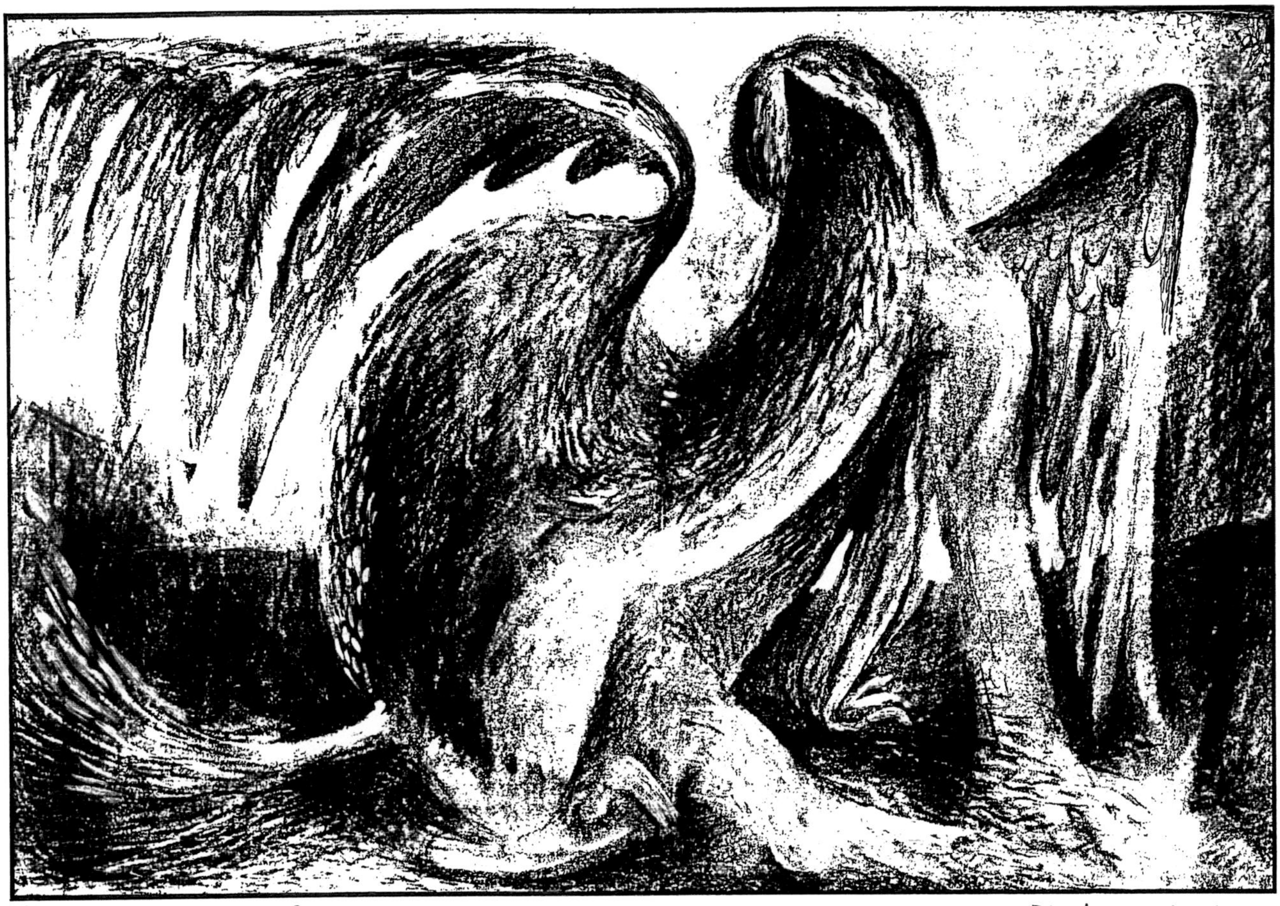

Fig. 391 Enigmatic Creature — Black paint, chalk

Above: 'Enigmatic Creature'

The posture and the manner of spreading its wings is heraldic, as if proclaiming a family crest. It seems it is also some indeterminate creature between land and air, with a head which could be seen either as pointed like a bird's or, it has its face hidden in a deep shadow cast by a helmet.

This creature has the body of a beast and wings of an angel — it could be a dragon.

Right: detail from 'An Eruptive Landscape' (see page 260)

The birdman tentatively finds his way across the volcanic zone of North Island, New Zealand.

Right: Fig 392 detail from 'Eruptive Landscape'

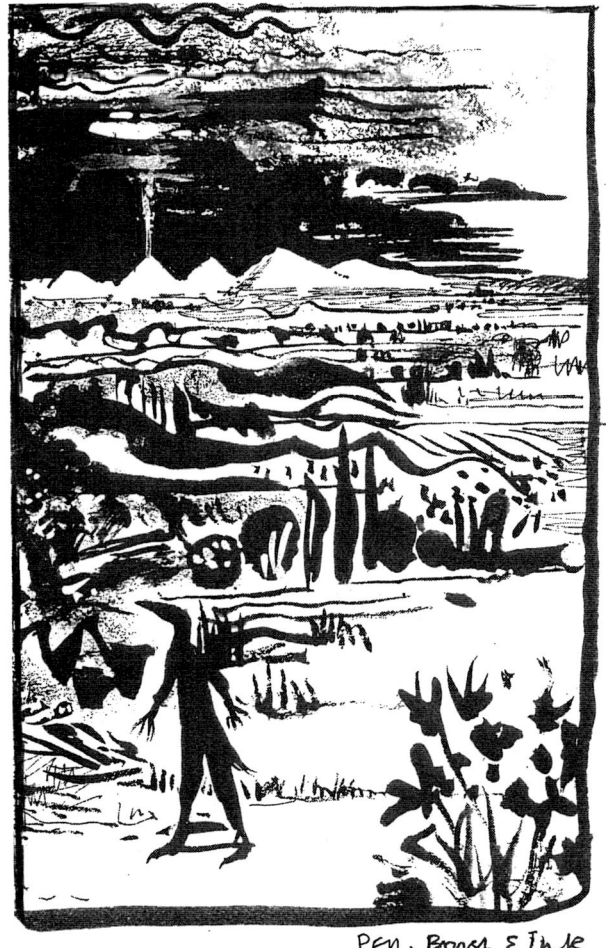

PEN, Brush & Ink.

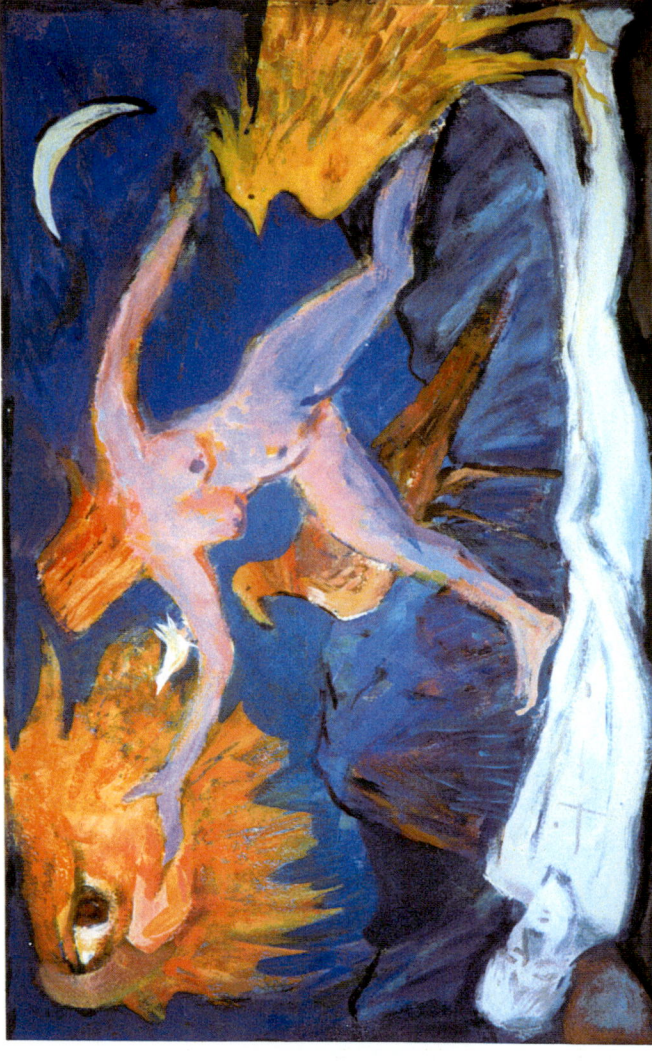

Fig. 394   A Possible Revival   Oil on Board

Aspects of the Earth Goddess – Three mythological scenes

above: 'A Possible Revival'

A male nude lies below. He could be dying or just asleep, or perhaps recuperating as he rests his head on a rock and an orange bird perches on his foot.
A leaping red-headed goddess stretches out a hand to greet the sun. She might revive the man by landing on his chest - or finish him off. A small white bird also stretches its neck expectantly towards the sun, whilst a bird in the centre stands passively watching the drama unfold.

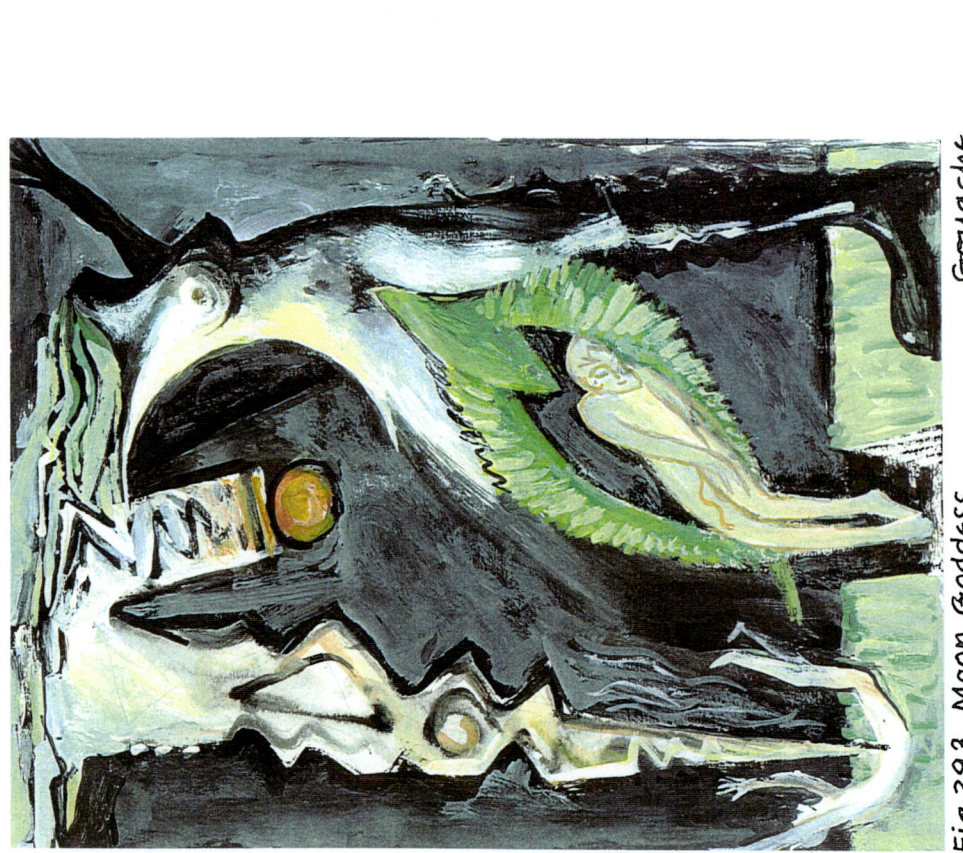

Fig. 393 Moon Goddess   Gouache

above: 'Moon Goddess'
A sinister aspect of the goddess, her side shaping into a new moon, her left foot enclosed in a jackboot. Yet this goddess of the night gives birth to a bird who holds an unconscious male figure within its wings. The green bird acts as an intermediary.

232

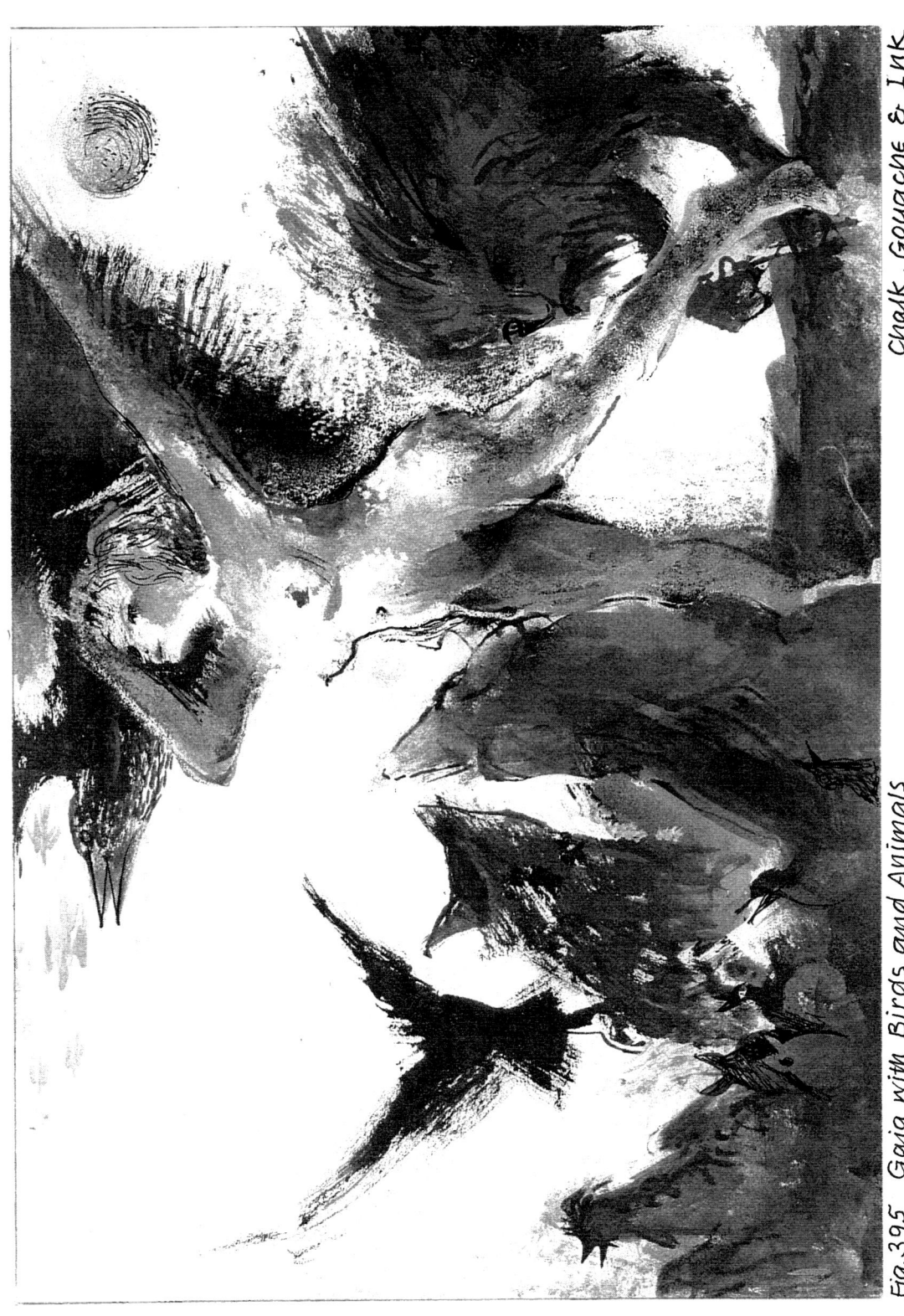

Fig. 395 Gaia with Birds and Animals   Chalk, Gouache & Ink

'Gaia with Birds and Animals'
A freestyle drawing which developed into this primal landscape with figures. Gaia, earth mother strides forth together with many birds and animals. A new day beckons......

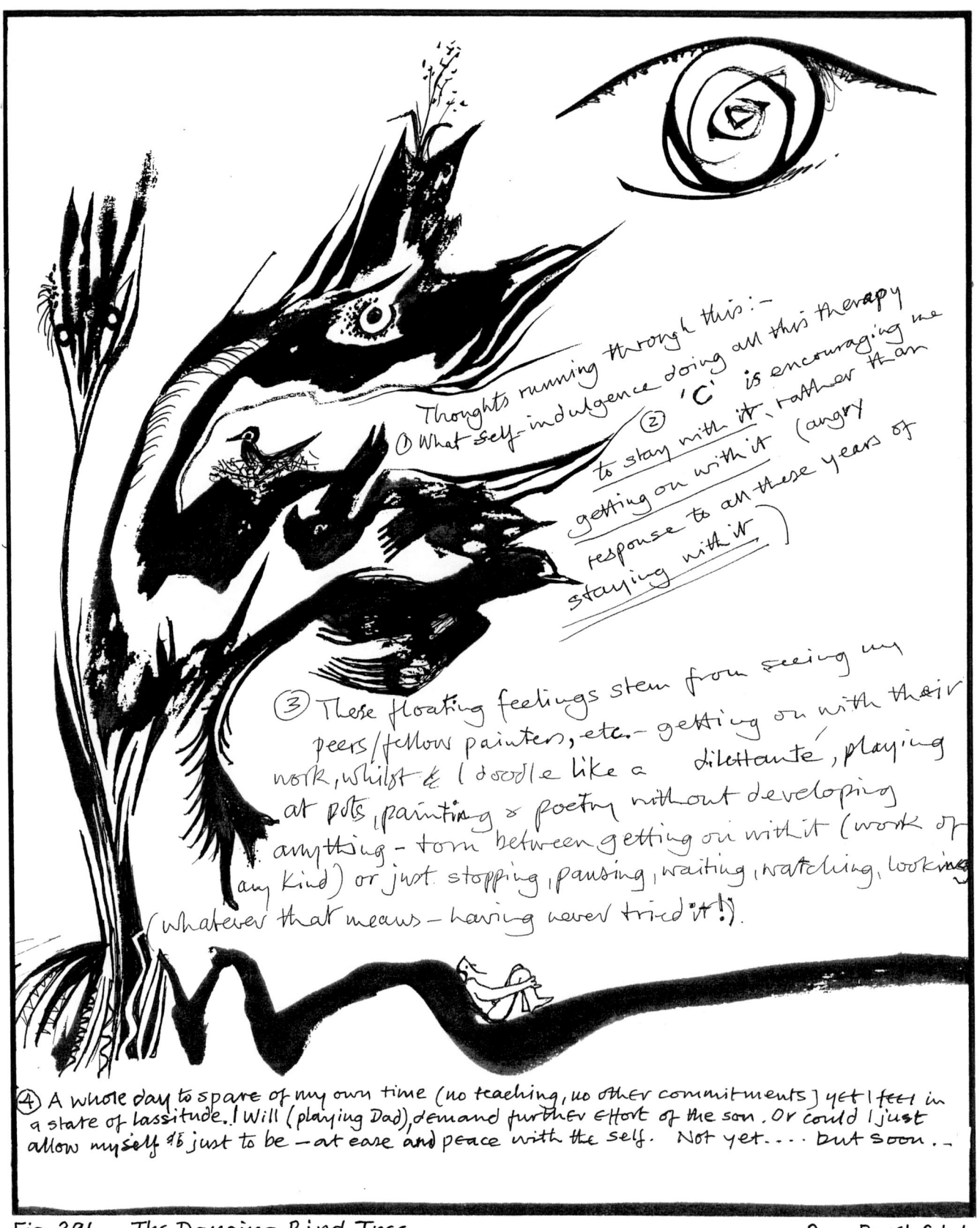

Fig. 396 The Dancing Bird Tree   Pen, Brush & Ink

above: 'The Dancing Bird Tree'
 A freestyle brush drawing with incorporated writing which complements the drawing. Doubts predominate - this was the time when I had thoughts about giving up the art therapy and just doing straight painting again.
 I sit pondering near the base of this great swaying tree form fashioned from parts of birds.

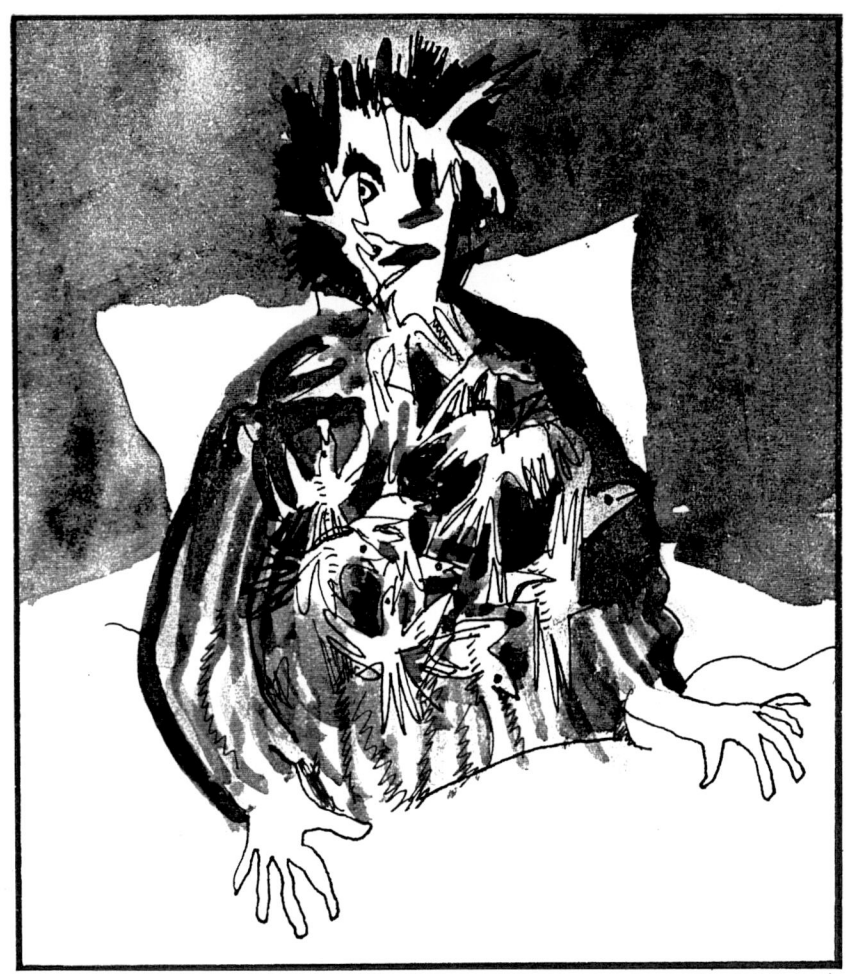

Left: 'Invaded by Birds'

A drawing based on a dream (N° 165 from 'Dream Journal').
On waking, some earlier anxieties (during morning depressions) accumulate and turn into heart flutters. These are transformed into an invasion of flapping birds.
Gripping the bed linen I will them to reduce their movement.
Eventually they disappear.

Fig. 397   Invaded by Birds   Pen & Wash

Right: 'Self Portrait'

My hands cover my mouth and chin. I look perplexed. This freestyle pen and brush drawing has two aspects – the portrait as shown and, by turning it through 90 degrees, two birds confronting each other – perhaps another way of feeling the internalised fluttering birds.

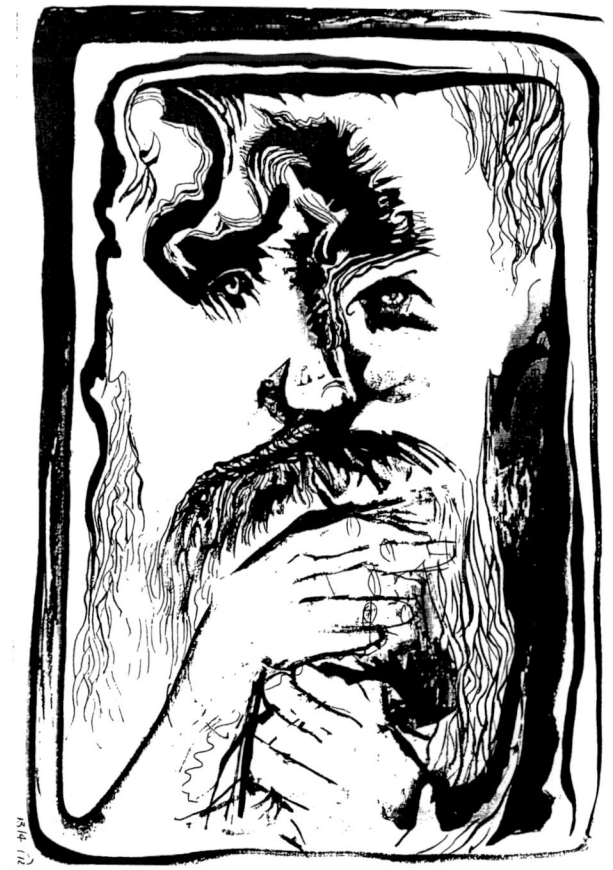

Fig 398   Self Portrait   Brush, Pen & Ink

The Fall of Icarus

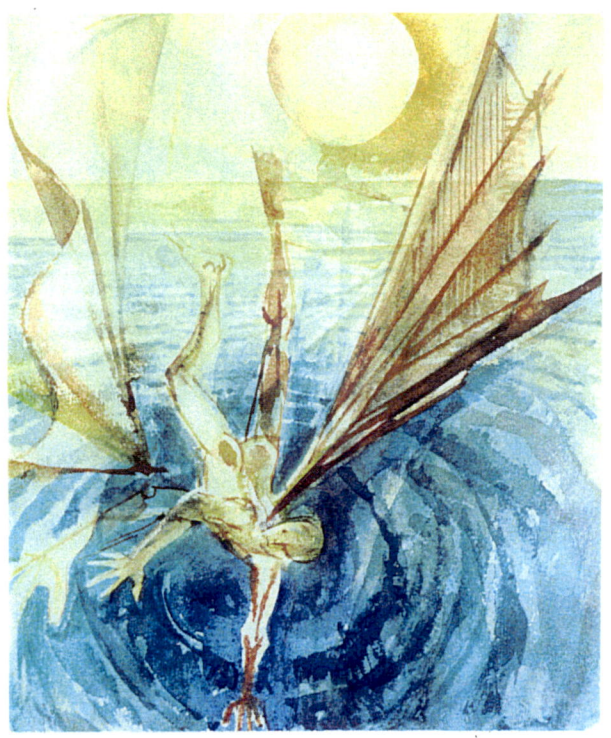

Fig.399 The Fall of Icarus N°1   Watercolour

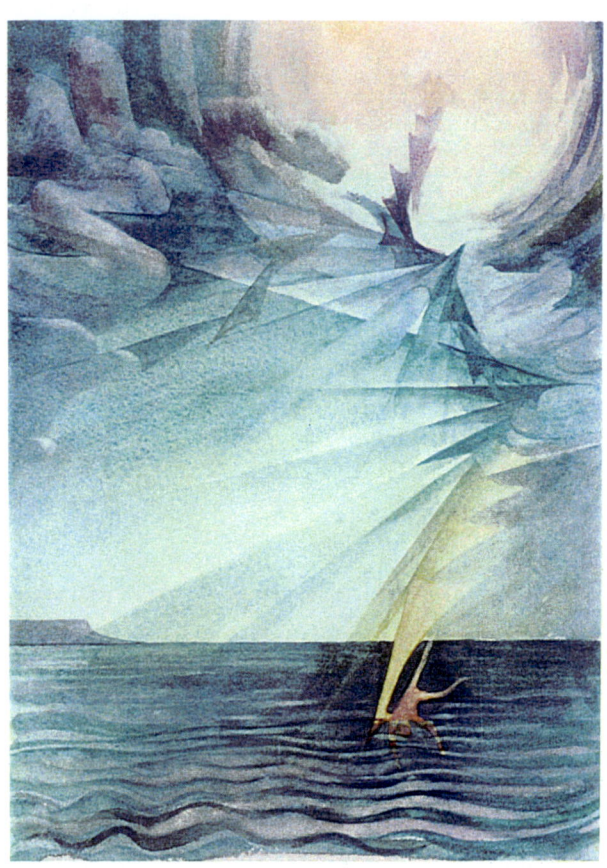

Fig.400 The Fall of Icarus N°2   Watercolour

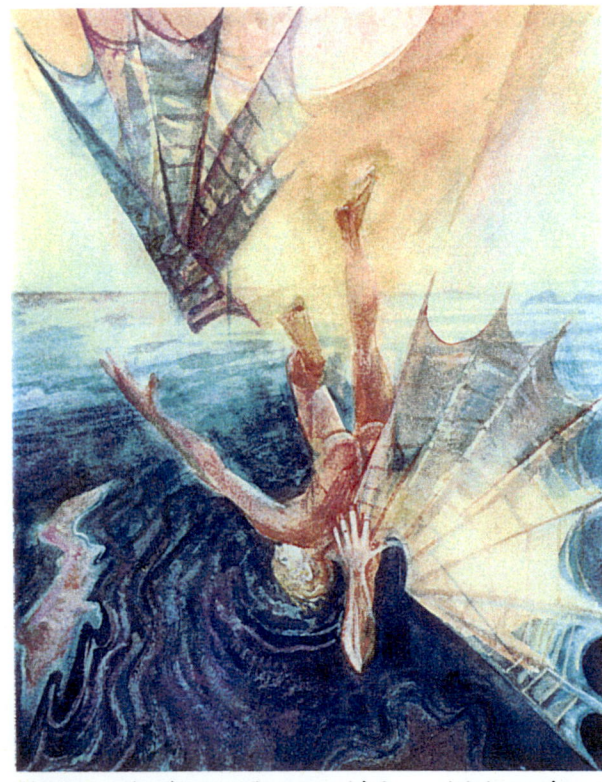

Fig.401 The Fall of Icarus N°3   Watercolour

Daedalus makes a pair of wings for himself and another for his son Icarus, to escape from Crete and King Minos. As the feathers were fixed with wax, Daedalus warns Icarus not to soar too near the sun lest it melt the wax. Icarus disobeys and flies towards the sun, falls into the sea and drowns.

Fascinated by this Greek myth I attempted some illustrations of this moment of falling and related them to the 'freefall' paintings in Part One.

Later I came to realise the internalised father had finally to be ignored (disobeyed) if I wished to aim for a more spontaneous approach – whatever the risks.

Ironically these three paintings aren't free or spontaneous but rigid and stylised – not quite what I was searching for!

A Miscellany of Bird Images

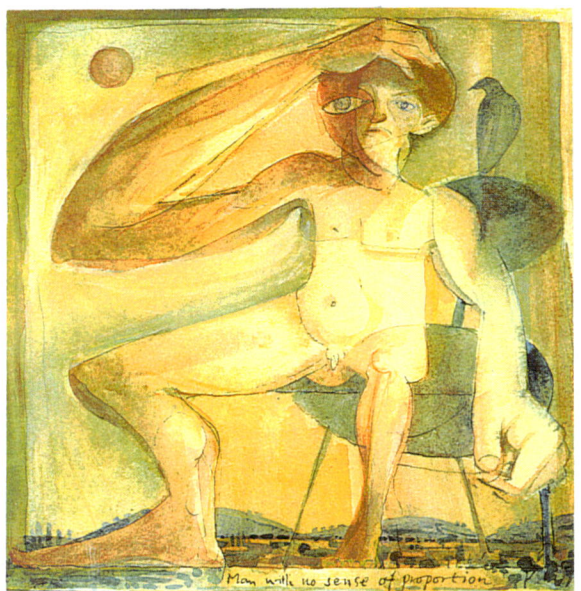

Fig. 402 Man with no sense of Proportion
Pen and Watercolour

The interest lies in the bird perched on the chair. It is offering new directions for the perplexed seated figure.

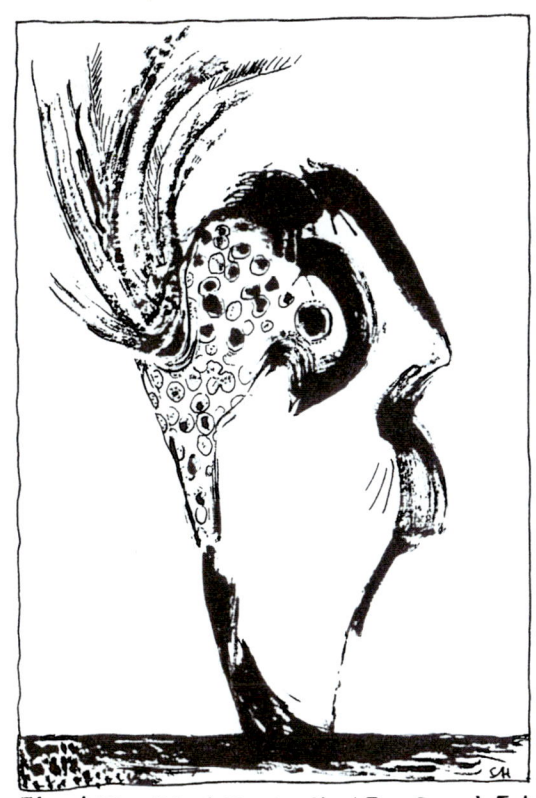

Fig. 403   Bird Portrait.   Pen, Brush, Ink

A moustached head with a feather in his cap - or a spotted bird taking a bow. In each case, showing off & seeking attention.

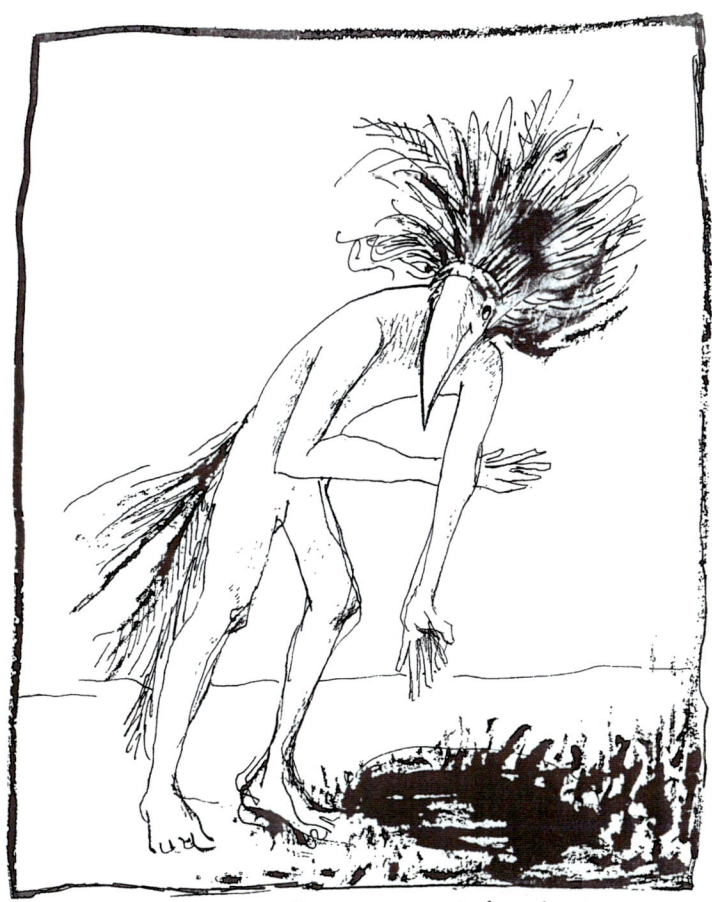

Fig. 404 Birdman finds a Waterhole - Pen, Brush, Ink

A early sketch for 'Healing place for a birdman'. (See page 152).

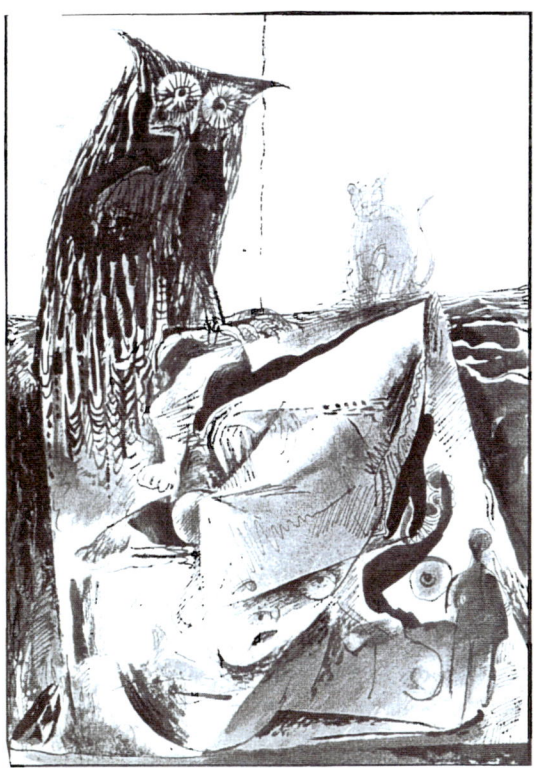

Fig. 405   The Owl   Pen & Wash

Amazed at the chaos below, the owl tries to understand what it's all about. A faint silhouette of a cat sits behind. A assorted fragments lie below.

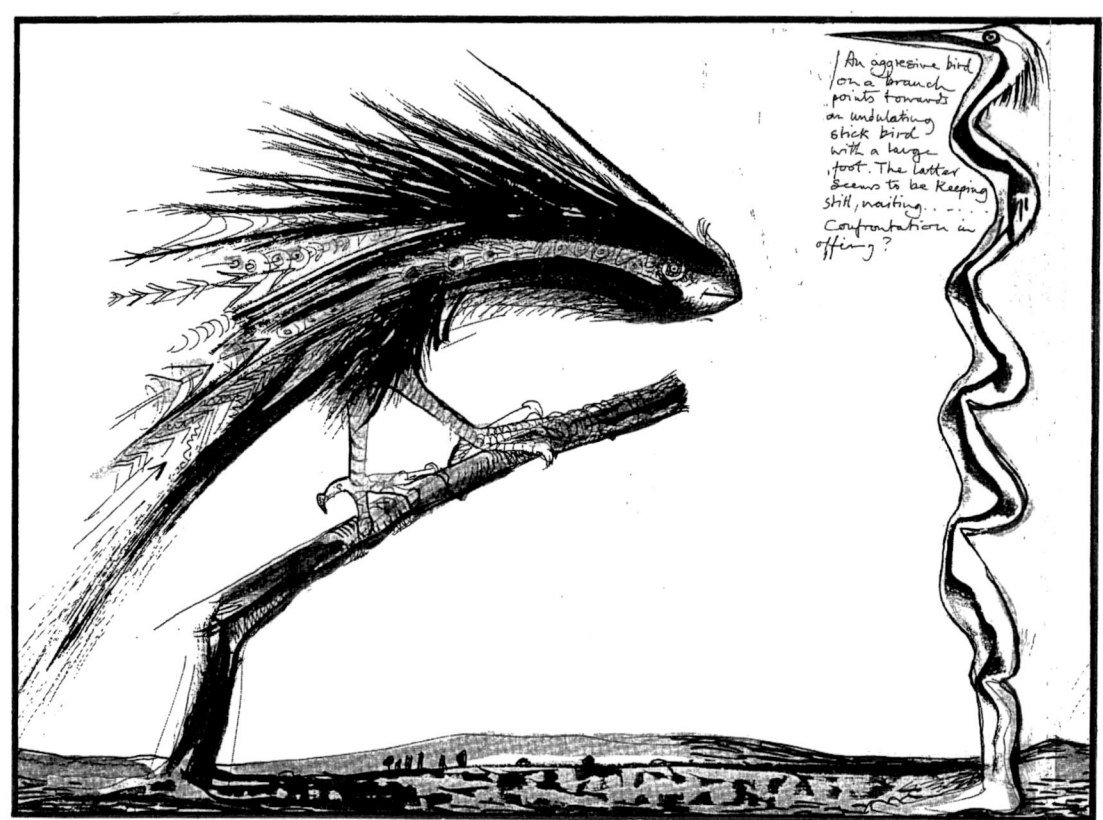

Fig. 406   Confrontation between two birds   Ink & Wash

A thrusting bird on a branch points aggressively at an apparently timid bird with a heron's head and a zigzag body, yet it too is potentially a threat. Its body may strike like a coiled spring.

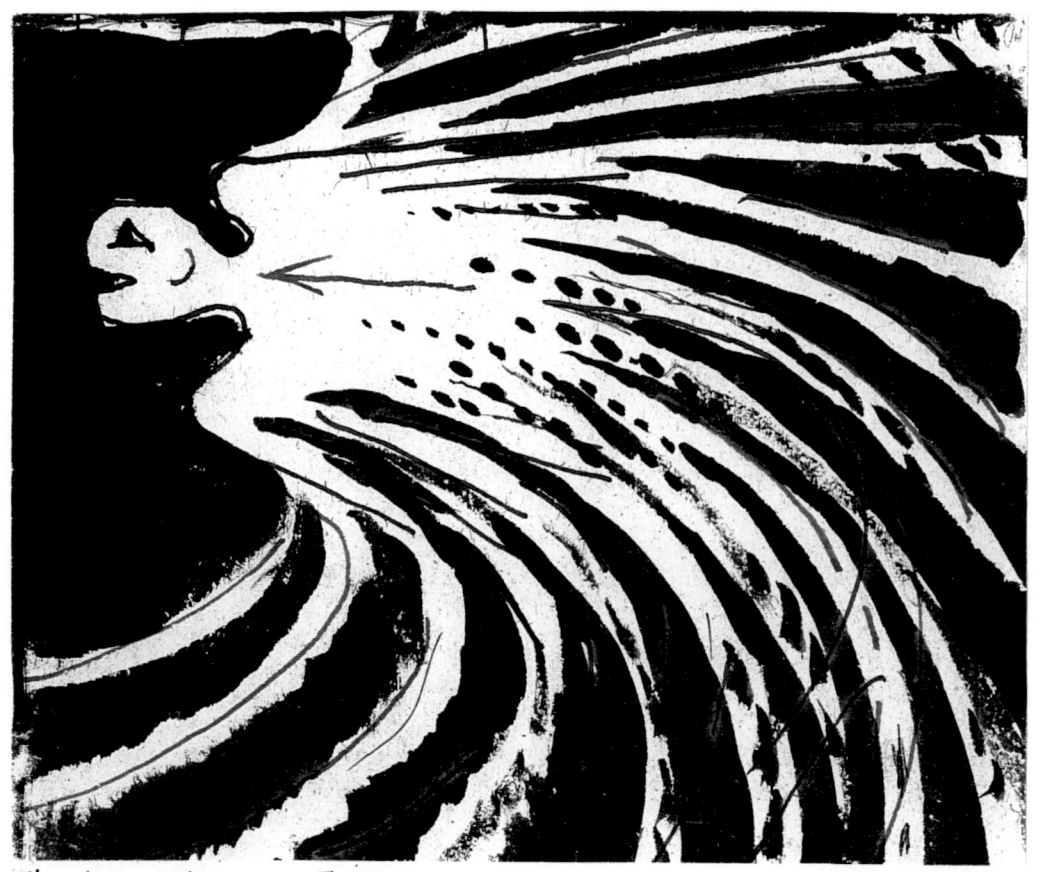

Fig. 407   Birdman Flying   Brush, Pen & Paint

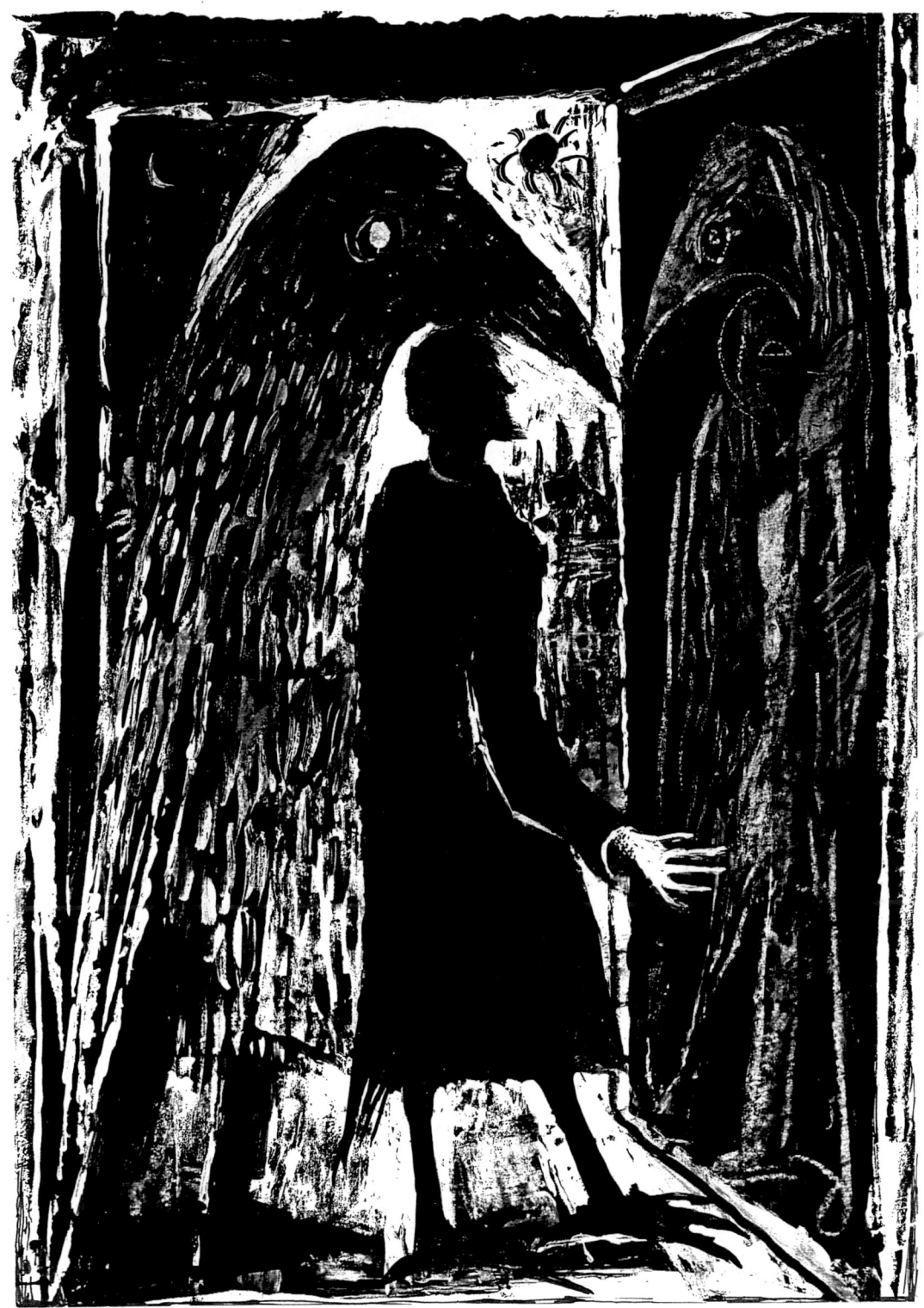

Fig. 408 A Mirrored Image   Brush & Paint

A large bird and a man face a mirrored reflection showing them as a combined Birdman. The transformation was inevitable, as both had already acquired parts from each other, the man claws, the bird trousers.

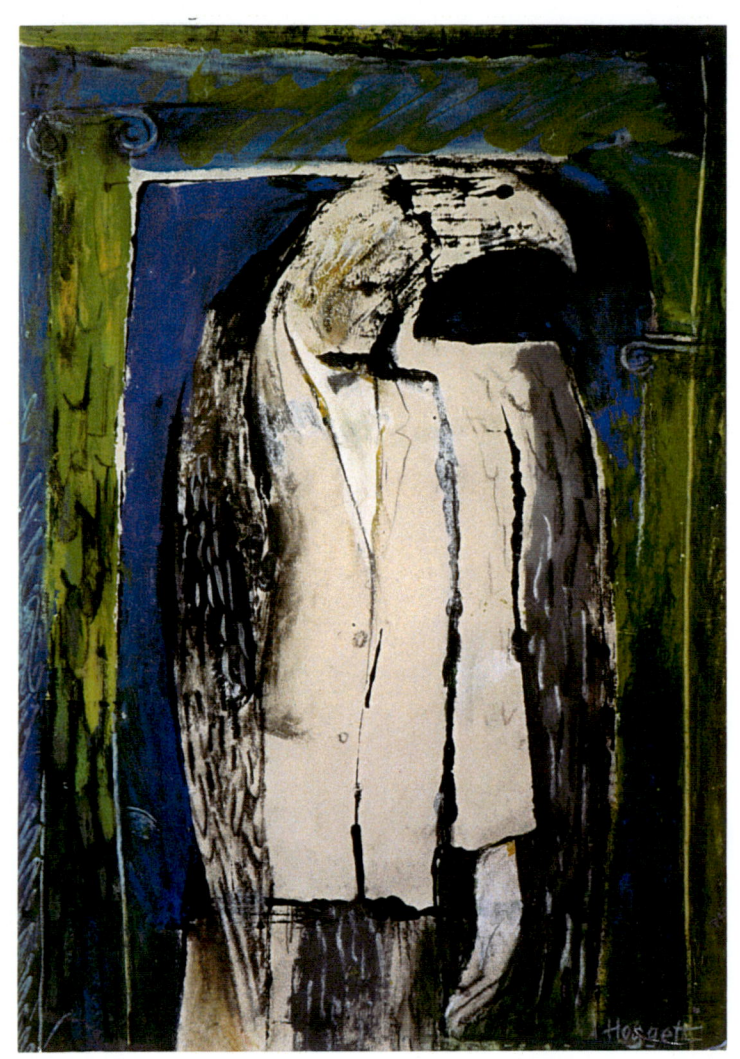

Fig. 409　Birdman　　　Finger Paints, Pencil

Birdman

A man in a white suit stands within a columned doorway. He pauses and meditates on change — of occupation, or lifestyle.
Gradually an eagle's beak extends from his head and a wing replaces his arm.
A new job opportunity perhaps?

* Footnote: Peace Sculpture (page 215). Designed in mid 1980s for Bradford University 'Peace Studies' library as a focal point.

PART FOUR

Finding One's Own Way - Tour of New Zealand

LAND OF THE LONG WHITE CLOUD	243
NORTH ISLAND	245
SOUTH ISLAND	252
STEWART ISLAND	262
Return to SOUTH ISLAND	267
Return to NORTH ISLAND	278
MAP	282
RETURN HOME	283

LAND OF THE LONG WHITE CLOUD

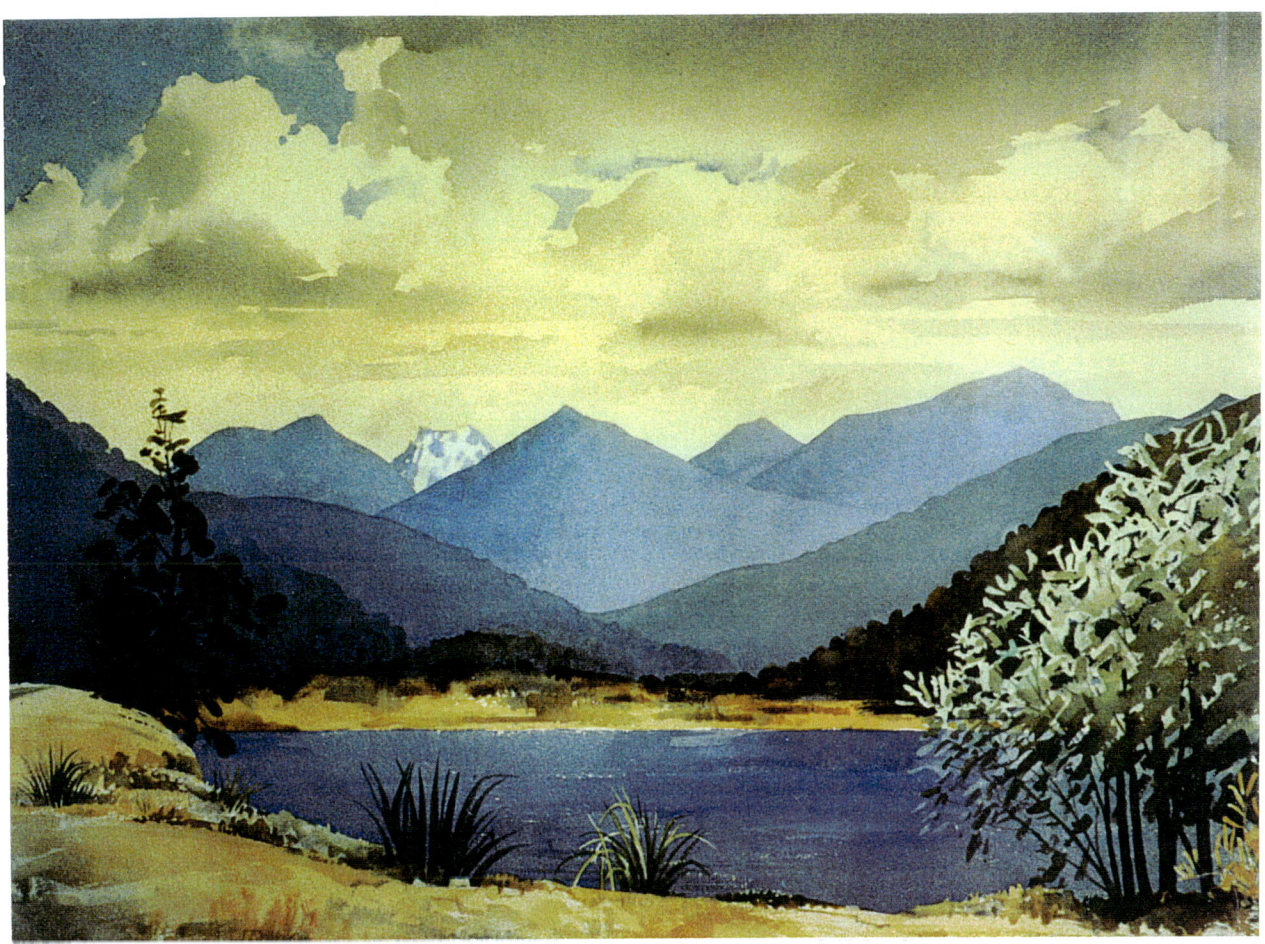

Fig. 410   The Southern Alps   Watercolour

'AO TEA ROA' – The Land of the Long White Cloud

The release of pent-up repression expressed in 'Thinking the Unthinkable' was the natural outcome of some five years of art therapy. It had felt not unlike a swollen river finally overflowing its banks, whilst further downstream it burst through the retaining dam of fear, to spew forth a mass of emotive fragments over the once calm and ordered valleys of my past. The effect was twofold – an aftermath of considerable energy followed by a period of lassitude.

During the therapy, working with my surrogate mum, I was sustained by her searching queries about the past; observations on dream material and, most crucially for me, her perceptive comments on the artwork. Yet eventually I began to recognise an impelling need for this dependency to be lessened. The very nature of my 'freestyle' work was forcing me towards a need for more independence from the curative processes of therapy.

In 'Stretching the Wings', the winged creatures, mainly birds, were offering clues which pointed in this direction. They were symbols which implied movement, both forwards and outwards – 'Take to the Wing' and 'Find your own way'.

I decided, therefore, to try to gain my independence by visiting New Zealand for five months, where my daughter and her family were living.

There would be the opportunity to paint during travelling and ample time to gather together most of the loose ends of my long curative process. Also, there would be the possibility, during long solitary trips, to slay the remaining monsters I'd conjured up, the remnants of my fears of women seen as predators, and other distortions

243

carried through from childhood into adolescence and finally into maturity. Also the fears of the inner darkness and 'aloneness' in isolation (easily put to the test in these circumstances). And finally, the quest for the inner child I'd so often ignored or neglected and never truly known. This journey to the antipodes could become a long-delayed initiation rite — an attempt to find my own way.

Before studying a map of New Zealand, I'd assumed that there were just the North and South Islands, overlooking a smallish dot at the bottom of the map. The dot, Stewart Island, was to play an important part in my curative tour, and the discovery of a legend about the country was a stimulus towards my search for origins, whether of lands, peoples or my own interior history.

Myths and legends often seem to fill the vacuum where simple explanations are not forthcoming. Being an inveterate mythmaker myself, I'd re-created all kinds of stories and fantasies surrounding my childhood, people I'd met, girls and women I'd loved, all of which compensated to a large degree for my lack (or fear) of true self-knowledge. I think I quickly made connections with my own mythology and this lively, imaginative Maori explanation on the creation of 'AO TEA ROA', the land of the long white cloud, NEW ZEALAND.

The map below, shows Maui's story and the places of the legend.

Considering the Maoris could have had no knowledge of the aerial viewpoint of the country, it's remarkable how closely the descriptions in the legend fit the shapes of the three islands. North Island is basically like a large flatfish with a tail, South Island bears some resemblance to a log canoe and Stewart Island is not unlike a stone anchor appropriate in scale to the canoe. Even the fish-hook and the canoe seat have accurate representations in the particular pieces of land.

I intended, during the tour, to take in all the islands, including Maui's seat (Kaikoura peninsula) and his fish-hook (Mahia peninsula).

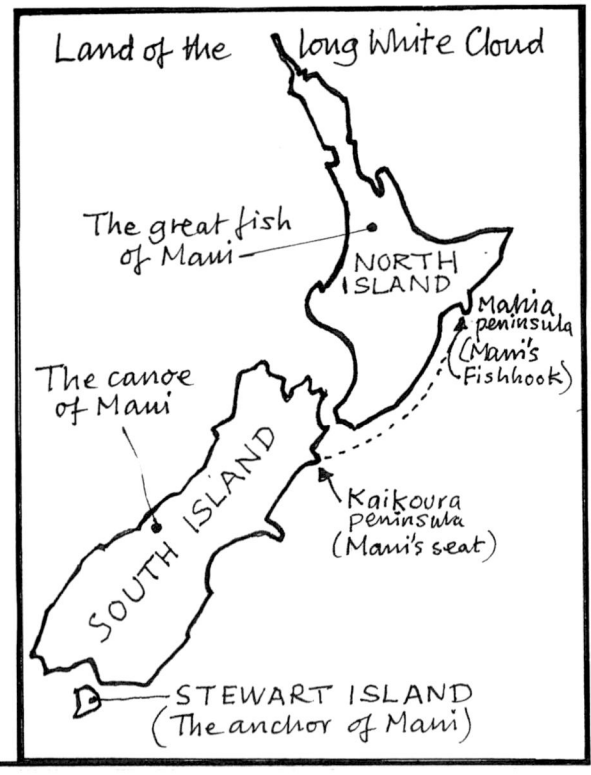

The Maori Legend on the Creation of New Zealand

Long after the creation of the world the demigod Maui, who lived in Hawaiki, went out fishing with his brothers.

They went further and further out to sea, where Maui took out his magic fish hook (the jaw of his sorcerer grandmother), tied it to a strong rope, and dropped it over the side of the canoe.

Soon he caught an immense fish, and struggling mightily, pulled it up. This fish was the NORTH ISLAND of New Zealand, called in ancient Maori 'Te ika a Maui' (the fish of Maui). The Mahia Peninsula, on the East coast of North Island was known as 'Te matua a Maui' (the fishhook of Maui), since it was the hook which caught the giant fish.

The SOUTH ISLAND was known as 'Te waka a Maui' (the canoe of Maui), the canoe he was sitting in when he caught the fish. The Kaikoura Peninsula on the Northeast coast of South Island was the seat where he sat. Another name for the South Island was 'Te wai Pounamu' (the Water Greenstone) since much greenstone (jade) was found in the rivers there.

STEWART ISLAND, south of South Island was known as 'Te punga a Maui' (the anchor of Maui) which held the canoe as Maui fished.

Fig. 4.11 Map and Maori Legend of New Zealand

A footnote on some journal extracts

Throughout the journey daily notes and sketches were entered into a journal. Much of the material touched on feelings and reactions to events and occasional inner turmoil underlying the practicalities of travelling. Some of the comments and observations seemed pertinent to the nature of this book and are entered here in smaller handwriting enclosed in outlined 'boxes'. These extracts seemed to me to act as a counterbalance to the retrospective record of the more mundane and practical facts of the long journey.

A dream before departure - diary 7 Nov.'95

'Leaving the company of others I swim out from the shore, only to find myself swept rapidly out to sea. I know I'm about to drown, yet seem philosophical about it, yet cursing my stupidity, saying, 'What a waste!' And then instantly I spot a vessel nearby. I hail it and am quickly hauled aboard.

DEPARTURE: 15th November 1995

Notes from a Journal. AUCKLAND 17 Nov.'95

After an exhausting twenty-four hr. flight, touch down, meet daughter and g'child. Later meet rest of family and settle for a quiet few days. Read local newspaper reports about Mt. Ruapehu eruption - "Pilots' reports of ash clouds prompt CCA to extend danger zone west of mountain". I carried memory of eruption weeks earlier in U.K. No doubt 'eruption' and 'inner turmoil' are closely related.

As the above journal note showed, I was quick to relate this geothermal event with my own 'outpourings' and, although the volcano had by now quietened down, I was keen to find a more active volcano elsewhere. Much later I was to paint my own interpretation of an eruption in a freestyle manner — (the first picture in Part Three, page 200).

Journal. Auckland 23 Nov. Recall waking from dream yelling 'Help, Help!' a number of times and am surprised the family aren't asking why I am shouting. In the dream a vicious older man tries to 'put me down'. I'm unable to confront him, but manage to struggle free. When I wake up I think about the dream imagery. Knowing I'm in N.Z. to allow 'my child' free rein, I suppose the internal dad disapproves, wants to maintain the past repressive life. As I view journey as a break from the past, I'm not too surprised internalised dad might wish to retain status quo.

After nearly two weeks to acclimatise myself and enjoy the family, it was time to organise a departure. Already I'd bought an old 'banger', a 1973 Hillman Hunter which, hopefully, would get me about for the next five months. I'd also registered with a bank using a cash point system, thus needing no traveller cheques, and the car boot was packed with necessities for a short tour of the central volcanic zone, before a return to Auckland for the Christmas festivities.

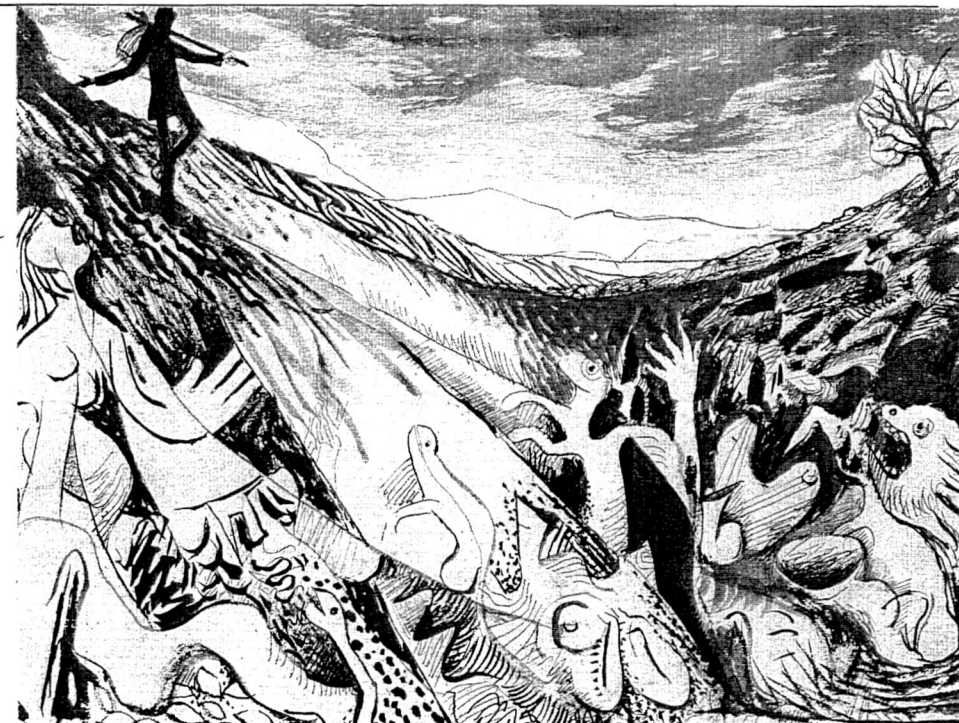

Journal 30 Nov. - On the road

Travelling south I glance at flattened lumps of extinct volcanoes - some higher ones glimpsed briefly between trees and hedgerows and intervening hills.

I wonder what interior might await a visitor on reaching the rim of the crater.

Later I draw my traveller venturing down into the abyss. The mood seems light and jaunty as he approaches a melange of beasties, etc., as if to make acquaintance with all his apprehensions.

Fig. 412
Entering the Abyss
Pen & Wash

NORTH ISLAND - Rotorua

I had arrived in the city of Rotorua, the geothermal centre, and settled into my first 'Backpacker' hostel (relatively cheap and self-catering). Here were the geysers, mud pools (spluttering, boiling, burping), hot thermal baths and, not too distant, an active volcano. But firstly, I joined a guided tour to visit an extinct example, Mt. Tarawera, in a 4WD truck. This was the volcano which, in 1886, had erupted and buried the village of Te Wairoa in two metres of mud killing 153 Maoris.

When we reached the edge of the crater we sort of slide-walked our way down a sixty degree slope to the base 250 metres below, observing crimsons and siennas (iron) and cool whites (rhyolite). Afterwards I visited the site of the buried village and

made a sketch. Here I read a notice, "Some villagers crawled out alive after four days."
Tohunga, the Maori High Chief was one of those who survived the four day ordeal but was to be banished later by his own people. He had prophesied the eruption some days before but was later considered to be in collusion with the devil in the mountain.
Prophets seem not always to be appreciated in their own country.

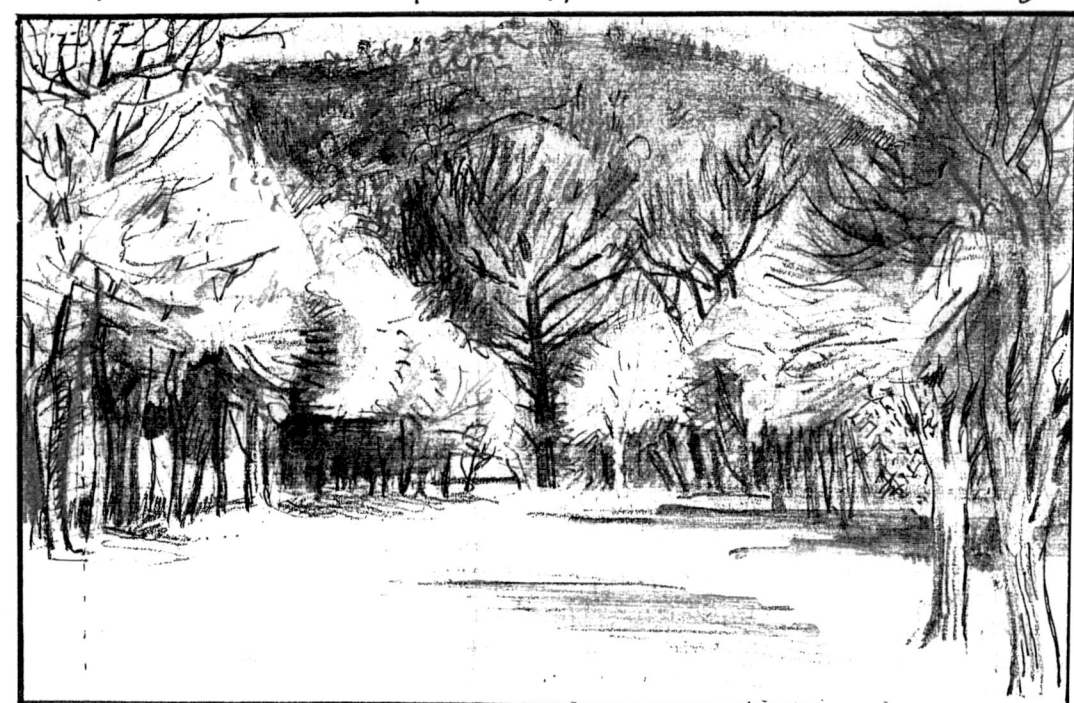

Left: Fig. 413

Site of the buried village of Te Wairoa, Nr Rotorua.

Black aquarelle pencil.

Roadside Breakdowns

What became both irritating and occasionally entertaining was the pattern of breakdowns with my ancient Hillman. So far, since leaving Auckland I'd experienced six. The annoyance lay in time lost and the sketches which never materialised as a result. The entertainment came from meeting locals, wayfarers or whoever, people I would never have seen otherwise, and places where I was sometimes towed for repairs, far off my itinerary. On a few occasions I felt slightly threatened — would I be attacked and/or robbed — but usually I had interesting talk about the district, the best (i.e. cheapest) place to stay, eat and drink. After many months of travel the car 'packed up' fifteen times and I was grateful to be a paid-up member of the AA! Perhaps it was also relevant, and a reminder, that things are constantly 'breaking down' if not attended to. This thought also reminded me that I was given the autobiography of the New Zealand author Janet Frame. I was reading this about this time, near the start of my travels and found that we shared a lot in common from our childhood days.

> Comment from Journal 28 Nov. Rotorua.
> 'Well into reading N.Z. author Janet Frame's autobio'. Her description of her childhood rang a number of bells. "I did my best to smooth the surface of life, to be, in a sense, invisible, to conceal all in myself that might attract disapproval or anger".
> Unfortunately, I felt I'd carried these repressive instincts well into adulthood.

Having seen many geysers, hot springs and boiling mud pools in and around Rotorua I thought it time to see an active volcano. This was White Island, some 50 kilometres off Whakatane on the east coast. I made a brief entry in the journal that day, made a photo-realistic painting and a photo or two.

> Journal. 6 Dec. White Island. Take a fast catamaran (an hour's bumpy ride) to this chokingly sulphurous island peak, rising out of the Pacific, its other half submerged under the ocean. The small party of six leap across a wide gap between boat and jutting rock with aid from Maori guides' hands. No place to secure a rope, and boat is taken out and anchored off shore. Many smoking fumaroles greet us, steam rising in irregular puffs and 'phuts', brilliant sulphurous yellows, acrid limes and lemons at their bases. As we advance over packed, baked mud and yellow or white streams we slowly approach the main crater. As we climb slightly to the edge we get a glimpse of boiling green sulphurous water....

Journal (continued)
....chokingly unpleasant between clouds of steam and fumes, some smelling of chlorine — the whole place seems highly toxic and a living prescence. This is a total 'breakout' environment and I feel very much in touch with nature's 'expressiveness'.
Later, I paint a larger than usual scene of an explosive volcano, an imaginary traveller and his feline companion watching an eruption, a baby evolving from within the cloud of ash above — and a single eye of the mountain watching the watchers.

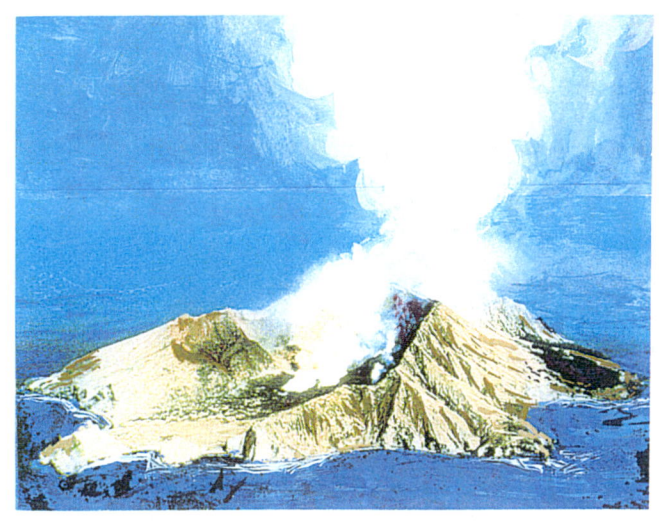

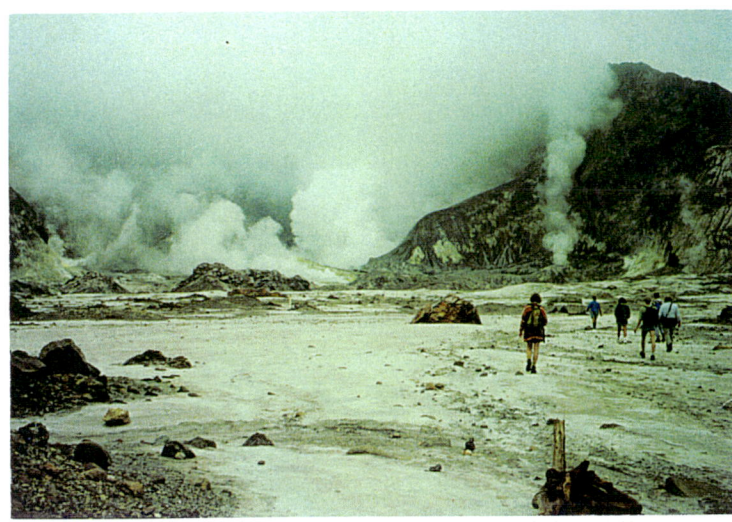

Above: Fig. 414   Gouache

'Photorealist' painting of White Island.

Left: Fig. 415   Photo

Our party with the guide leading us towards the crater.

Below: Fig. 416   Oil

Watching the Volcano (Freestyle painting)

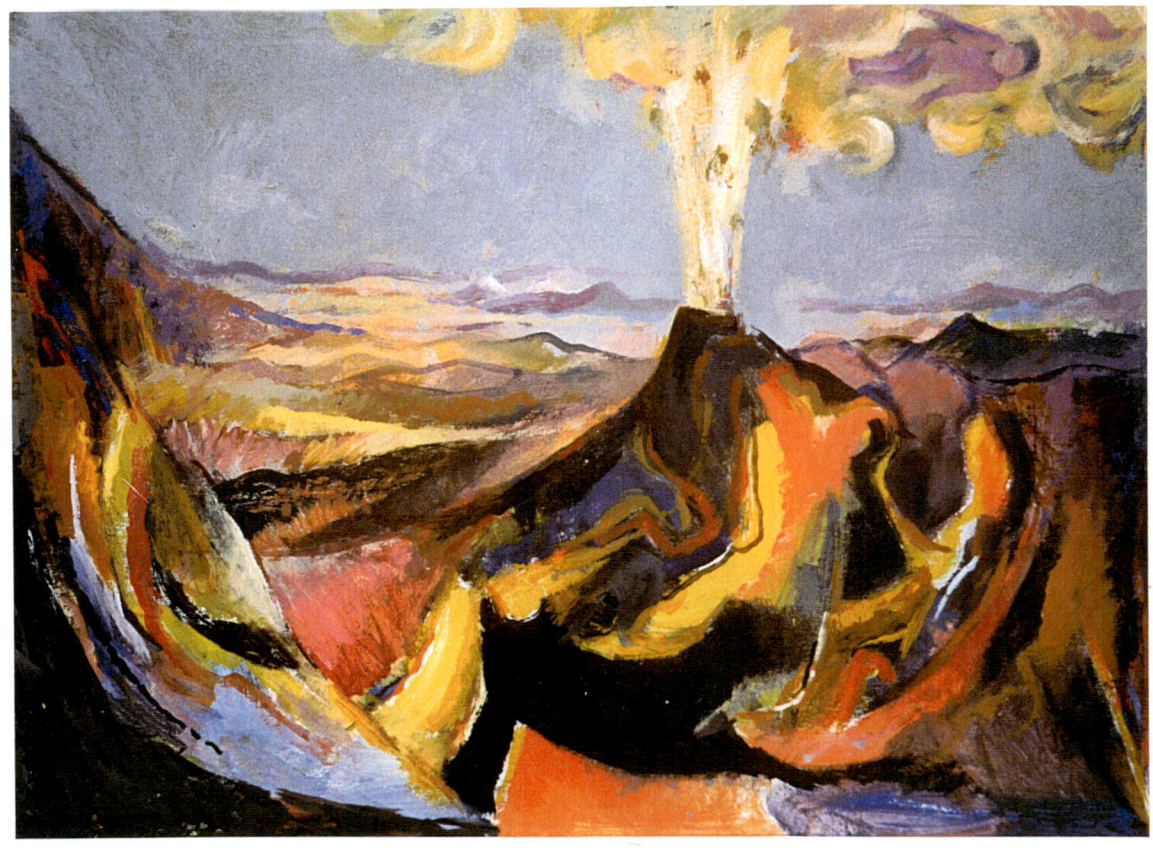

Napier

After about a week in Rotorua, it seemed time to visit the place where an earthquake occurred in the 1930s, Napier. So, after another car mishap while passing through enormous tracts of forest (could the U.K. have once looked like this?) and yet another two or more hours waiting, I finally found myself on a sunny seafront overlooking the Pacific and registering into a small 'Backpacker' almost at the water's edge. Put my feet up for a while and read a bit more from Janet Frame:

> Journal 7. Dec. Napier. J.F. biog:- "... never forget that a writer must stand on the rock of self, and self's judgement, or be swept away by the tide, or sink into the quaking Earth...."
> Here was someone expressing feelings about writing in relation to nature's 'quakes and storms. It seemed appropriate to this particular place I'd just arrived in.

Severely damaged in the 1931 earthquake, Napier had been quickly restored in the prevailing Art Deco style of European architecture. It looked like most of the buildings were ready for eating — a decorator's confection of pinks, lemon, tints of blue, greys, salmon — all light-hearted, jolly, especially in the intense brightness of the sun here (something I was only just getting accustomed to).

That evening I tried to imagine the darker side to all the colour, what the quake might have looked like (in a freestyle interpretation), a sort of stage drama:

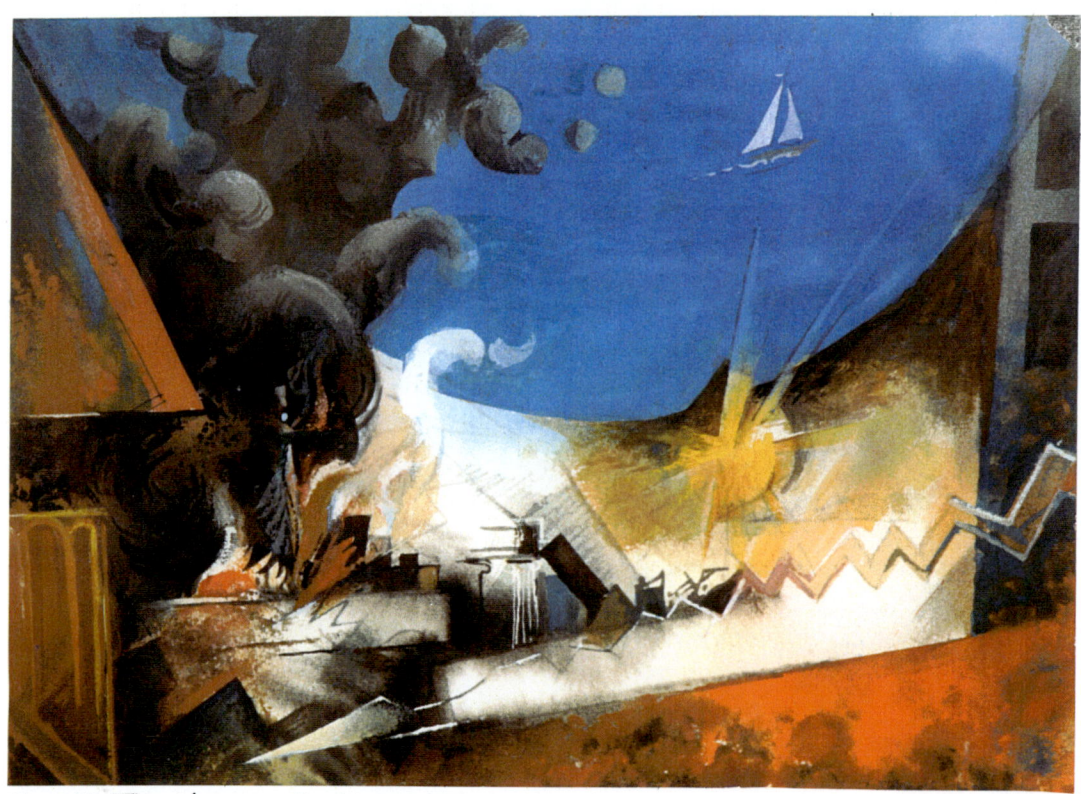

Fig. 417 The Napier Earthquake of 1931 — Gouache

The next day I met someone in the city who offered me a place aboard his racing yacht. For two hours we waited patiently at his club, hoping a race was about to start, but an approaching storm cancelled the event. I filled in the following hours sketching a boat in the harbour and was soon approached by another member, Charles, who wanted a watercolour of his boat. He rejected my price as too high but was prepared to offer in exchange four nights with full board in his luxury lodge overlooking the bay.

(This bartering later became the pattern during my travels, for I made a number of paintings and one drawing — my 'bread and butter' work — in exchange for accommodation and/or board, thus eking out my savings considerably).

During my stay at Charles' lodge I found myself overlooking Hawkes Bay with a view towards the Mahia peninsula across the far side (this was Maui's Fish Hook from the legend described on page 244). I sketched a storm which swept us all out to sea.

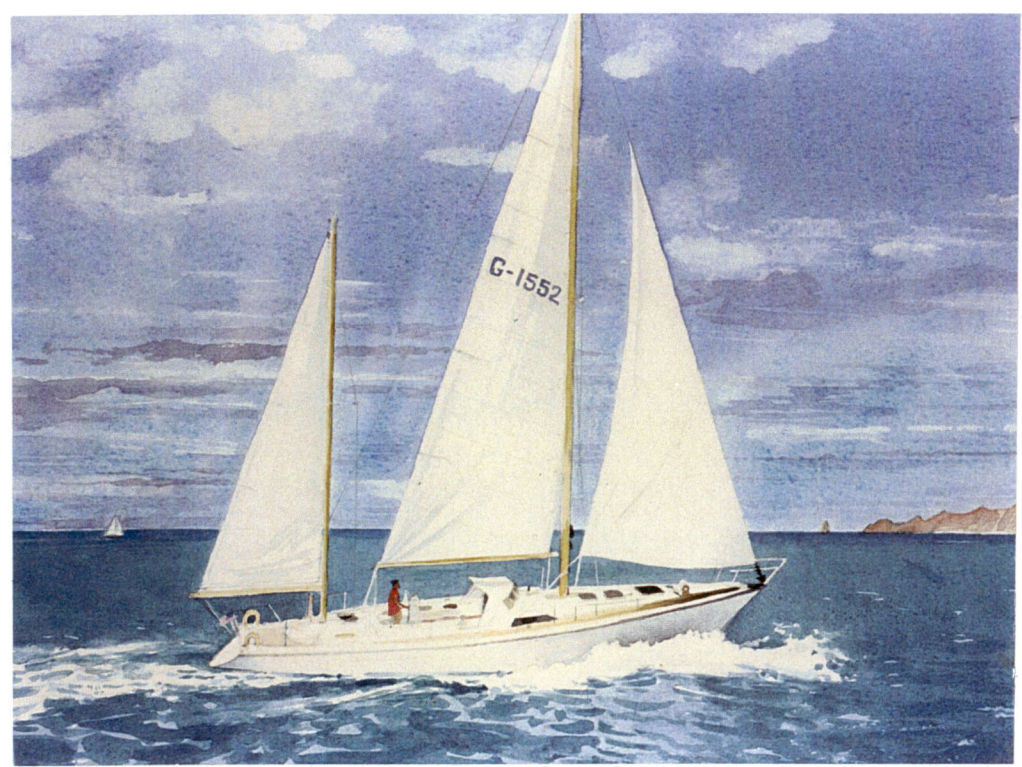

Fig. 418   Charles' boat 'Candida'   Watercolour

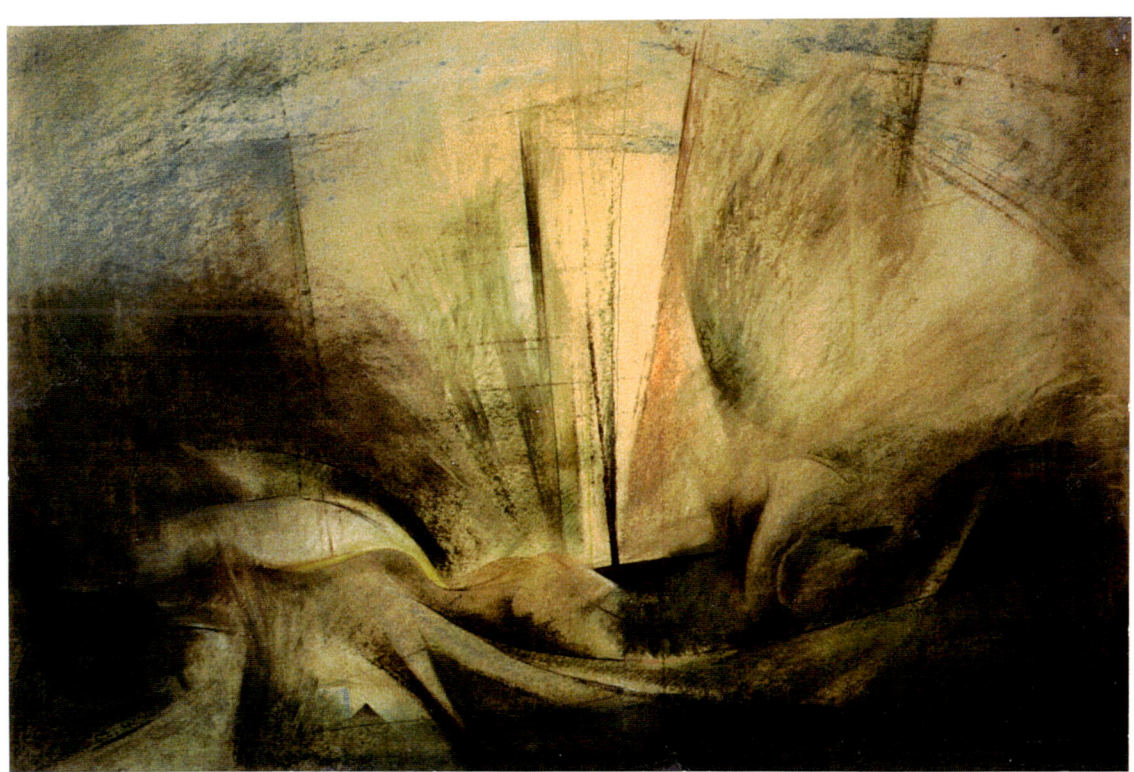

Fig. 419   Yacht in a Storm off Napier   Pastel

Journal - 18 Dec - Coromandels.

Although my AA membership allows free service from the local AA, I could do without all the breakdowns, costs and time wasted. In what sense wasted I need to ask myself as I become increasingly irate, and sometimes anxious about what all the fuss is about. I begin to feel this is something I didn't leave behind in the U.K., this tendency to rush, to get from A to B as if I had to get along as quickly as possible. Perhaps buying this old banger had a hidden purpose — to make me exercise more patience, to watch, look and listen more intently. Nevertheless, the nature of my anger due to these 'exterior' breakdowns could well be related to my own repressed rage from the past — and now fully expressing itself.

The Coromandels

I'm here to visit a cousin of a friend living in Coromandel township on the Northeast of the peninsula. I overshot her address along a side road, climbed a very steep and dusty mountain, reached up, over and windingly down to the other side of the peninsula before I'd realised my mistake. Finally I arrived back, having clocked up some extra fourteen kilometres and, looking more closely this time, discovered a lively middle-aged woman, Margery, standing by her gate amid various animals. After a generously large meal, I turned in exhausted and awoke to another hot day.

We then visited old Gold mine workings and equipment and later a stamping machine which nearly deafened me. Later I met Margery's son who took me out deep sea fishing, where I achieved a 'first' - catching four small snappers (all returned to the deep) and a couple of mackerel I offered later to her cats.

After three days I realise I'm not able to paint, and, with hindsight I found I was unable to draw or paint until the New Year. This extract from the journal indicated the change of mood:

Journal - 20 Dec - Coromandel Township

Depart early morn. after farewells to Margery and son Graham. Follow coast road to Thames and head over to other side of Coromandel bay to Miranda. Seascape so full of tonal contrasts: feel compelled to do watercolour of intense white shell-strewn beach. Vast numbers of waders on mudflats further out whilst gulls and cormorants mingle. All a range of neutral tones from the whites, then blue & ochre greys down to deep Indigo, gathering storm clouds.

Buffeting winds become so severe I lose a brush and sponge to distant sand and am forced to pack up. Not everything goes to plan - but looking forward to the Christmas festivities with family.

Auckland

22nd-31st Dec. A busy ten days preparing for a long tour of South Island I remember, and also a jolly time during the festive activities. I booked a ferry crossing for the New Year and got the car fully serviced yet again, then tested out the camping equipment and tent - and tried sleeping out in the garden. I'm a softie as a camper - most uncomfortable night ever! Prepared and sorted out the art materials. A disaster when my new automatic camera broke down and wouldn't be available until at least a month after Christmas. Got a premonition that the crossover from North to South Island would prove psychologically as well as physically testing.

Taupo

Journal - New Year's Day. Taupo 'Backpacker' Hostel

Farewells from the family before the three month tour of South and Stewart Islands. This afternoon stood by the great Lake until early evening. A local described the spectacular sunsets during and after the Ruapehu eruption on the far side of the lake - the result of ash particles. Tonight I experience a dream, stronger in imagery than any other I can recall:-

"In the city the dreamer enters a large building, possibly a church, whose watery environment seems to waver, expand and then shrink. With others I float upwards through an opening high in the wall into a dark cavernous tunnel steeply rising into a flight of stone steps. Strewn across the steps, litter of all kinds impedes our progress as we try to race up the stairway. We have to clear a way through rubble in order to find a way through a wall, and then rush breathlessly ahead. The pace quickens and I gain a clear lead towards my escape. Unfortunately this turns out to be a gallows with an attendant hangman who wastes no time in placing a rope over my head and pulling it tight. Now I hang in space (there is a huge chasm beneath me), gasping for breath and in great agony, knowing I've only a short time to live, wishing it would all be over quickly.

My companions, who I'd beaten in the staircase race, now grant my wish, grasping my ankles firmly and swinging me down into darkness and oblivion."

How appropriately the subconscious self uses my very last day in the 'North' (my rational side), reducing its controlling influence, and offers me insight towards the 'South' (my intuitive body/heart), confirming the direction I had wished to follow. In hindsight I now think I was influenced by Auden's long poem 'The Age of Anxiety' which, at the time of reading, seemed very much about this obsession of mine.

Later I attempted two pen and ink drawings illustrating the dream (fig. 420).

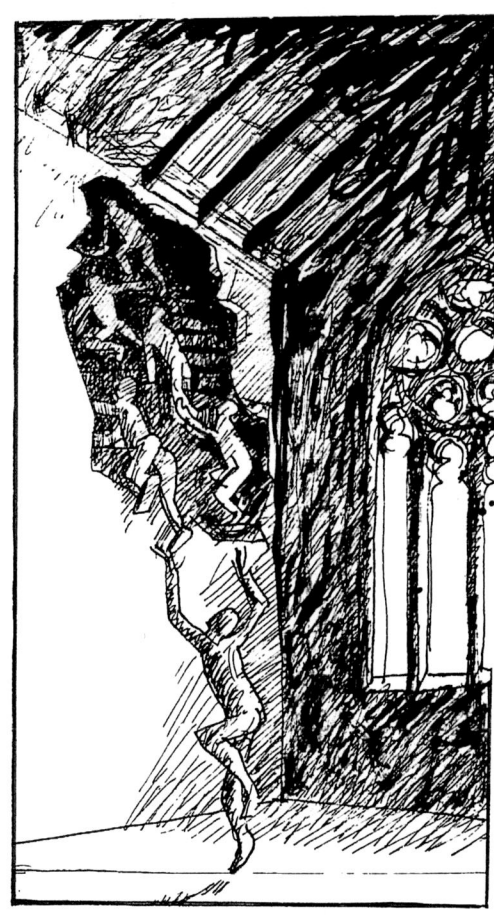
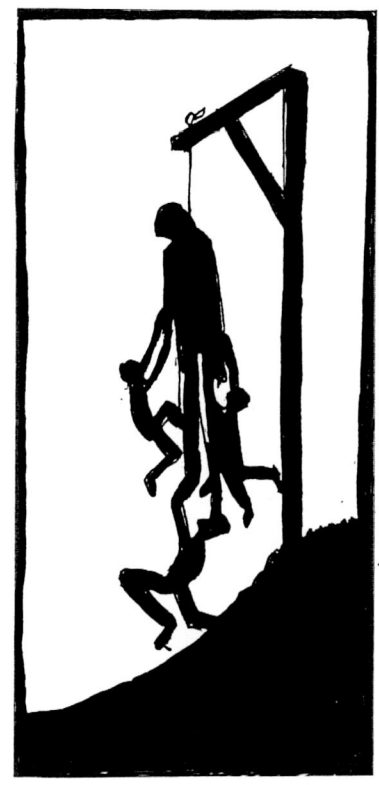

Fig. 420 : 'New Year's Day' dream.
Illustrating the text from the
Journal entry on page 250.
Pen & Ink

Wellington. 2nd. January 1996

I'd departed from Taupo early, crossing the desert road, seeing a landscape of ancient lavas, pumice — perhaps a smattering of ash from Ruapeha just a few kilometres away. Everything was lifeless except a small stream near the road.
Everything else seemed to conspire to heighten the dream of 'death' I still carried in the mind — yet it was now a totally upbeat mood of something prophetic I'd experienced. Travelling on through miles of solitude, with an army base somewhere in the middle I'd eventually reached Wellington in the afternoon and sought out the Backpacker booked in advance, close to the ferry terminus.
In the afternoon walked around part of the harbour where a Russian three-masted training ship was inviting everyone aboard. The crew of the 'Nadezhda' from Vladivostok even allowed a few youngsters a little way up the rigging. Something which, in my present mood of that day, I felt at least mentally agile enough to attempt. Instead I walk into the Art gallery to a Robert Mapplethorpe Retrospective — and all his fetishes/obsessions — and brilliant photography.
Much more to see, including a wide variety of sculptures and many fine historic buildings. Obviously I wasn't going to be able to do justice to this city.... perhaps on the return journey....

Journal. Wellington Backpacker - Ferry Terminus 3 Jan.

Enjoyed a good breakfast — one was catered for in this large hostel — formerly a grand hotel of the Art Deco period — and had packed everything back into the car boot.
Everything seemed fine before switching on the ignition and ready to leave for the terminus. I'd just half an hour to spare and, as I pulled out from the kerb, sensed something was wrong and realised I'd a flat tyre in the middle of busy traffic, unable to find anywhere to pull over. I drove straight to the ferry, got out and emptied the boot, exchanged the flat for the spare, just made it to the boat.
Slowly the sense of rush and anxiety lessened as the ferry pulled away from the city. The sea was shimmering with sun and many gulls circling about added to the gradually lifting mood. The crossing of Cook Strait in warm sunshine to Picton in South Island was a real tonic, just what I needed before the drive to Nelson.

SOUTH ISLAND - Nelson

Journal Jan 3rd NELSON Sth. Island

I had fears that the drive from Picton to Nelson might include yet another blow-out, so I was happy to give a lift to two young Bostonian Backpackers whose condition of entry was to help me to push the Hillman to the nearest garage, or Nelson, should this trauma arise. I was becoming road-wise. Two hours later I dropped my companions in Nelson and went in search of the Hotel I'd booked for a few days.

Custom House Hotel was by the quayside and an ideal spot to look at the shipping. Having settled in, I was soon to meet Willy, a young Maori who was literally painting the boats but was also about to start painting on canvas, joining the local Art College later in the year.

After lack of sketching for past three weeks it was a relief to find myself keen to work again, and taking Willy off to Cable Bay, near Nelson on his day off, loaning him some of my equipment. On route to the bay I found an ideal camp site by a river - should I feel the inclination. Whilst Willy painted the shore I found myself doing a small picture of cabbage trees surrounding a Bach ('an 'historic' 1900s, or earlier) bungalow of wood with corrugated tin roofing)

Jan 4th What the hell is happening? Yesterday was tyre trouble and later, the loss of a half-filled sketch book. Today I lose my favourite Oz hat with a wide brim, then a lot of dollars in a dud phone box and now, a few hours ago I break a tooth which will need dental attention. This isn't all - to add to my increasing irritation, I find that the driver's door lock has been tampered with and I can no longer lock it. More hours are lost getting a repair. I begin to wonder how many coincidences might add up to a conspiracy!

Jan 5th Today I get dental advice (can leave tooth until my return) and go out painting, when my folding canvas chair seat tears and collapses under me. I ask myself if someone, somewhere is giving me a message, as my entry into this 'new' life in the South seems to be becoming a disaster. Deciding to calm down I make innumerable visits to appropriate professionals until every problem has been solved, including a new radiator for the car (apparently the cause of most of the car traumas). One thing I now know for certain - I do need to relax! That gut feeling of impending trials, following the ferry crossing now seems justified.

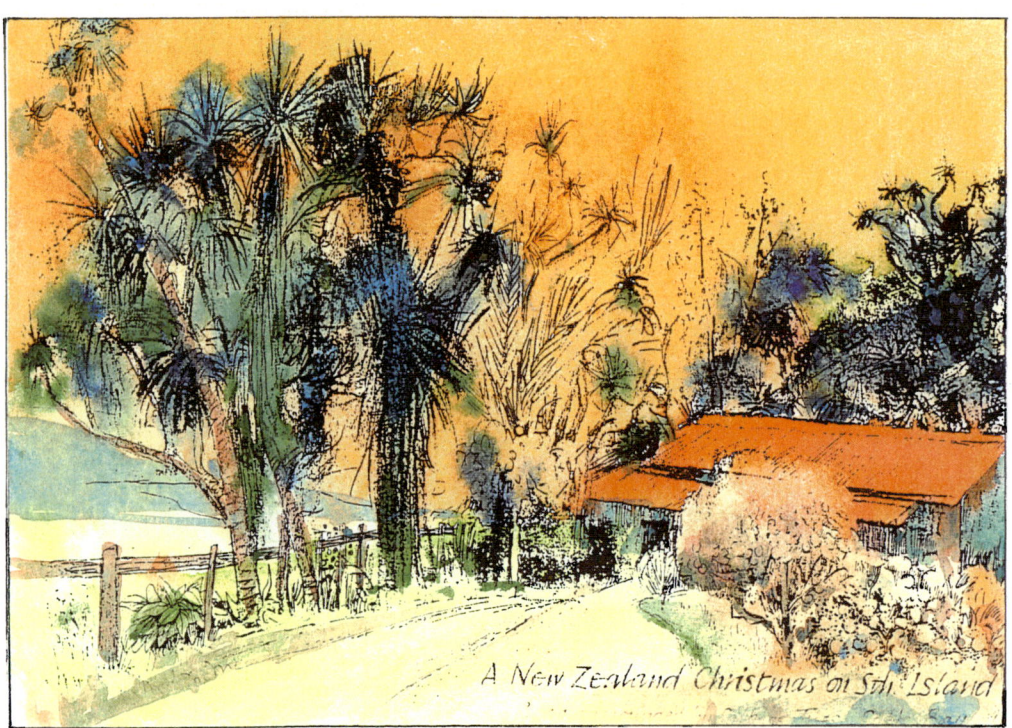

Fig. 421

A Bach, surrounded by Cabbage Trees, Cable Bay, Nr. Nelson.

[Bach - An early type of wooden bungalow with corrugated tin roof]

Pen & Water-colour.

Despite the 'setbacks', I had enjoyed Nelson, the high standard of Ceramics in the city, the 'Arthouse' cinema offerings and the city itself. Then, after five days, I decided to pitch the tent on the site near Cable Bay, having met the farmer of the flat (valley) who allowed me to stay as long as I wished.

Journal 7th Jan. Wakapuaka River Camp Site.

Early evening, after a visit to Maori Burial site — after reading account of local Maori heroine in Nelson Library. I'd painted a view of the estuary close to my camp from a cliff above when the tide was out. I was interested not only in the shapes formed by mud and water but also by a spit of land separating the sea from the estuary. A passing stranger told me briefly the story of one Huria Matenga and her burial site at the end of the spit. For a change, here was a true story, rather than a legend or myth.

In 1863, Huria Matenga, a Maori Princess, together with her husband and a friend, swam out to a stricken wreck, the brigantine 'Delaware', close to her Pa (or camp). All three were powerful swimmers and frequently re-entered the sea during the storm to bring all ten crewmen to shore, bar the first mate, who was later found drowned. (Later was known as the Grace Darling of N.Z.)

Intrigued with the story which related to the scene I'd just painted, I set off next morning to find the site (having first sought permission, as the sites are strictly for Maori use), and walked over a mile along the long spit only to find that the cemetery was so well hidden that it took a long time to discover. Eventually the enclosure revealed itself in low-lying shrubs. It contained varied headstones and two substantial Victorian marble memorials - of Huria and her husband. My somewhat romantic attitude found these incongruous, as most of the other graves had simple wooden or stone headstones, 'ethnic' in character. Then I recalled Huria was a Victorian heroine and it made sense.

The next day I returned to the bluff and completed the painting of the estuary (below). The burial ground is in the centre of the picture. To the right is a much larger Maori site.

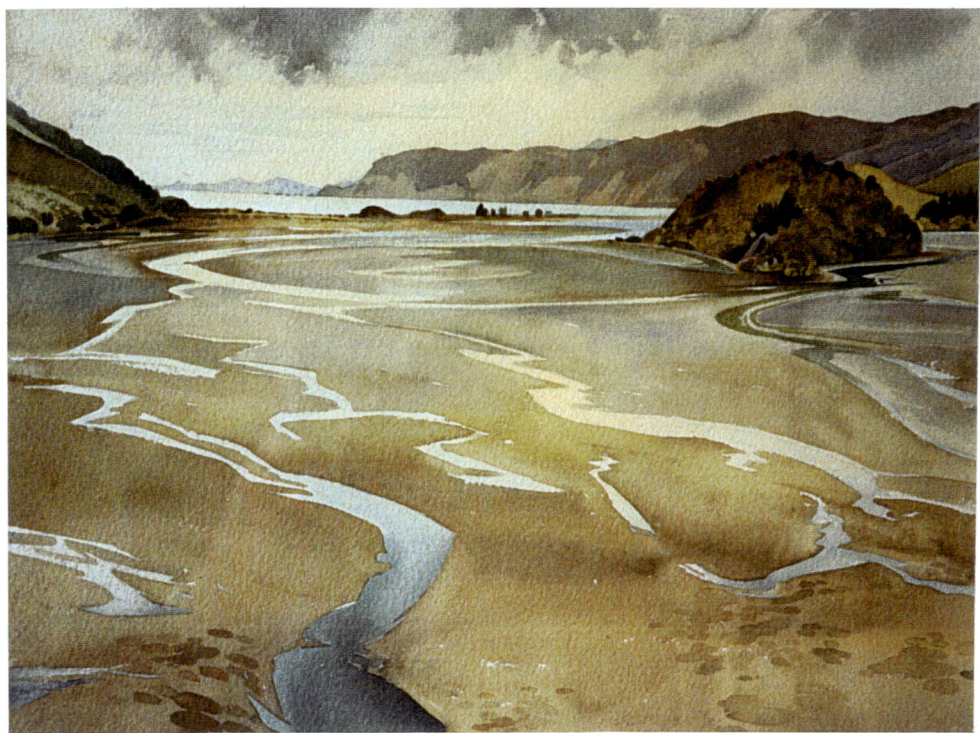

Fig. 422 Estuary, towards Delaware Bay   Watercolour

By the fifth day on the site I was accustomed to a routine — thousands of cicadas shrilled me awake very early each morning and continued throughout the day. Climbing out of the earth around the roots of the native kahikateas, they discarded their red carapaces near the base, warmed themselves then started rubbing their legs together...... I tried to sketch them quickly, and the great elephantine roots of the trees.

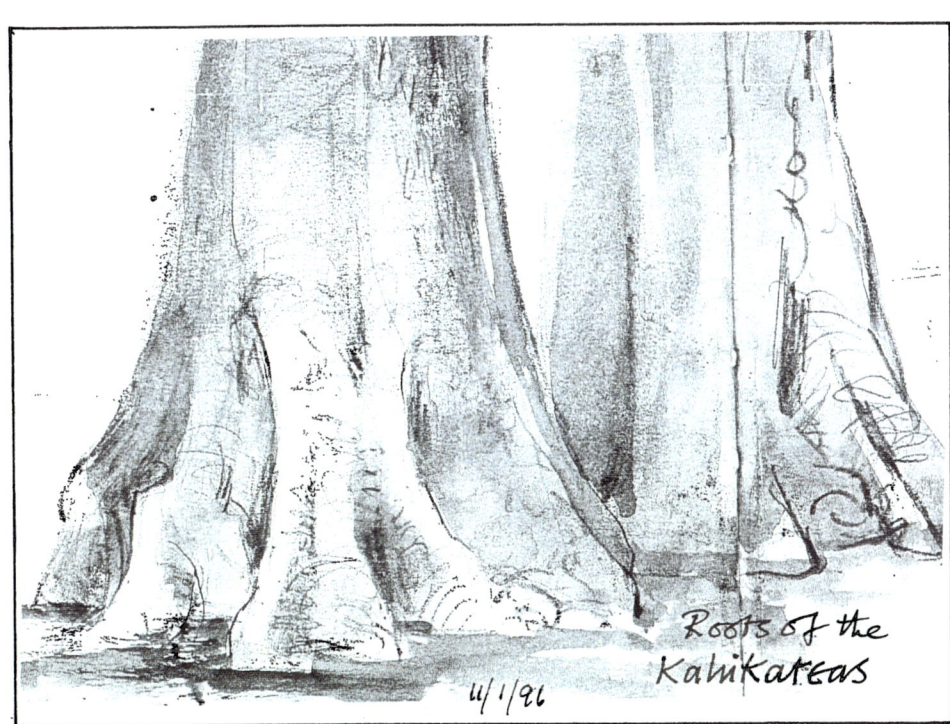

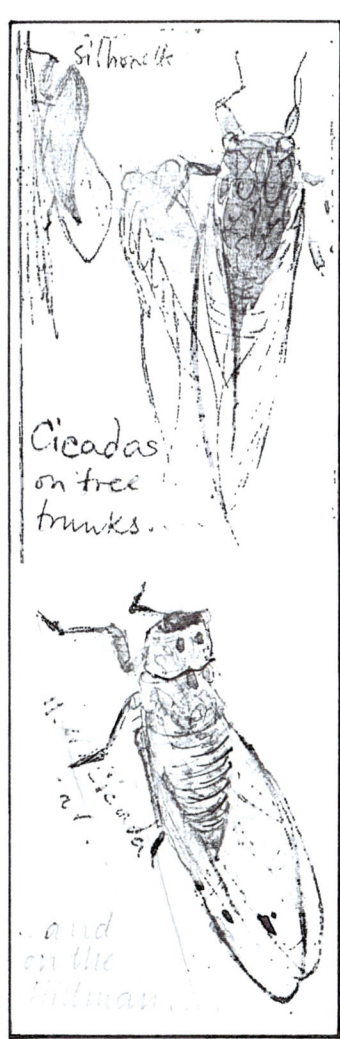

Fig. 423 Roots of Kahikatea Trees   Pencil & Wash   Fig 424 Cicadas   Pencil

253

Journal - Campsite Jan 11th.

Days of camping alone - a few distant figures swimming in the river, an occasional passing truck rattling along on a distant unsealed road.
The Sony walkman packs up - a low battery and no news. Begin to find effort of continuing tour alone daunting (obviously I've little tenacity!) Very wet all day and I'm writing this under canvas, horizontally, in this shallow single tent. Solitude most painful when not able to communicate about visual splendour around me. Reflecting on huge exterior world just beyond this thin membrane - feel I'm indulging in a momentary luxury of feeling sorry for myself. Off soon to see a foreign film at Nelson Arthouse cinema - and get some more provisions. That should cure the malaise. Meanwhile the cicadas shrill on....
Do one further drawing along riverbank through tent opening - a lively line of willows, going into battle like a charge of horses....

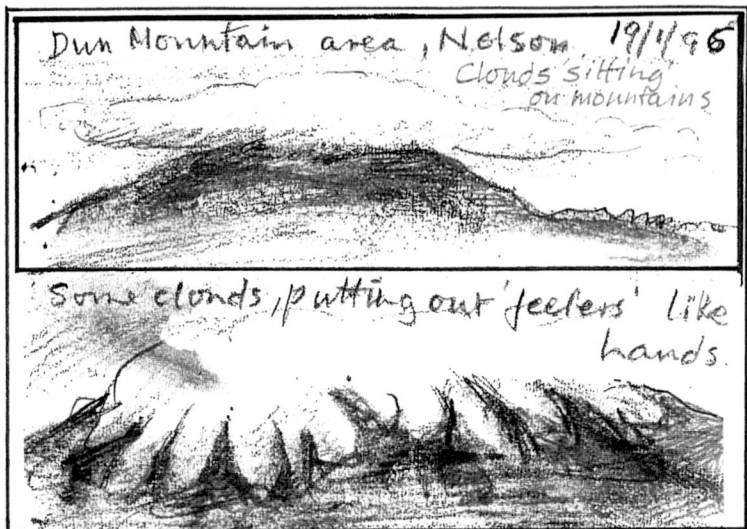

Fig. 425 Dun Mountain Clouds, Nelson Pencil

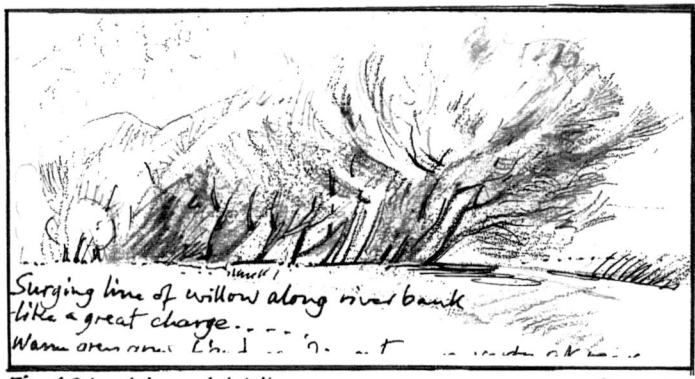

Fig. 426 Line of Willows Pencil

Journal Sat 18th. - Custom House Hotel

Sudden departure from camp. Late evening I'd been running a fever so settled down before it was dark. Suddenly I'm aroused by sounds of a truck and shouting. "Get up, get out, you'll be flooded out within an hour". The farmer was giving me just time to clear everything away before the river overflowed its banks - he was here to clear his flocks onto the higher ground.
It seems the river had already swollen six feet within last two days of heavy rain, with water pouring off the surrounding mountains. So nature confronts me, insists on immediate action - or possible drowning!
Now in the comfort of a warm bed - and a ton of very damp and dirty washing.

Nelson 18 - 24th.

During the camping I also enjoyed drawing the native trees (below) and the way clouds often clung to mountain tops (above). I got tablets from a pharmacy for 'Travellers Gastroenteritis' (probably didn't boil river water long enough), and took it easy for a few days before moving on down the East coast to Kaikoura.

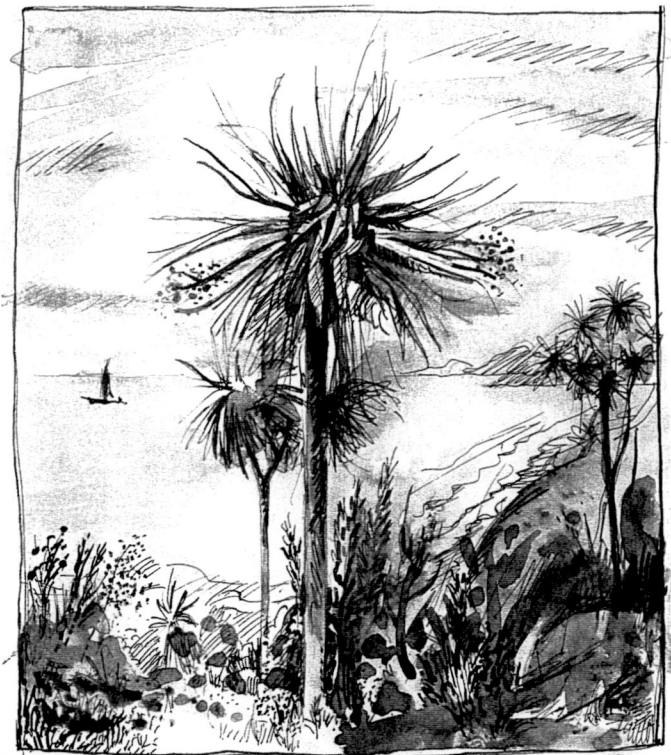

Fig. 427 Cabbage Trees, Cable Bay Pen & Wash

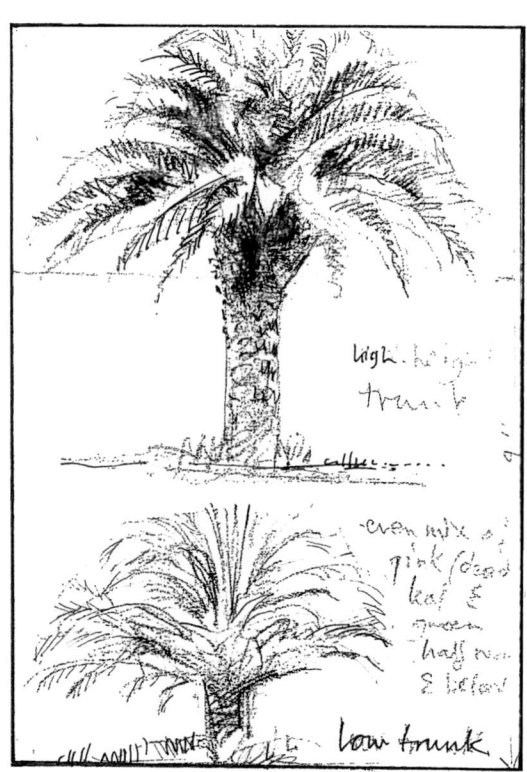

Fig. 428 Palms, Nelson Pencil

Kaikoura

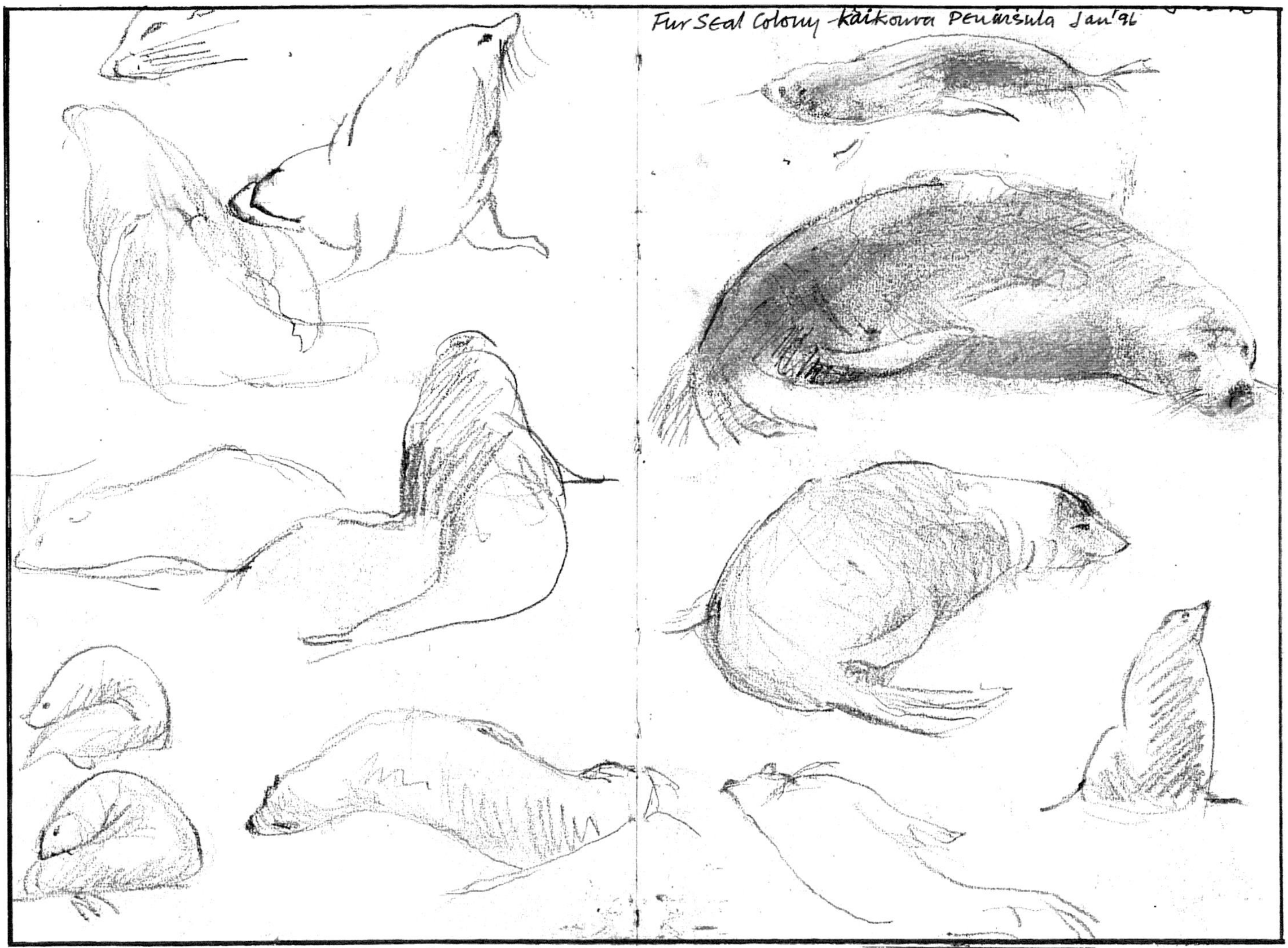

Fur Seal Colony Kaikoura Peninsula Jan '96

Fig. 429   Fur Seal Colony, Kaikoura   Aquarelle Pencil

Journal 24 Jan. Backpacker Hotel Kaikoura

The whole district, the town and peninsula, so visually attractive I register into the very shabby accommodation for a week. Walk up to the beginning of the peninsula (Maui's canoe seat - legend page 244) and have to sketch a colony of fur seals immediately - in case they go away (they rarely do).

Then climb onto the cliffs above. The views are superb and this becomes a productive time with pen and ink sketches, colour notes, paintings and a few 'freestyle' pictures.

In the meanwhile I need to renew a half-year car licence and buy a 'fun' camera (my automatic has yet to arrive).

Have first meal out with any quality - decide to try rock lobster (crayfish) Great!

The sea and coast is alive with creatures - Whales (see three), Dolphins, many fur seals and great swathes of white across the sea - thousands of sea birds picking krill above the great sea trench where the whales dive for giant squid - or whatever..

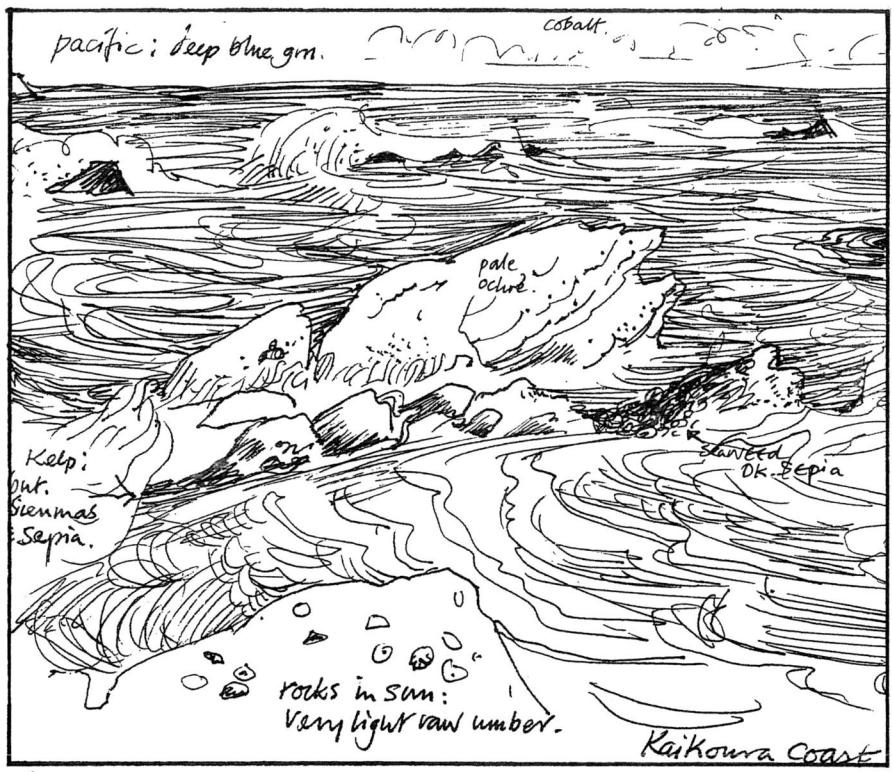

Fig. 430 Sea, Rocks, Waves, Shells & Colour Notes.   Pen & Ink

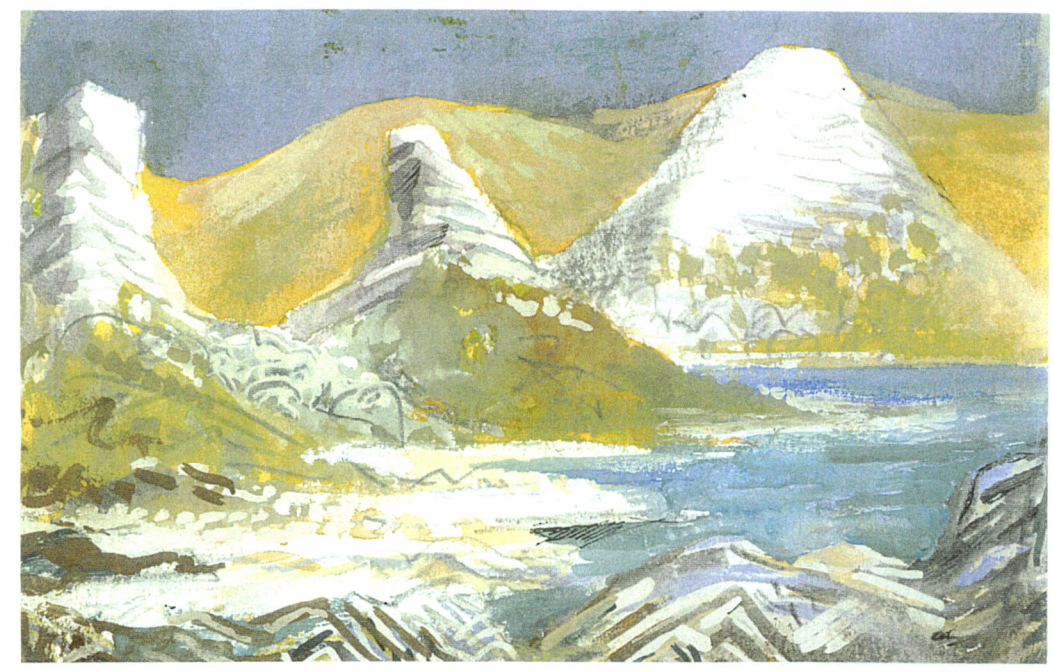

Left: Fig 431
One of a series on 'Rhino Horns', trying out various media – this in gouache.

There were cliff formations in fantastic contortions on one section of the peninsula. This group of eroded forms was known as 'Rhino Horns'. They seemed to echo the shapes of seals which reared up as they turned their heads.

Right: Fig. 432. A picture incorporating rocks and seals.

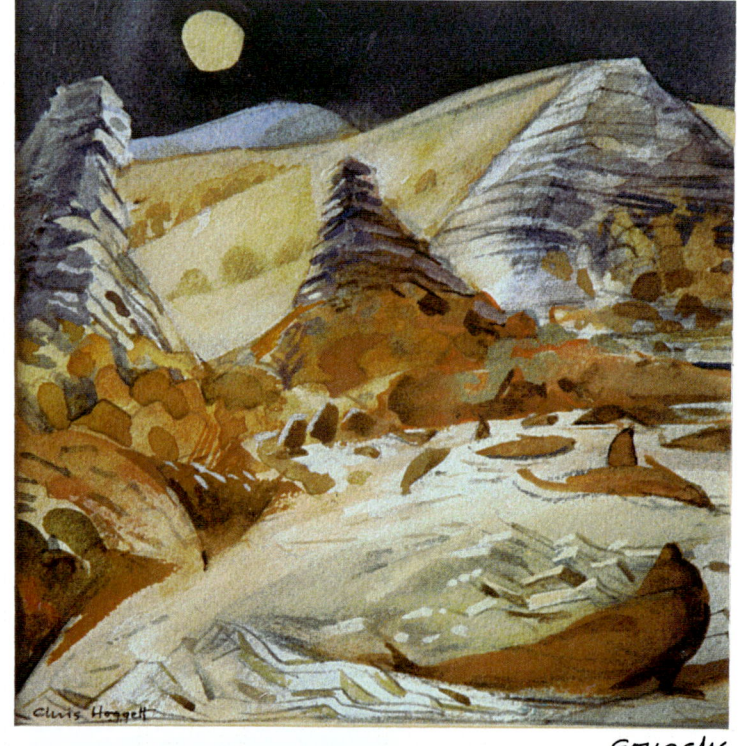

Gouache

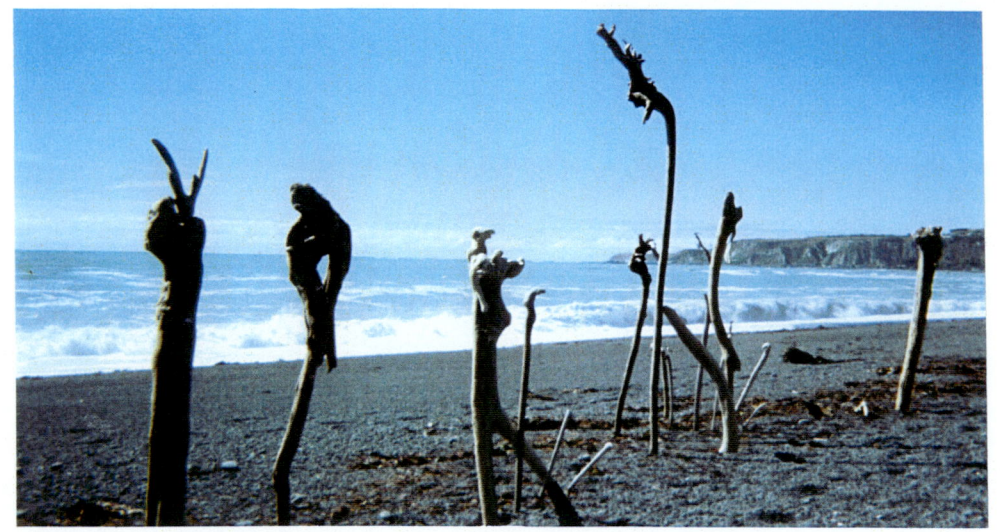

Left: Fig. 433
The sea throws up driftwood and someone sees possibilities in arranging a kind of sculpture show.
(The first snap using the 'throwaway' camera)

Views from the cliffs stimulate one to paint, small scalloped bays, the 'Rhino Horns', remains of an eroded cliff, the distant mountains pointing the way towards my next destination down the East Coast - Christchurch.

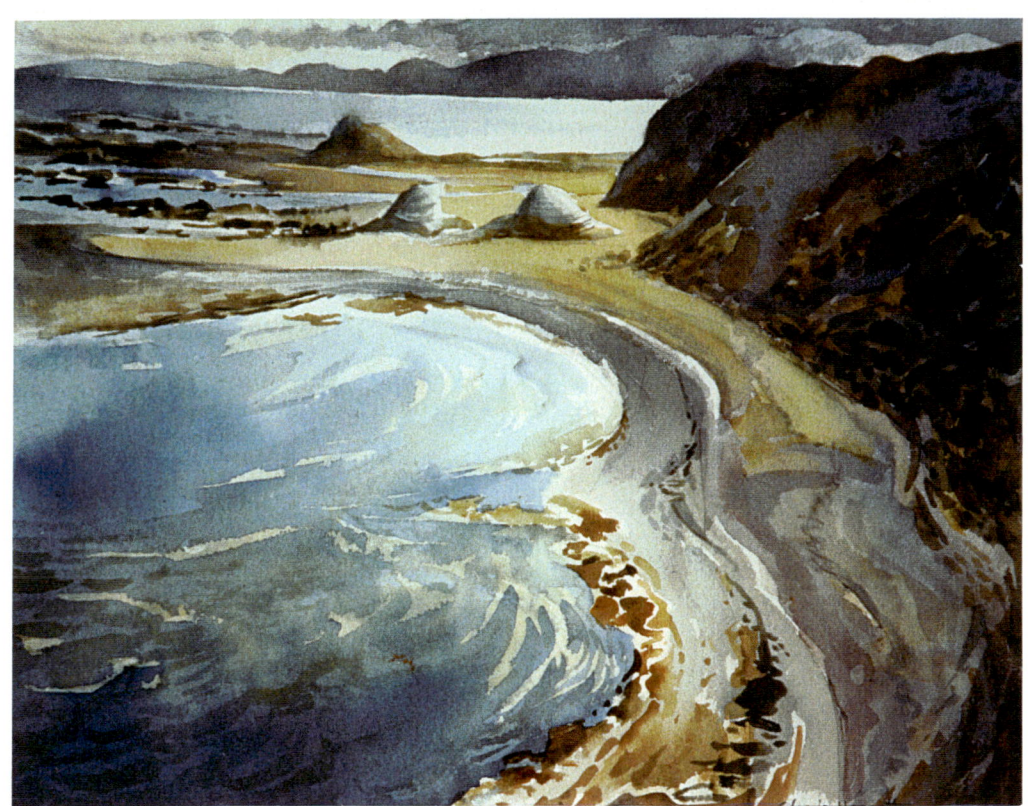

Fig. 434 Kaikoura Peninsula   Watercolour

Recall that this is Maui's Canoe seat, where he cast the hook which landed the big fish (see Maori legend, page 244).

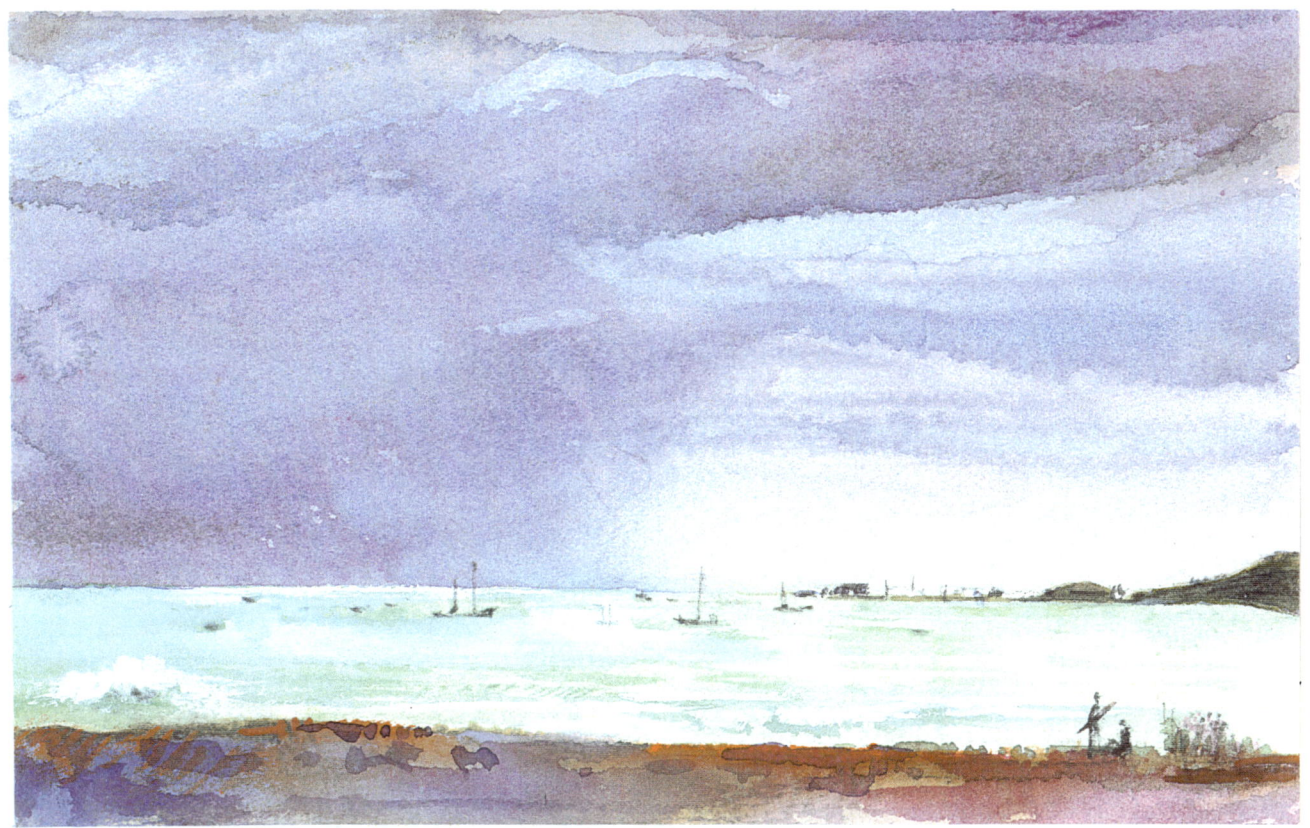

Fig 435 Kaikoura Harbour - Purple sky and Opal sea   Watercolour

257

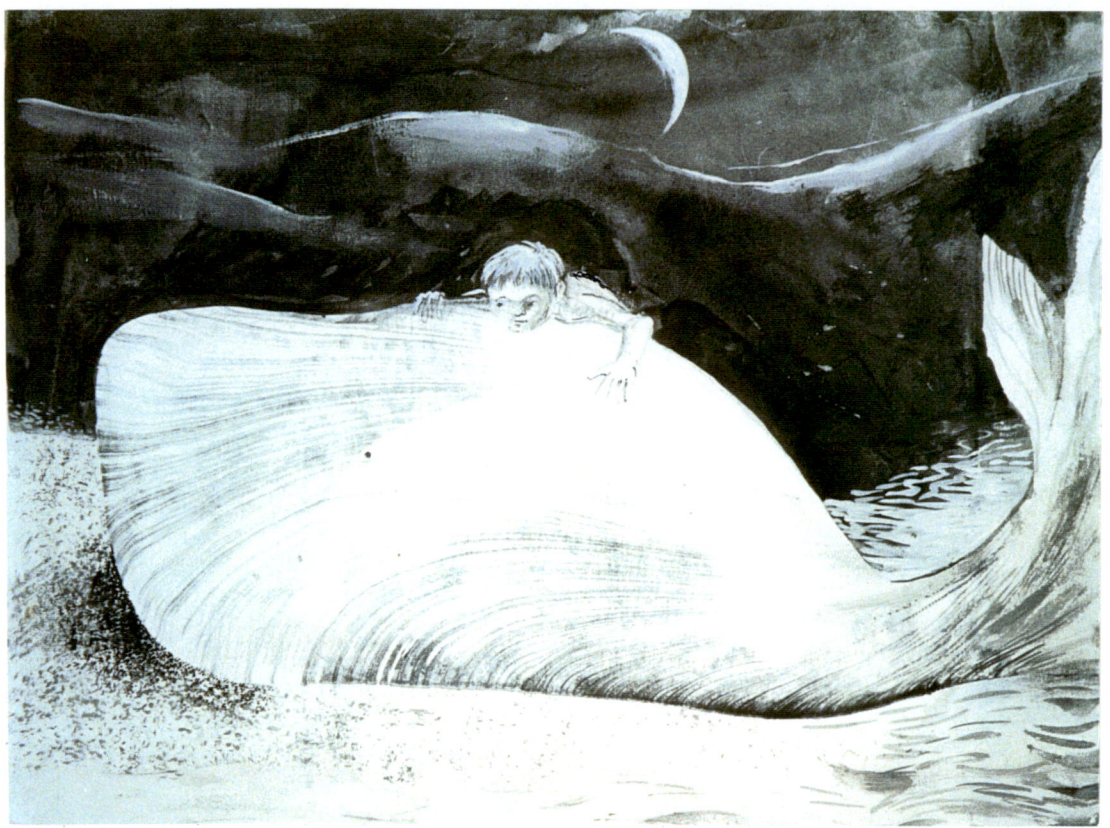

Fig. 436 Boy on a Whale   Pencil & Wash

To round the week off in Kaikoura I took a trip on a whale-watching boat and saw three of these great mammals surfacing for fifteen minutes or so. Later, to my surprise, I found I'd made a child-like freestyle version of a beached whale — with a boy hugging its back. Totally unrealistic yet somehow appropriate. The boy is in possession of his dream.

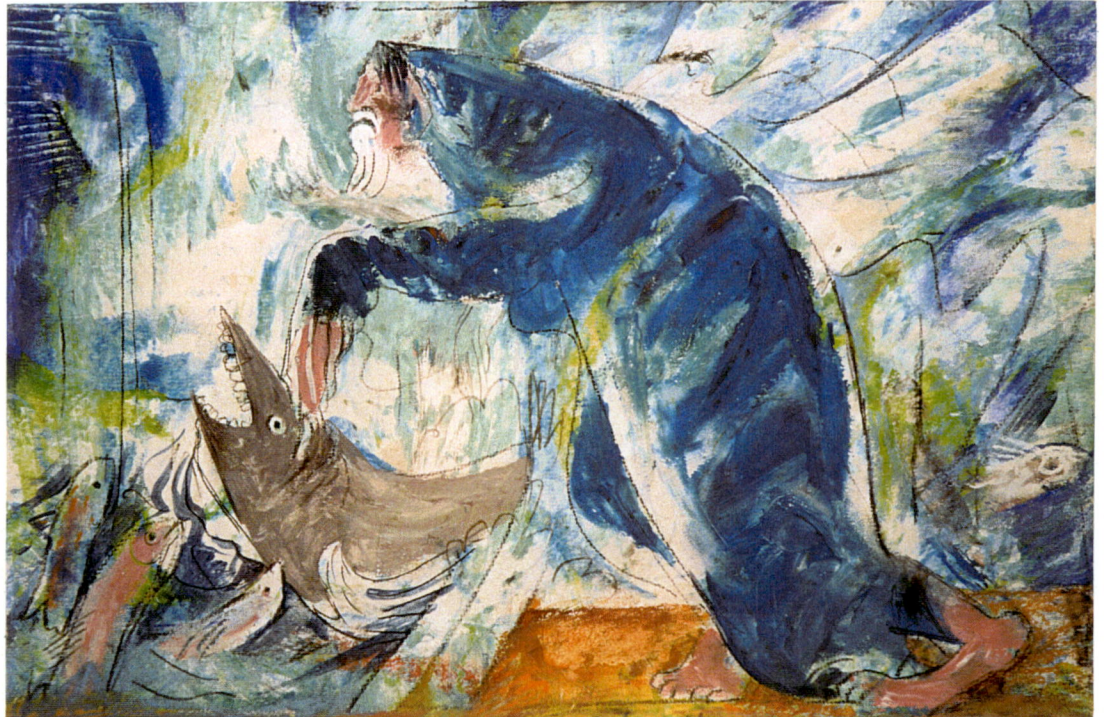

Fig. 437 The Old Man and the Sea   Pencil & Fingerpaint.

'The Old Man and the Sea'. This elderly character robed in deep blue, touches a large fish and others leap up to greet him. His flipper-like hand and rounded form suggest empathy with the life of the sea. Perhaps he will metamorphose into a marine creature.

Christchurch

After a week of comparative solitude it was a change to follow this with a week of 'culture'. I found a hostel in the centre of this most English of cities — a large Anglican Cathedral, punting on the river, etc., — and opposite the Arts Centre. It was also festival week with a surfeit of exhibitions, foreign films and music. An interesting Max Ernst show was on and some fine paintings by Francis Hodgkins, and finally I went dancing with a lively Japanese girl who banished the solitude for a week. Between all these events I had made constant visits to the Botanical Gardens, sketching a fine array of trees (Fig. 438 below).

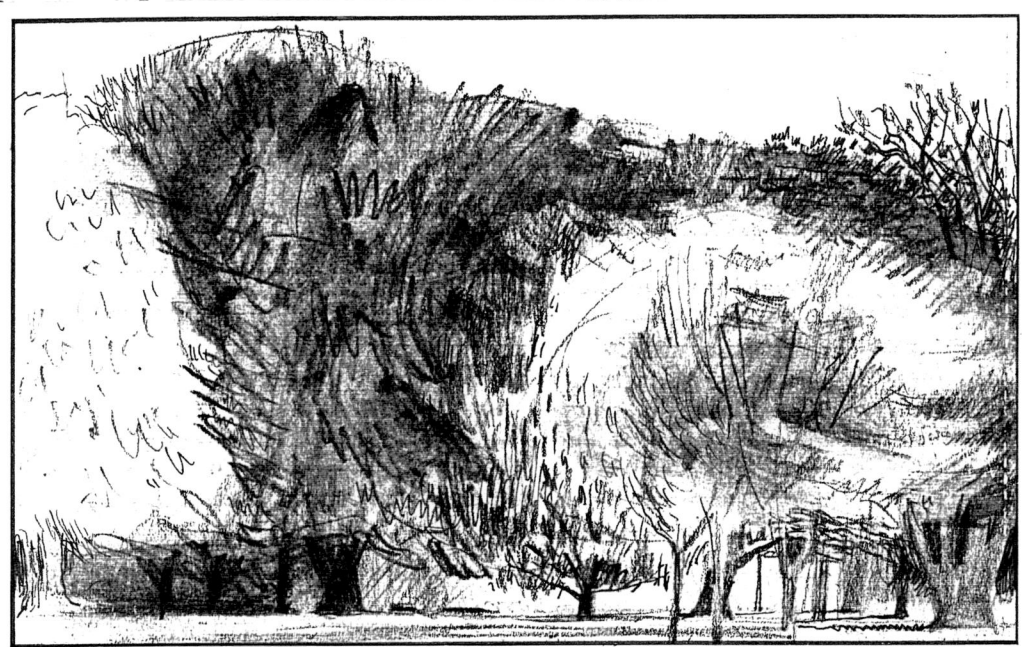

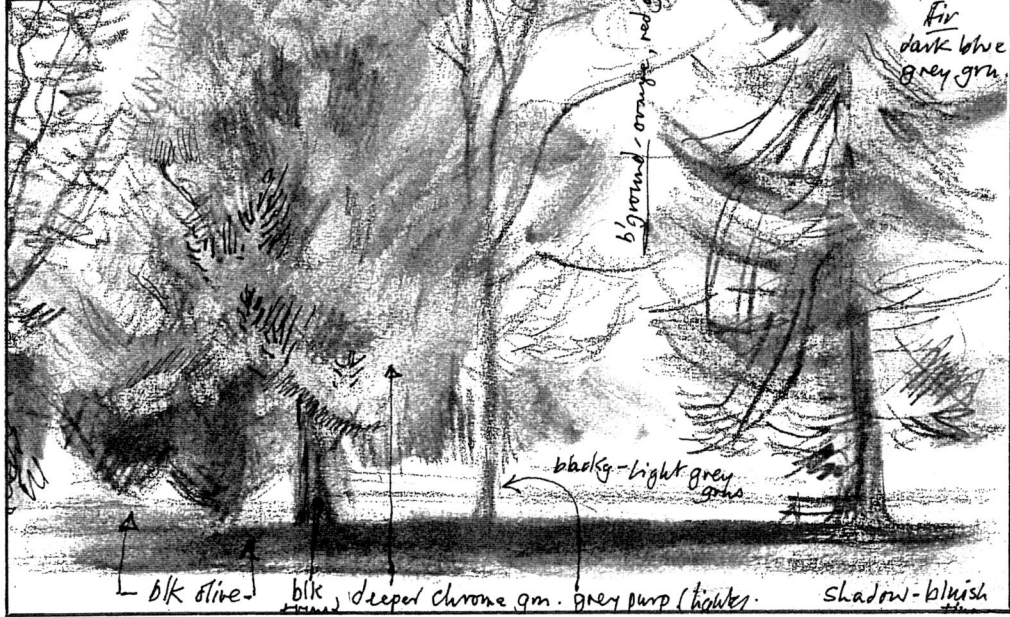

Fig 438   Two studies of Christchurch Botanical Gardens   Acquarelle Pencil

---

Journal 7 Feb. OAMARU

Travel down in torrential rain from Ch.Ch. to this city of fine classical facades along its main street. The city is known also for being the Penny-farthing capital of N.Z. and I see two of these early bicycles on the streets. There's also a colony of the rare Blue Penguin which I visit at dusk, when they wade ashore to their prepared 'nests' – the wardens here take great care of the birds.

This afternoon I follow a 'heritage trail' in exceptionally hot weather to visit Janet Frames' childhood home. Arrive on the site to find her home was destroyed by fire and is now only a narrow strip of fenced-off burnt grass – the only indication of the house, although the surroundings evoke some of the atmosphere from her biog... Leaves somehow a sense of desolation – until I recall the dancing the other day – a sort of enchantment, and the inner child holds his breath with pleasure – until the fantasy passes. Find I don't wish to sketch, so take photos with another of the throw-away cameras – wonder when my own camera will arrive – should be by courier in Dunedin later.

Dunedin

I remember looking westwards, travelling south from Oamaru, seeing the Southern Alps, which must have been some 150-200 miles away and felt I could have touched them, so clear was the atmosphere. It was this fact which made watercolour painting so challenging over here, for there were little or no signs of haze, mist or fog conditions which frequently added mystery to English landscape. There was no sense of aerial-colour distance, only a hard-edged clarity to rocks, hilltops and so on. I found it impossible to paint this particular view and so later drew my own mountain range, with an erupting volcano and also a birdman searching for a retreat or nesting place. (fig. 439 below).

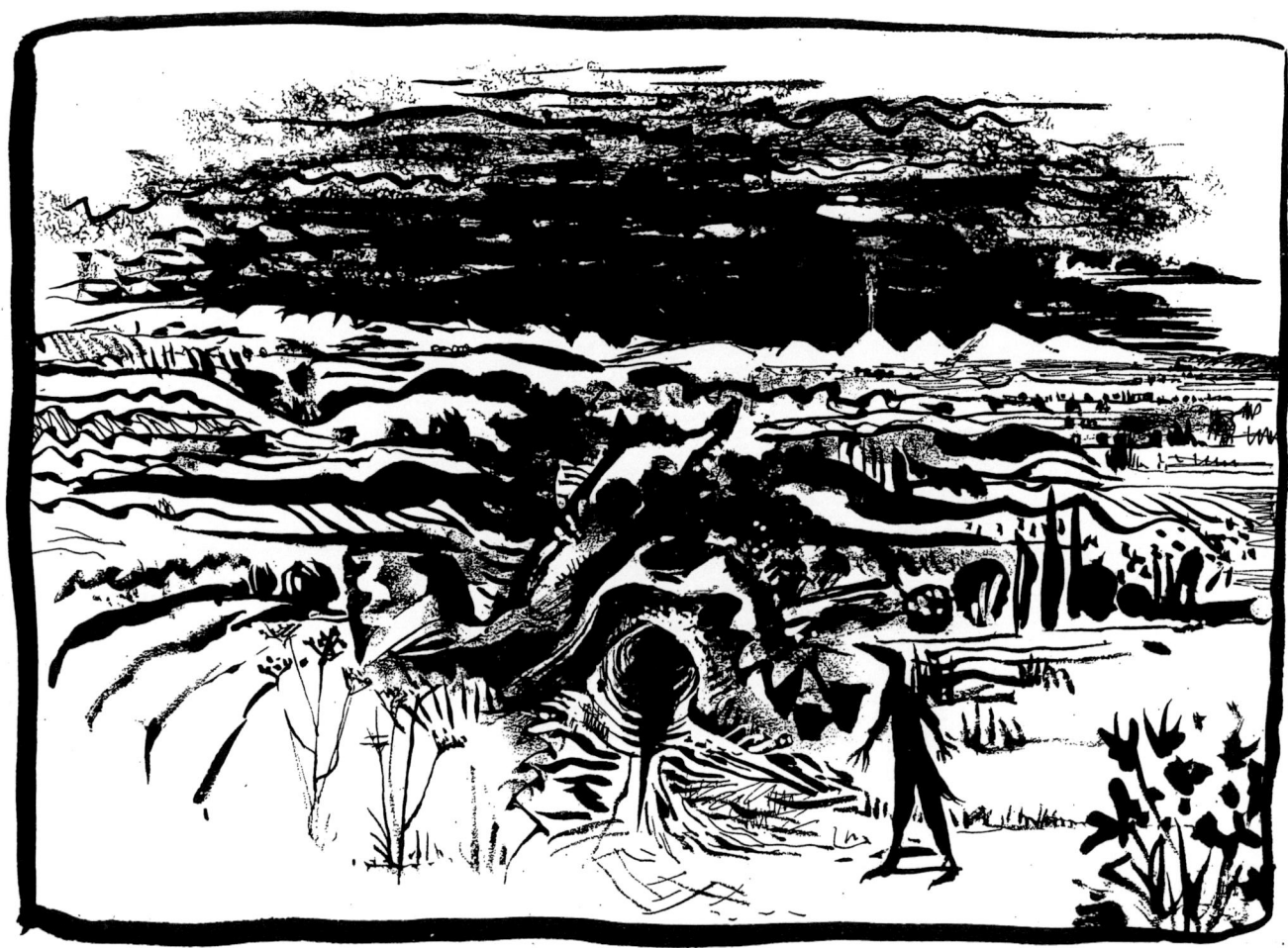

Fig. 439   Birdman in an Eruptive Landscape   Brush and Ink

Notes from the Journal - 9 Feb - 16 Feb. Dunedin

Find the most attractive and welcoming 'Backpacker' of them all with a high viewpoint, above this substantial Scottish and European-styled city, overlooking the harbour. As it rains the first few days I find myself in the library, holding Paul Klee's diaries and enrolling as a temporary member for a $50 deposit - I now have reading material for about a fortnight.

Next morning put car into garage for check-up and service (now a routine practice), and spend a few hours enthusing about, and sketching the wonderfully inventive sculptures of Pacific Islanders and the Maori culture. I even find an equivalent for my 'Joker'. (fig. 441).

During the stay I watch massed bands of pipes and drums competing with each other in the city centre - am informed this city is more Scottish than its sister city Edinburgh (from which it acquires half its name - Dun-Edin).

Later, a visit to the Albatross colony on the peninsula. The parent birds are sitting on chicks as large as themselves!
Little drawing or painting ....
But much sight-seeing and reading Paul Klee's enthralling diaries.
Klee makes an observation about his inner voice ..... "It seemed to me that I had no strength of character whenever I heeded the inner voice more than orders from outside." I'm only too well aware of this struggle.
Suddenly decide to book a flight for Stewart Island after seeing advertisement in the hostel. Although I'll be missing last stage by road to Invercargill, savings in time and money seem more important.
Another quote from Klee - "The more I build things up, the more they tumble down". I feel he's advocating the freestyle approach here - intuition over classical structure.

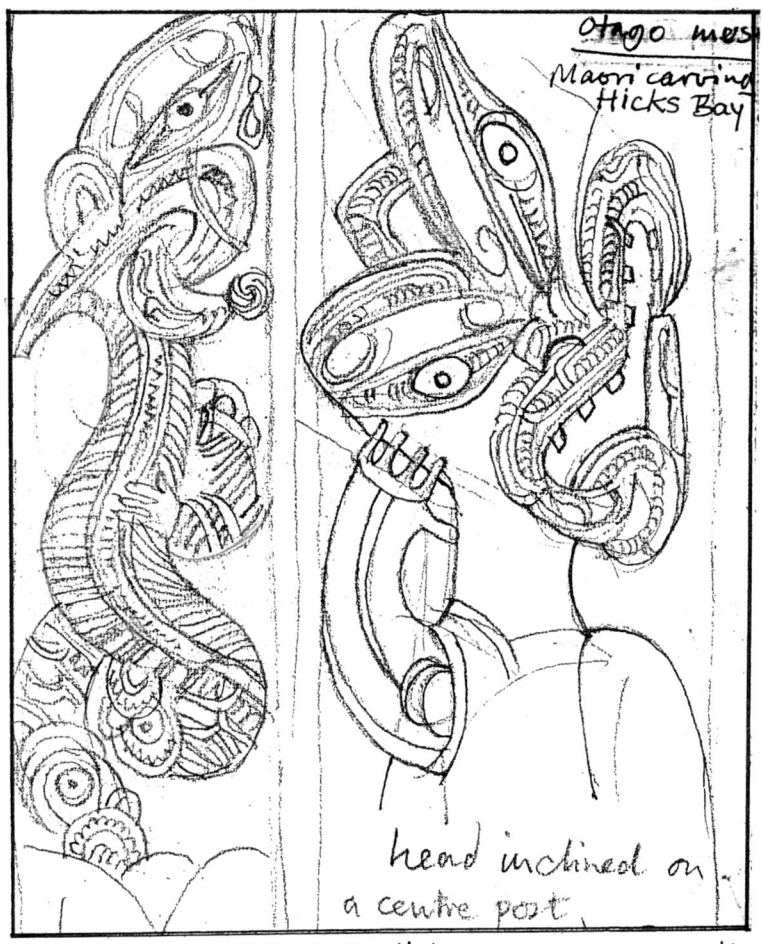

Fig. 440 Maori Carving - Hicks Bay   Pencil

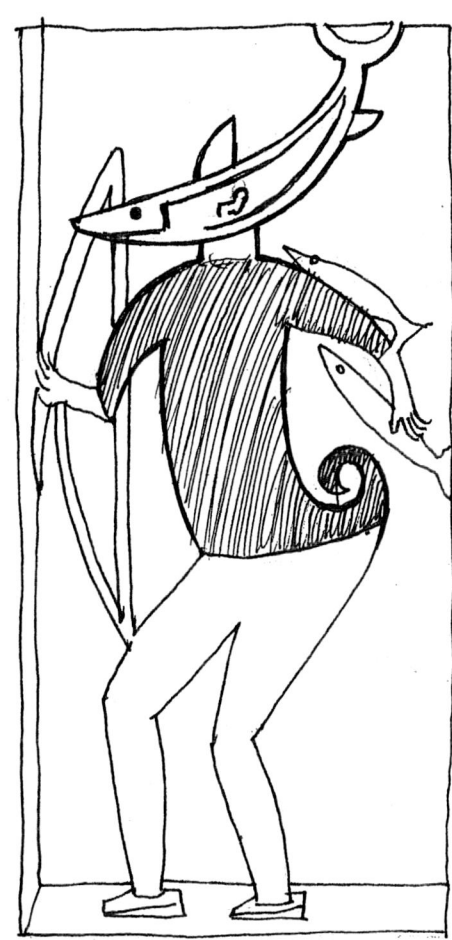

Fig. 441 Roaring Bravado
Sth. Solomon Isles. Sea Spirit
Pen and Ink

Drawings at Dunedin - Otago Museum

Before the flight I saw a little of the province of Otago, including a visit to the town of Lawrence and a look at 'Gabriel's Gully', the site of the first gold rush of the 1860s. The possibility that my maternal grandfather may have made his fortune and then lost it in N.Z. (a family legend!) drew me to the site - now a mass of grassy humps. I found registrations of his surname in the local museum but nothing conclusive.

Whilst painting, I was sheltering from direct sunlight in the car, leaning slightly over the steering wheel when an elderly Maori stopped his car, and came up to enquire if I was ill - a kindly act.

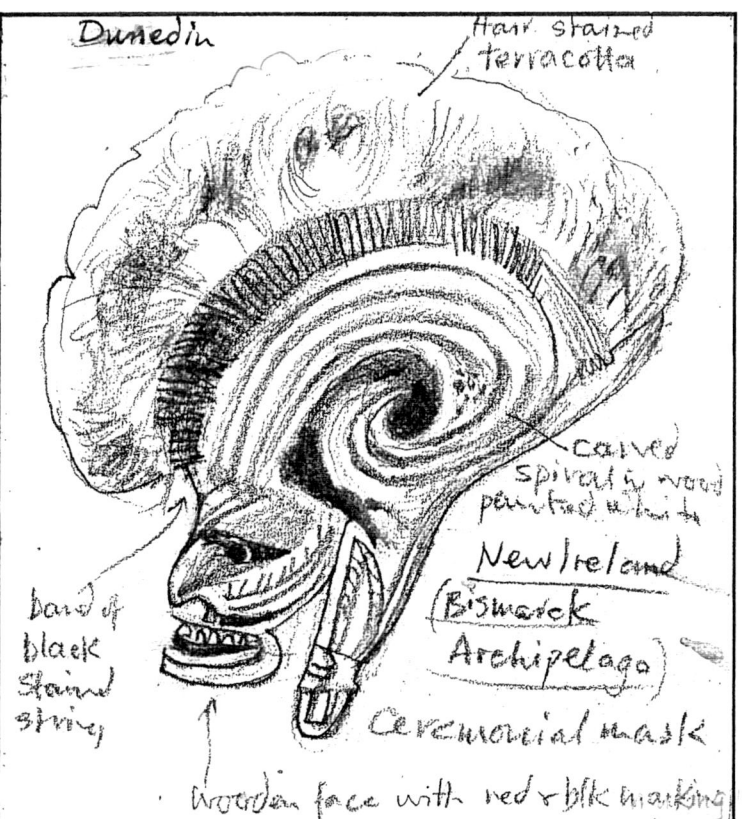

Fig. 442 Clay and skull mask   Ink.   Fig. 443 Ceremonial Mask - New Ireland.   Pencil

STEWART ISLAND

> Journal 16 Feb. Stewart Island. The Shearwater Inn, Oban
>
> A 200 mile flight in a "string-and-sealing-wax" monoplane (or so it felt, with thoughts of Icarus) from Dunedin to Oban, the only town on Stewart. (Maui's Anchor - legend page 244).
> Having come all this way to be at this southernmost place, I feel suddenly as if I'm in a vacuum wishing to resist any kind of transformation at all costs. I feel as if I'm about to relinquish past skills, 'classical' ways of working ('of tumbling down' writes Paul Klee). Know this is the journey into unknown inner self and find it initially too daunting. The great explorers in this field of search - Klee, Redon and Debuffet for example - they found the courage, tenacity and ruthlessness which is essential. Could I.?
> Have registered into Shearwater Inn on Halfmoon Bay and visited Information Centre where I glean a few facts about the Island. Only two per cent. is habitable, bush and mud take up the remaining space. This still leaves enough kilometres of road to trudge along for the next week or so. Seem to be about a dozen vehicles on the road, including one old taxi. If one wants to see more of the island, this is accessible from a boat - provided you register in what and where you're going and keep to marked tracks. There is no immediate means of rescue here I'm informed.

After a long sleep next day I started walking along the coast road towards Horseshoe Bay, visiting the local store, enquired about fresh fish at the quayside and ended up in a fernery, a forest section mainly of varying ferns and a few native trees. (fig 444).

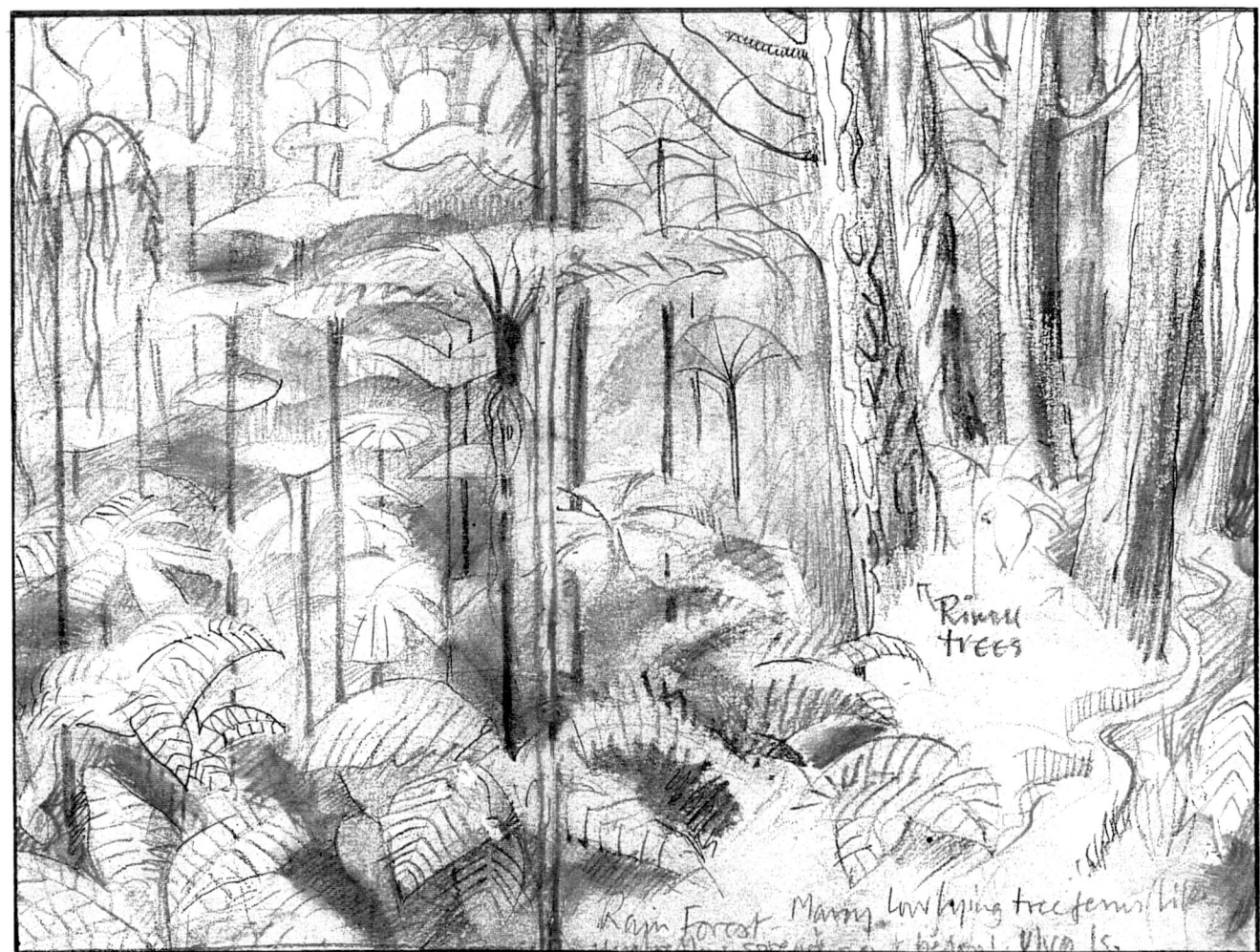

Fig. 444. A Fernery with native Rimu trees   Aquarelle Pencil

The following day I walked all the way to Horseshoe Bay and found a coffee shop on the ground floor of a red house, centred on the middle of the horseshoe. The owner Val, offered crystals also, and full board at a price I couldn't afford. But when Val knew that I was painting my way around New Zealand she offered full board in exchange for a drawing to advertise her 'Retreat'. I transferred here for three full days before her next group of guests arrived, making an ink drawing for a new letterhead. (fig. 445). Later Val also asked for a sunrise in watercolour (fig. 449).

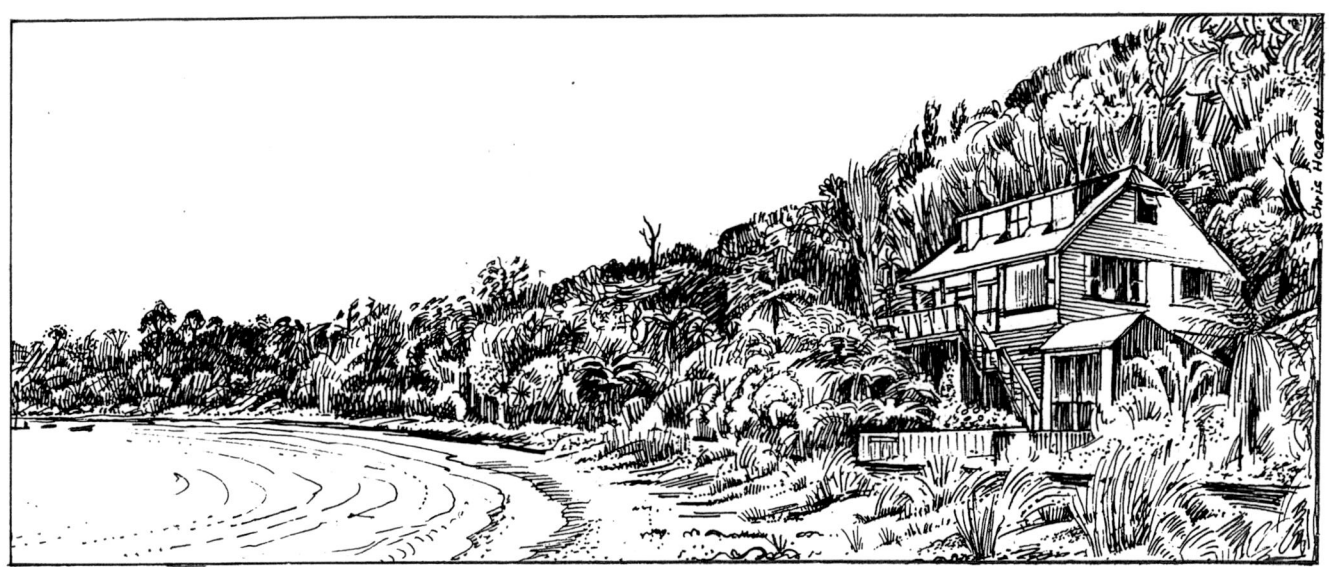

Fig. 445 'The Retreat', Horseshoe Bay, Stewart Island.   Pen & Ink

A day out on Ulva Island close to Oban. It was mainly rain forest, where I enjoyed seven hours listening to marvellous bird song whilst sketching along the shore and in the forest. A quote from Delacroix came to mind — "The true subject of painting is yourself — your impressions, feelings, your need to look inside — not outside yourself." I was reflecting constantly on my inner reactions which is much easier when alone!

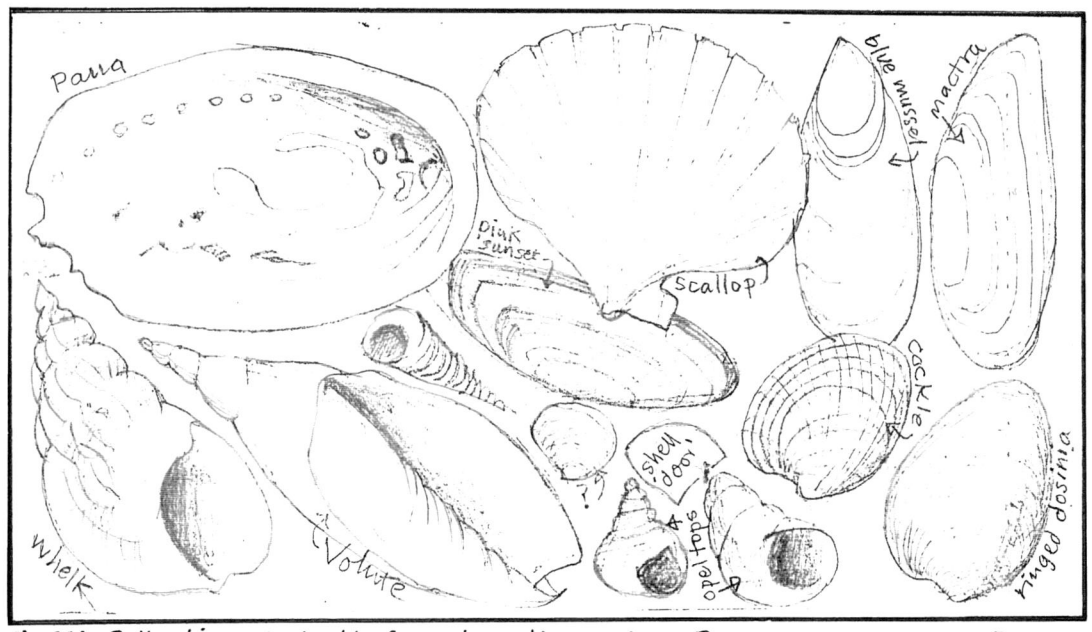

Fig. 446 Collection of shells found on Horseshoe Bay   Pencil

Journal 19 Feb — Val's Retreat

This evening after sunset I've found time to read another extract from Klee's diaries; "And now an altogether revolutionary discovery; to adapt oneself to the contents of the paintbox is more important than nature and its study". Find this very much in tune with my own mood, searching as I am for the essence of this place, rather than the visible appearance of nature (with the exception of my 'bread-and-butter commissions!')

A dream image last night emphasises this: "A train is nearing its destination and I'm required (by whom?) to leave, by jumping off, as I try to pacify someone who wishes to stay on board."

The link between the dream image and Klee's observation becomes clear — to leap out fearlessly (take a new route) using any means available — tools, paintboxes, whatever...

I've looked across at islands further out to sea, Val tells me these are the 'mutton-bird' Islands, belonging to the Maoris. The birds are Australasian shearwaters which nest in holes in the earth, said to taste like mutton and used as food by the Maoris.

Draw selection of shells found on the beach

Aspects of Horseshoe Bay, Stewart Island

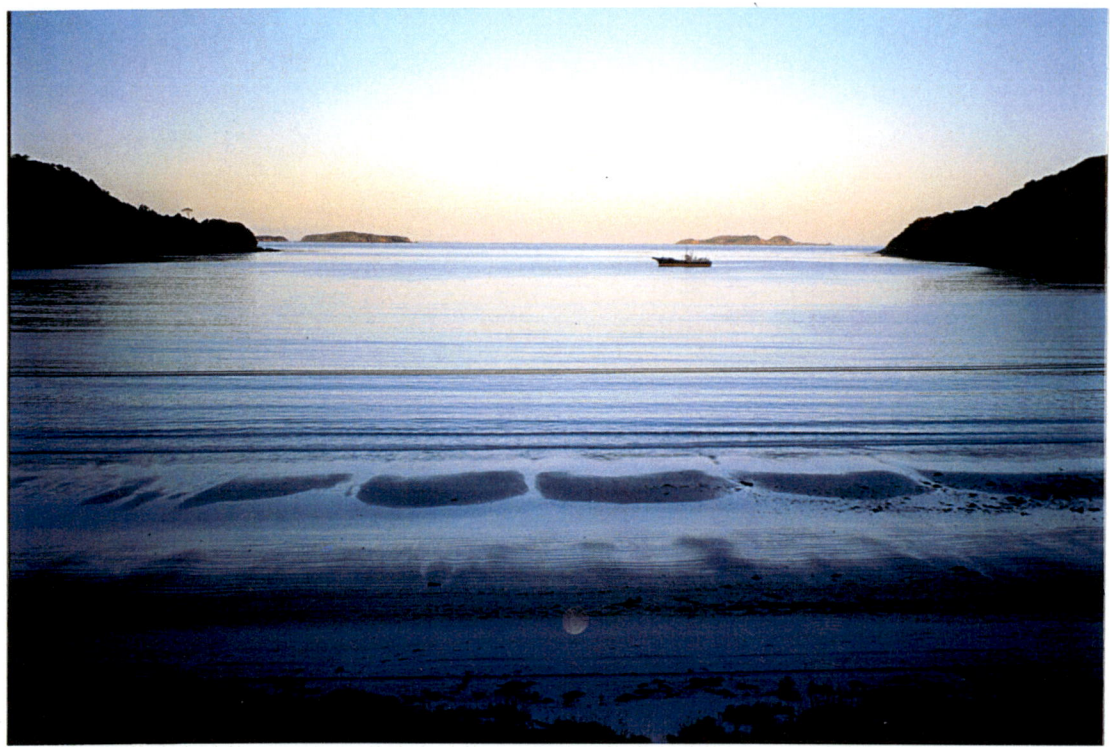

Fig.447 Horseshoe Bay and the Muttonbird Islands.

Above: Photograph of the bay near sundown.
The Muttonbird Islands are on the horizon. A Japanese fishing vessel is anchored in the bay.

> Journal 19 Feb · The 'Retreat'
> I'm overwhelmed by the incandescent sunsets over the bay. Sitting, looking out of a large picture window each evening I'm mesmerised by the slowly-changing colour combinations reflected from the sea. This is the place I've been waiting to discover.
> Paradise on earth – for a colourist.
>
> 21st Last full day at Val's Retreat. Become so intoxicated by Nature's magic I can't draw or paint the bay — I've tried, but scrapped each attempt. Take photos instead. Do one watercolour of a sunset for Val, but its only a ghost of its actual self.
>   Klee again :– 'Looking for new ways.. ...this is the essential thing; becoming is more important than being"
>   This third day in this bay is pivotal to the whole journey – sense some deep change underway.... the true centre to the tour.
>   Make freestyle sketch of bay with surrounding ferns and palms. Know it's important – will get C. to comment on it when I return.

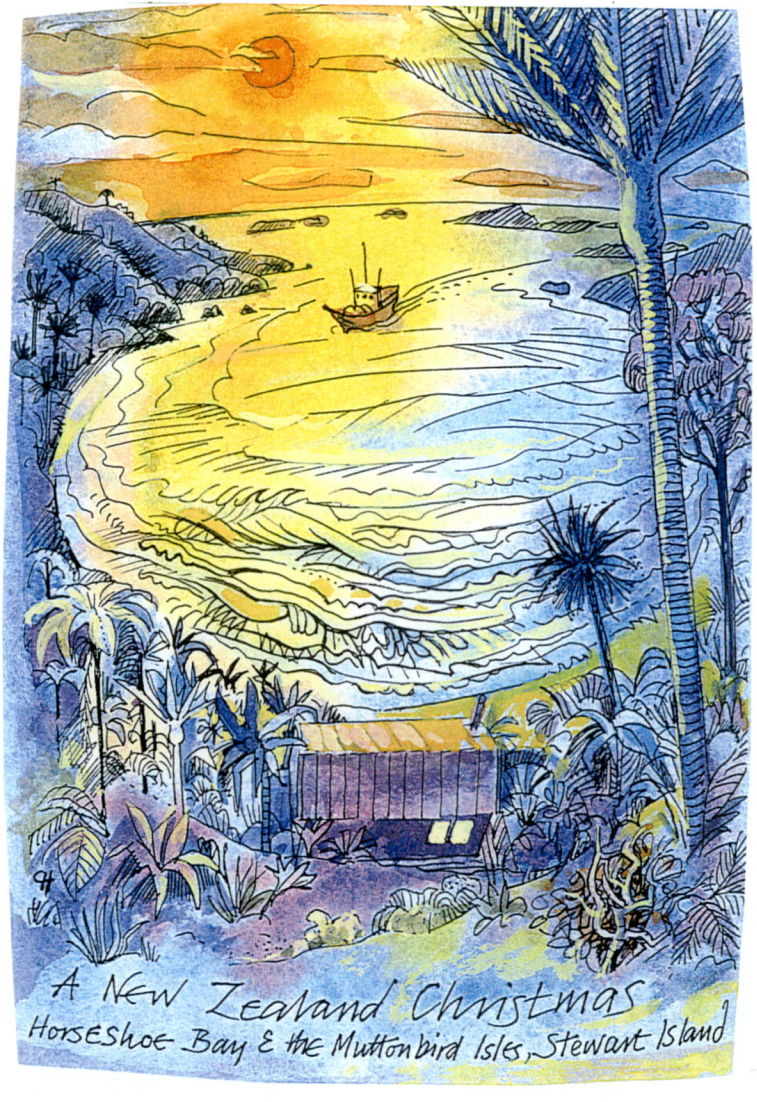

Right: Years later I use the bay as a subject for a Christmas Card, taking a high viewpoint to emphasise the horseshoe shape. Val's retreat lies surrounded by palms and ferns.

Right: Fig 448 Horseshoe Bay Xmas Card
Watercolour, Line & Gouache

Right: Fig. 449

Sunset over Horseshoe Bay. Watercolour

(following the 'Retreat' drawing (fig 445) my second commission from Val).

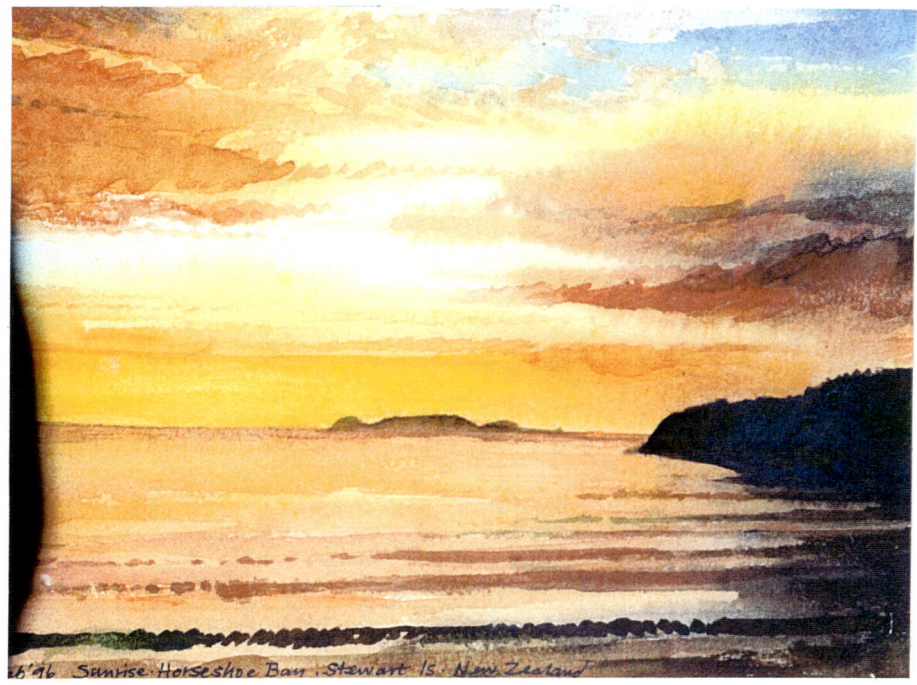

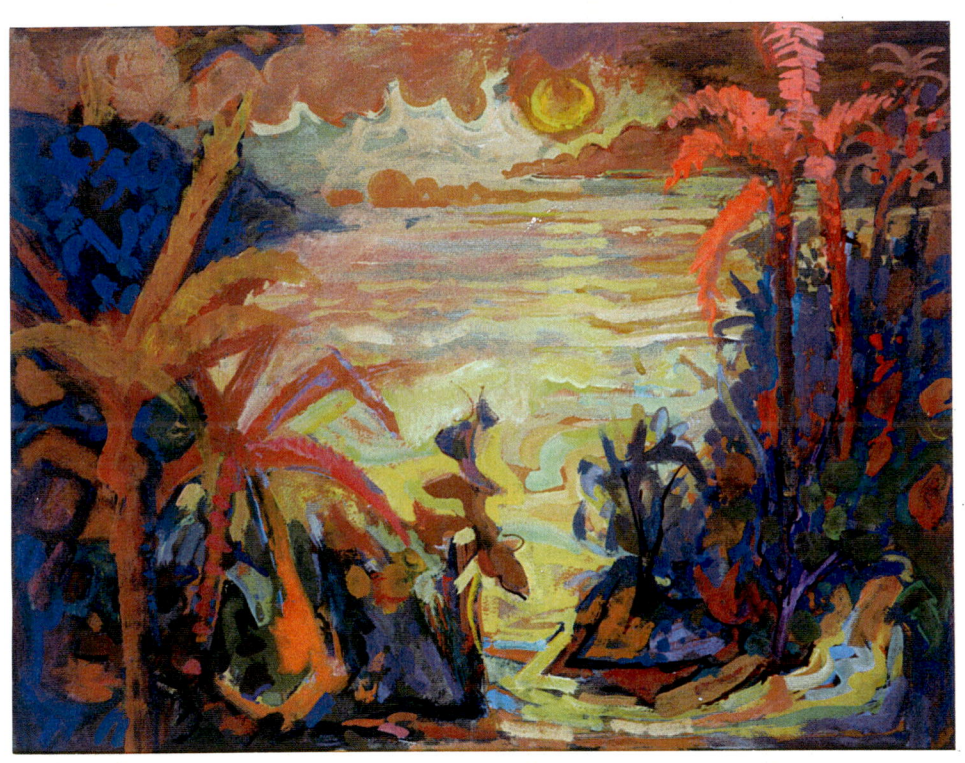

Left: Fig. 450

Evening at Horseshoe Bay.

Gouache

(painting of the bay - late evening).

(see text below).

Return to Shearwater Inn reluctantly, feeling I could have stayed at the Retreat indefinitely if it had been available - I thought everything would seem like an anticlimax. During the last complete day in Oban I realised a certain structure underlay the Stewart Island episode, rather like some symphonic work - A:B:C:B:A
i.e.: A - City   B - Village   C - Outback   B - Village   A - city
    (Dunedin - 7 days) (Oban 3 days) ('Retreat' - 3 days) (Oban 3 days) (Dunedin 7 days)

(The last 'A' was only a projection, but I had thought I'd stay about another week there).
  The quest for the South was the essence of the journey, the desire to find the creative child. I realised that despite any possible adventures ahead, emotionally I'd found a cure for the years of depression and repression. The painting 'Evening at Horseshoe Bay' contained the embryo, about to leap through the birth channel, and held the moment of rebirth. It was the moment also when I could retrace my steps. Everything else would later be 'coloured' by this revelation.

The Stewart Walks

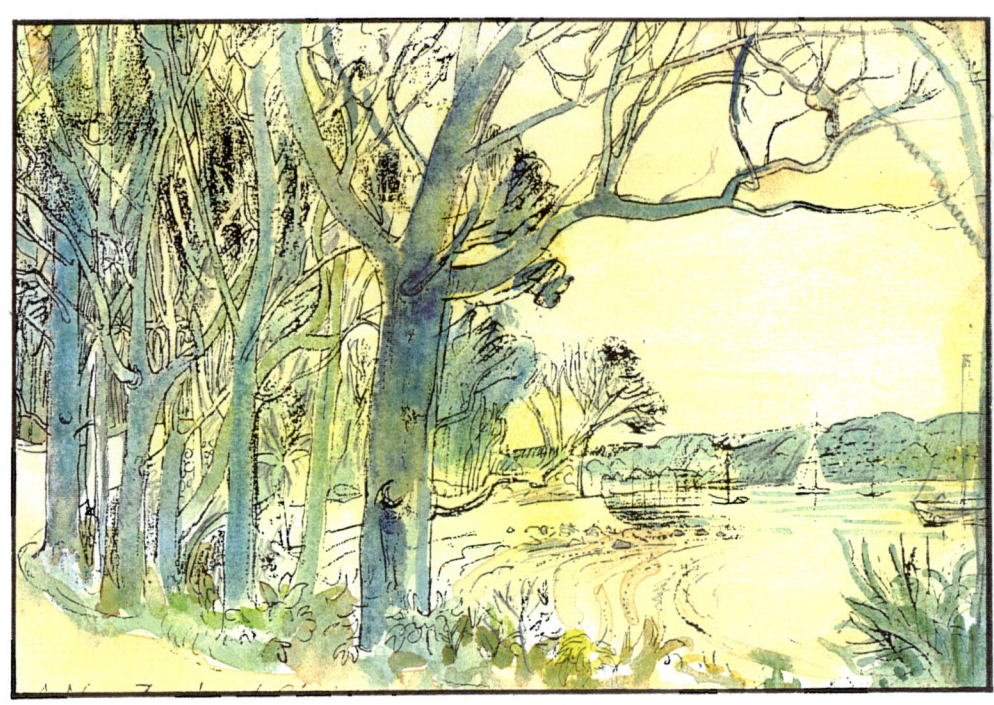

Right: Fig. 451

Blue Gums on Lonnekers Beach Oban

Ink & Watercolour

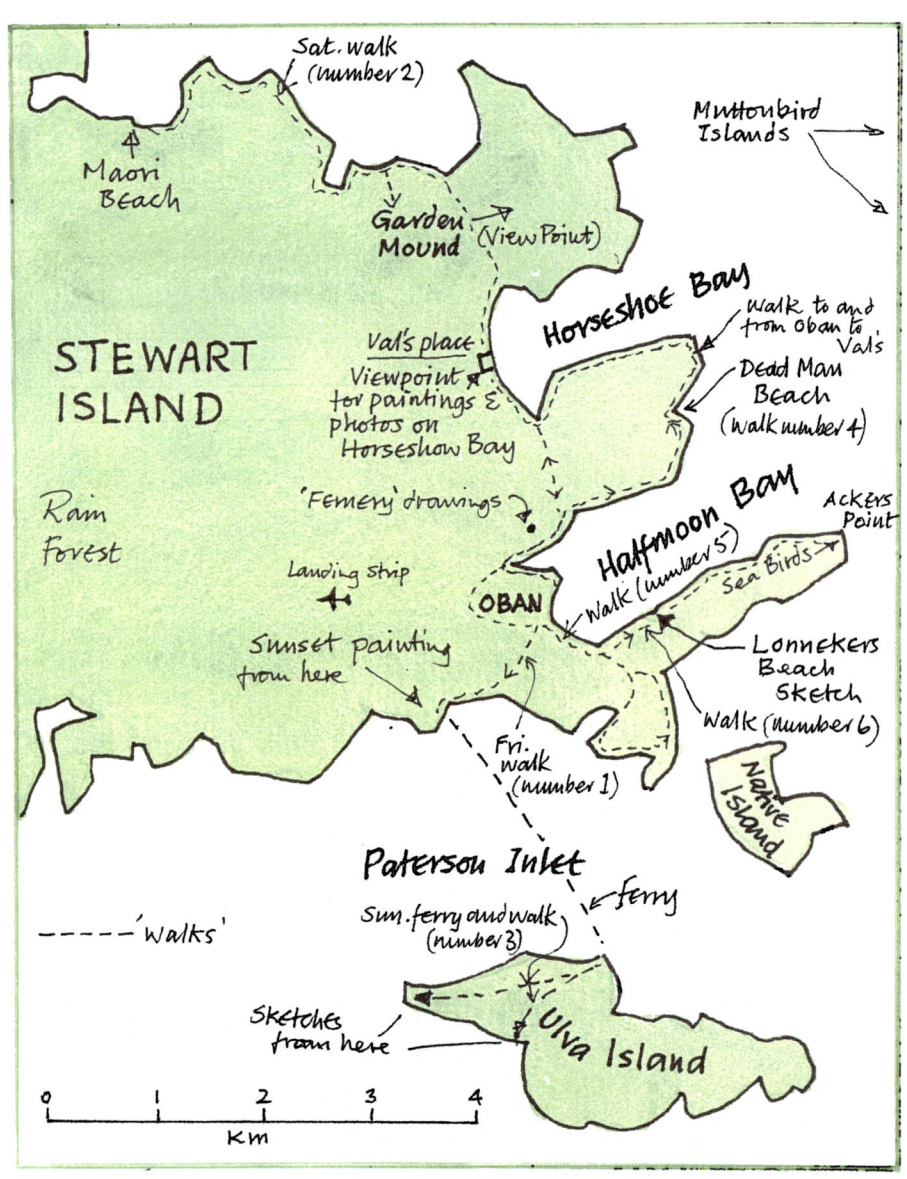

Journal 24 Feb. Oban.

Penultimate day. Walk to see Blue gums (Eucalyptus) trees along Lonnekers Beach near Oban - lovely scene, so compelled to do small w'colour.

Interested in Department of Conservation signs showing distinctions between walks, tracks and routes:-

WALKS - Easy going strolls of 'horizontal' nature along well prepared pathways.

TRACKS - For vigorous walking with steeper climbs, and a higher degree of fitness.

ROUTES - Tough treks through the bush for the very fit and able. Usually lasting between three to eight days duration.

Decided to list my walks on local map as memory aid - all are truly 'walks' except number 2 when I made 'a track journey - very energetic - steep and hard going.

Left: Fig. 452

Drawing based on local Tourist map of Northeast coastal area of walks and sketching points.

Dunedin - Te Anau - Queenstown - Arrowtown - and the Sounds

Journal 25-28 Feb. Stewart back to Dunedin

25th Flight back in brilliant sunshine - look out over Horseshoe Bay and see Val's red house. I'll long remember the few days there.

26th Hillman safe and sound outside hostel. Seems to run well, so will risk not going in for 'check-up'. Check provisions needed for next part of journey West. Return the Klee Diaries and reclaim $50 deposit.

28th Final full day. See 'Underground', Balkans film with savage, humorous overview of man's darkness and war, treated like a circus act. Felt film pertinent - a study in 'freefall' creativity - I often resist, yet know it is attainable if one takes the risk. Resistance to change always remains, so powerful sometimes, like sloth creeping up on one like a drug. Perhaps constant travel isn't conducive to concentrated picture-making. Its time to move on - towards Te Anau tomorrow

Journal 29 Feb. (Leap Year!)
Pick up a couple of hitch-hikers at Dunedin and drop them off at Balclutha, then halfway into Otago pick up a couple of young Germans and we decide to share journey for a few days they contributing towards the fuel.

March 1st.
Visit Doubtful Sound (Fiord). Heavy mist and rain create the equivalent of Scottish Highlands - full of atmosphere and mystery. One of wettest places on earth we're informed, on sea-going catamaran - see Dolphins making big curvilinear leaps out of water. Next to Milford Sound which is visually less interesting (despite the hype) but people much more so. Meet a Canadian who works on Keck telescope, Hawaii - his area of research is the study of black holes. Rather different to my own kind!

March 3rd - Arrowtown.
Drive Northwards with my German companions leaving them at Queenstown. I miss their company, as I decide not to stay - too 'glitzy' and overcrowded. Instead drive North a few miles to Arrowtown, an old gold-mining town. Book in to 'New Orleans' hotel, finding very cheap, large 26 bunk basement all to myself. Reserved mainly for N.Z Rugby teams!
Built in early 1800s and now a historical centre of timber buildings along the main street. Check at local museum about my Gold Rush Grandpa where I'm offered a form asking for more details - perhaps I'll follow this up!

March 4th Visit Queenstown.
Return to Q'town to watch some local sports like bungee-jumping and para-gliding, and a hair-raising jeep ride along narrow hair-pin bends down mountain side with an acquaintance met near Dunedin. All these activities I don't need - instead I take ride in a Gondola to high point and settle down to watch and draw an instructor and pupil paragliding from some 3000 ft.

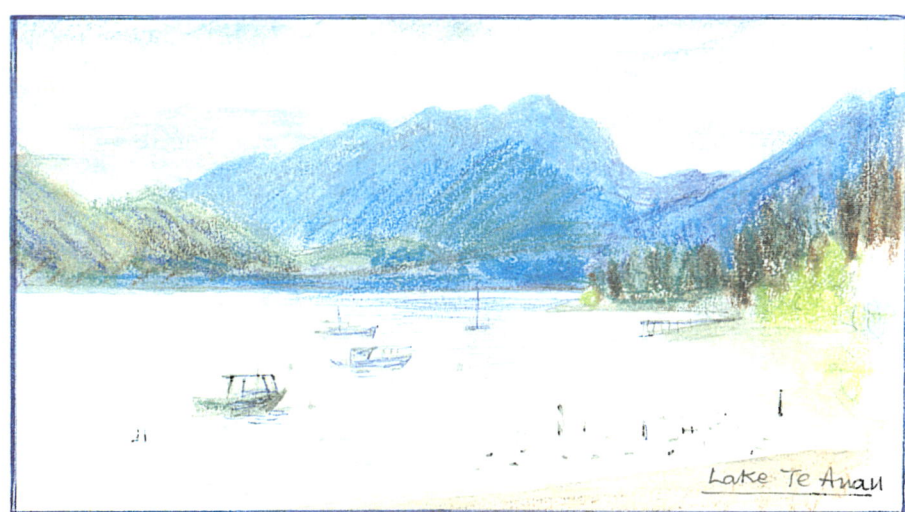

Fig. 453 Lake Te Anau Coloured Crayons

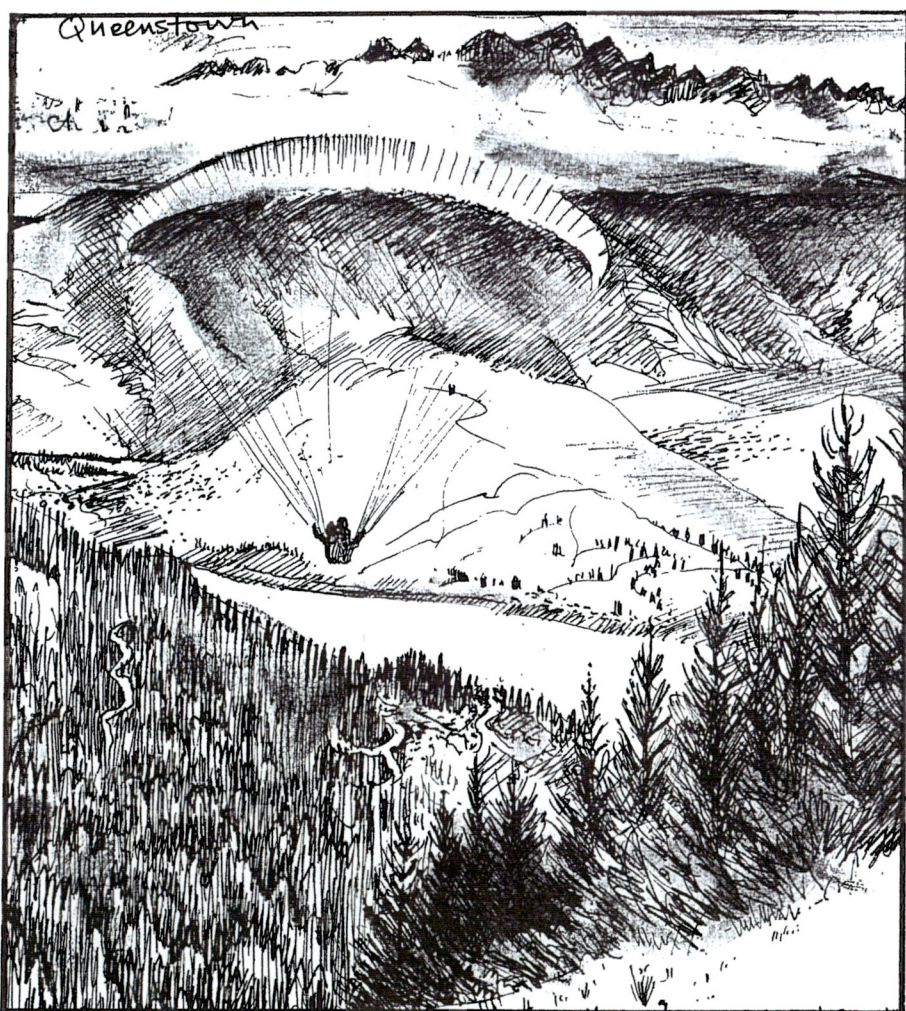

Right: Fig.454 Paragliding at Queenstown Pen & Ink

Wanaka and district

After three days in Arrowtown I felt a sudden need to move on, probably because of the empty bunks in the basement of 'New Orleans' – and 25 ghosts to remind me of my solitude.
On the drive towards Wanaka in the Hillman (now a remarkably reliable vehicle after the fitting of a new radiator) I stopped at the Kawarau Mining Centre and enjoyed an hour panning for gold. My net gain was $00.03 (about 3 cents worth). I wonder how long it took my maternal grandpa to make his fortune (see March 3rd entry in Journal, page 267). Later, I stopped overnight alongside a beautiful lake which reflected the mountains. Walked up Mount Iron, a modest 546 metres, but offering expansive views over a schist valley with long windbreaks of Lombard poplars (fig. 455).
Later that day I took a long drive along an unsealed road, following the Matukituki valley, finding a view of Mt. Aspiring (3030 metres) in the Southern Alps (fig. 456). It's a very rough, rocky road towards the end of some 30km where I saw a cloud of dust in my wing mirror. I pulled over just in time to see a bunch of gunmen, rifles raised, fly past in a battered truck and many large dogs. I suddenly realised I was in the outback – with men hunting wild boar. Realised also I was running low on petrol and the Hillman's suspension was taking a battering – and I did need a sale when I returned to Auckland!

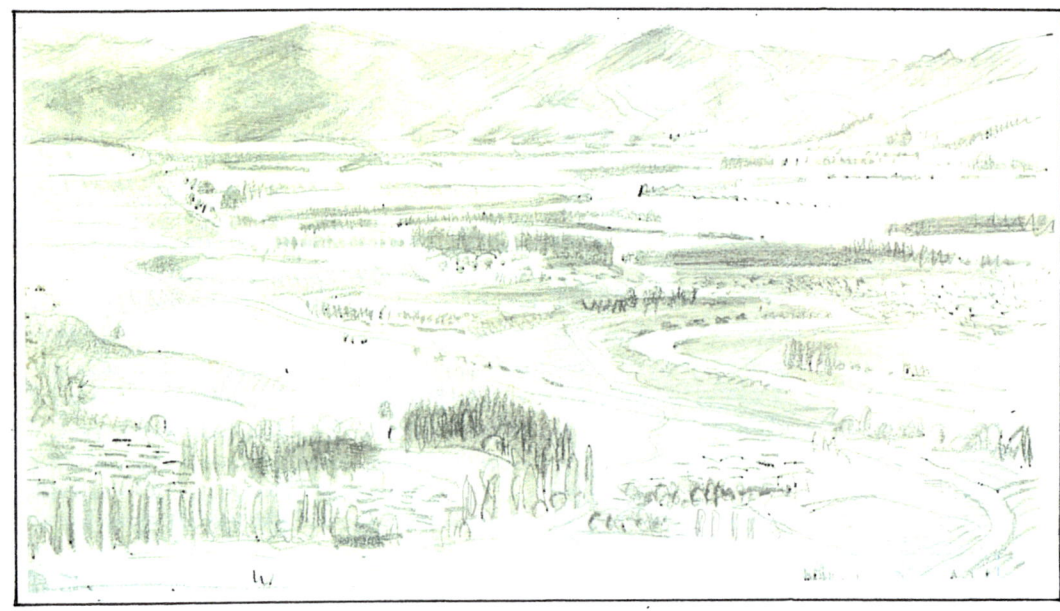

Fig. 455
View of schist plain from top of Mount Iron

Pencil

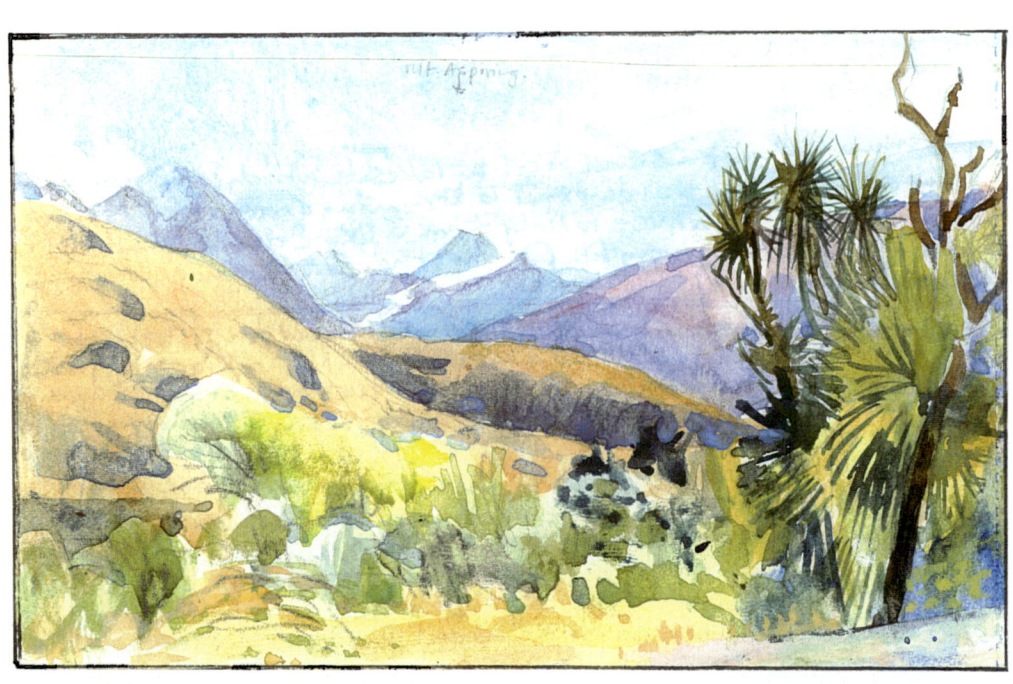

Fig. 456
View of Mt. Aspiring from Matukituki Valley, with cabbage trees.

Watercolour

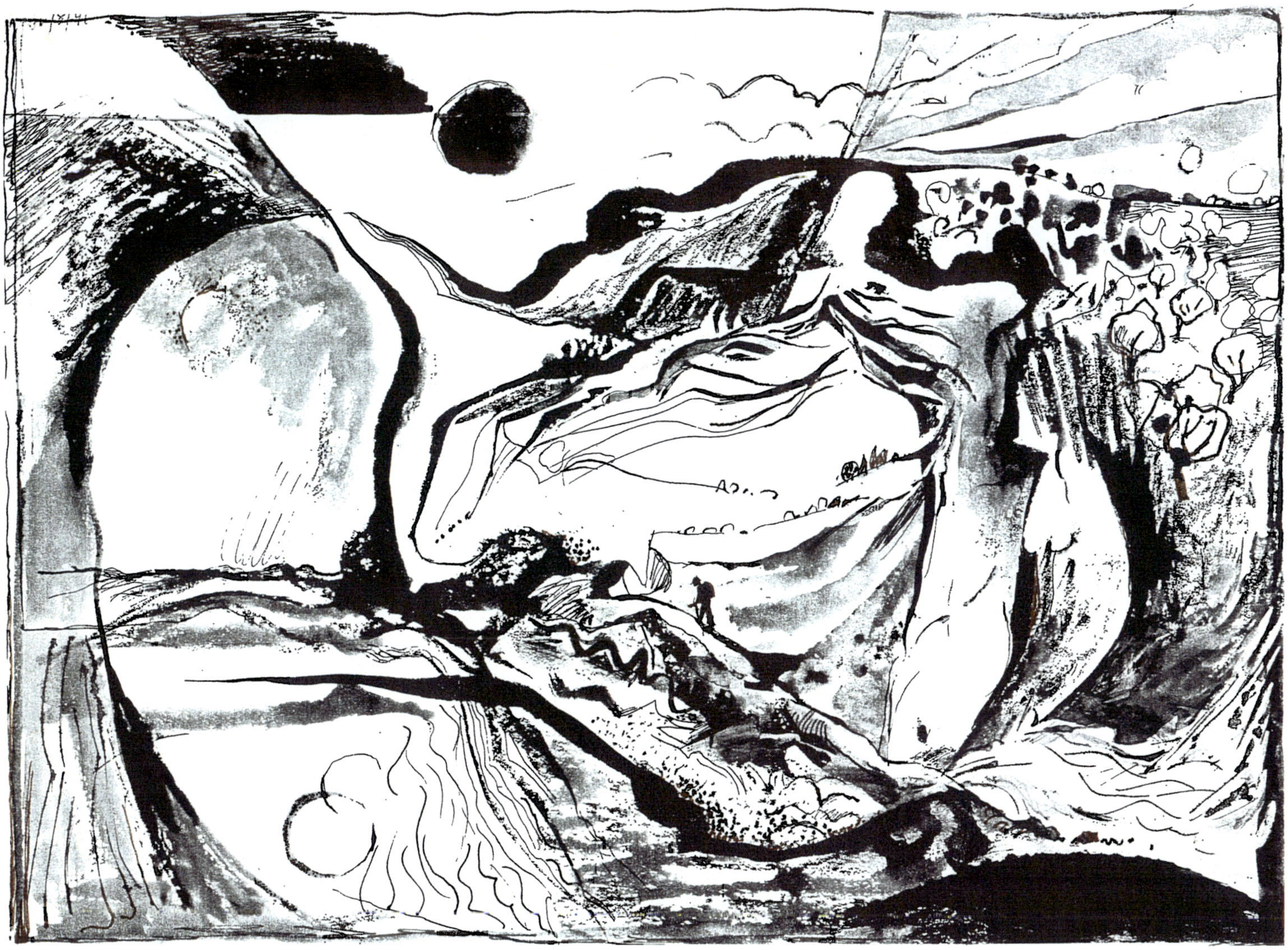

Fig. 457　Backpacker in Hilly Country　　　Pen, Brush & Ink

I walked more frequently now between car journeys, sometimes climbing to higher levels than usual, often finding stunning views. Later a pen and brush drawing developed, attempting to show the spaciousness and timelessness of this mountainous region (fig. 457).
One afternoon I saw a surprising sight - Mount Aspiring was sending up smoke signals. As the white low-lying cloud drifted towards the summit it separated into small puffs - like a Red Indian sending smoke signals (fig. 458).

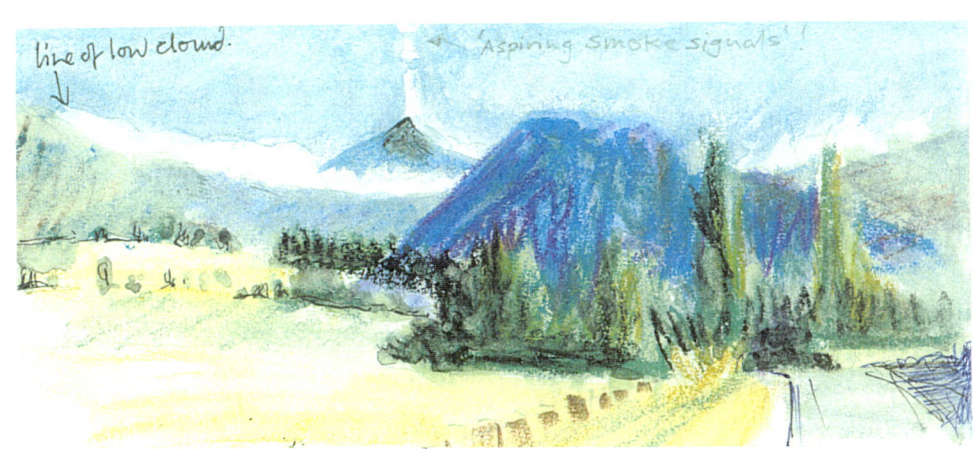

Fig. 458

Mount Aspiring sending smoke signals
　　Coloured Chalks

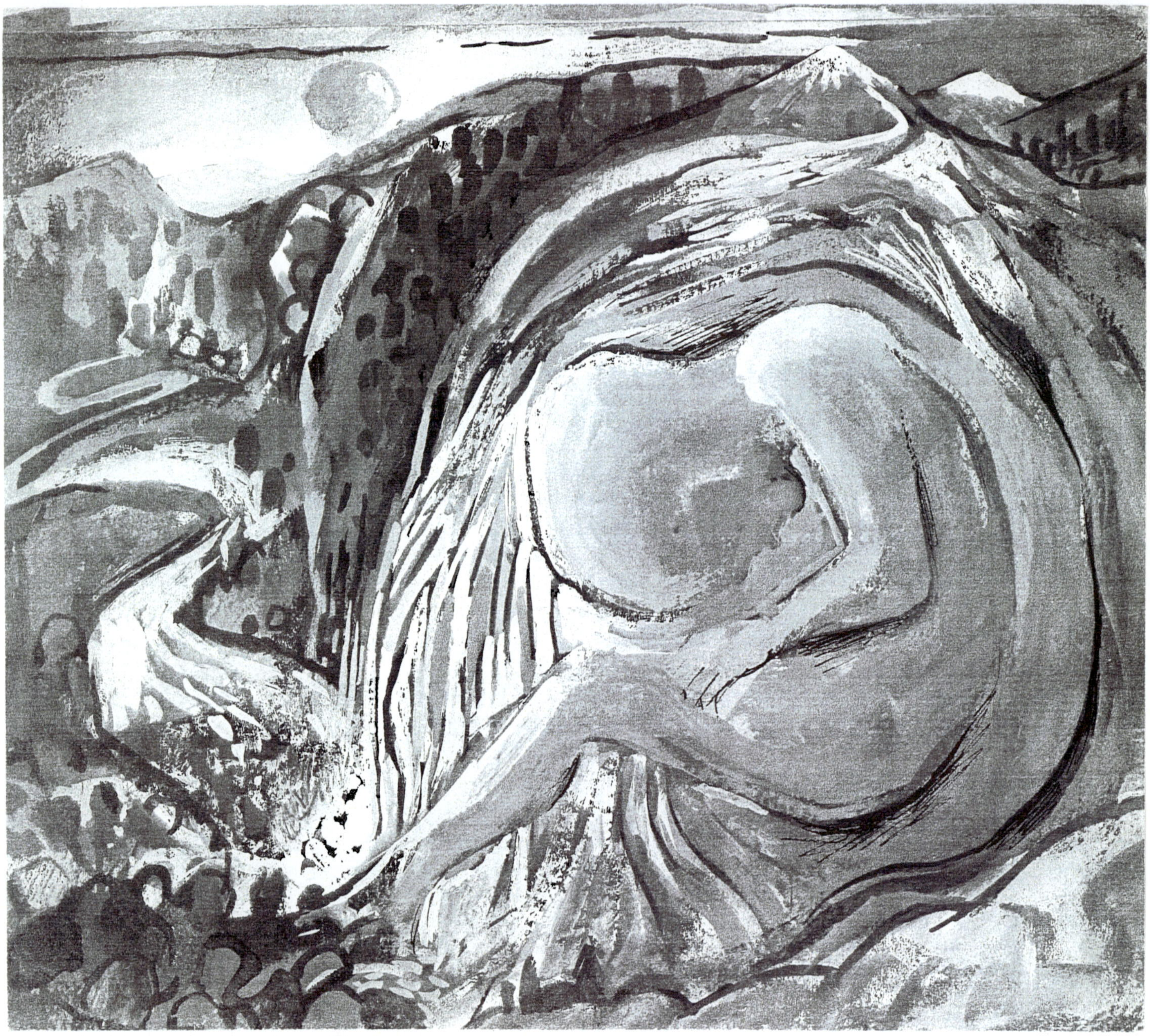

Fig. 459 Haast Pass Renaissance   Gouache

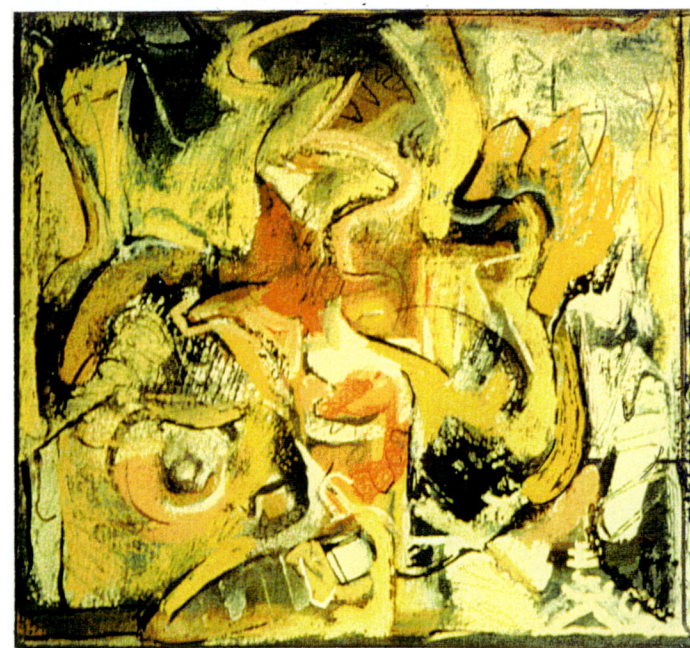

Fig. 460 Fragmentation   Gouache

Perhaps because of the great scenic contrasts in the Haast district, mood swings became more apparent - this certainly showed in my freestyle paintings - relative calm (fig 459) to angry chaos (fig 460).

One visit to Jackson Bay I met my match - a cloud of sandflies thwarted me as I tried to sketch.
The flies drove me away in minutes and I felt totally distracted, rather like the figure writhing about in the sand-coloured abstract painted later.
The re-birth figure seems also to make a re-appearance.

The Haast

Journal 7 March - Haast Pass
The most spectacular part of journey so far. Starting from Wanaka early this morning along a road with two large lakes on either side (Waera and Wanaka), many waterfalls, rain forests and scenic reserves.
 Arrive midday at the Haast and book for one night in hostel. Decide to take coast road south as far as it goes - to Jackson Bay. The beach which extends for miles is crowded with many thousands of trees, uprooted and torn. I stop for a while and paint a few of them. (fig. 462).
 I discover that these represent but a fraction of uprooted forest off the mountains where local weather conditions cause massive tree avalanches which occur regularly, sliding down into swollen rivers, sweeping the debris out into the Tasman Sea. The tides then bring them onto the beach.
 Think about the way nature is constantly destroying parts of itself, taking 'risks', so to speak - and compare with my own puny hesitation to do likewise. If only one could 'offload' like an avalanche the rooted fears of change, of challenge.
 On return to hostel, paint some of the tall Nikau palms which proliferate around here in the rain forest.

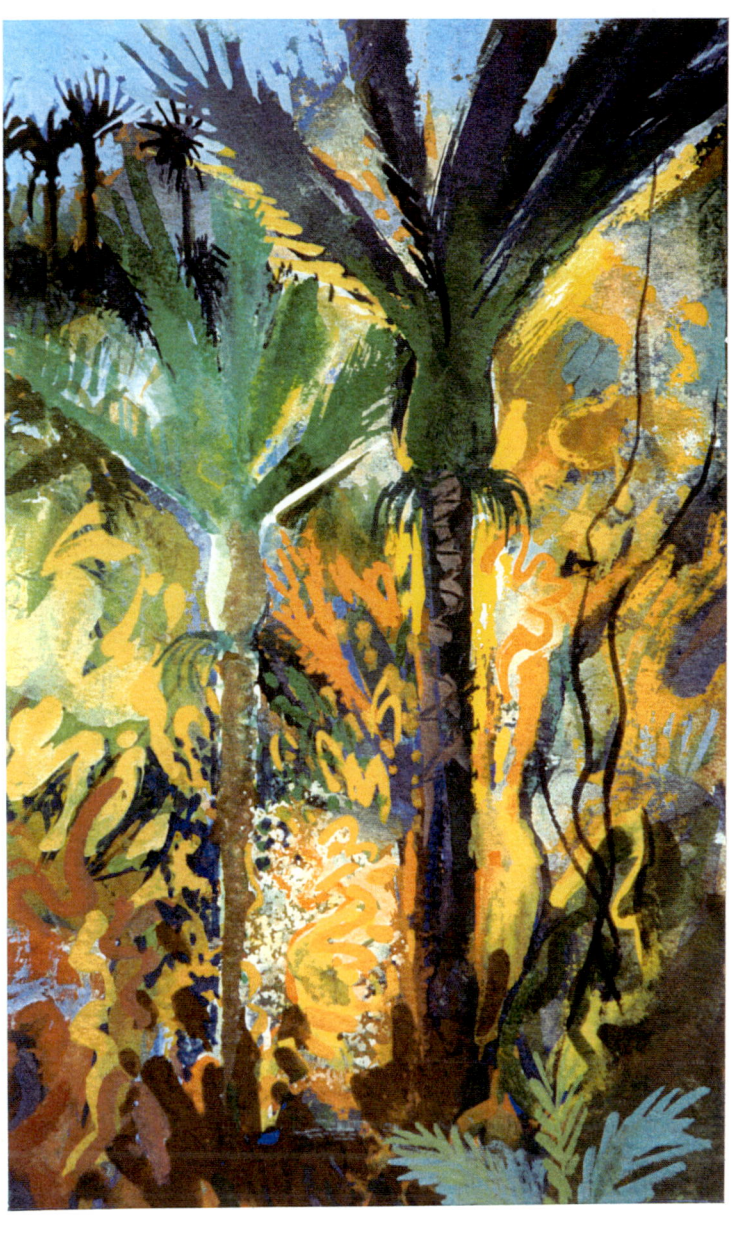

Right: Fig 461

Colourful rainforest on the Haast, tall Nikau palms overshadowing ferns   Gouache

Below: Fig. 462

A few of the many uprooted trees on the Haast beaches.   Watercolour.

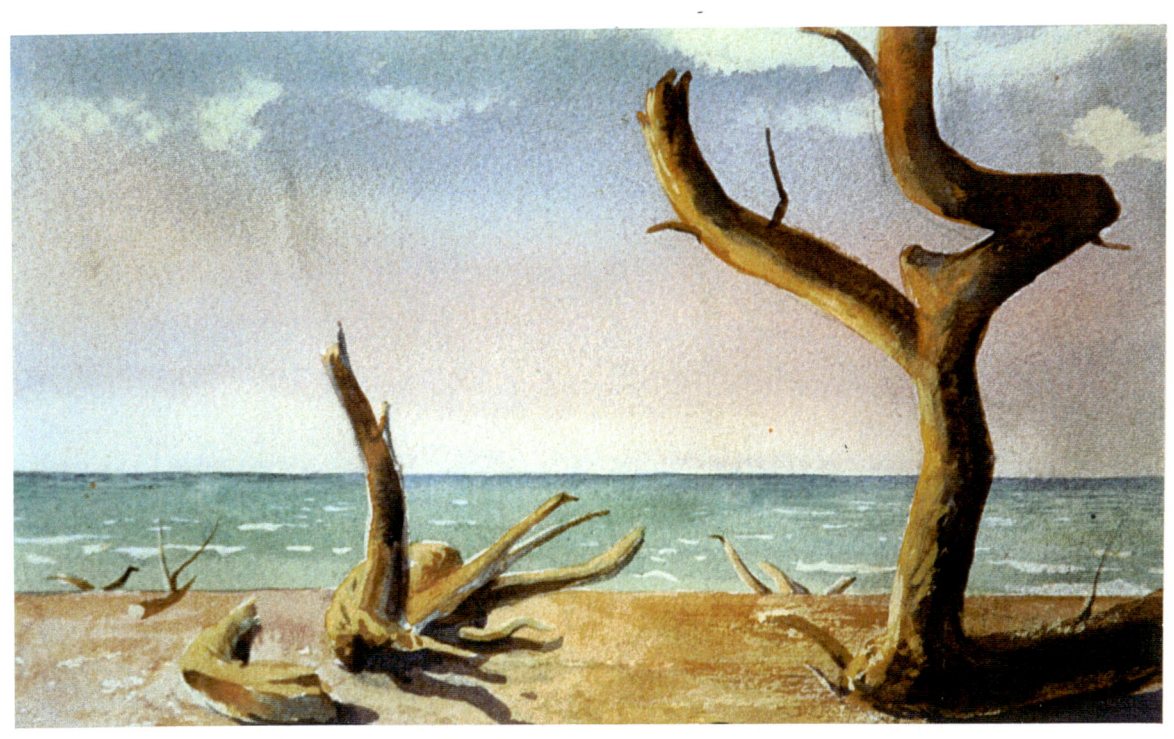

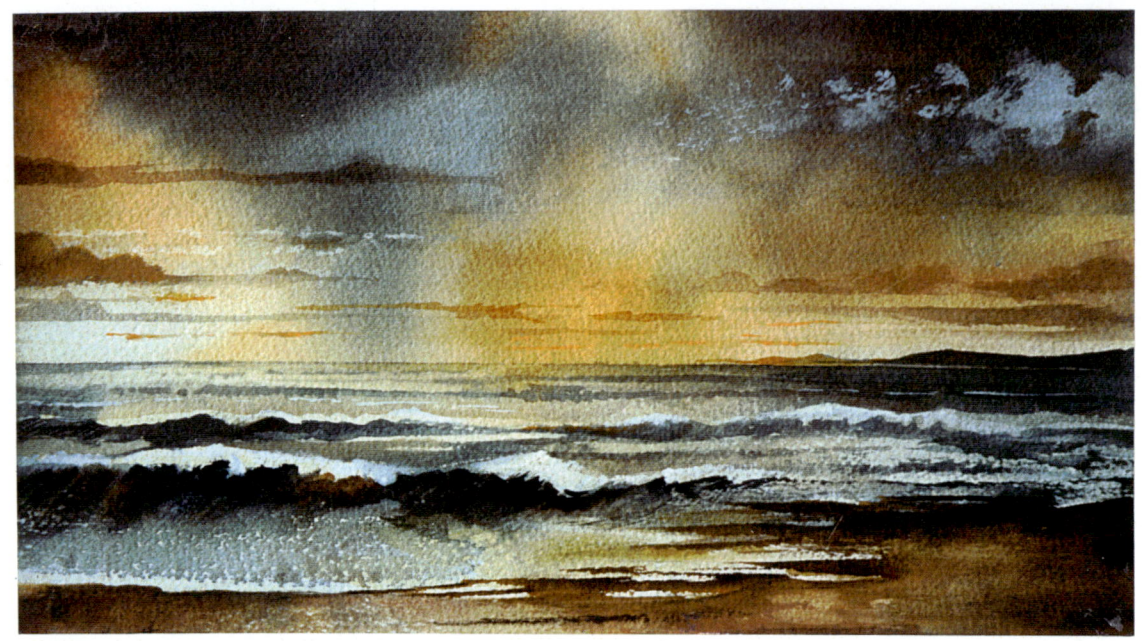

I drove North up the coast, the Tasman sea continually surfing on my left. I stopped to make a quick colour sketch and complete it later (fig 463). Just before I reached Fox township I turned a bend to find a magnificent view of the Alps, Mt. Cook snow-peaked near its centre. - so another sketch for later development (fig. 410 at the beginning of this section).
When I reached Fox, I walked up close to make a drawing of the swinging rhythms of dark lines mixing with the pale blue greens of ice, moving hammock-like across great pinnacles. At the base lay large ice boulders, broken away from the main mass of ice.

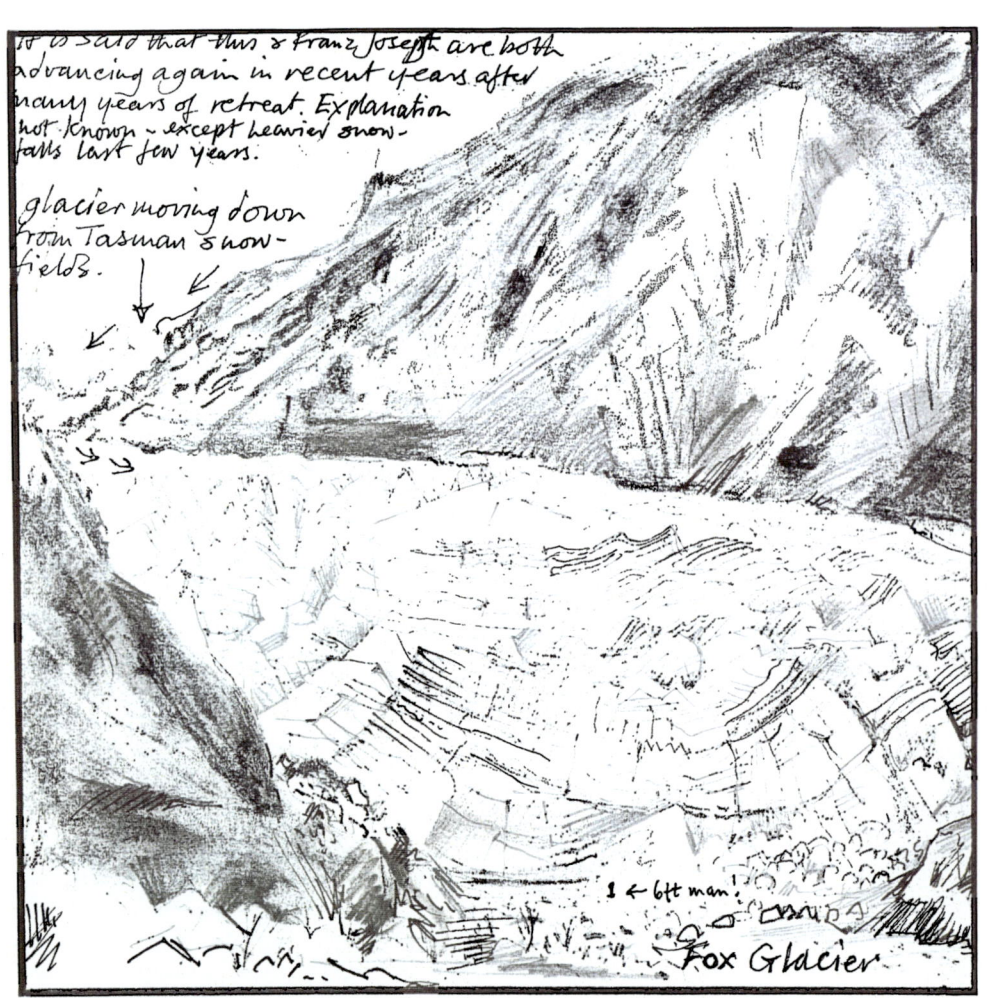

Above: Fig. 463
Tasman Sea, Evening
Watercolour

Left: Fig. 464
The Fox Glacier
Pencil & Ink

The Tasman Sea, Fox, and Franz Josef Glaciers

Journal 8 March – Franz Josef Backpacker.
Settle here for one night. Aware of young exuberant coach groups lodging here – somewhat overwhelmed as I cook my supper. Make an effort to strike up some conversation with a Scot and a couple of Oz students, but for the moment become an 'old fogy' – until I find Rob Morton, someone of my own age. Then discover he's cycling down the whole length of the West Coast – and feel an old fogy again!

Morning – 9 March.
Decide to walk on glacier. Learn a basic technique – our instructor teaches the party I've joined, the Franz Josef 'Shuttle'. This entails climbing or descending sideways on the narrow ice ledges, with the 'free' leg always passing behind the supporting leg. Doing this the body remains vertical – important on ice.
Impossible to convey the sense of scale, it's so vast on the brilliant brightness of the icefield. Less cold than I'd expected and always very jolly and entertaining company.
Write this up before setting off early tomorrow.

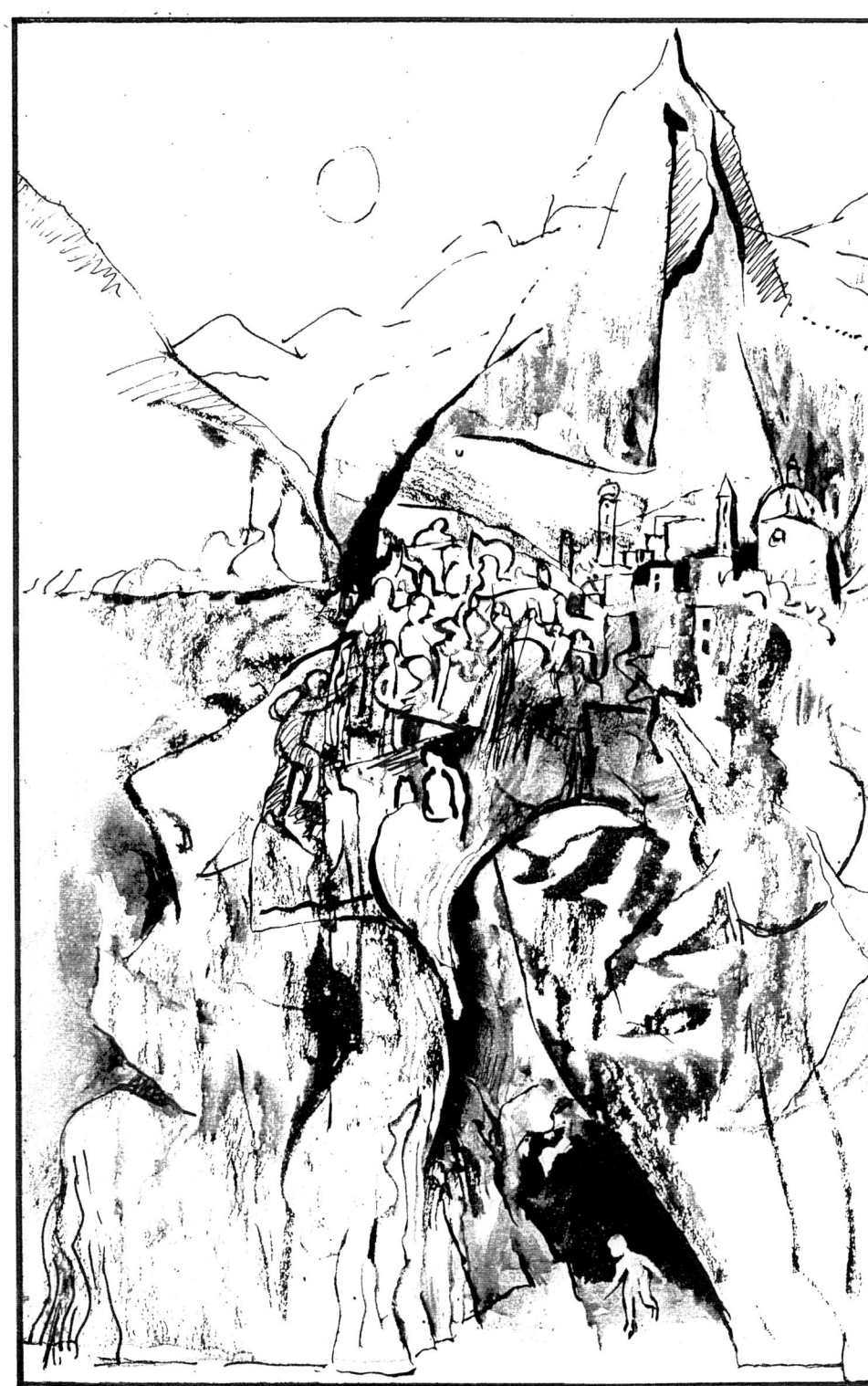

Fig. 465
The Mountainous City

Later draw this city of imagination, a child emerging from a cave, intent on climbing up to the glacier heights.
A large head encompasses the scene.

Brush & Ink

Inchbonnie

I journeyed on again to Hokitika to see this surfing centre, then briefly at Ross, another Goldmine town. On the drive North I had been surprised how many dead possum I had passed, one at every kilometre in some parts, often picked clean by the large harrier hawks here. One particular bird was engorging himself with such ferocity it was reluctant to move as I approached.

I continued towards Greymouth when I recall feeling a sudden urge to turn inland until, in late afternoon, I saw a lake with a cluster of small farms. This was Inchbonnie, a district surrounded by tree-covered mountains. I had stopped to paint the mountains and ancient Kahikateas with sheep grazing when a young farmer and his family drove up and asked to see what I was doing. He asked if I'd do a painting of his farm and I found myself arranging another deal — two smallish watercolours for a week's accommodation.

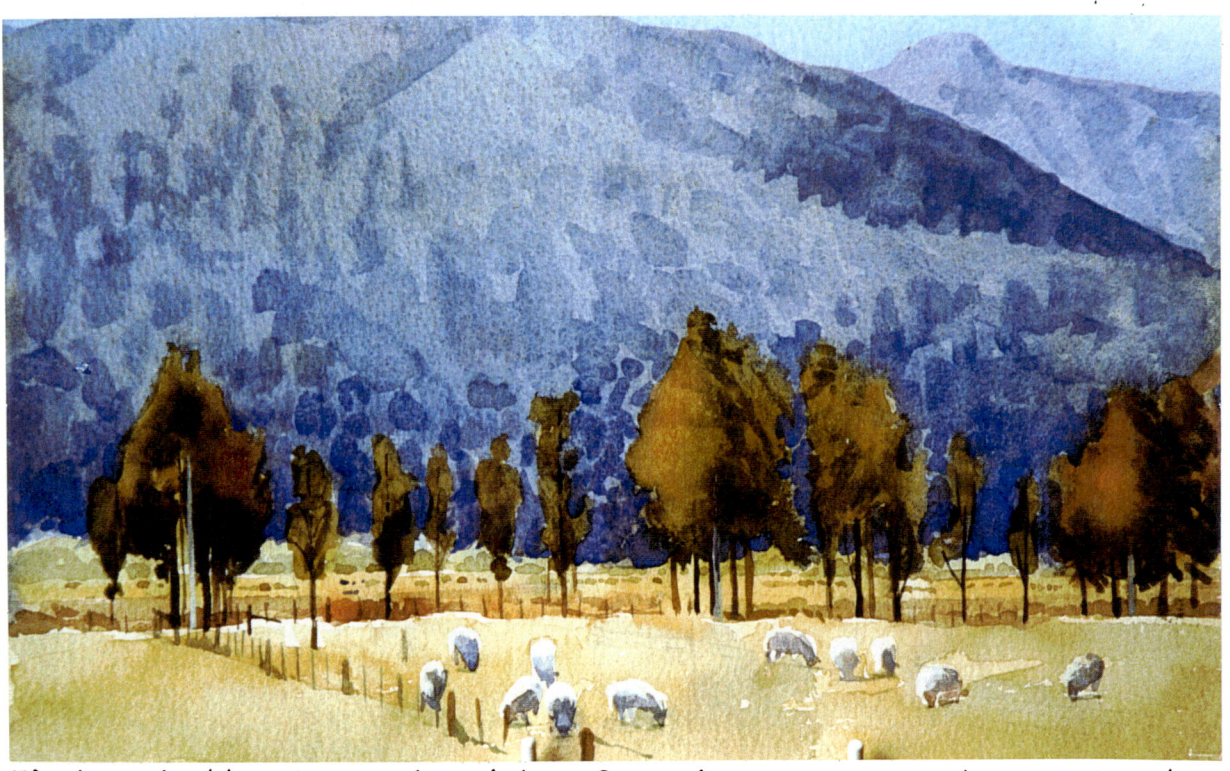

Fig.466   Inchbonnie Flat (the picture Grant found me painting).   Watercolour

---

Journal 10-16 March. – Sheepshed, Inchbonnie.

Delighted by my sleeping quarters in this converted sheepshed. This place offers the calmness I need, the perfect counter to the excessive rush up the West Coast.

Here, amongst ancient trees like Kahikatea and the willows near Lake Poerua, a place to recoup and develop the artwork. I'm asked if I'll draw a favourite pony for one of the girls and for Grant a landscape with his prize Hereford Bull.

I'll leave two watercolours for the family and take photos before I depart.

I cook in a makeshift kitchen with a view over the flat and the narrow end of the lake – many birds fly across the scene. There's been a downside to all the pleasures during the days – a total sense of isolation after sunset, as the shed is some distance from the farmhouse. Also I can't get radio reception in this valley. On the other hand it becomes possible to adjust as the nights pass and I usually see the family in the day. Another factor adds to the loneliness at night – the occasional hoots from the Trans-Alpine Express which passes close by.

Grant, the farmer, has recently bought an old abandoned Catholic Church and is having it transported a few km up the road for conversion into a fishermen's lodge. I give him colour sketch and take another photo.

Fig.467   Grant's 'Catholic Church'
Watercolour

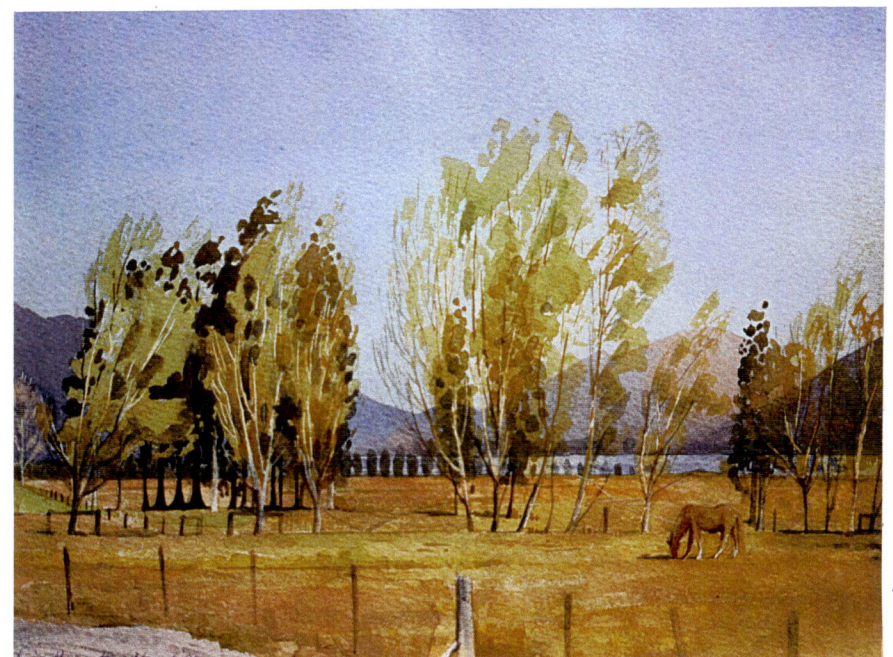

Right: Fig. 468

The flat, Inchbonnie. Willows, with Lake Poerua beyond. 'Sandy' the pony in the foreground paddock.
watercolour

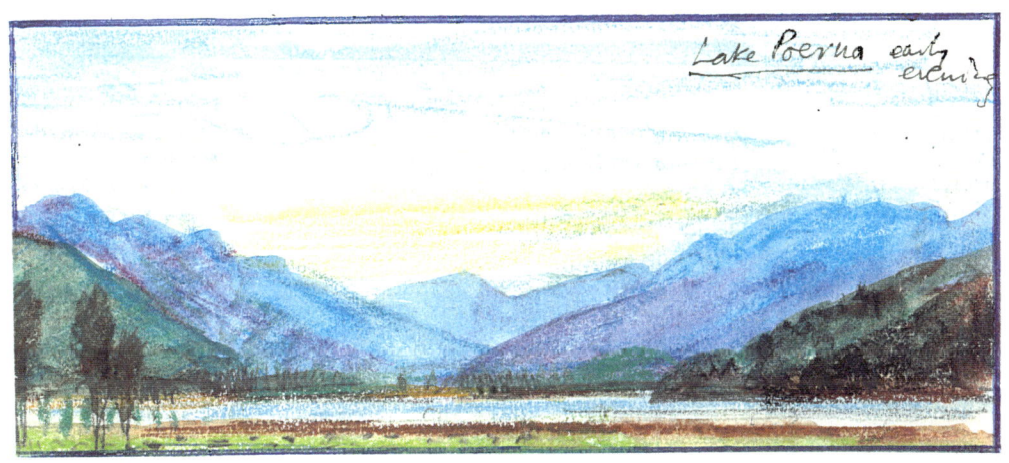

Left: Fig. 469

Lake Poerua – the view I took at each evening
watercolour & chalk

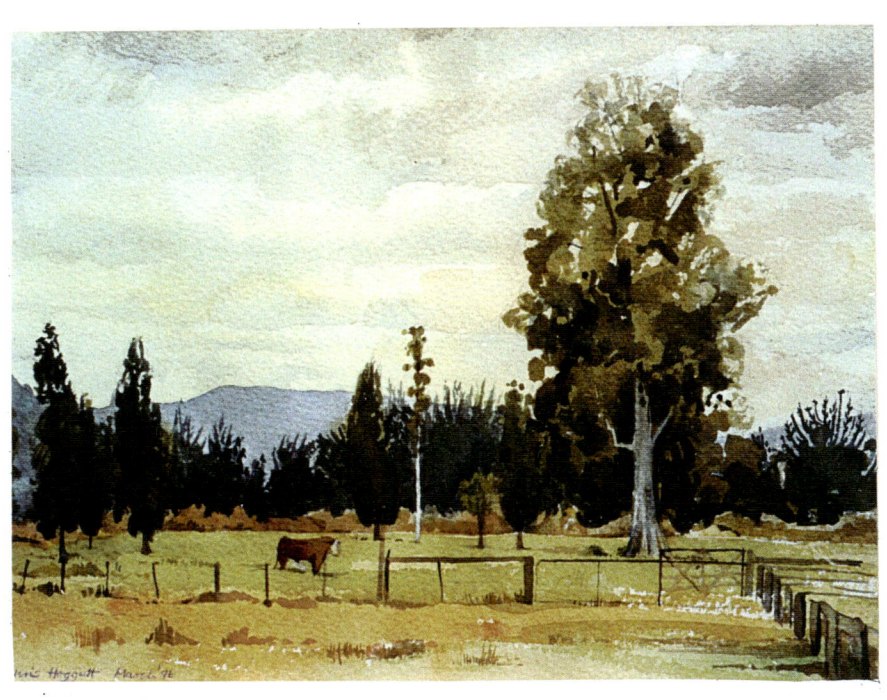

Right: Fig. 470

Some of the ancient Kahitatea trees which remain from the original forest that covered this flat, mostly cut for timber. Grant's Hereford Bull stands in the paddock.

watercolour

Murchison, the Nelson Lakes and Nelson

After a 'rest' period of a week at Inchbonnie I wanted to drive North again, not knowing where I might next stop overnight. I returned to Greymouth, following the coast road towards Westport and noticed an interesting variation on the dustcart — here similar looking vehicles are used for collecting avalanche fall-outs, sizeable rocks being hauled into the truck to keep the road open. (Roadsigns up the West side of South Island warn of closures on many routes in mountainous terrain)

After a day's driving and a stop-off at Punakaiki to see and listen to the monstrous sounds shouting from the blow holes there, I finally reached the township of Murchison.

Journal 17 March - Murchison

Find there's much less planning as travel continues. Whereas I always booked days ahead at the start of the tour, now I take my chance and ask around — there is always somewhere and, as a last resort, I can always pitch my tent (although after my swift departure from rising waters, I'm less enthusiastic about that).

This afternoon I decide to make a long drive to see the Nelson Lake district and on the way have to photograph the interesting patterns caused to the countryside by logging and replanting, especially on hillsides. When I arrived at the Lakes the weather was very unsettled. I'd intended painting but the constant changes of atmospheric conditions made it impossible — but it was good to study the transformations in the mountains and lakes just by looking and taking the occasional photo. Gradually as the day wore on these very steep, deep concealed valleys and their dark lakes became oppressive and I need to get away.

The weather worsens and it feels necessary to move on and return to Nelson, so I stay only two nights in Murchison.

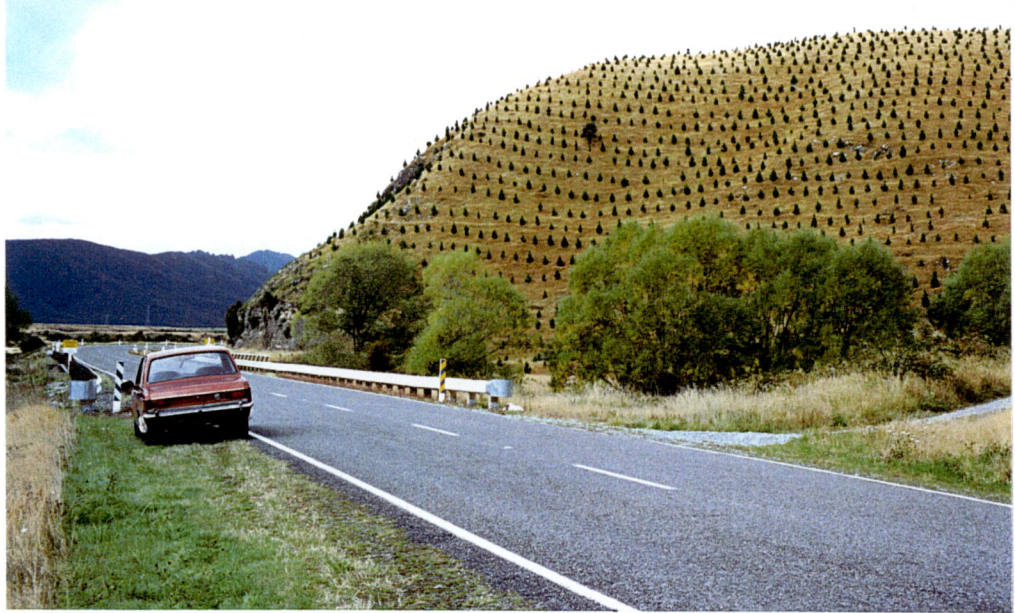

Fig. 471

Between Murchison and the Nelson Lakes. Patterning on a hillside of a new plantation. My old Hillman takes a rest

Photo

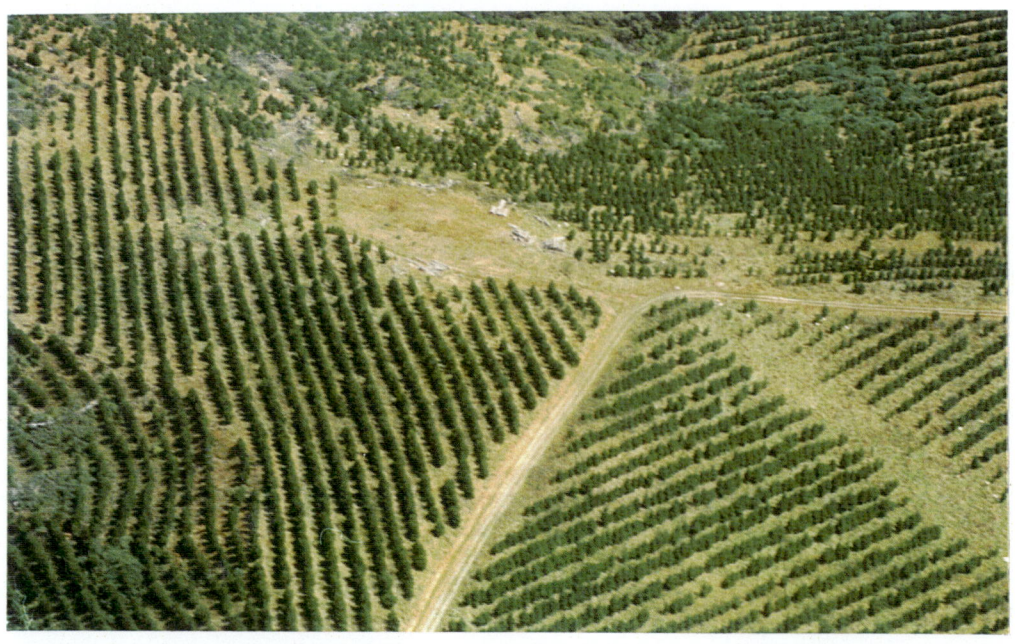

Fig. 472

A photograph taken on the flight from Dunedin to Stewart Island, showing patterning of the land.

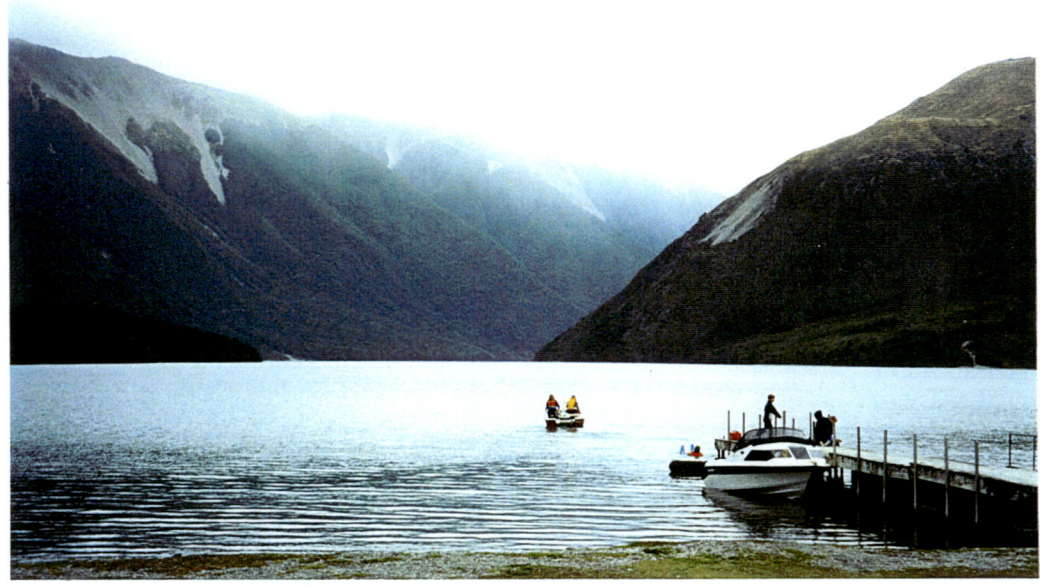

Fig. 473

Lake Rotoiti, the Nelson Lakes. The nearest feeling I got to that experienced at Wastwater in the English Lake district.

I returned to Nelson after the three-month tour and this time settled into another part of the city. I'd decided to re-visit the camp site I'd been forced to abandon and thank the farmer for his timely rescue with a watercolour of the estuary. In return he and his wife offered me a large plate of hogget (my namesake and, out here, a yearling sheep) for dinner. And then came the letdown - the river never flooded the flat and I could have stayed on, but it was a near thing. Nevertheless the romantic aspects of escape from near-drowning were truly squashed!

On the return across the flat I passed by the camp site and recalled a sense of nostalgia for this quiet place. Quiet by then because the cicadas had gone.

Journal 20-21 March - Nelson and Picton Ferry.

Booked ferry crossing for 21st, get a haircut to control the 'wildman' appearance and yet again for the umpteenth time have another check-up on the Hillman.

21st.

This morning, I've just finished packing and happen to glance through the window of my room and see not Nile Street, Nelson, but my own street in England. This weird experience makes me look for structural similarities in the architecture and I find a few salient shapes - but could the inner-self be longing for the return home?

From Picton the crossing of Cook Strait is calm and sunny, the gulls screeching and perching on the superstructure above deck on the lookout for scraps. The ferry docks at Wellington midday so I contemplate travelling for most of the day until I reach New Plymouth.

At this point, re-reading the journal, I notice a strange omission - I'd failed to write up any mention of Mount Egmont. From the start of the Southern tour I'd intended to visit and hopefully part-climb this vast symmetrical cone of an extinct volcano, which was said to offer spectacular views around the South west seaboard.

Yet on my drive up from the ferry, when I should have turned west towards New Plymouth I deliberately turned due North. I recall feeling apprehensive as I approached the fork in the road and now thought of the many reasons why I wanted to avoid the district. I remember dismissing excuses for tiredness, wanting to move on, and having already seen too much, and realised I was fearful about the mountain itself. It was partly to do with its sheer size and its symmetry but also because I had been advised not to venture onto the higher levels alone.

Finally I drove on to Taupo, and promised myself that one day I probably would attempt the climb - in company.

Journal 22 March - Taupo 'Backpacker'

Return again to this much used staging-post, and visit the nearby geothermal site known as 'Craters of the Moon'. The craters are partially concealed by plant growth around their perimeters but dark steaming holes appear occasionally, emitting strange howls, squeaks and groans from deep fumaroles and steam vents. A strong sulphurous smell prevails. This is a highly active landscape, bubbling and exploding with life. This turbulent site mirrors a feeling of some active time ahead, and a return to Auckland.

Auckland

After the long tour of South Island I was going to have a lengthy period of recuperation with my family – or so I thought, for as soon as I arrived there was an eruption of another kind. A visit to a dentist revealed inflammation across the lower jaw and I was given a choice – either an extraction which was expensive, or antibiotics until my return home which was much cheaper. I chose the latter.

In the meantime all the travel equipment was sorted and an array of sketches spread out with a view to developing the most promising pieces.

Journal 23 March – 1 April – Auckland.

25th – Family all away today, so opportunity to work in 'studio' conditions. Looking at and developing some earlier sketches – or so I hope for I can't find the energy or inclination to begin. Decide to wait until a little later which turns out to be a little too late, the evening closing in and inspiration fading with it. Realise there never was an appropriate time ahead – its always in the here and now. All the space I'd allotted myself frittered away, looking for some insoluble dimension, lying within some 'hidden fold of time', just at the periphery of things. What do I mean? Perhaps that there is some sense of order within the chaos.

I take one small abstract which I can't understand. It allows no interpretation, is pre-verbal, has no apparent meaning, and I decide to continue with it regardless...

27th – Work is dire today. There's no breadth of life and I tear it up. Perhaps a period of transition?

28th – Negative feelings, seem insurmountable. Could this be, in reality, a glimpse towards a breakthrough?

29th – Awake from a heavy 'downer' – try to paint my way out of it, enlarging one of my hilly landscapes, a bit of imaginative drawing concerning an old 'backpacker', a few creatures, an encouraging gesture in the sky... Some hopeful stirrings....

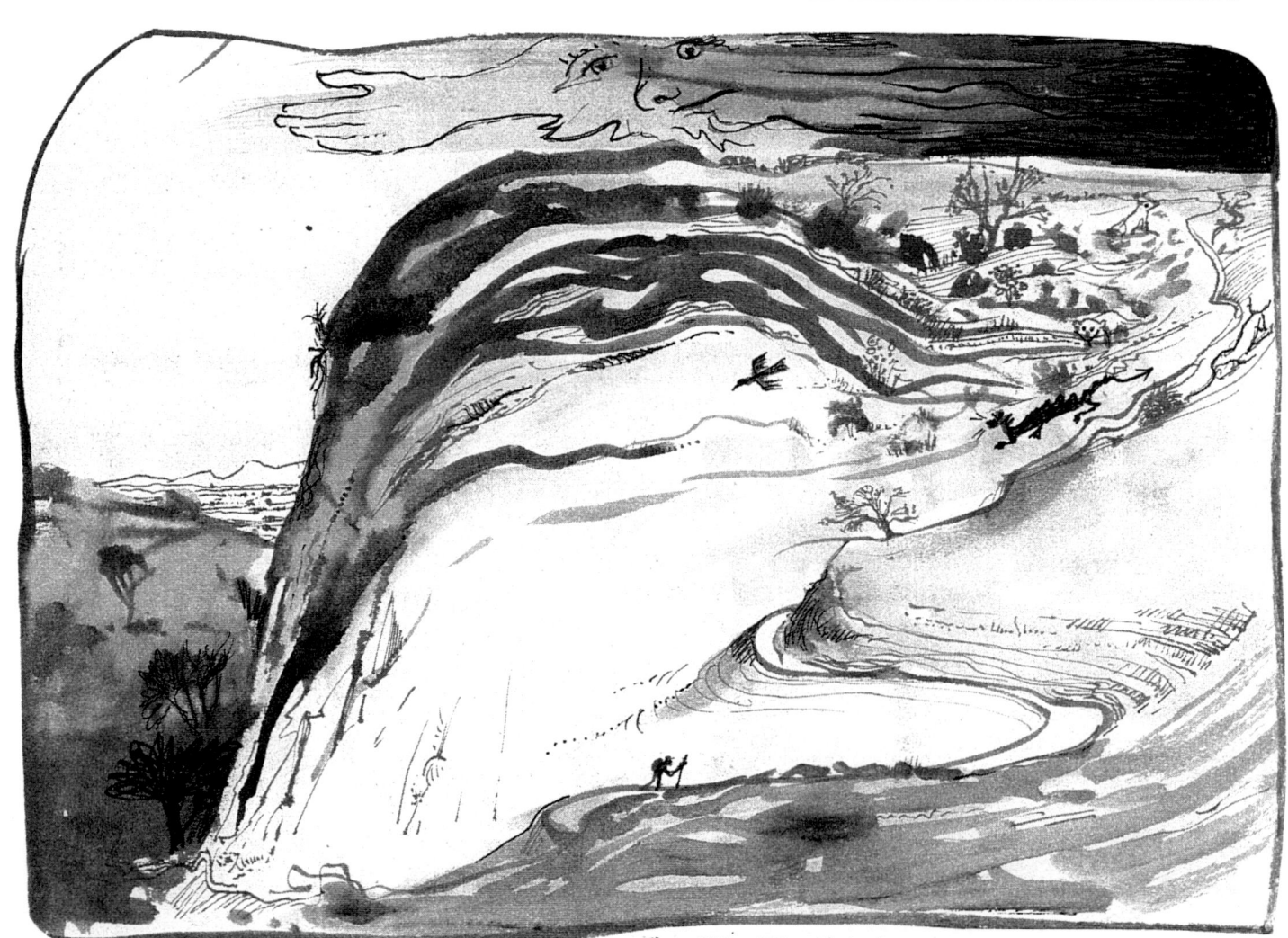

Fig. 474 *The Helping Hand* Pen & wash

Attempting to overcome the angst of the past few days I made myself useful about the house, responding to requests to construct a shelving unit, a garden table and a fender for the fireplace. These activities lifted the mood – and postponed creative struggles ahead. Realising that only three weeks remained before the return flight I decided on one more journey: return to Coromandels on East Coast that I'd yet to discover. I arranged to stay in a bach at Tairua.

Tairua, Coromandels

> **Journal 2 April - Tairua**
> After the people-filled days of Auckland here's the antithesis - total isolation in this timber shed - an early bungalow (1880?) or bach. Facilities simple - 'long drop' outside; an electric frying pan for all cooking needs. Throw back on one's own resources for as long as I can endure it - possibly five days.
> Unloading all the equipment from the Hillman and the bare minimum of art materials.
> I see a small mount only a mile away and drive up as far as possible, then walk to the top - a long view across a straggle of small islands and rocks into the Pacific.
> I note the presence of a couple looking over my shoulder and feel very resentful.
> Aware that solitude is essential when working.
> It's now April and I'm aware that Autumn has arrived - it's getting dark around 6.30 p.m.

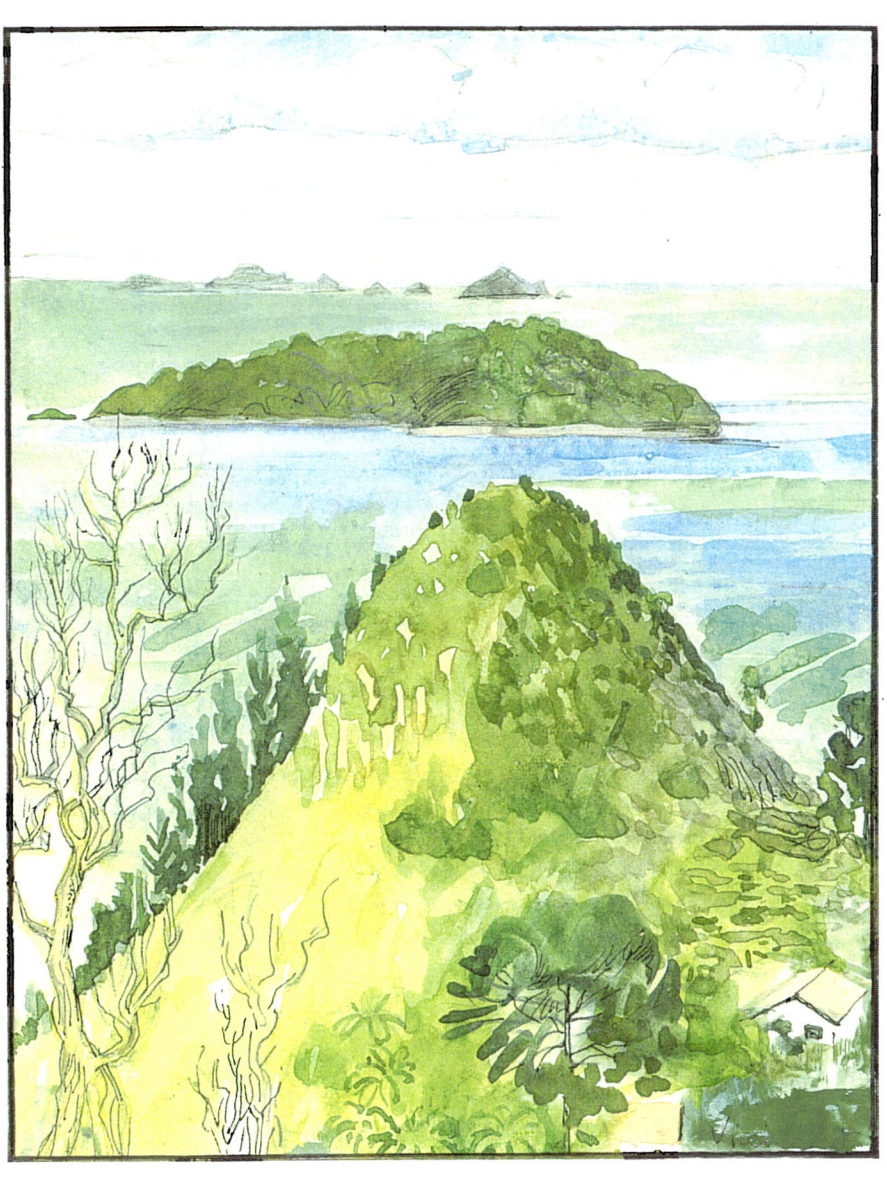

Right: Fig. 475

Paku Mount, Tairua.

Watercolour

After I bypassed Mount Egmont on the return trip North, I'd considered that to be a psychological defeat, or at least a retreat from the intended visit. What next occurred seemed recompense enough:

> **Journal 3 April - Broken Hills**
> At the entrance to 'Collins Drive' Golden Hills Mine.
> The legend on the sign outside the mine read "This mine tunnel goes through 500 metres. To enter, torch, hardhat, and warm clothing should be taken - WATCH YOUR HEAD"
> As I'd brought none of the listed items I chose to stay outside and draw the entrance. As I was completing the work I saw tiny points of light and heard voices advancing from within, until three warmly dressed people emerged.
> One of the group enthused about an interesting side shaft some 50 metres in - would I care to look? He'd lend me a torch. Hesitantly, partly because not kitted up, but more because I still feared dark holes, I somewhat reluctantly accepted his offer.... it was only 50 metres inside....
> Advancing with a pale beam of light I looked out for the side-shaft but, after some five minutes, became aware I'd missed it for I sensed I must have covered at least 100 metres.
> It was at this point I knew I'd subconsciously made a decision to advance as far as I dared and found myself pressing on, knocking my head a few times and getting steadily wetter from constant drips and trickles of water from the roof. Becoming more nervous because I loathe confined spaces, I glanced back to see a pinprick of light - the entrance from which I'd entered. I'd heard mention of another shaft further inside and, despite more dripping of water forming in pools underfoot I felt I'd try just a little further.
> I decided I needed to have seen at least one of the two side-shafts and I made a few extra steps to be greeted by a marvellous starry sky of phosphorescent points. The colony of glow worms had me transfixed and transformed my fear into delight at finding this glow of light in the grave of darkness.
> At the same moment I discovered also the deeper shaft and returned with all my fears allayed and even found the shaft I'd missed earlier. I think the owner of the torch was relieved to have it back - I'd been inside for longer than he or I had expected.

Broken Hills

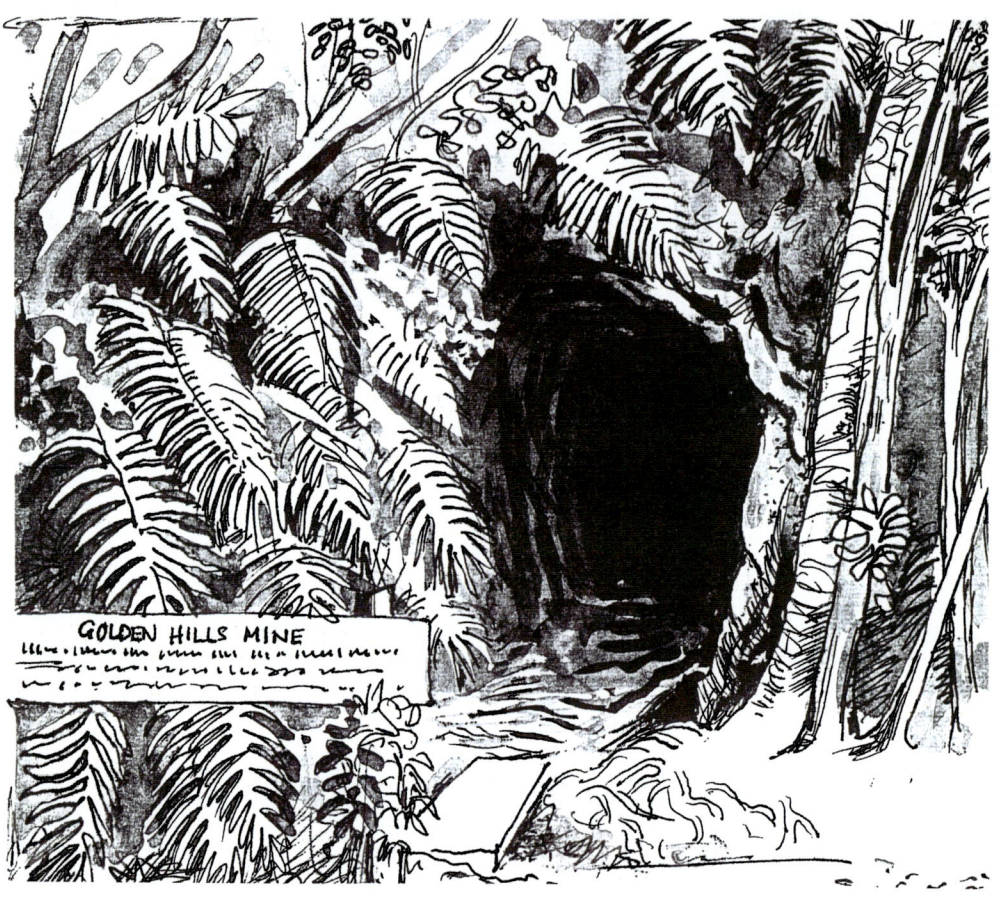

Fig. 476

Entrance to Golden Hills Mine, Coromandel.

Pen, Ink & Wash

Journal 4 April - Tairua.
Elation follows yesterday's experience - feeling I've overcome most of my nervousness about the dark. Also some 'insight' into the darkness - finding the light within. Who said 'Only within the inner dark will one find the light'?
5th (Good Friday) All the stores closed and people seem to have left the township. The place seems deserted, although I can see some boats on the inlet nearby.
Still exhilarated after the mine exploration - perhaps now I could endure the pain of concentration long enough to develop some of my sketches?
Perhaps one form of endurance can metamorphose into other areas - like perseverance. Whatever, the vision of light in inner blackness - order out of chaos.

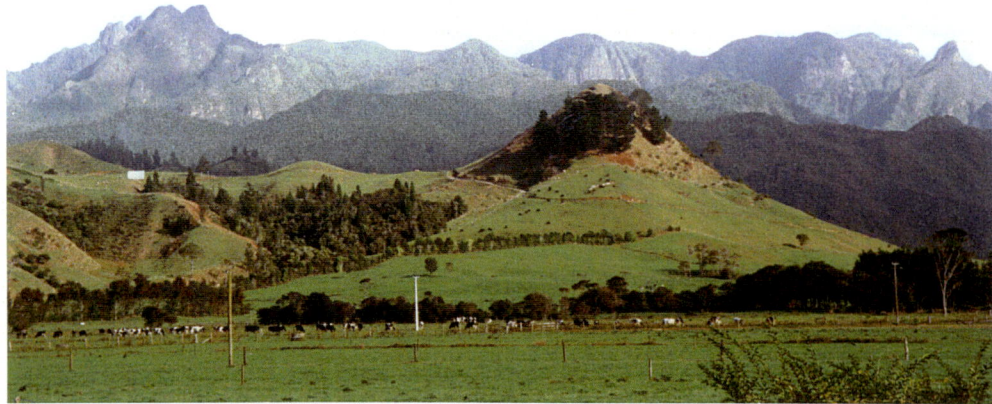

Fig. 477

Photograph of the Broken Hills district, close to Tairua - such a contrast to the gentle Cotswolds I know.

The following day, everything packed away, I headed back to Auckland but via the Martha Hill Mine - a misnomer now-a-days, as it's a vast hole in the ground. Started in 1878, when gold was discovered, it was a hill. This commercial mine will eventually reach a depth of 200 metres.
At Paeroa township I see great stacks of old tree trunks in the fields adjoining the road - all ancient native trees from old silted up valleys which once swept down towards the sea. They are now dug up for their valuable timber, used for carving and fine joinery and furniture. Like archaeological finding, discovering and using the old to enhance the present.....

Auckland

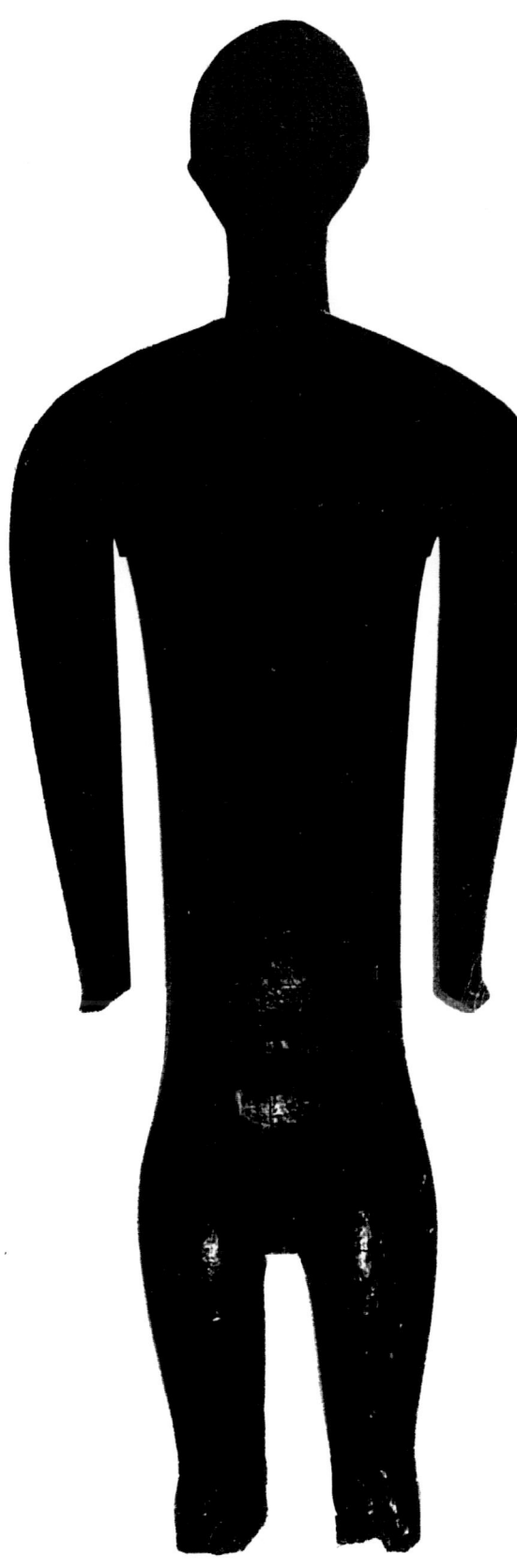

Fig. 478 'Kava de Hine Aligi' - Carved wood goddess. Auckland Museum.

The very first and last man-made image I saw in New Zealand. On my last visit I photographed this silhouette of this Polynesian giant goddess, approx. 9ft. high. (From the Nuknoro atoll in the Caroline Islands).
Overleaf: An annotated map I kept in the journal, reminding myself of dates and corresponding place names throughout the tour.

Journal 6 April. Auckland.

Easter Sunday! Manukau Car Auctions - $16 entry into a large car park where one attempts to sell one's own car. Given a printed notice with spaces for you to fill in relevant details. - I write in $1100 in the hope of getting $1000. I sit about, walk, chat to prospective buyers.... and someone looks under the bonnet for the third time, and I have a sale for $900 which is only ten less than my purchase price. Even with all my services and replacement parts, it worked out much cheaper than a five month hire rate.

Sunday Evening. An evening with my Kiwi in-laws. We talk about Maori fortifications used during the New Zealand wars with the Brits. Apparently the Brits were so impressed with the Maori trench systems that these were adapted by the army in World War One.

There was also interesting talk about the Maori language - their use of metaphor to replace adjectives which are not used, hence their ability to create myth and their skill in oratory - the spinning out of long descriptions of people and things.

Everyone showed an interest in my trips - explained it was as much about a search and self-testing as discovering the country. My daughter thought my long tour South was an achievement for an 'oldie', which felt very reassuring. Even now, I begin to sense a psychological strengthening.....

A Dream - 9th April - I'm a teacher/therapist on a weekend course somewhere. The purpose is to get information about the arts. A modest list of students enrol to start with, until numbers increase as weekend approaches, then I need whole place to accommodate everyone. As course starts I'm **constantly interrupted** by older members of staff... the gist is, 'What are you proposing to teach?' I walk out, searching for a loo which I then find is the subject matter for a painting class. As I don't intend exposing myself I search elsewhere. Another teacher is dealing with technical painting matters, and I suddenly become inadequate.

When I wake I realise the 'older' voices continue to question what I'm about - there's still opposition to change...

Journal 13 April

Reflections on the journey. This country symbolises change, contrast and movement. In the movement of the land itself - earthquakes, the explosive force of its geysers and fumaroles, the avalanches of trees and the destructive force of its rivers.

Then the great contrasts - the heights of the Southern Alps and the depths of the sea trench off Kaikoura - and not forgetting the eruptive power of an active volcano and the stillness of an extinct one.

Also the hidden depths behind the surface appearance: the compression of plate tectonics which cause the upheavals of land and the 'quakes in Westland'.

All these natural phenomena mirror the interior happenings, bringing together many loose strands concerning the curative aspects of the past few years.

16 - 20 April:
Last few days around town with family; Sold three pics!
An Island Dream: 'An Island, quite small, surrounded by a vast ocean. The land has many deep valleys, fiords and mountains with a tendency to be either threatening or welcoming. Voices whisper into my ears about eradicating something but I'll have none of it, for I know these mysterious places with their ancient past contain the wisdom I seek. I keep travelling the valley slopes which can be dark and forbidding, but I observe rich colourations which hold great promise and potential peace'.

This dream is a summation of my N.Z. experience; conflicting inner voices - overall optimism about the journey.

281

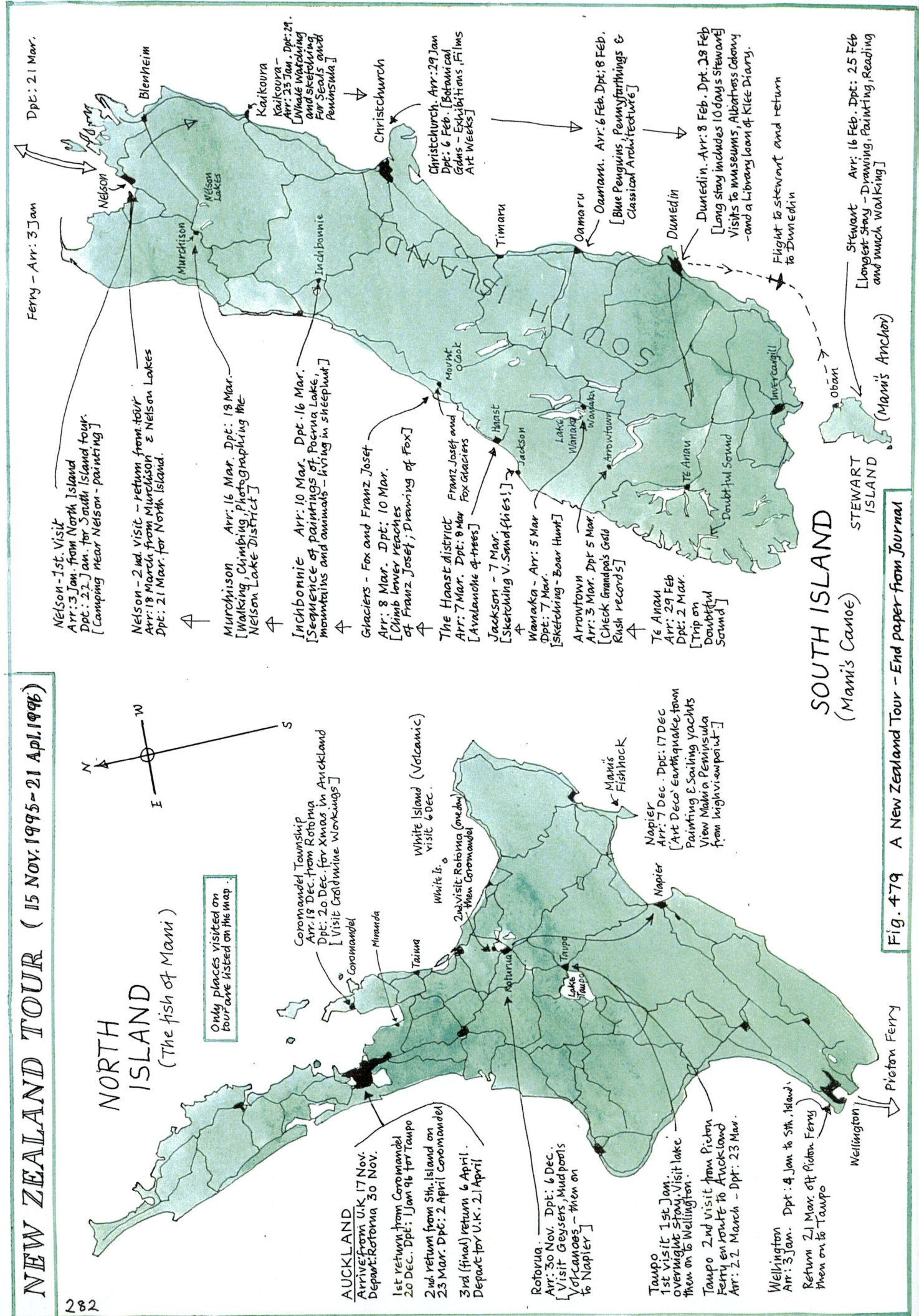

Fig. 479 A New Zealand Tour – End paper from Journal

Note

I departed from Auckland for Sydney, then Bangkok and arrived back home nearly thirty hours later. Gradually, after a few weeks, I gathered up the notes, sketches and paintings and reviewed what had occurred. With the artwork I didn't feel I'd achieved very much. Large paintings hadn't materialised, visions and developments culled from the trip seemed uninteresting.

On the other hand, the search for regeneration and insight into the therapy years seemed most fruitful, real feelings of creativity were established, even if not often shown in the artwork.

Many months later however a number of freestyle paintings began to reflect the stored-up imagery from the journey. In particular the few illustrated here summed up the essence of the places I'd absorbed. The paintings shown below and overleaf suggested for me the expansive and optimistic nature of Otago (South Island) landscape.

In retrospect, the benefit of long, stored-up memories expanded and helped to develop the visionary imagery for the final sections of this book.

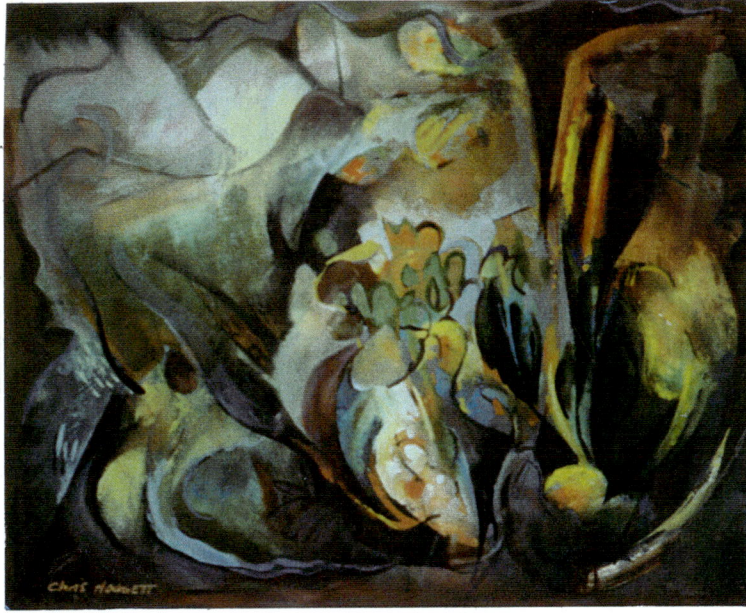

Fig. 480   Near the Southern Alps   Gouache

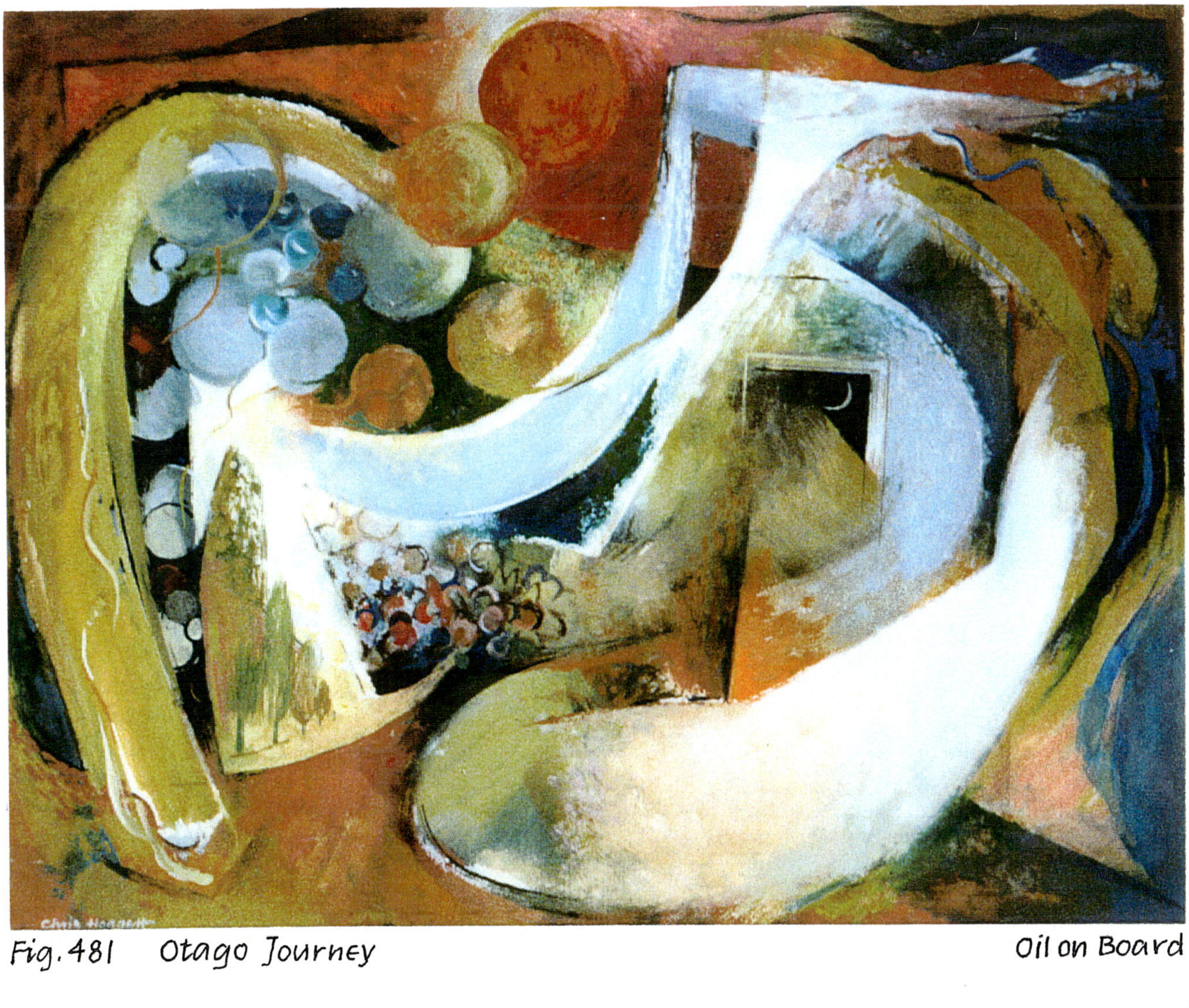

Fig. 481   Otago Journey   Oil on Board

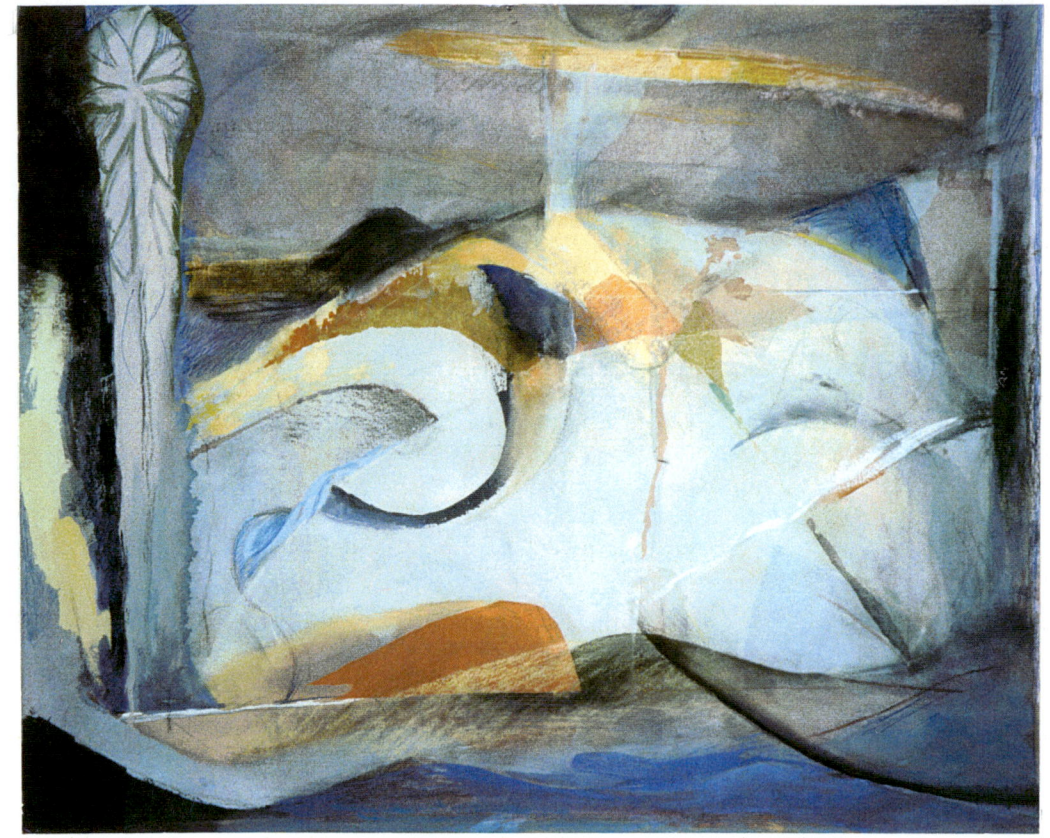

Fig. 482 Antipodian Memories   Gouache & Collage

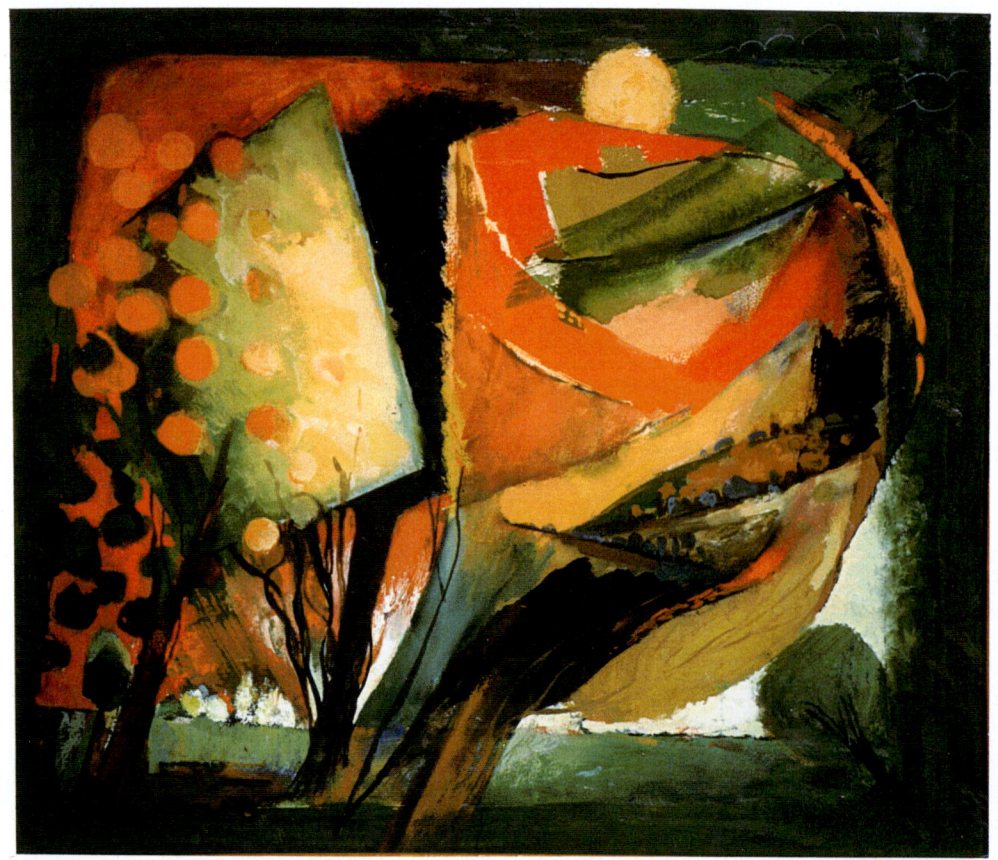

Fig. 483 The Orchard   Gouache

PART FIVE

Five Visionary Landscapes

CLEEVE COMMON AND UFFINGTON RIDGEWAY	287
1 UFFINGTON WHITE HORSE	289
Gaia, the metamorphosis of the land beneath the White Horse, known as 'The Manger'	
2 BELAS KNAP - LONG BARROW	297
Earth Mother, connections between Neolithic tomb and a Babylonian Epic	
3 JURASSIC WESTWOOD	307
Finding the feminine through painting and its manipulation reveal a vision	
4 THE STONE PIT	315
The 'Hero' and its supporters; a number of discoveries in the rock face of a disused quarry	
5 POSTLIP WARREN	325
Earth Woman, another discovery in the valley below the quarry	

CLEEVE COMMON
AND UFFINGTON RIDGEWAY

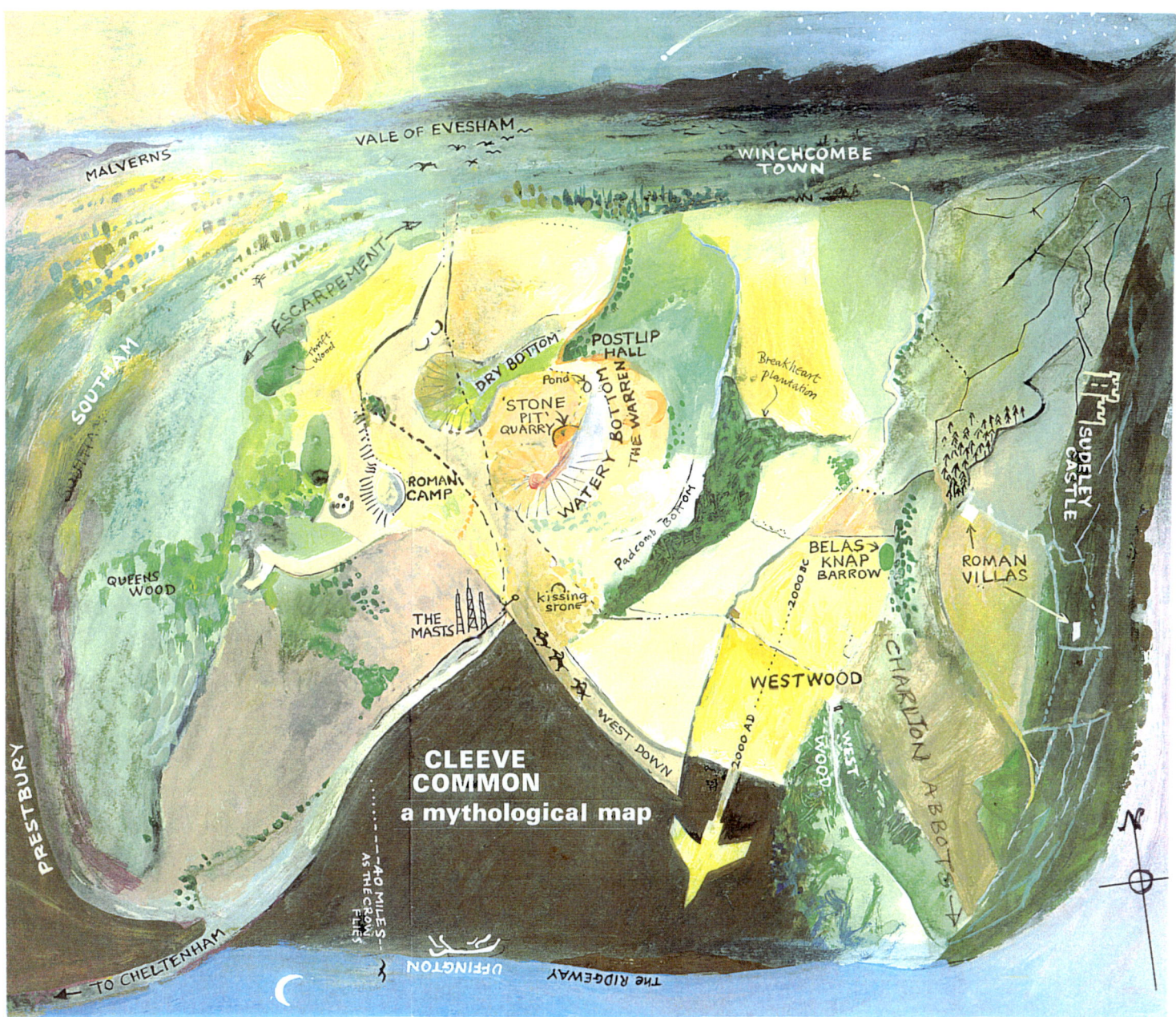

Fig. 484   A Mythological Map - Cleeve Common   Gouache, Pen & Ink

This great limestone piece of common land on Cleeve Hill in Gloucestershire is the highest point of the Cotswolds, rising to 330 metres, with a periphery of about ten miles containing 1000 acres of land. An escarpment along part of the western edge overlooking the great Vale below offers views of the Malverns and the Welsh mountains and, to the north, the Vale of Evesham. Having also three low valleys it has for me the ingredients of the perfect walking place. It has also many ancient building sites including a Neolithic barrow, Roman Villas, medieval Castle and a Hall; an early Hill Camp and many old quarries — and in this century, three radio masts.

The myths described on the following pages were engendered within this hill-top and valley site (except the Berkshire White Horse) and helped transform a repressed personal history into a 'breakout' of expressive art work, and an affirmation against the years of depression.

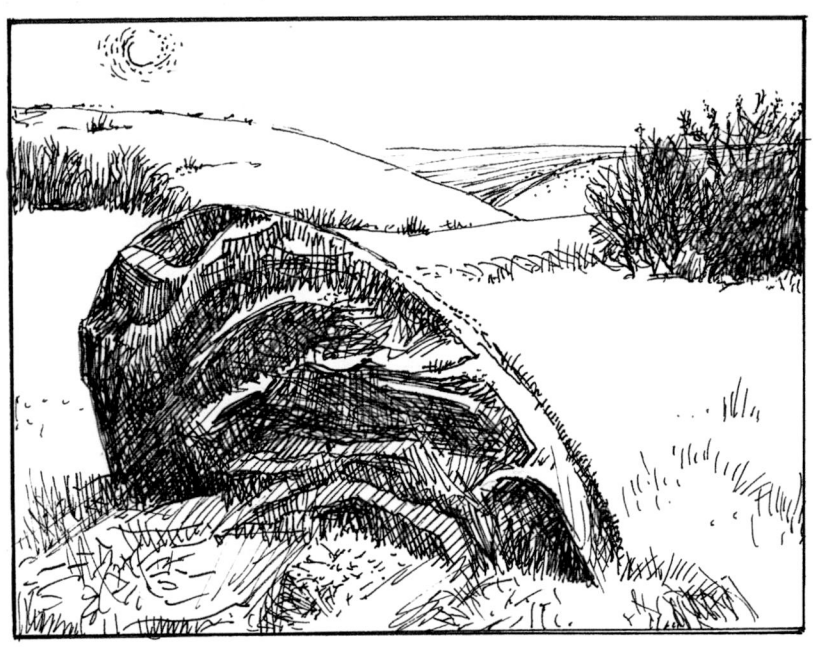

Fig. 485   The 'Kissing Stone'   Pen & Ink

This singularly isolated semi-circular stone stands sentinel just North of the Masts, leading to the approach to Watery Bottom and, to the right, Belas Knap and Westwood areas.

It became a touchstone, icon, an entrance to a world of something 'other'.

Occasionally, like a Pope, I bent forward to kiss it, acknowledging that perhaps I had just arrived in this new country.

Perhaps its my personal Cotswold 'Blarney Stone'.

VISIONARY LANDSCAPES

1993 to 1998 were, in hindsight, what could be called the visionary years. During this period four Earthmothers or Goddesses were to reveal themselves, and a group including a Hero and his Warriors were also to make their presences felt.

All these projections (some might prefer the term myth or fantasy) were a necessary response to the stressful and depressive upheavals due to working with 'C.' on so much repressed subconscious material.

I decided to encapsulate each visionary sequence of work within separate sections, treating each as if it were an isolated episode, when in fact each experience overlapped and intertwined with the others in the course of these five years.

Uffington White Horse was first seen in August 1993, Belas Knap Barrow in February 1994, Westwood Valley in March 1994, the 'Stone Pit' quarry in May 1994 and the Postlip Warren, May '97.

Although the particular piece of landscape or its man-made re-shaping was the source of a 'revelation', each place had its own unique voice — or I felt that it did. For example my projection into the Uffington land formation was strong enough to produce a 'fantasy' response (figs 490 to 498). Whereas the countless drawings and paintings of the Westwood site only gave up their secret within the last few paintings in the studio, almost four years later, long after I'd worked at the location itself. The mirage here lay not within the land but in the use of paint itself, through a process of evolution with the brush on the canvas.

The 'Stone Pit', or quarry, was different again. Here the rock/stones were dumb — (had no voice) for a long period as I made various studies of the place in a very realistic manner until, quite suddenly, five apparitions were activated by two particular dreams and a free-style drawing. One final character showed up nearly four years later (pages 315 to 324).

The Postlip Warren experience came not so much from the place itself but from a painting of a painting I'd done much earlier (fig. 547).

Belas Knap was the odd one out as there was nothing to reveal, given that its builders had conceived a Goddess shape for themselves, and yet, by lying face down on her great belly, 'she' it was who quickened some intuitive sense to uncover the subsequent finds.

(Although Uffington was first seen in 1993, it wasn't until a year later that the vision occurred — some months after Belas Knap).

1 UFFINGTON WHITE HORSE

The first sighting was from below, an oblique viewpoint with long thin lines of chalk sweeping across the soft green just below the ridge. Momentarily losing sight of it on the climb I caught sight of gliphs of white as I reached the Ridgeway path. Here were wide swathes of chalk no longer recognisable as a complete creature — was this part its back, that part of a leg?

I found parallels with the strange geometric forms known as Nazca lines in Peru which could only be appreciated fully if viewed from the air, and wondered if these ancient tribes had something in common — the ability to visualise shapes as if seen from above whilst working only on the ground.

Perhaps they had made preparatory designs and then scaled them up on some sort of grid system. Or could they have conceivably have discovered a method of becoming airborne using great taut animal skins sewn and fashioned into kites to view and direct the layout below?

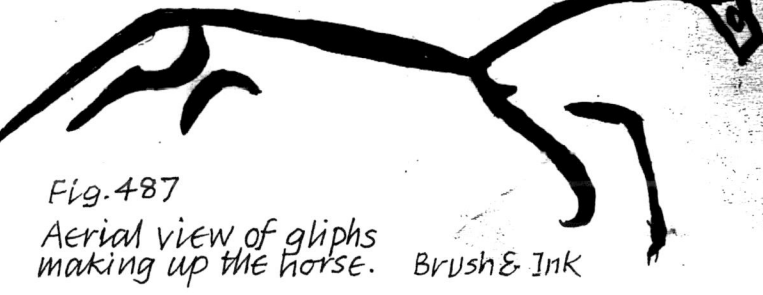

Fig. 487 Aerial view of gliphs making up the horse. Brush & Ink

Fig. 486 Freestyle abstract pen drawing based on gliphs of horse.

Right: The first colour sketch after third visit to the site.

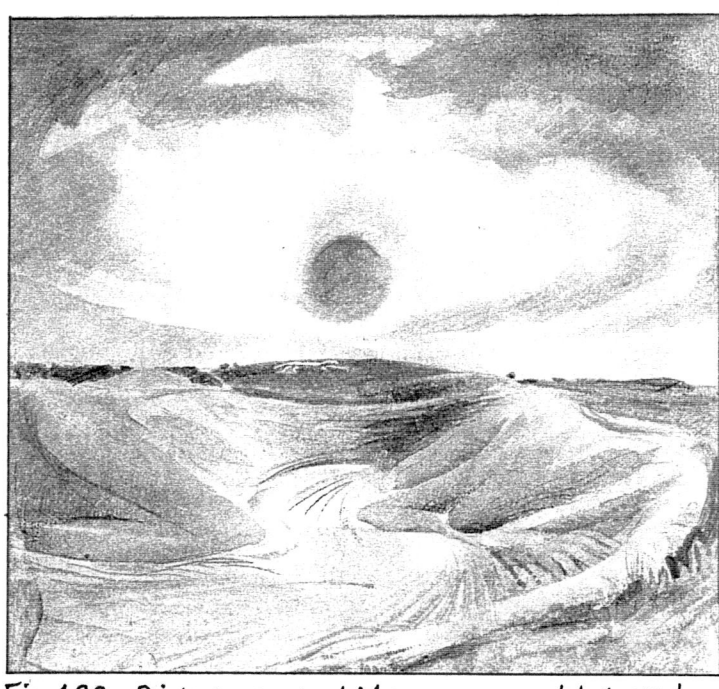

Fig. 488 Ridgeway and Manger. Watercolour

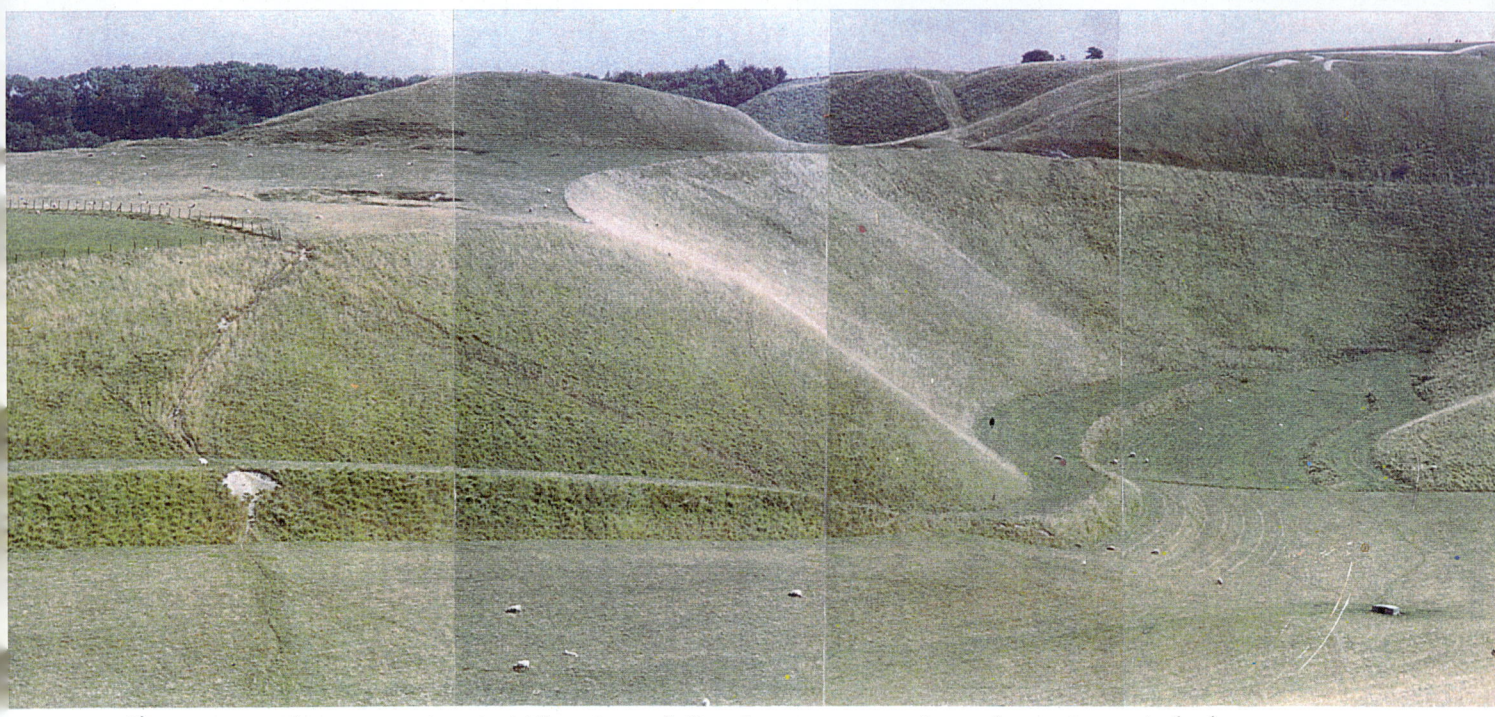

Fig. 489 Photograph of Uffington White Horse area (see text top right).

These meditative thoughts grew out of the first visit to Uffington in August 1993 and it would be some months before returning again with a friend who observed a few things I'd overlooked — the viewpoint from the small flat-topped tump of Dragon Hill. Just below lay the flat hollow known as the Manger. Unaccountably I was intrigued by the name. A holding place for sheep and horses?

Having seen this shape, had the Iron Age tribe chosen this site where a lively, youthful creature (perhaps a dragon or horse) might leap up from its feed below to settle on the ridge above? From where sprang this idea about this piece of ancient Wessex countryside?

With hindsight I must have been projecting feelings and ideas into something I knew nothing about and it wasn't until a visit about a year later that I was to uncover a possible explanation for these early musings.

In the summer of 1994, walking across a lower level to view the Manger again, I found my interest drawn more to the surrounding forms which shaped this flat hollowed space — a curious mix of undulating folds and slopes.

After a few hours, having nearly completed a painted study of the scene I became subliminally aware of some underlying form just beneath the surface of the land, and was suddenly jolted into a realm which could not have been anticipated — where only Gods or Goddesses reigned. In empathising so closely I now glimpsed parts of something so monstrous it caused a sharp intake of breath.

First the head, face down, partially covered by a folded arm. Then a suggestion of another arm leading towards a wrist with long fingers brushing through the dry grasses to settle close to where I sat. Then in a rush, a rudimentary breast, a belly hugging the rear of the manger, a thigh enclosing the left side before fading into the grass, then a further line hinting at a calf.

The scalp tightened in a moment of fear and I felt unnerved. Keeping very still, with some minutes of reflection on what had occurred, the impossibility of what I'd seen, led to a momentary calm and I gathered up the painting gear.

I turned and started back to the car at the far side of the meadow — and felt a sudden chill rise within as if a vast shape had obscured the light of the sun.

Now in the car I waited. This had been empathy with a vengeance, the inner child's demands meeting a huge response. Much later I felt that some deep crying need for contact with this vast earth mother and her breast must have surfaced that day.

It also called to mind many visionary works by painters, particularly the landscape visions of Van Gogh and Paul Nash, the Freudian dream and reverie material used by the Surrealists and the cosmic anxieties of Matta and some of Gorky's later work — to take just a few examples.

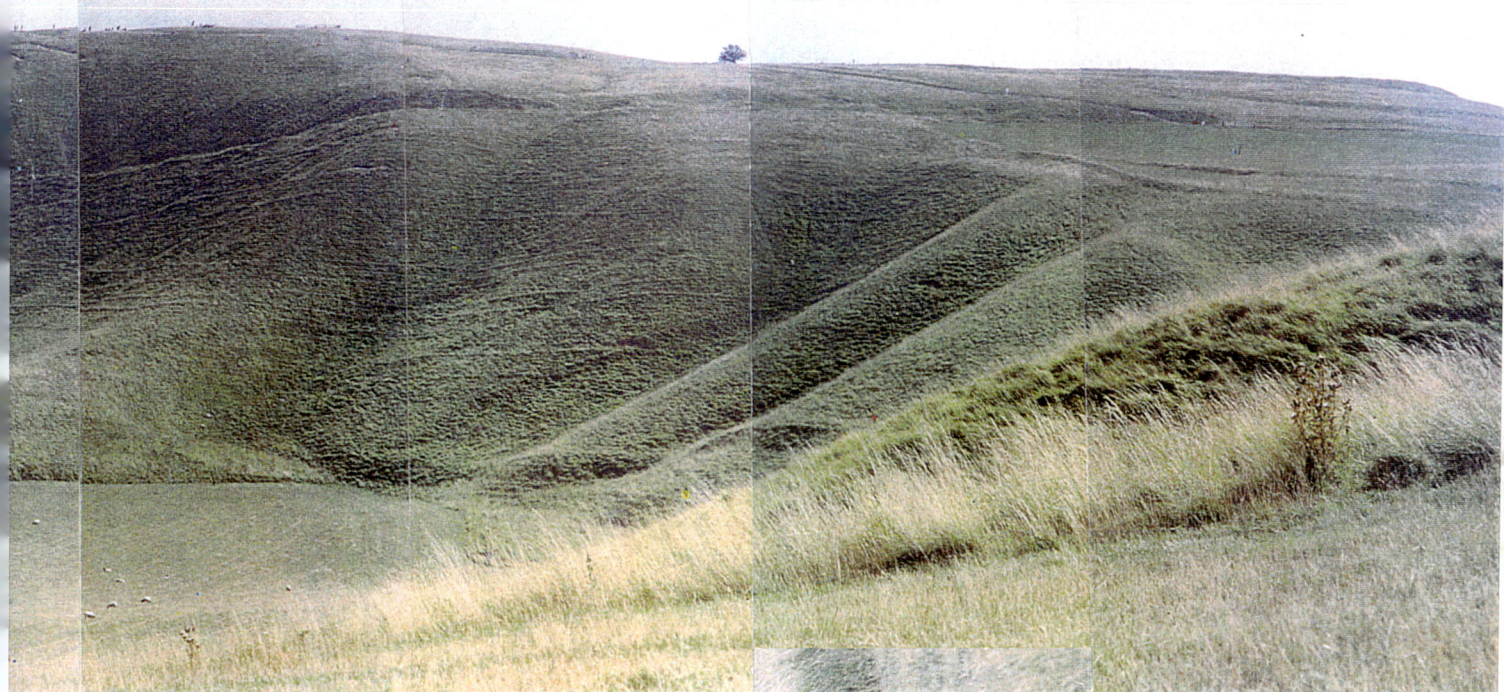

Above: A series of eight photos making up the landscape surrounding the Manger below the White Horse. Top left is Dragon Hill and top far right is the Uffington Castle area. Taken some months after the experience described here.

Below: Pastel drawing recreating the scene above, taking a higher viewpoint to help visualise the image found there.

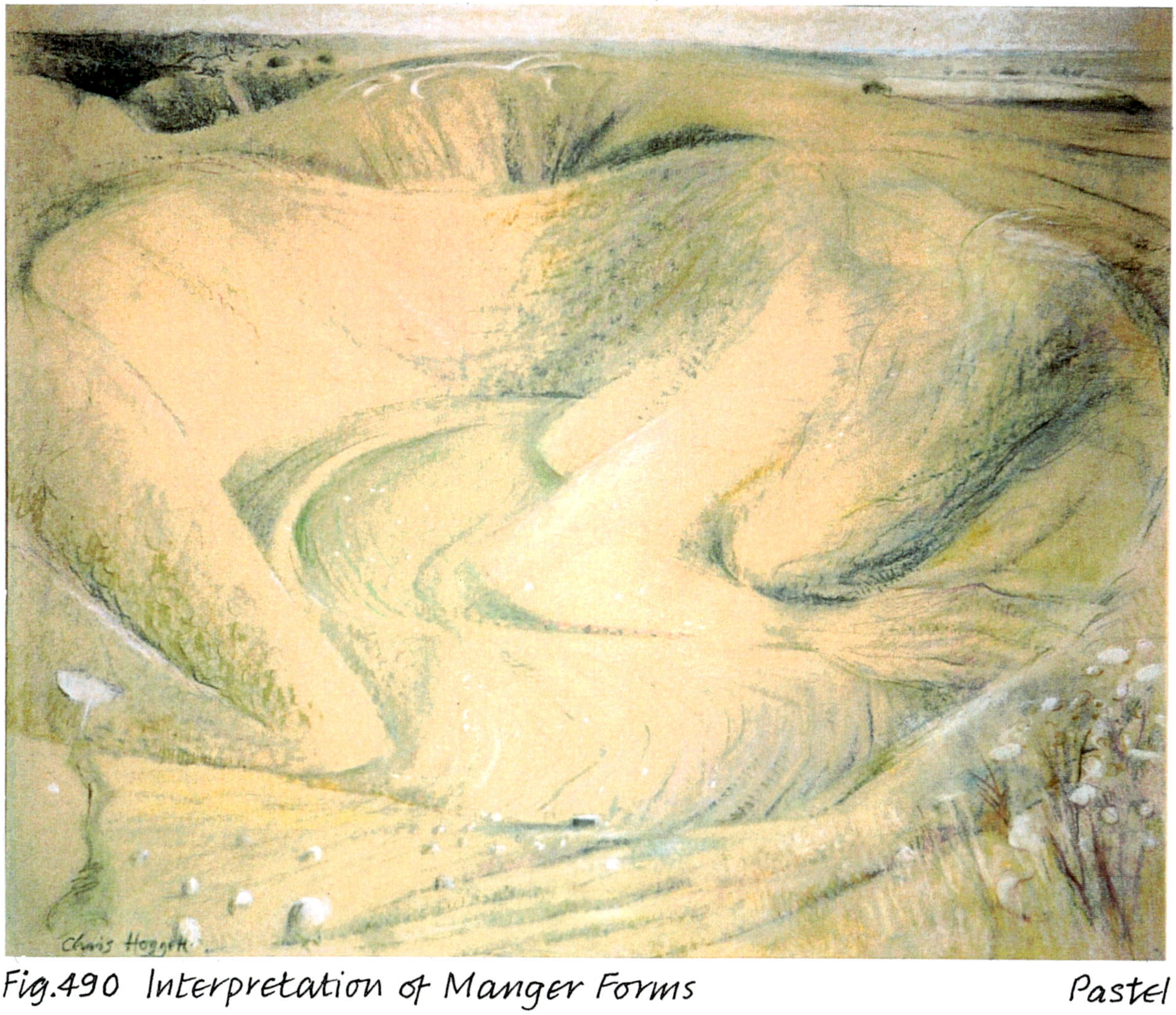

Fig.490 Interpretation of Manger Forms   Pastel

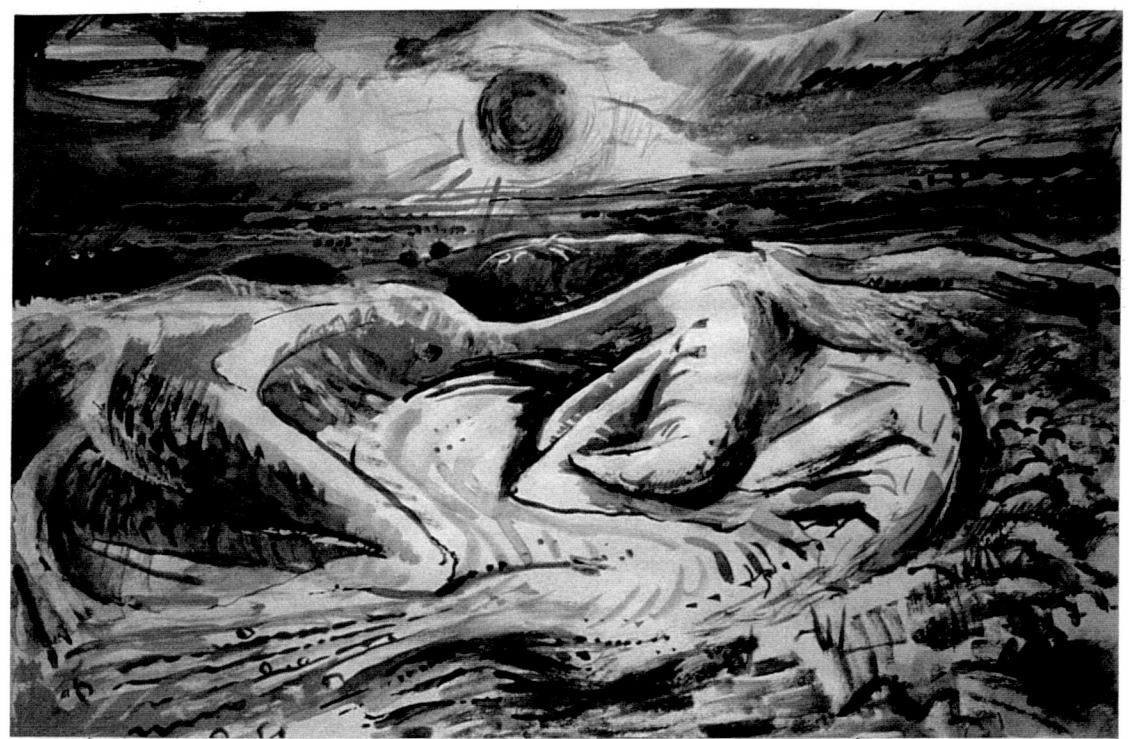

Fig. 491 The Sleeping Goddess - Uffington   Gouache

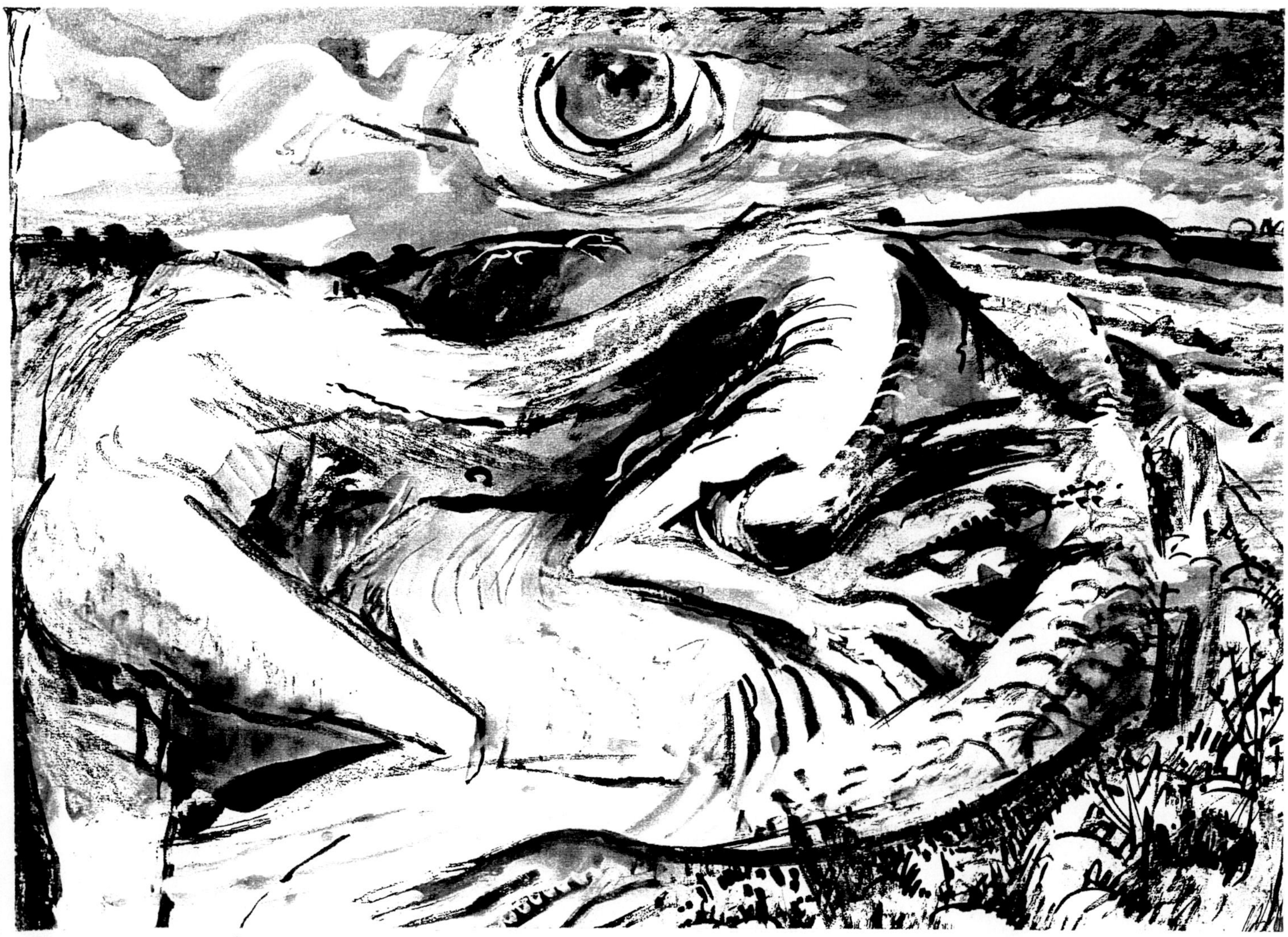

Fig. 492 Sleeping Goddess; Eye of the Sun - Uffington   Brush & Ink

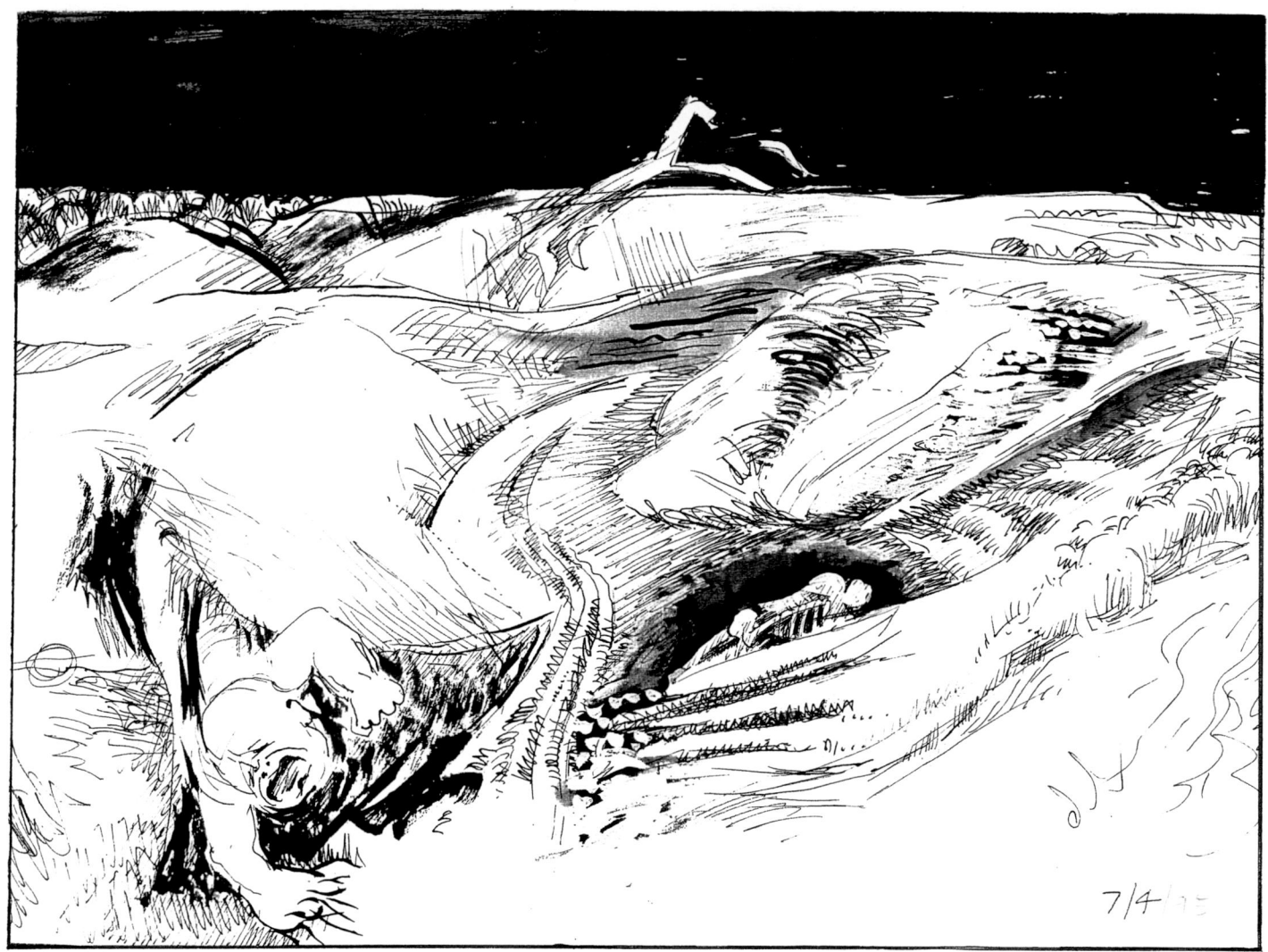

Fig. 493   A Womb-Tomb Place   Pen, Brush & Ink

Over the next few years a series of drawings, paintings and photographs described and developed this initial experience of Uffington. Although the figure seemed to possess human elements I nevertheless always tended towards the horse and occasionally a bird head and claws. The two drawings opposite show all three, or combinations of these. The lower ink and brush drawing with the 'eye of the sun' expresses most fully the apprehension of the day.

The drawing above (fig. 493) is an exploration into further feelings conjured up by this place — that of birth, life and death. Showing the birth of the babe and a skeletal form being nudged into a pit by a giant hand it now registers as a Womb-Tomb place with a life symbol above — the horse leaping into the sky.

Overleaf are further variations on the Uffington Earth Mother theme. The introduction of the monkey attempting to wake the 'goddess' may relate to a childhood memory — Mother and others saying 'He's a little Monkey' when I was probably trying to gain her attention. (Fig. 494). Other drawings with combinations of creatures followed until I worked on a painting of a triple-breasted figure arranged rather like a life model on a rostrum, her sheer scale emphasised by the manikin painter. This sleeping form recalls a faint memory of the many-breasted Goddess Artemis of Ephesus — an ultimate symbol of fertility and fecundity (figs. 495 and 497).

The sequence was rounded out with a final painting showing a resting place for my demanding child who, after feeding, found a sleeping space in the manger. The 'Blue Pony' fits snugly within the mothers form and seems to be blessed by a winged father figure. (fig. 496).

I did end up pondering about the Iron Age folk. Did they decide that this great holding space, the manger, was the place to cut out the horse above?

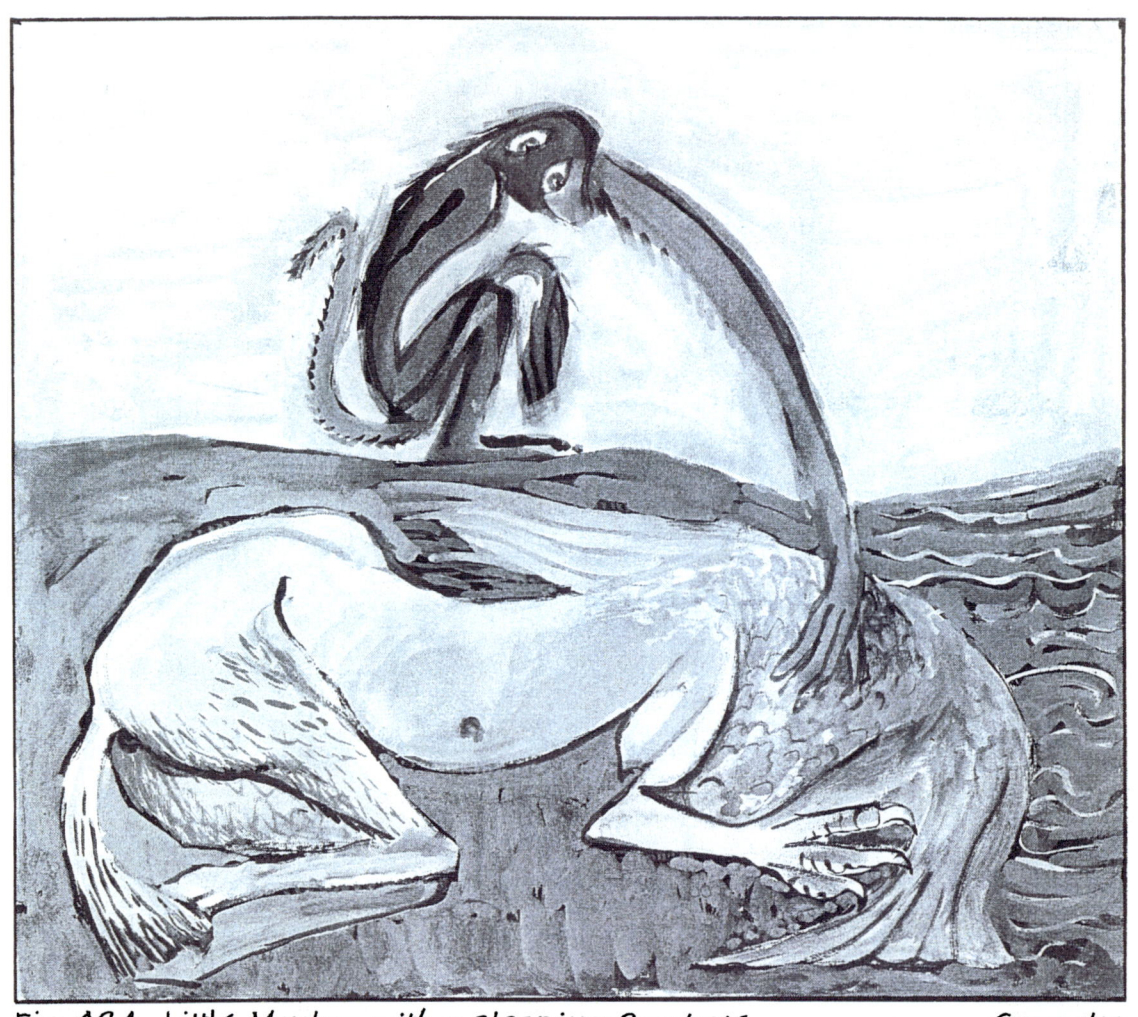
Fig. 494 Little Monkey with a Sleeping Creature   Gouache

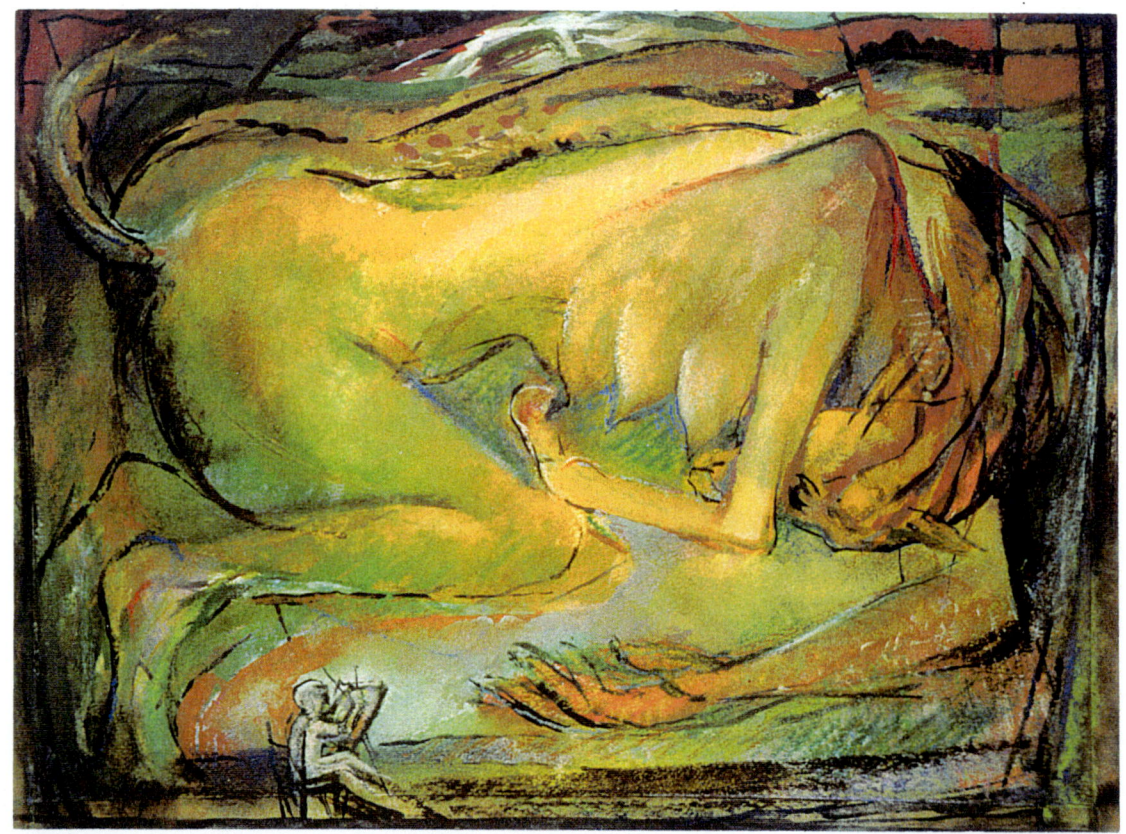
Fig. 495 Sleeping Earth Mother as Artist's Model   Gouache

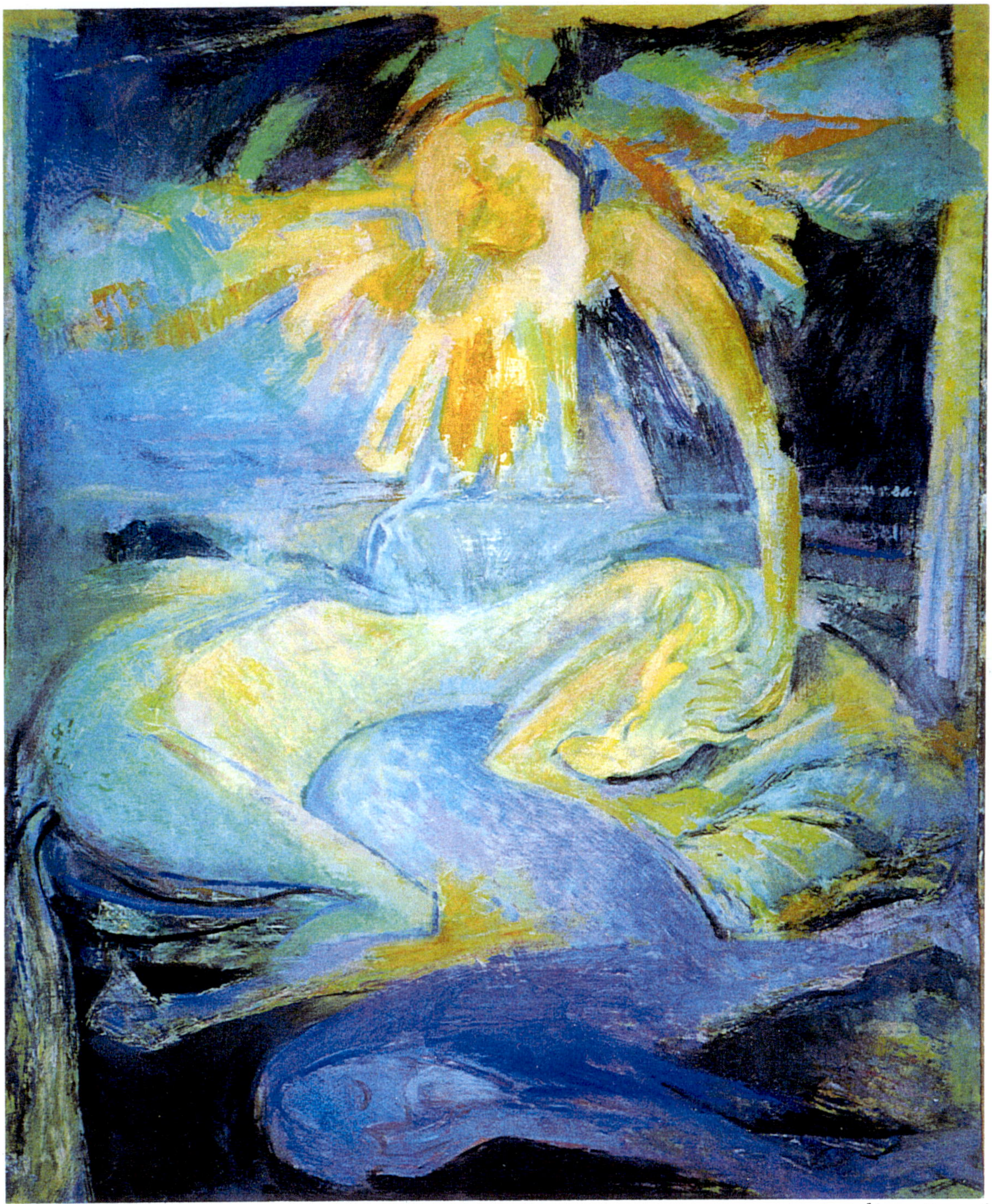

Fig. 496 The Blue Pony - Uffington   Oil on Board

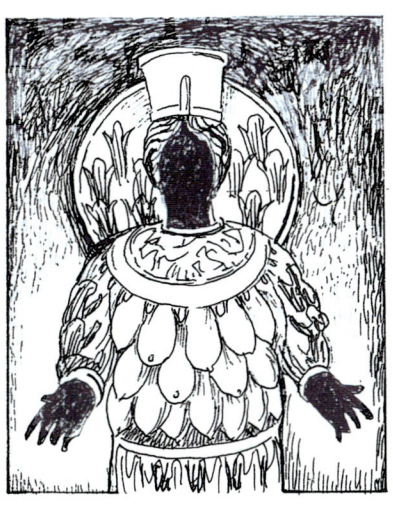

Figs. 494, 495 and 496
These three paintings attempt to capture an idealised nurturing, which I hadn't experienced.

Overleaf: 'Untitled'

There was a twist in the tail, so to speak, in this sequence of work. The calm and apparent peace for the blue pony was soon to be shattered by a metamorphosis of the horse/earth mother. Also the pony, now transformed into a vulnerable youth, seemed to be asking the wrong question and was being duly snubbed by the contempt of this monstrous image, showing her strong rejection.

Left: Fig. 497   Artemis of Ephesus   Pen & Ink

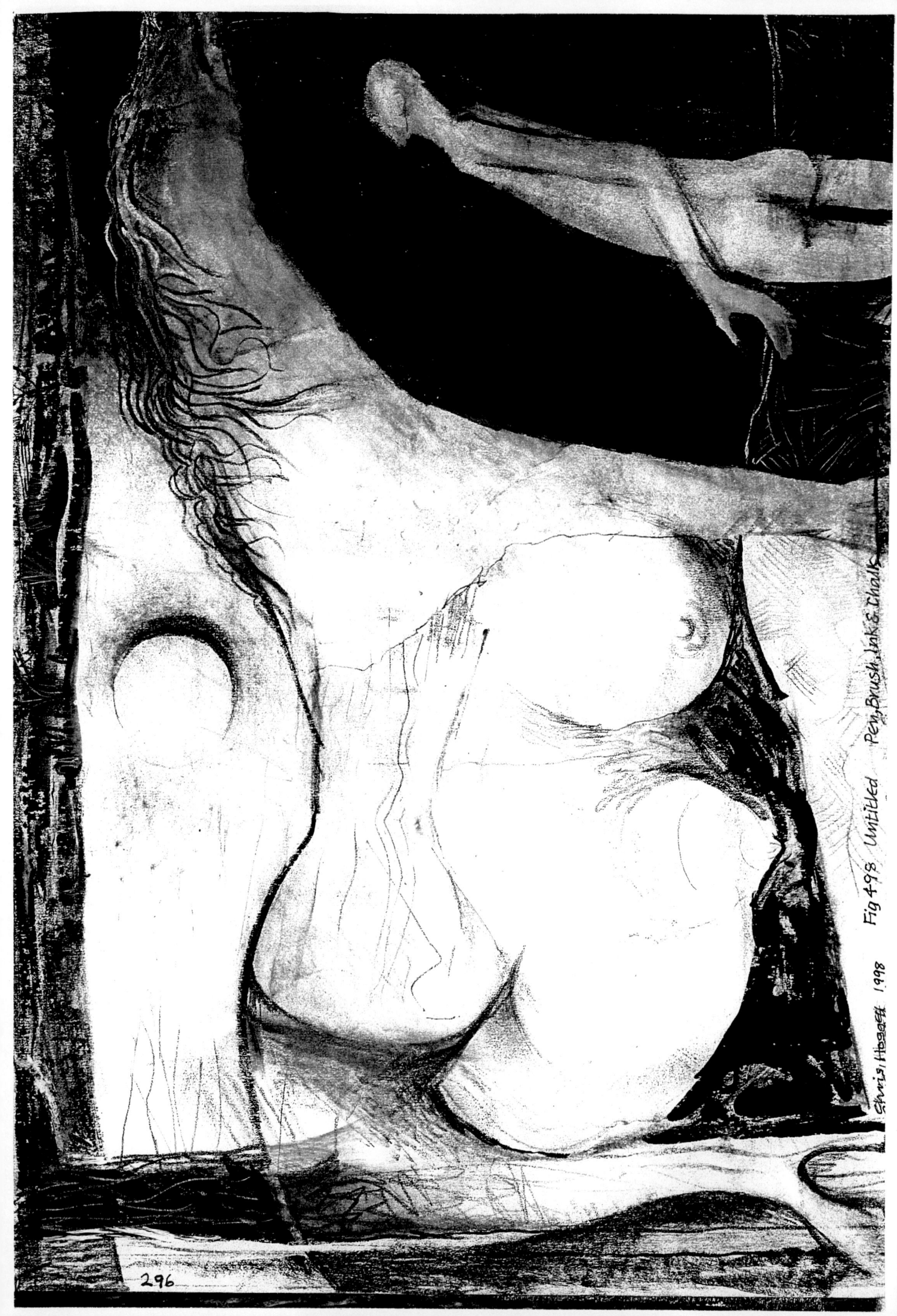

Chris Hoggett 1998 Fig 498 Untitled Pen, Brush, Ink & Chalk

2 BELAS KNAP LONG BARROW

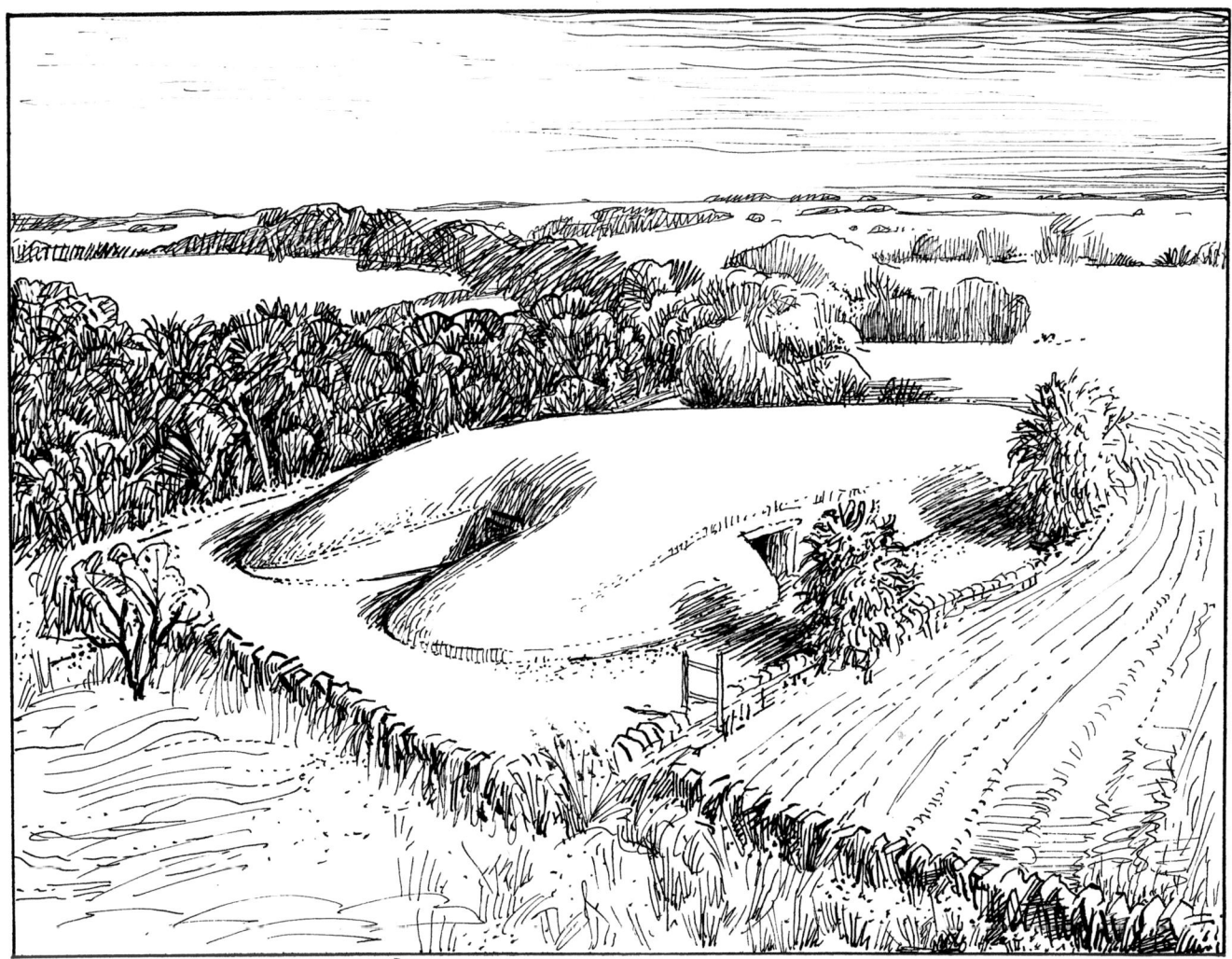

Fig. 499 Belas Knap Long Barrow, Gloucestershire   Pen & Ink

It was, for a February morning, remarkably warm, enough for me, feeling lethargic after the long walk, to climb up the long barrow and lie spreadeagled on its summit, staring into the sky. Maybe I was receptive to something, for when I turned and lay down, the great burial mound seemed to be humming. I tried to rationalise this strange experience. (Pressure on the eardrums, exhaustion after walking, etc.)

Possibly I'd slipped into a reverie of sorts, making connections with Gilgamesh, an epic I'd recently read, inscribed in stone at the same time as Belas Knap was being built in 2500 B.C. – Echoes across 4500 years between this hill barrow in Gloucestershire and a Babylonian story in Mesopotamia. It was not only the similarities of time. Lying on this Earth Mother tomb, I experienced the fear of death, of what lay beyond – the world of gods, goddesses, bulls and gazelles, a monstrous forest & heroes – these parts of the Gilgamesh Epic had left a strong impression.

I had ceased momentarily to be part of the 20th century, sharing instead an empathy for these ancient peoples – identifying their supernatural beings with some of my own dark fears. There was a particular empathy with 'Enkidu' (page 298).

A personal mythology developed around the idea of a protective Earth Mother on the one hand (Belas Knap) and a desire to overcome some imagined monsters on the other, until it dawned on me that the protective Mother and the Monster might be one and the same – that the creature I desired, I also feared.

A few drawings and paintings based on the Gilgamesh Epic emerged from these musings.

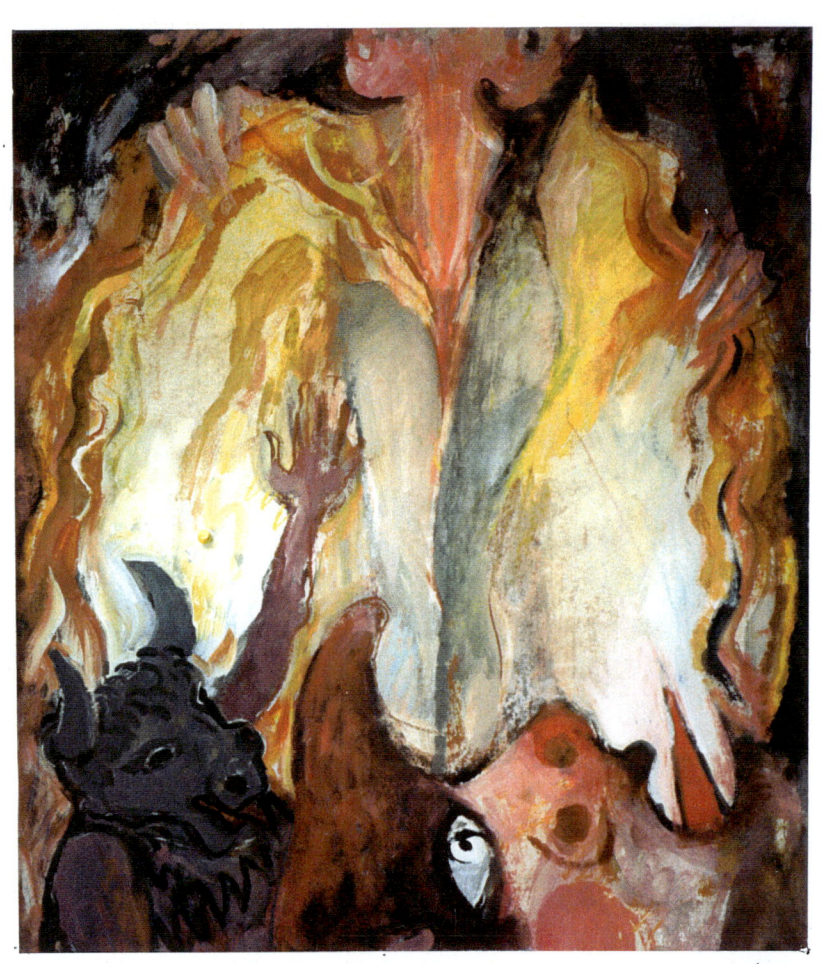

ILLUSTRATIONS FROM GILGAMESH

The aggression in human nature, the often destructive search for power, has been recorded in legend since time began. Gilgamesh (approx. 3000 B.C.) is a good example. In the character of Enkidu, the 'ministrations' of Shamet, and Gilgamesh's desire to win the fight (and also the loss of innocence Enkidu suffers) it was easy to empathise with the 'loser' — here was my own sense of inferiority, of subjugation to the woman

(see the end of this section for a summary of this epic — page 306).

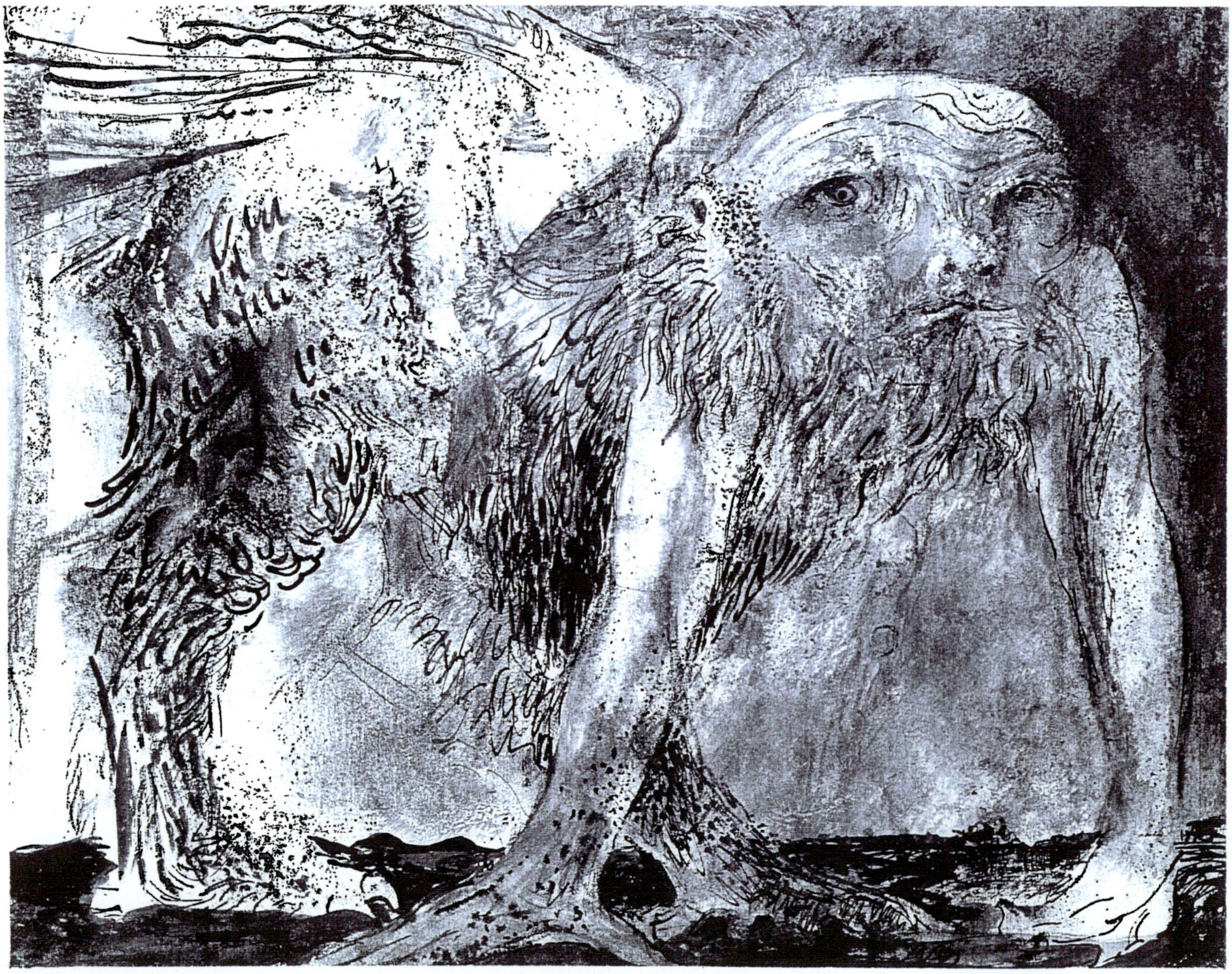

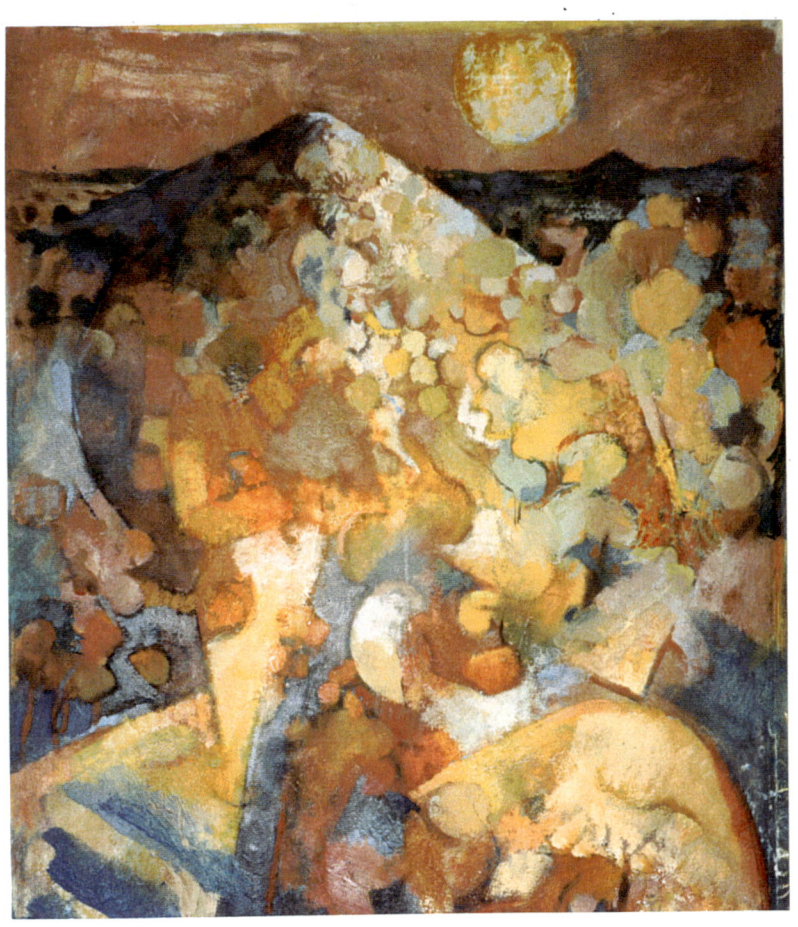

Left: Fig. 502
The Cedar Forest
Oil on Board

An interpretation of the monstrous nature of the Cedar forest where Gilgamesh and Enkidu must face a great challenge and subdue their fears within its great canopy.

The visual idea was to turn the forest into some form of giant portrait — the suggestion of a high volcanic skull and hill slopes below which hint at shoulders. Many trees obscure the fearsome face within.
The forest lies beneath a lowering sky and full moon.

Top Left: Fig. 500

Gilgamesh and Enkidu visit Ishtar, the Temple Goddess. (Other sources say Shamet the prostitute).

Pastel on toned paper

Left: Fig. 501

Humbaba, Guardian of the Cedar Forest.

Graphite Powder, Pen & Wash.

Right: Fig. 503

Gilgamesh and Enkidu become firm friends following their fight with one another.

Watercolour and Chalk

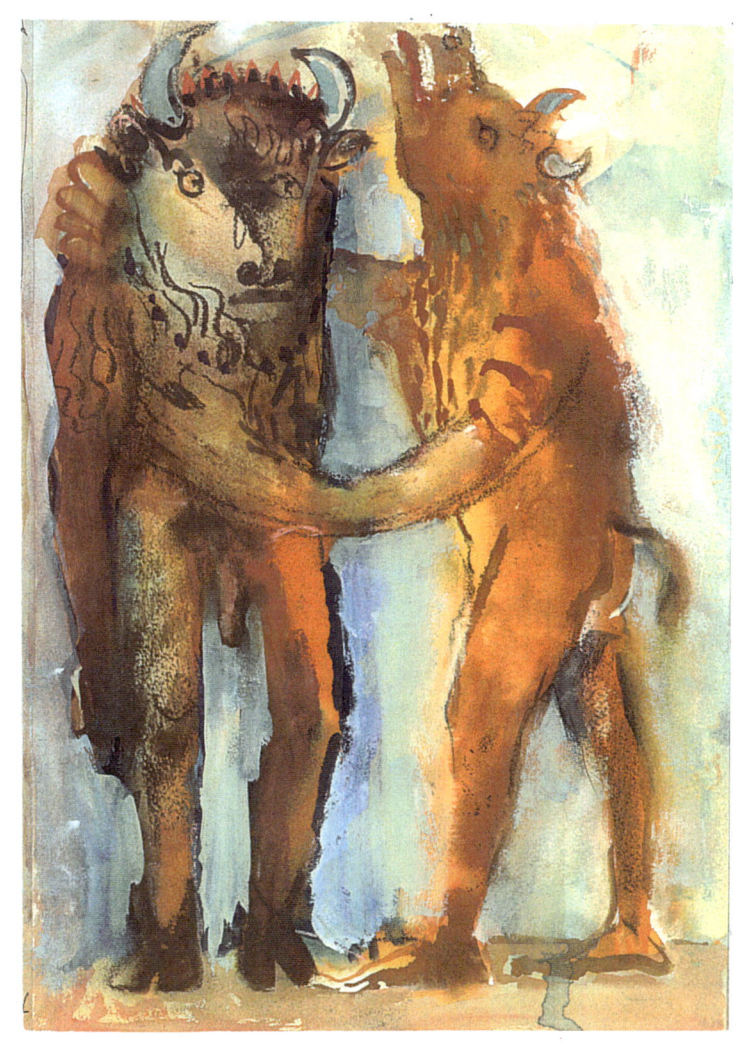

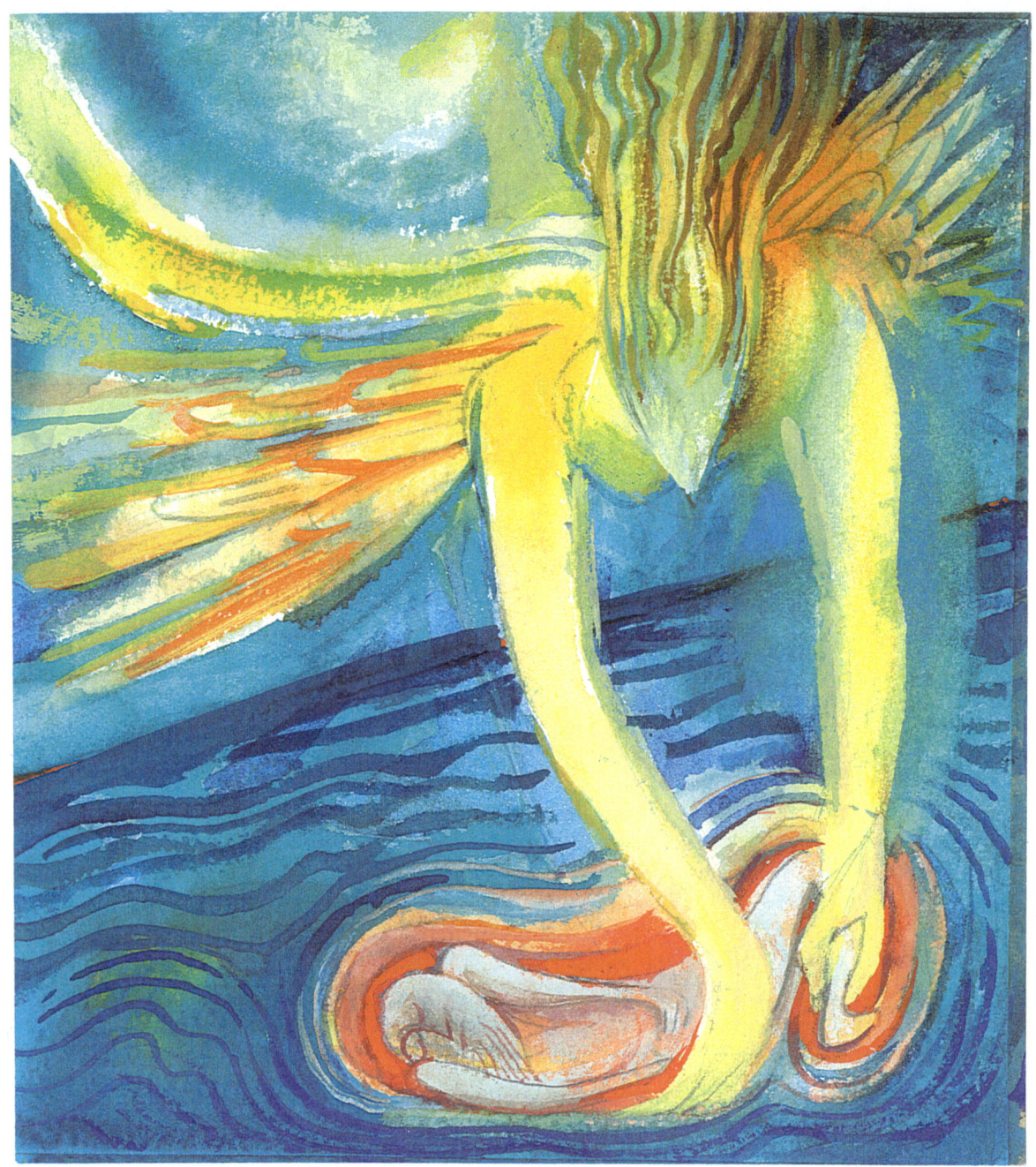

Fig. 504 Angel-Bird rejuvenates Elderly Man   Watercolour

RESURRECTION

This was possibly one of the most difficult times during the therapy years where so much of the work was accomplished and yet feelings of psychological weariness brought on yet more depression.

Fortunately some free-style work helped me through the later stages. One painting depicting a prematurely-aged and lethargic character being rejuvenated by an angelic bird-like figure helped to lift me out of the doldrums. This in turn reminded me of a drawing from the mid-1980s which I'd entitled 'Raising the Dead'.

This represented a disembowelled figure (a shade of the earlier skeletal work), leaning back, its skull-like head wrenched right back — curiously I felt the possibility of a revival, some hint of animation in the limbs.

These two potential re-awakenings had an enlivening effect as I now drew 'Awakening the Dead' with a bull-god (thoughts on Gilgamesh) leaping over a swathed corpse with such vigour I felt the figure would soon open its eyes and remove the bandages.

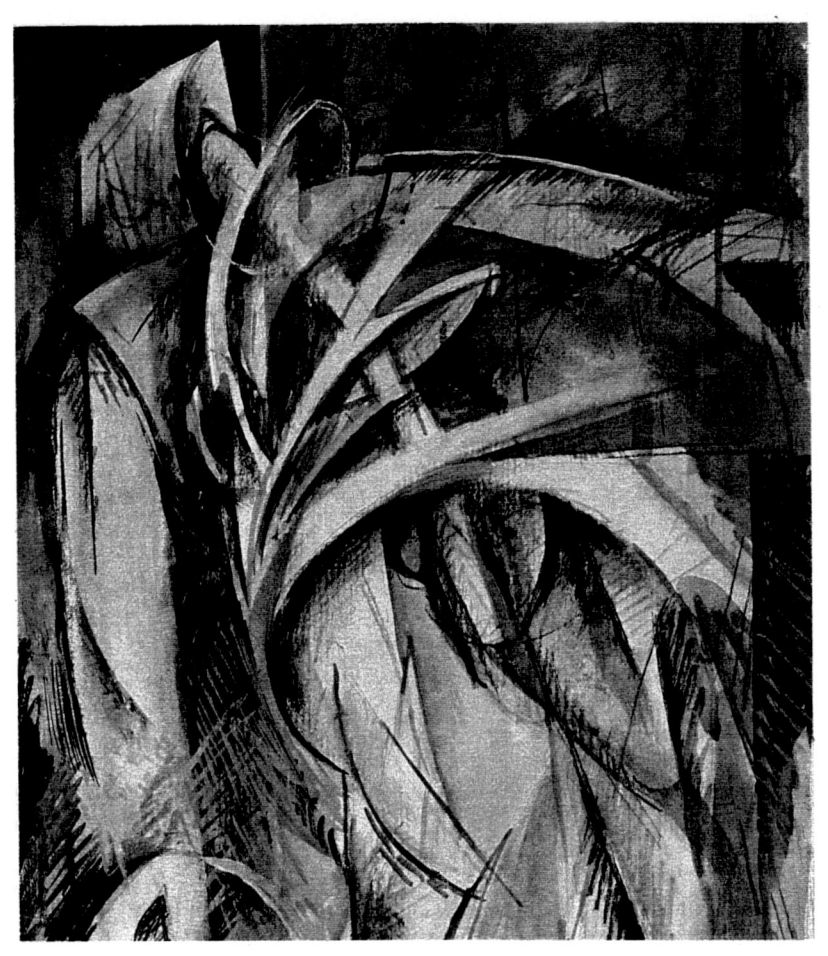

'Raising the Dead' (fig 505)

I was reminded of the sheep skeletons drawn in the early 1980s. The disembowelled figure appeared soon afterwards, rib-cage opened out, skull thrown back — a symbol of despair. The antithesis of regeneration — yet this drawing later became the source of a re-birth — a kind of dying to the old depressive feelings.

Left: Fig 505 Raising the Dead
chalk, wash, pen and ink.

Below: Fig 506.
Awakening the Dead
Pen and wash

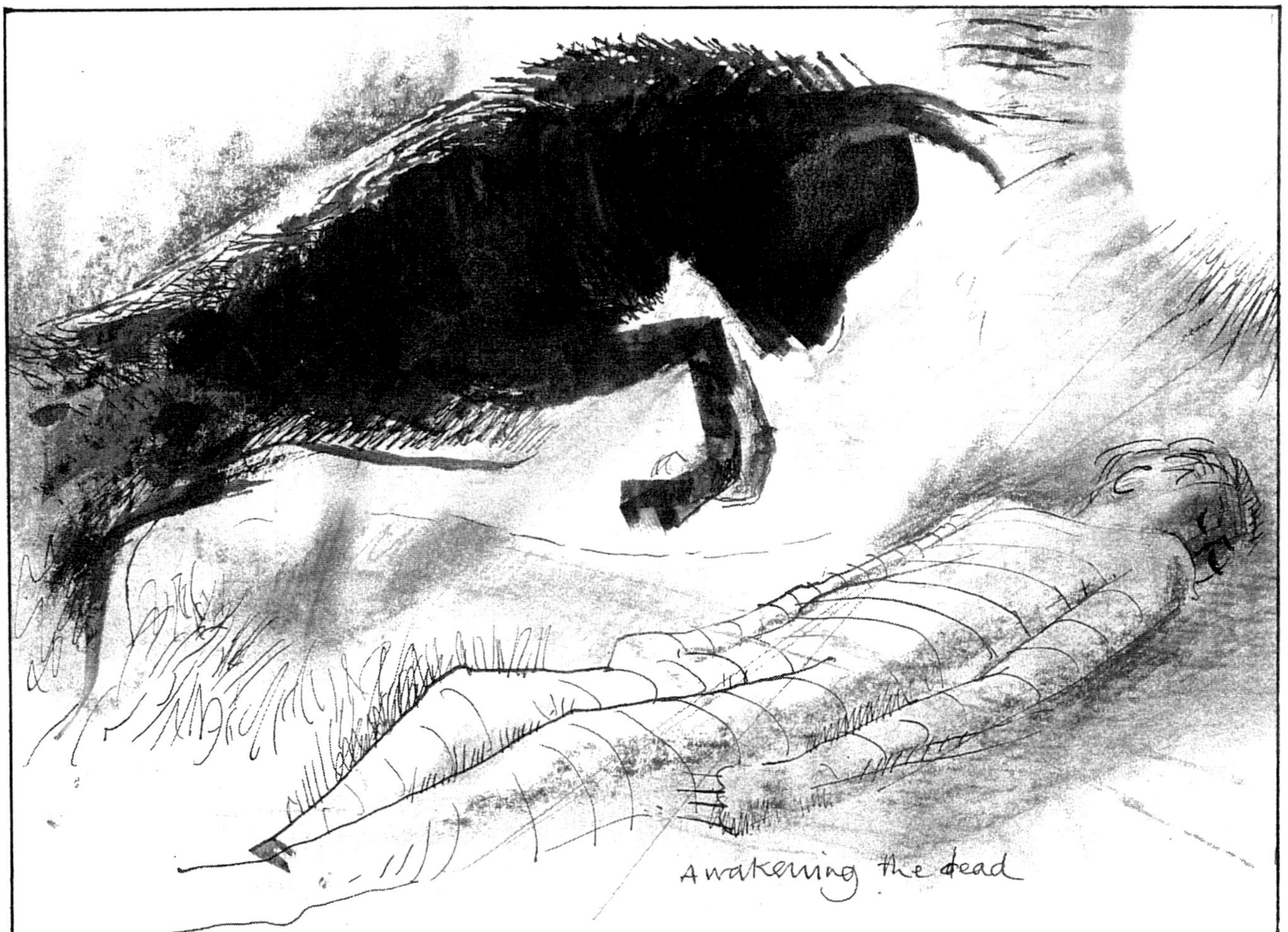

Awakening the dead

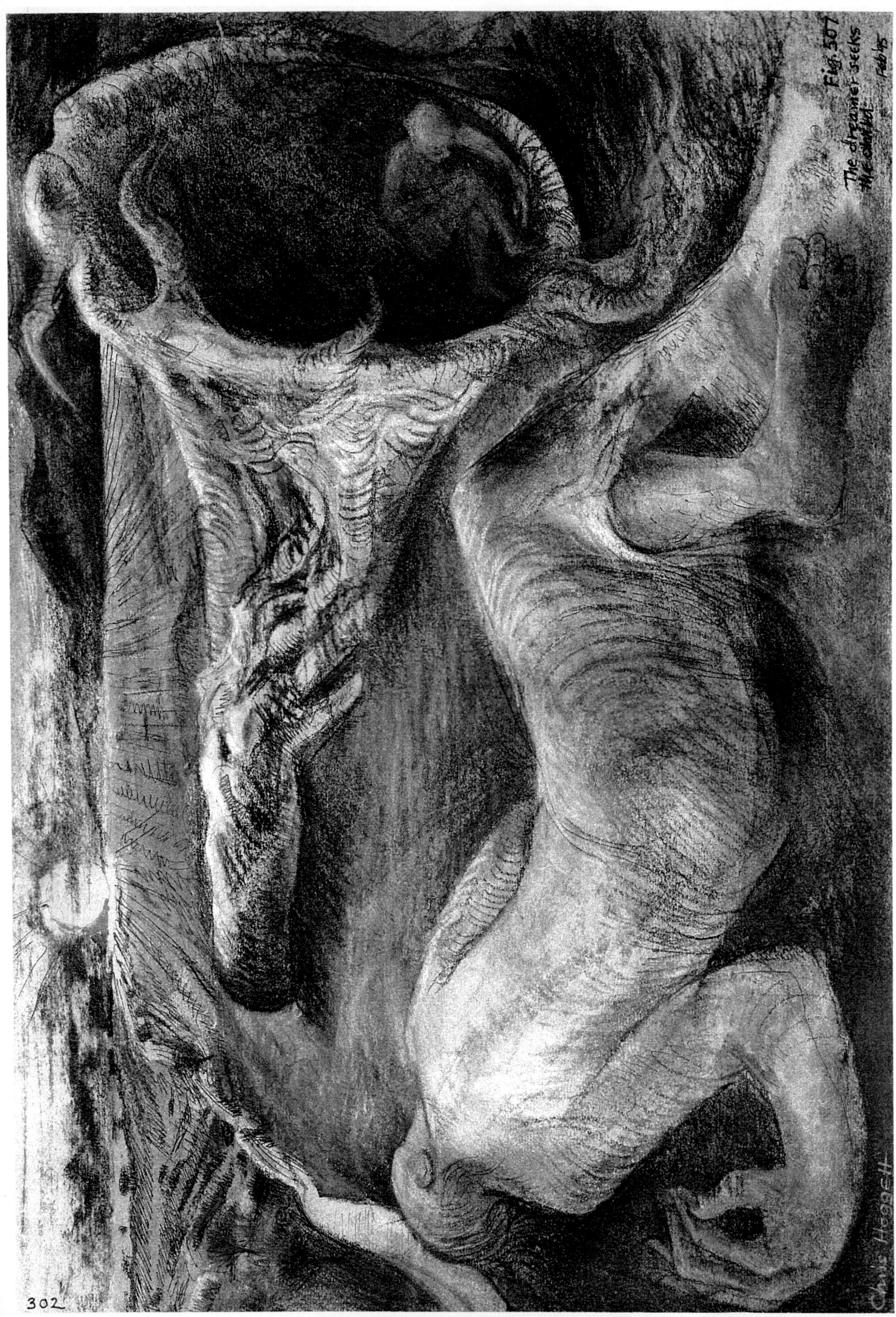

Fig. 507
The dreamer seeks
the centre
Feb 15

THE FATHER AND THE SON - Two Dreams and Two Drawings

The drawings relating to ideas on resurrection may have activated my subconscious, for not long afterwards I recall two vivid dreams:

Left: Fig.507 'The Dreamer Seeks his Son'   Pen & Chalk

'A small child waits behind the gates of a large orphanage. His father is about to arrive having heard a trumpet call. The father describes meeting a small creature, emaciated, grey and slightly rat-like standing before him, its upper front teeth missing. The father asks 'Are you sad'. 'Yes' replies the child. The father says, 'I've come to take you home'. The child whispers, 'I can't believe it, I can't believe it.'

Waking from the dream I recognised my own childhood with the broken front teeth, the result of a fall. I also felt euphoric, as if a powerful dream image of regeneration had offered itself up — for me to get in touch with the inner child.

The drawing which followed (fig.507, left) is a re-interpretation of the dream, the father resting on his journey to find his child. The father's anticipation is such that his right hand detaches itself to form the top end of a sawn tree trunk, feeling its way towards the child asleep within the hollowed out roots. The treetrunk suggests the trumpet with which the child summoned the father.

Below: Fig.508 'Sculpture in a Cemetery' Then I recalled a second dream:

'I had entered a cemetery with my students, looking for a subject to draw. Then we found a sculpture which resembled a cross from the back and had a male figure in front with a broken off left hand. Suddenly a winged manikin rose out of the stomach.

Another drawing illustrated this. (fig.580 below). The development from the previous drawing was striking — the child was not only 'found', but was now given its freedom.

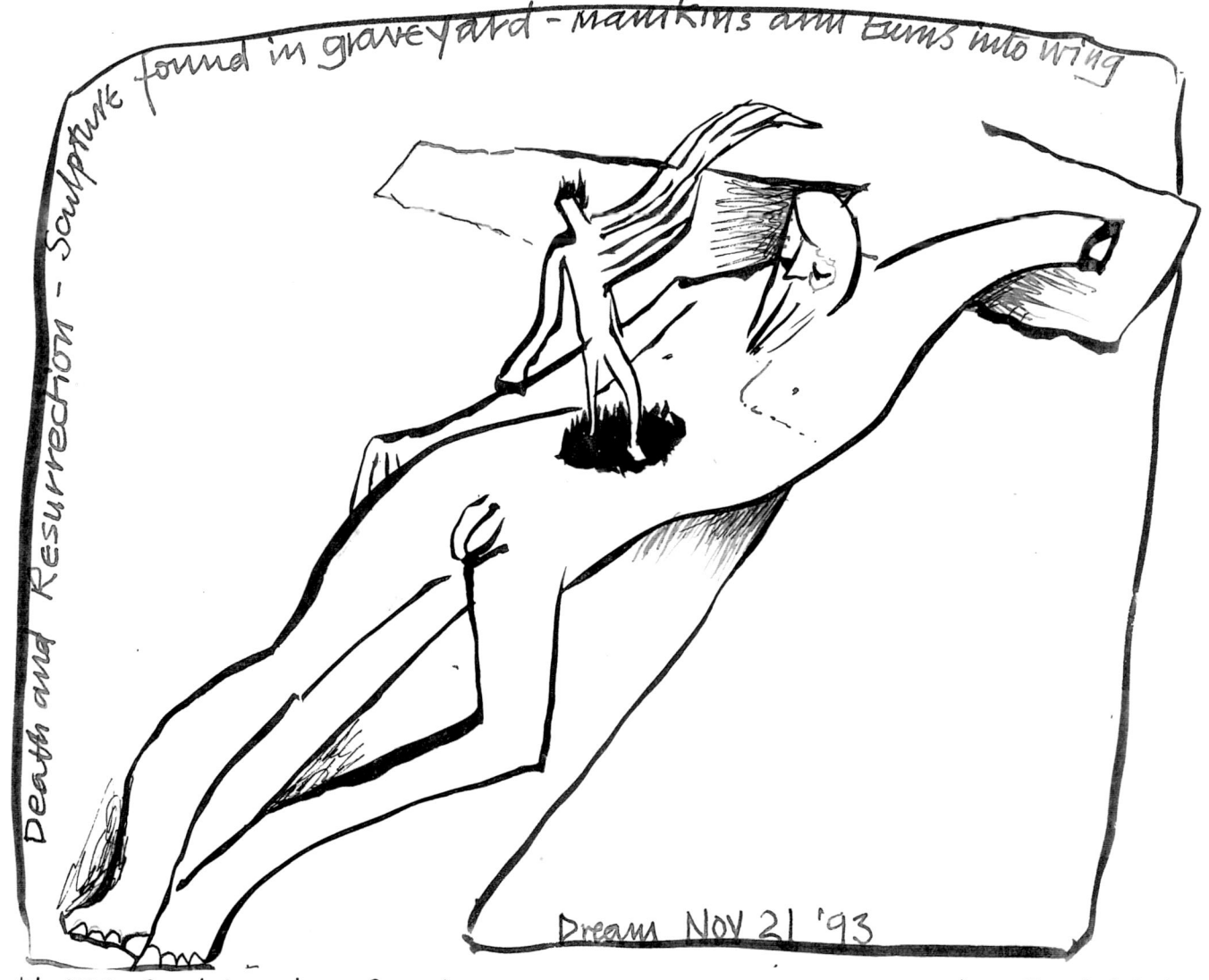

Fig.508 Sculpture in a Cemetery   Pen, Brush & Ink

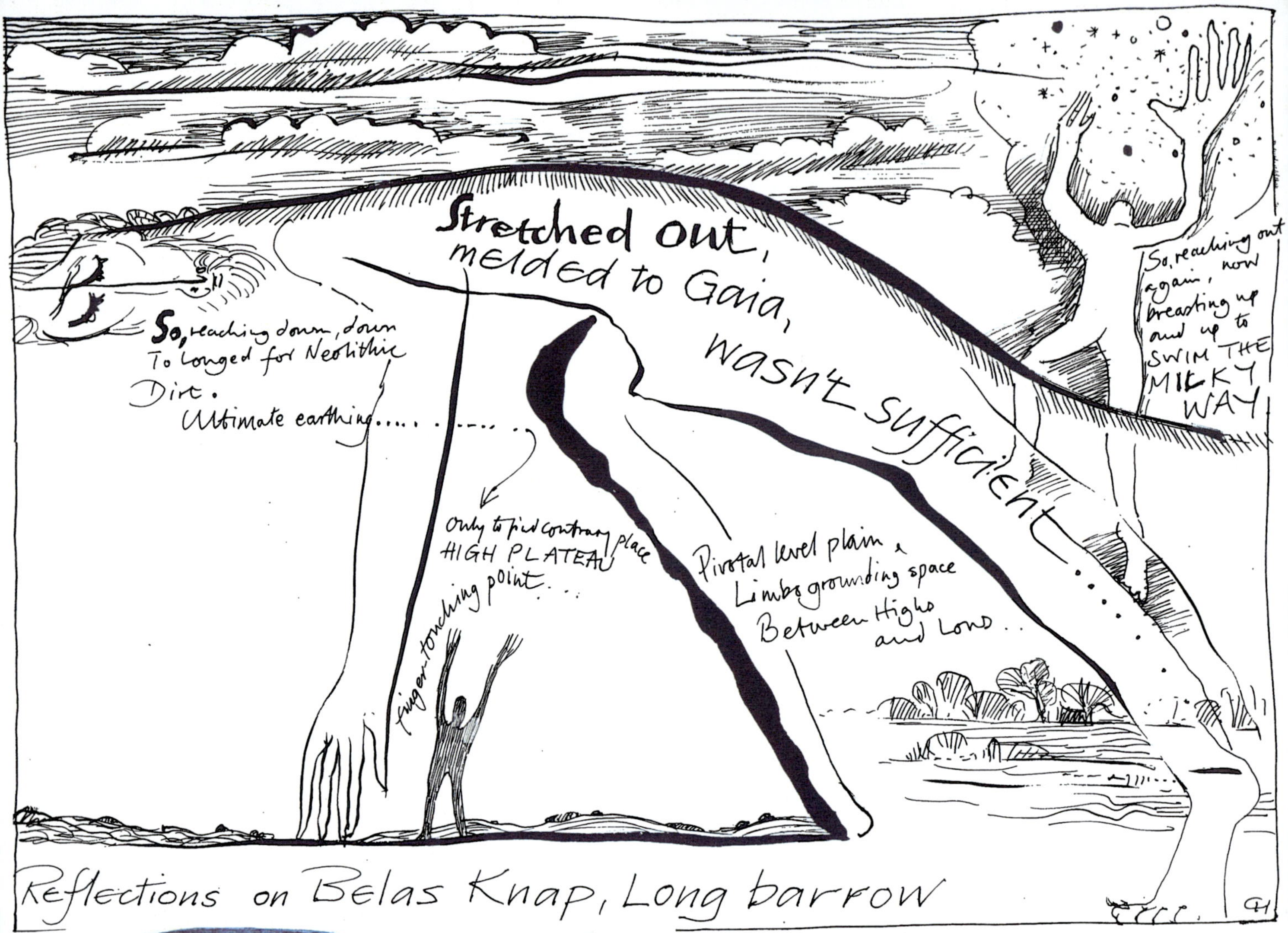

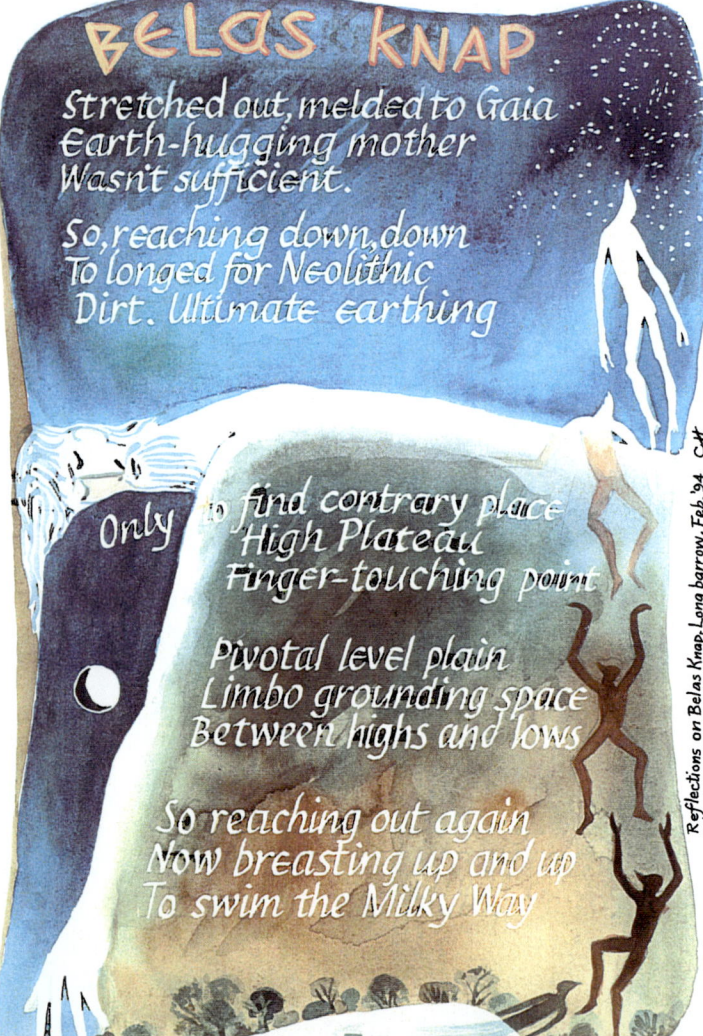

Above: Fig. 509 Reflections on Belas Knap No 1 Pen & Ink

A WORLD OF MYTH AND FAERY

More frequent walks to the long barrow loosened up amorphous and conflicting moods. Words and linear threads began to interweave.

I found myself making a drawing with an obscure poem entwined inside. 'Reflections on Belas Knap' was seeking to comprehend the confused feelings of seeming to exist on different levels simultaneously. Stretching out on Gaia NOW, thinking of Babylon THEN, hoping LATER for understanding, communication.....

Another version using gouache emphasised the 'reaching out and up' perhaps reflecting the manikin rising out the father figure in the cemetery. (fig. 508).

Left: Fig. 510 Reflections on Belas Knap No 2 Gouache

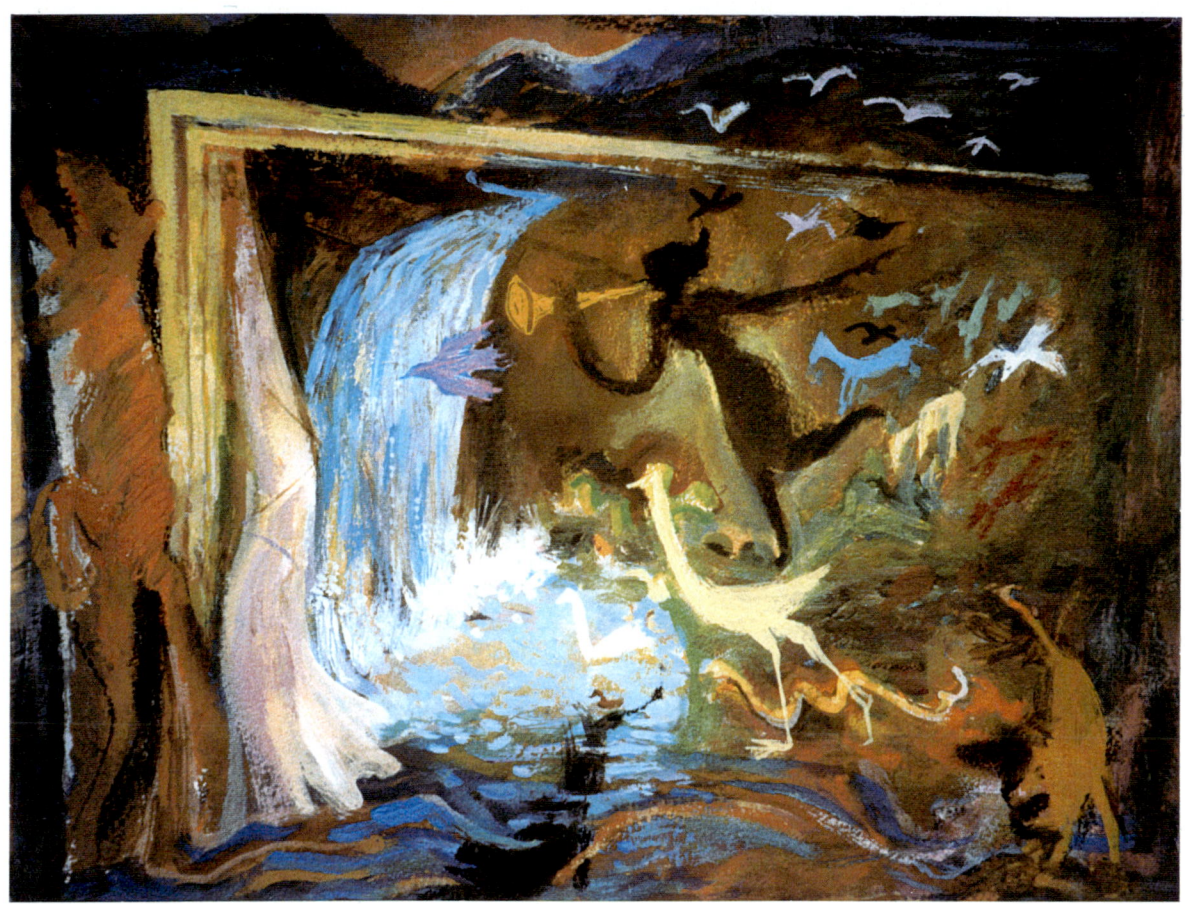

Fig. 511 The Trumpet Call – A Fairytale · Oil on Paper

Concentrating on mythology and dream work was a possible catalyst for a free-style 'fairy-tale' type of painting. 'The Trumpet Call' (an echo from the father-son dream - fig 507) revealed a monster, a princess/goddess blowing a trumpet, a range of creatures as if coming out of the Ark and a river/waterfall. I had some sympathy for the timorous creature who seemed to wish to remain concealed and uncommitted behind the proscenium curtain as the drama rushes forward to meet him.

The world of myth and 'faery' continued with this pastel drawing 'Life Vessel'. A large bowl fills the whole picture space with figures rising from the base, swimming skywards – reminiscent of the figures in 'Reflections on Belas Knap'

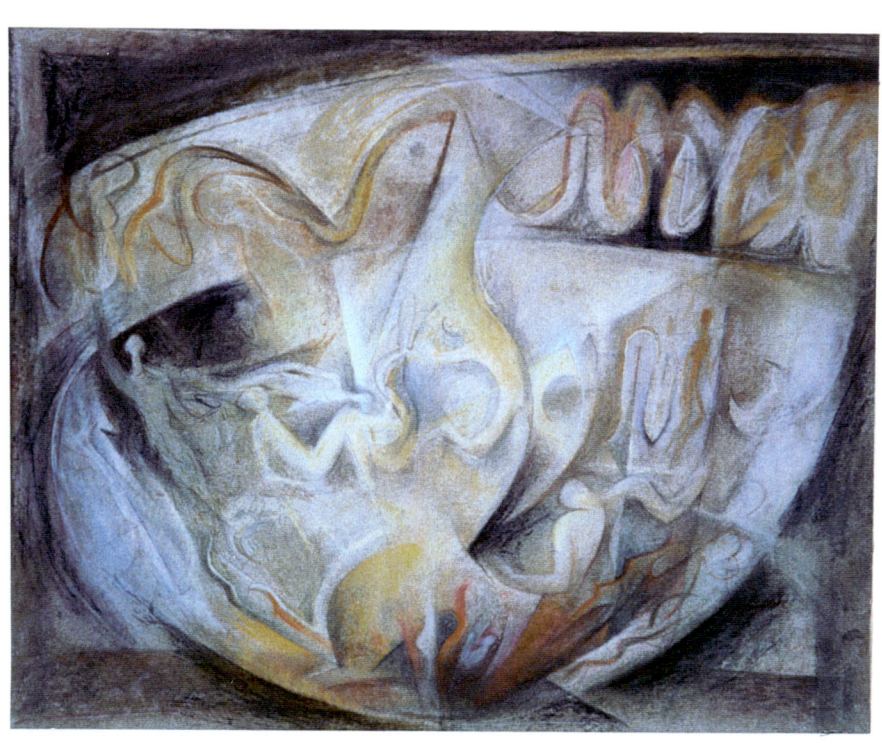

Right: Fig. 512 Life Vessel Pastel

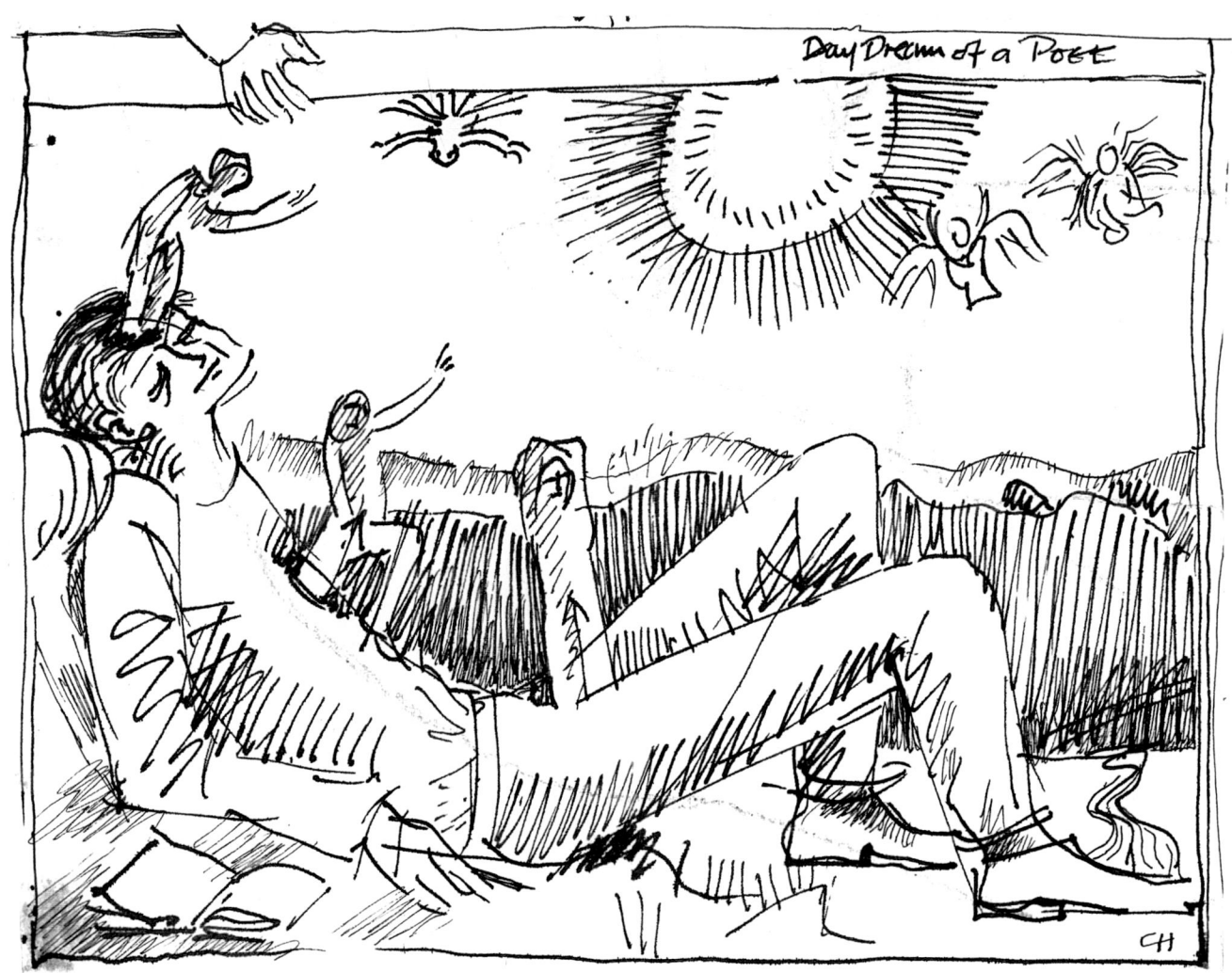

Fig. 513   Day dream of a Poet   Pen & Ink

Sometimes tiredness led to resting against a wall or grassy bank then musing on the direction my work seemed to be taking. From the visits to Belas Knap and these times of rest, I made this pen and ink sketch - 'Daydream of a Poet' showing the fruits of his fantasies spring from his head, heart and groin; his thoughts, feelings and creativity regenerated again. The overall expression of the drawing was of hope, exemplified by the angelic putti.

The Epic of Gilgamesh - a Summary

Gilgamesh, an historical king in Mesopotamia (2800 B.C.) later became a semi-divine being. He was a tyrant in Urak, whose citizens ask the gods to send a companion to entertain him, thus easing their lives.

Heaven creates Enkidu, part-animal, part human who lives with gazelles. He is parted from his wild life when Shamet, a prostitute, couples with him for six days and seven nights. His strength sapped, he meets Gilgamesh and they fight, an encounter which Gilgamesh wins. Enkidu loses his 'nature', is no longer able to stay with the gazelles, can only live with humans. He and Gilgamesh become firm friends and enjoy various adventures, one of which involves killing the monster Humbaba, guardian of the Cedar Forest. Later Enkidu dies, leaving Gilgamesh desolate and seeking the key to eternal life which is foiled by a snake who takes away the plant which would have endowed Gilgamesh with this great gift.

3 JURASSIC WESTWOOD

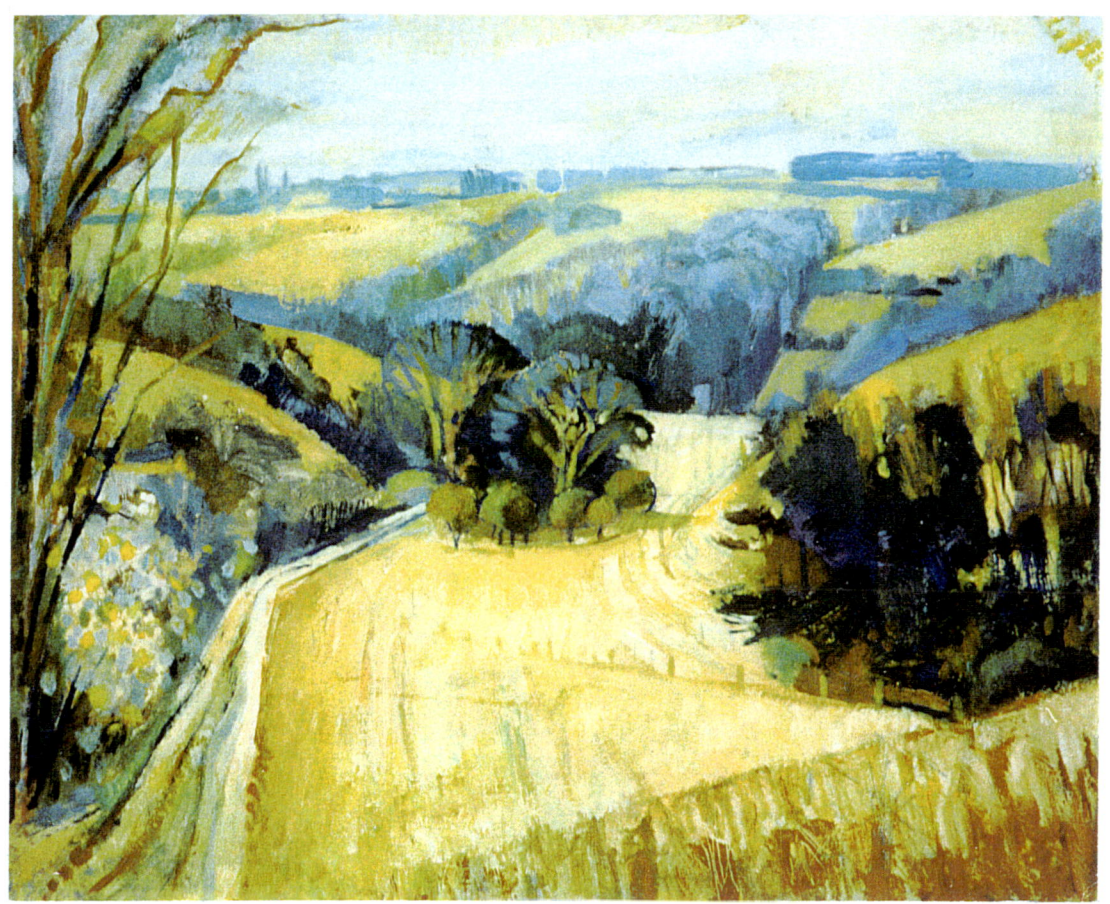

Fig. 514   Towards Westwood, Charlton Abbots   Oil on Board

Already the Ridgeway at Uffington, with its great White Horse and the Manger below, had offered an intimation of something just beyond my understanding. It would be another year before another metamorphosis within the landscape would bear fruit.

Now, some months later, just over the brow of the local Cotswold escarpment a new find offered further hints of something just beneath the surface of the land. This small wooded and gently sloped valley lay hidden in a fold of the hill — I call it Westwood after the wood in its centre. I came upon it one cold March morning in 1994 from a bridlepath along a ridge with a high viewpoint. Certain shapings of the wooded area defined the form of the land and caused me to pause, indeed almost hypnotised me.

Certainly I'd projected into it something I was unable to grasp. Could it be called the spirit of place? It did seem to be an ideal antidote to the grandeur of Uffington — it was much smaller in scale and suggested a place of rest, of contemplation perhaps.

There were to be no sudden revelations of this sort, only a slow unfolding of its essence

Psychologically, this period was a particularly low point of working through the therapy, with acutely depressive mornings, a sense of artistic inadequacy and an inability (I felt) to express my feelings about this place.

After years of unearthing so much personal history during the therapy sessions, I'd imagined the depressions would gradually decrease. On the contrary the reverse seemed to be happening. The constant attempts to lift oneself out of the condition stirred up things I'd been avoiding for years — and led me soon to some archaeological digging into seams of the subconscious and this particular landscape.

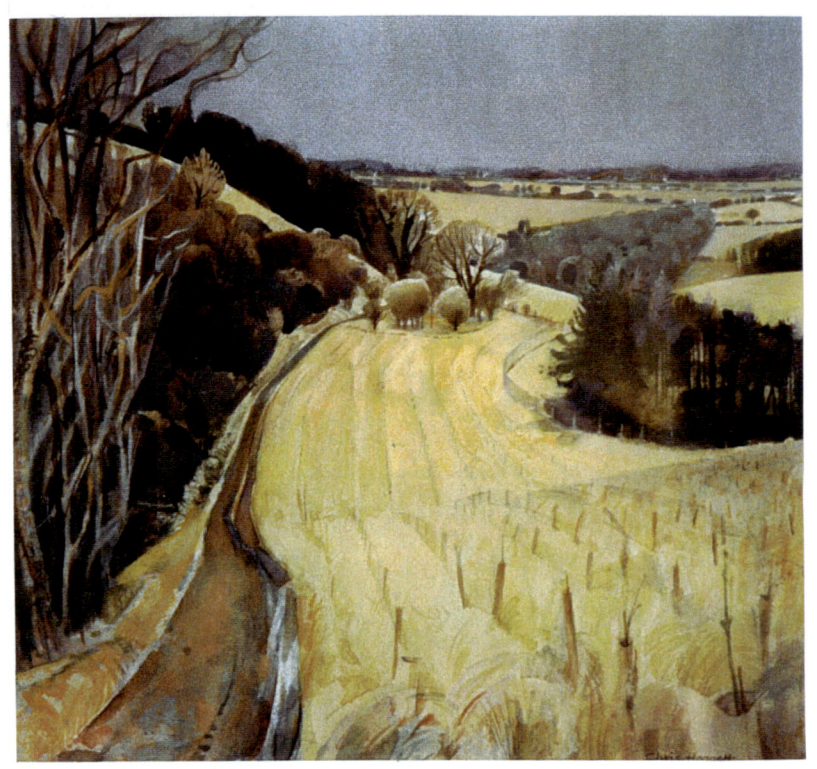

Incompetent Pictures

On this page are two paintings and a drawing I felt were 'inadequate', a result of the depressive moods at the period (1994-1995).

A number of other paintings of this landscape were later destroyed.

Above: Fig. 515
'View towards Westwood - Summer.' with a new plantation of hardwood trees.
Watercolour & Gouache

Right: Fig. 516
Viewpoint further to the right of above scene. Rough sketch with various notes.
Pen and Ink

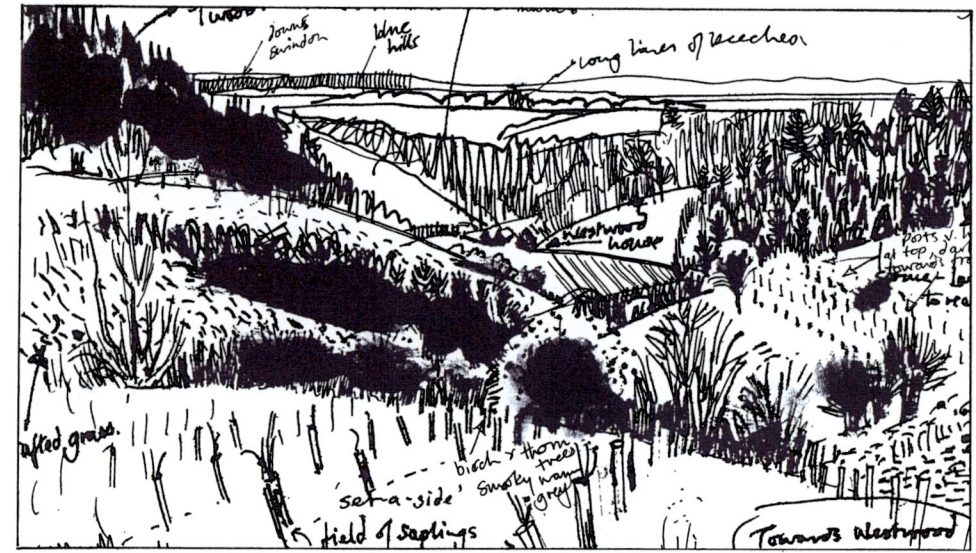

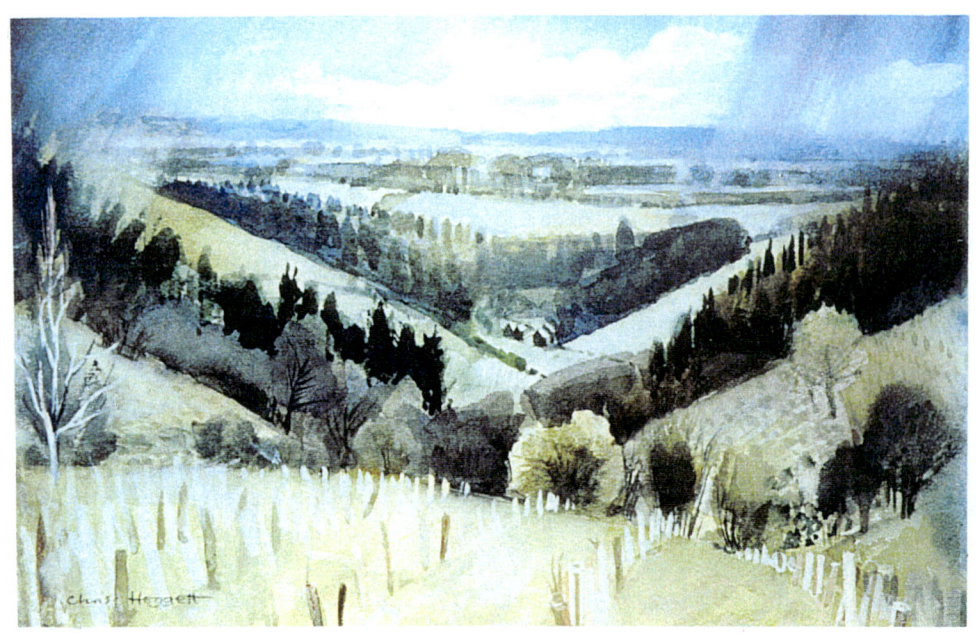

Left: Fig. 517
General view of the Westwood area with the wood in the centre of the scene.
Light showers falling over the Cotswolds.
Watercolour

FOSSIL DISCOVERIES

With the continuing depressions I was considering stopping the therapy. I could choose to 'unwind', retreat and tell C. it was time for me to cope by myself. Paradoxically it was thoughts relating to the archaeological aspects — the digging into subconscious elements — which caused me to hesitate taking a negative approach (I knew it was an escape from emotional pain) and to think more about the geographical aspects of this place. The discovery of a large fossil on the higher slopes of the valley transformed the emotional unearthing into practical digging of the upper landscape, the 'real' surface.

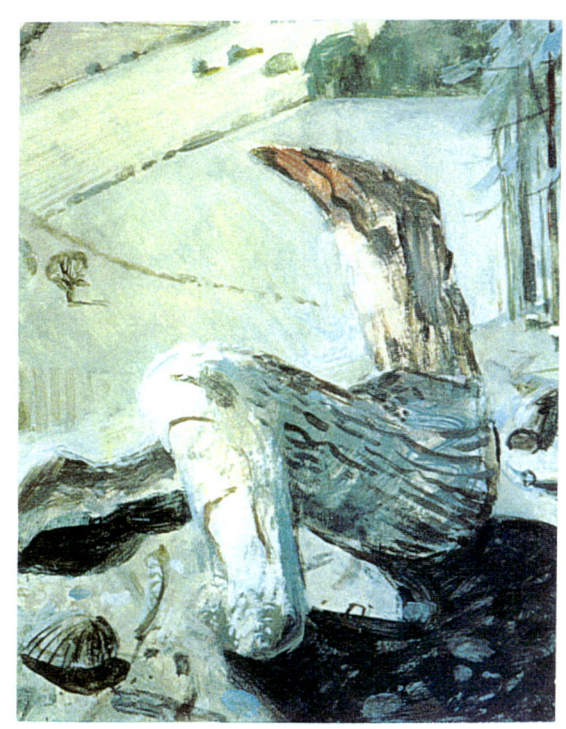

Right: Fig. 518 Log Figure. Found on slopes above the Westwood Valley   Acrylic

Below: The land now took on forms relating to the fan shape of a scallop, groups of trees would begin to float, fish begin to appear in the sky.

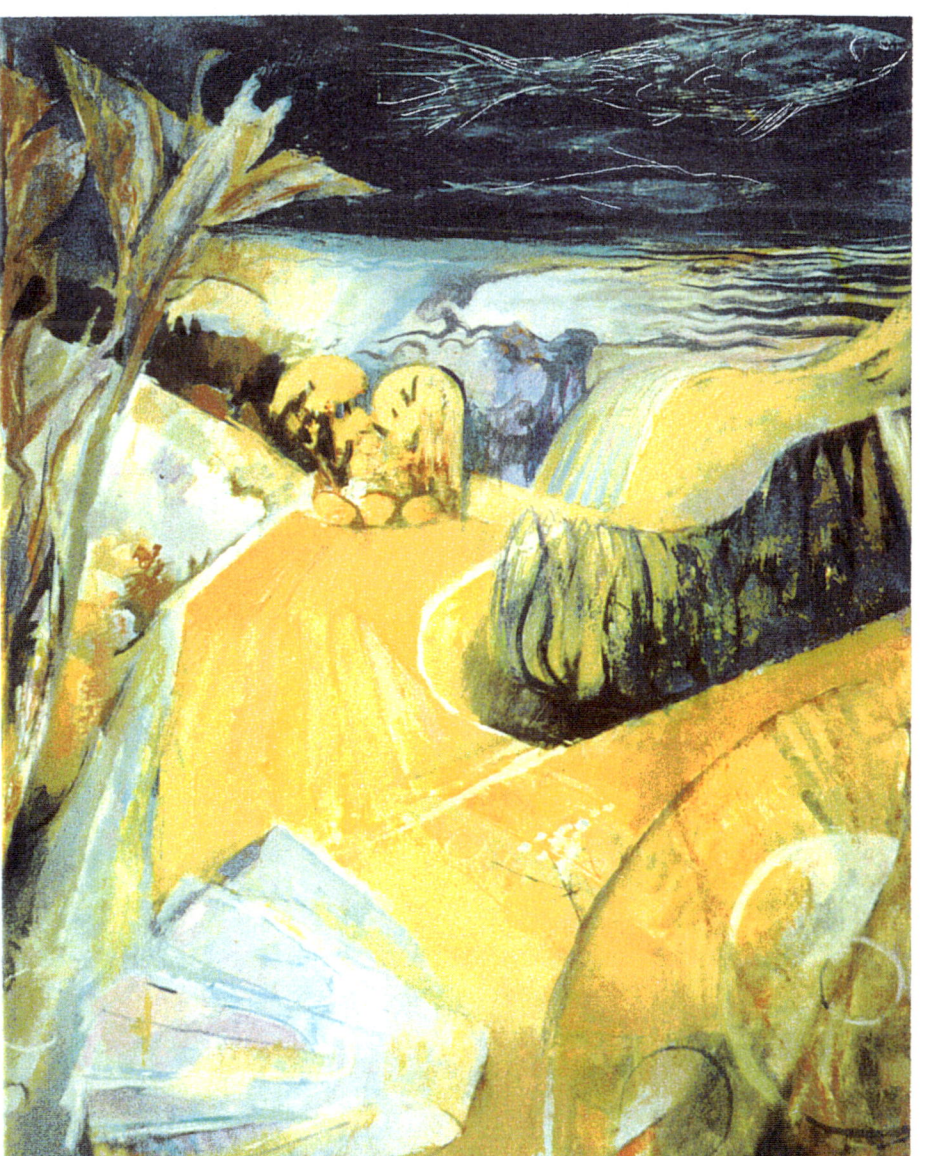

Below: Fig. 520
Pen sketches of possible compositions for paintings.

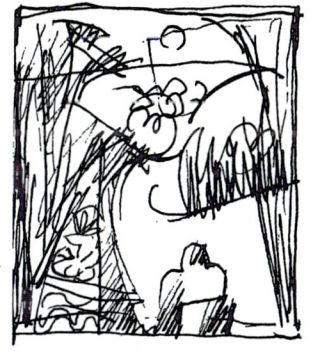

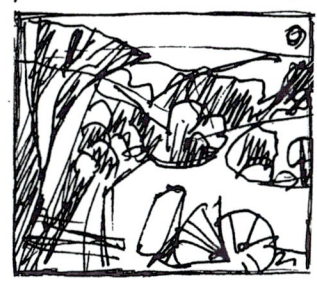

Left: Fig: 519
Jurassic Seascape Westwood transformed by fish and fossils.
Oil on Board

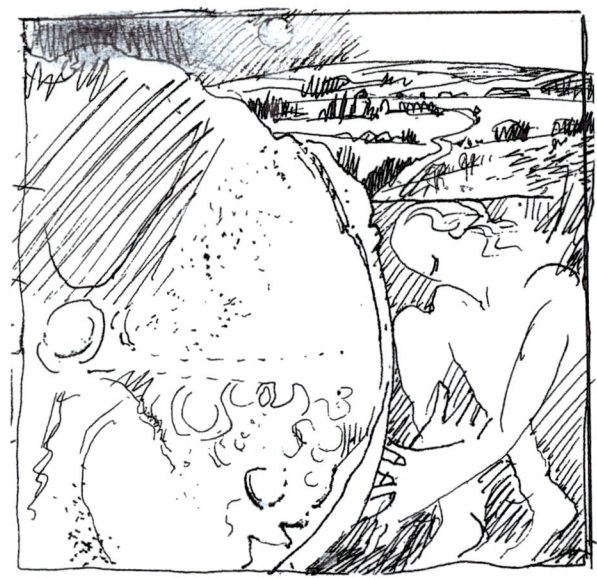 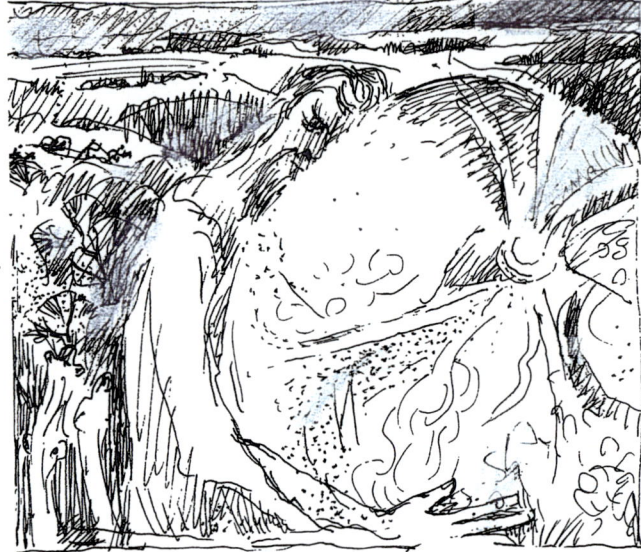

Fig. 521 Two of a series of pen sketches of self making contact with archaeological beginnings. A painting later developed was considered 'inadequate' - and destroyed.

Connections were made between conscious (surface) and unconscious (fossils beneath). I knew then that some active imagination would keep things on course with no retreat from the therapy.

The result of this fossil find, a large sea urchin, was to lead to many more discoveries. 'Devil's toe-nails', urchins, scallops and many others from this once living Jurassic inner sea, now an Oolitic limestone bed.

Further items were added to the collection - small logs, twigs, assorted stones (rough and smooth) and feathers. My work which had been directly representational since the discovery of the valley was now influenced by these finds — of what lay beneath the surface as well as things above. Overlooking the valley from the hill on the left was a large sawn log (see figs 518 & 524) from some earlier tree felling. Its anthropomorphic shape was so compelling I sketched and painted it in situ and later added a stone suggesting a seated figure.

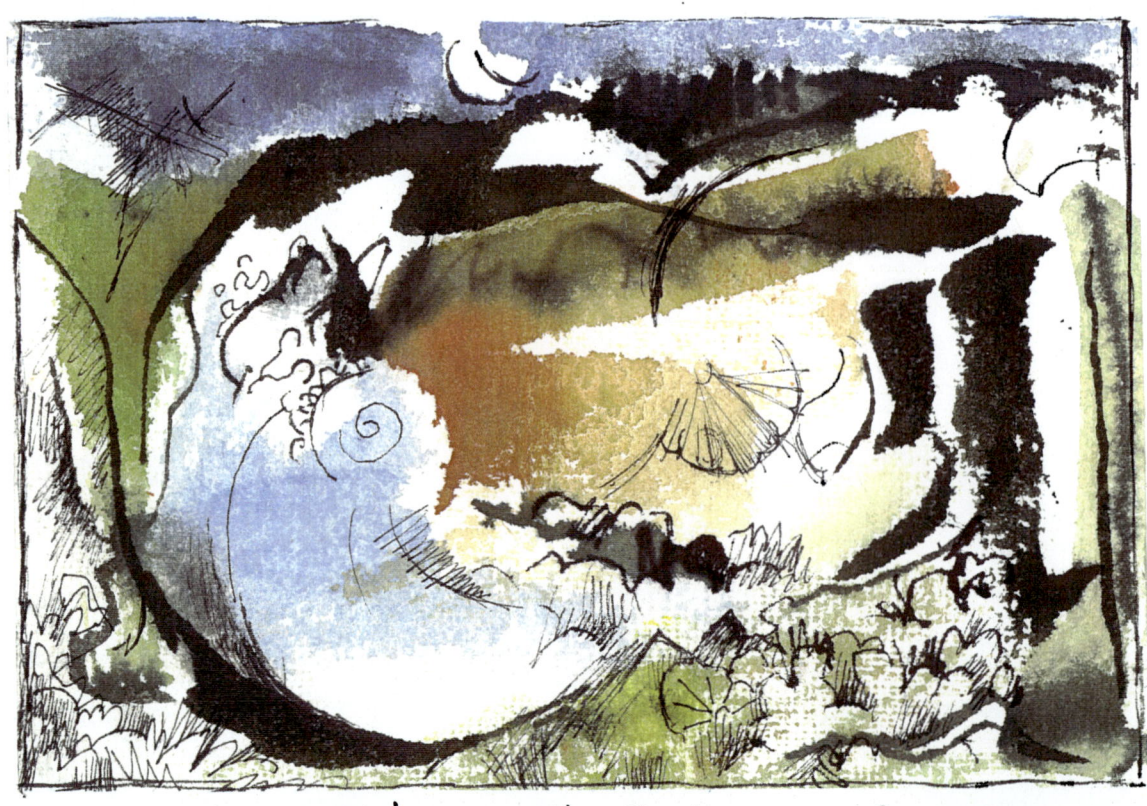

Fig. 522 Colour sketch incorporating Fossils   Pen & Watercolour

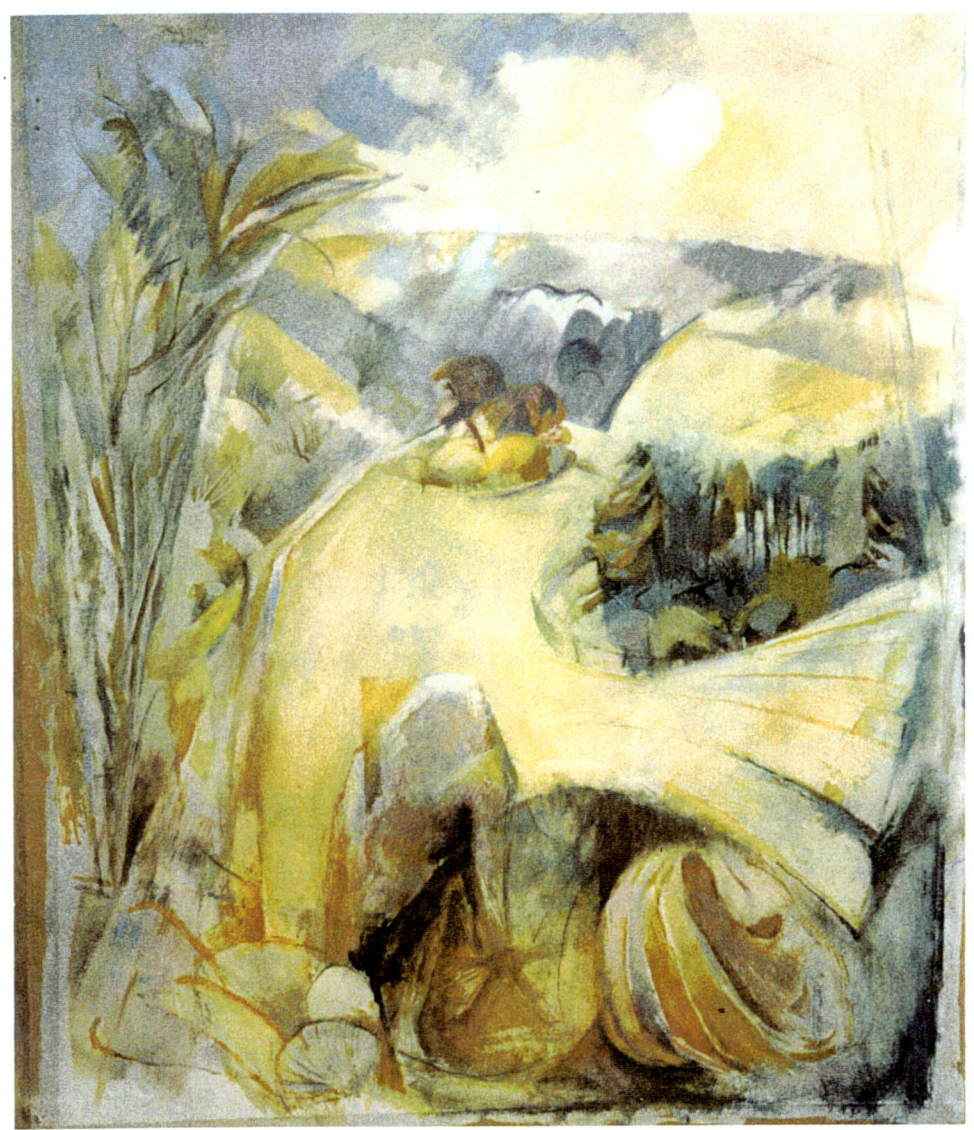

Fig. 523 Westwood Fossils   Sometimes the earth would rise up to reveal subterranean holes or tunnels.
Oil on Board

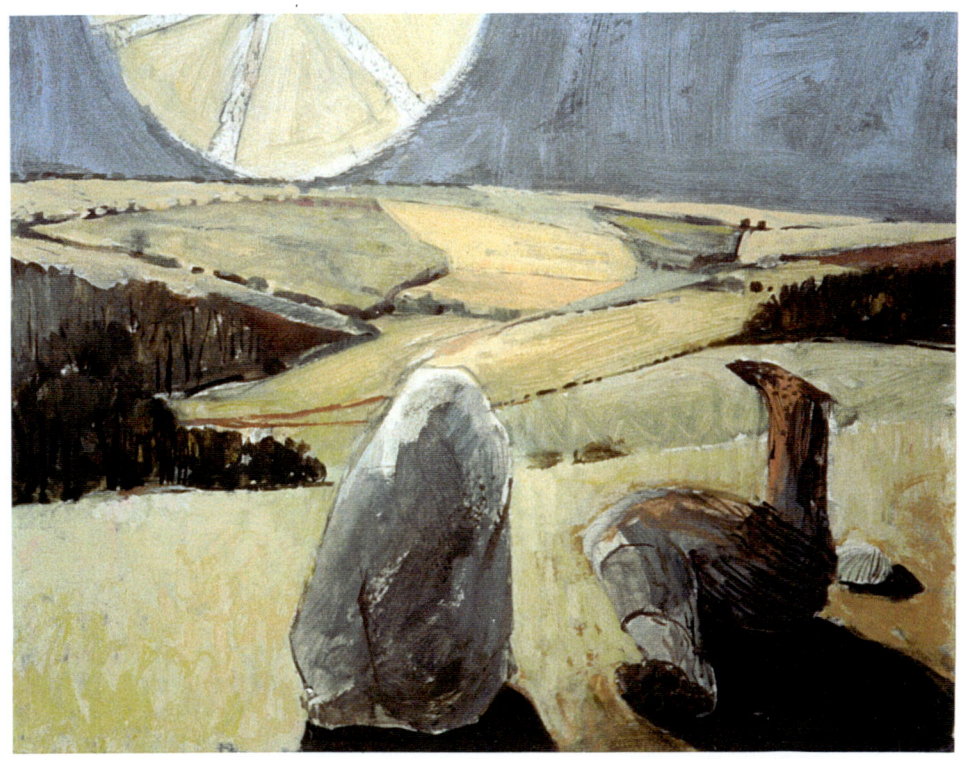

Fig. 524. Wood, Stone, Fossil, Earth — Above Westwood Found natural objects: a stone-like seated figure, a log as a reclining one — the two in conversation/contemplation overlooked by a fossil sun.
Acrylic

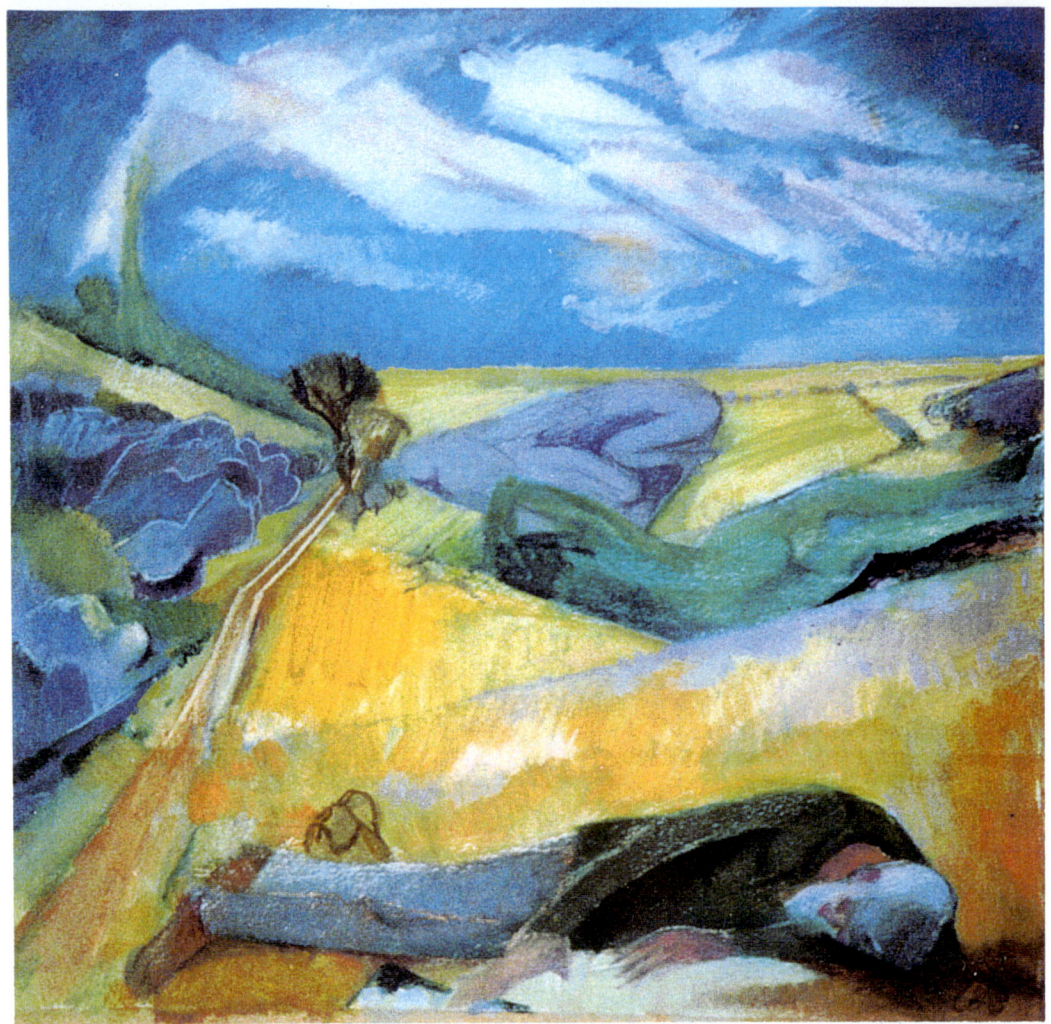

Fig. 525 Westwood Daydream Oil on Paper

A major change followed the fossil drawings and painting. One midday in the summer of 1995 I suddenly felt very weary after a morning drawing and nodded off after a snack. This was a unique happening for me, so I recorded the event as a reverie, dreaming about the wooded areas transformed into reclining nudes and the wind blown clouds into angelic hosts.

This painting was to effect another change following the exploration between levels above and below the surface. A series of pictures of figures as landscape, or landscape as figures.

Below: The landscape assumes a 'human' skin. The fields take on the colour and smoothness of flesh, the trees, of hair.

Fig. 526 Westwood Watercolour

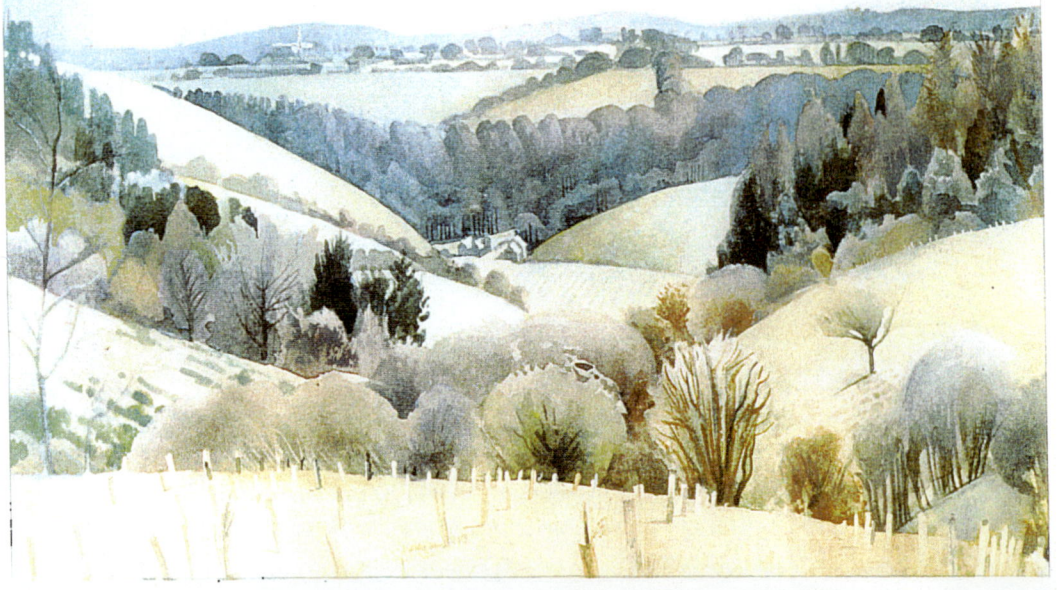

The Westwood scene continued to transform itself, the contour of the left-hand track now became the contour of belly and thigh of a dancer, a field beyond her raised arm, a line of hedgerow her hair and so on. By 1997 a number of sketches led to a large painting of a recumbent nude and then another (figs 529 and 530).

'Spring (fig. 531) seemed an appropriate title for a new found Venus, giving out a totally different reaction to the final Uffington drawing (fig. 498, page 296).

The Goddess was no longer in her rejecting 'mode' — there is a more positive, optimistic 'voice' — the depressive phase had lifted.

Below: Fig. 529 Westwood Dancer
Oil on Board

The small sketches (right) helped clarify and develop ideas for the paintings below and overleaf.

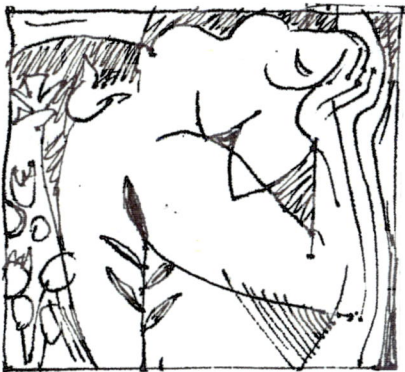

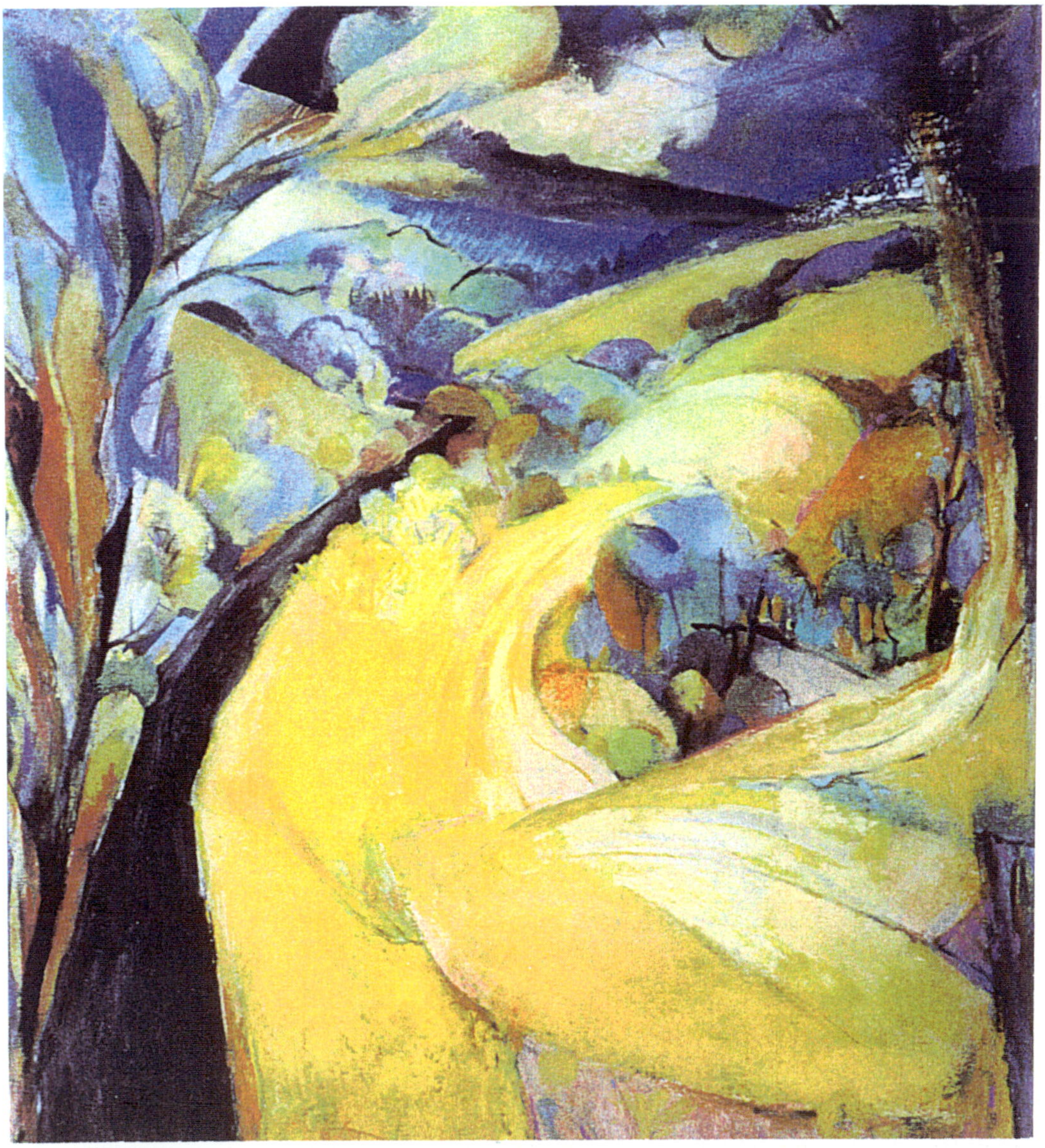

Fig. 527 Sketch for Spring, 1st. version   Pen & Ink

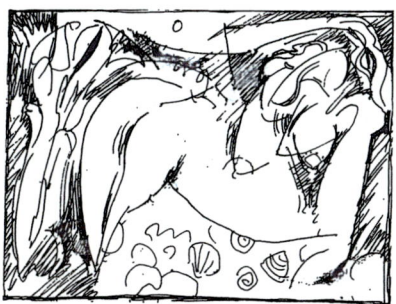

Fig. 528 Sketch for Spring, 2nd. version   Pen & Ink

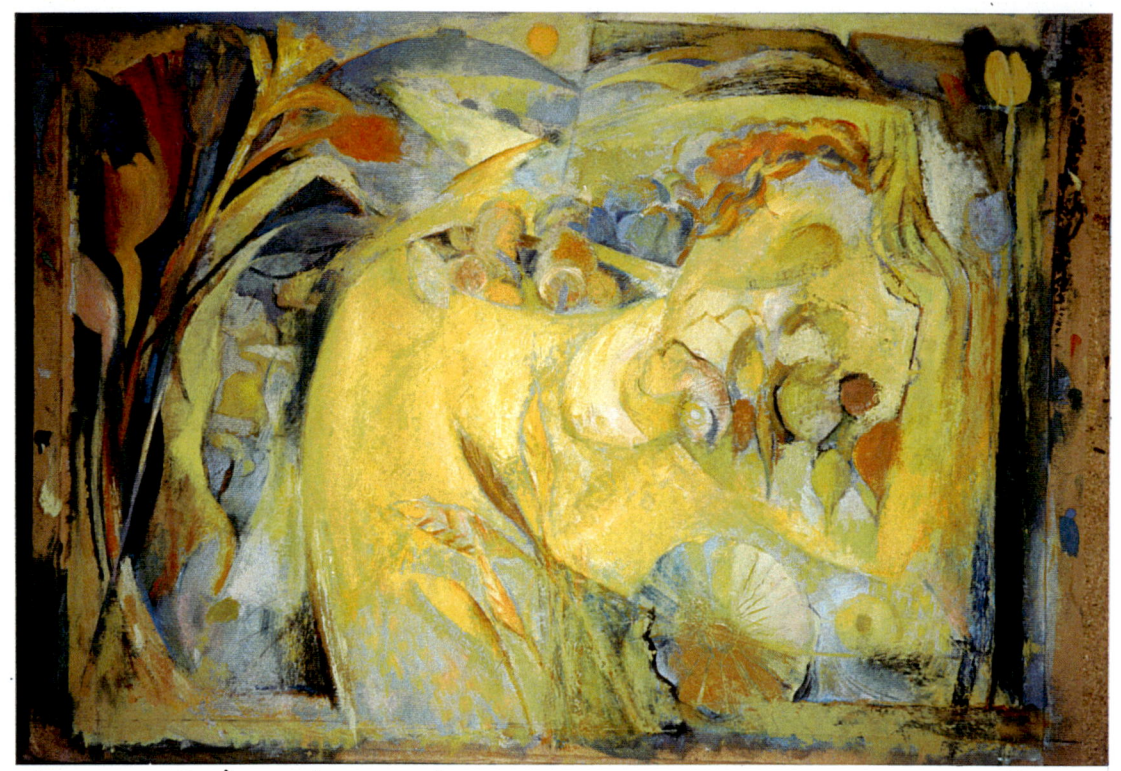

Fig. 530　Spring　1st version　　　　　　　　　　　Oil on Board

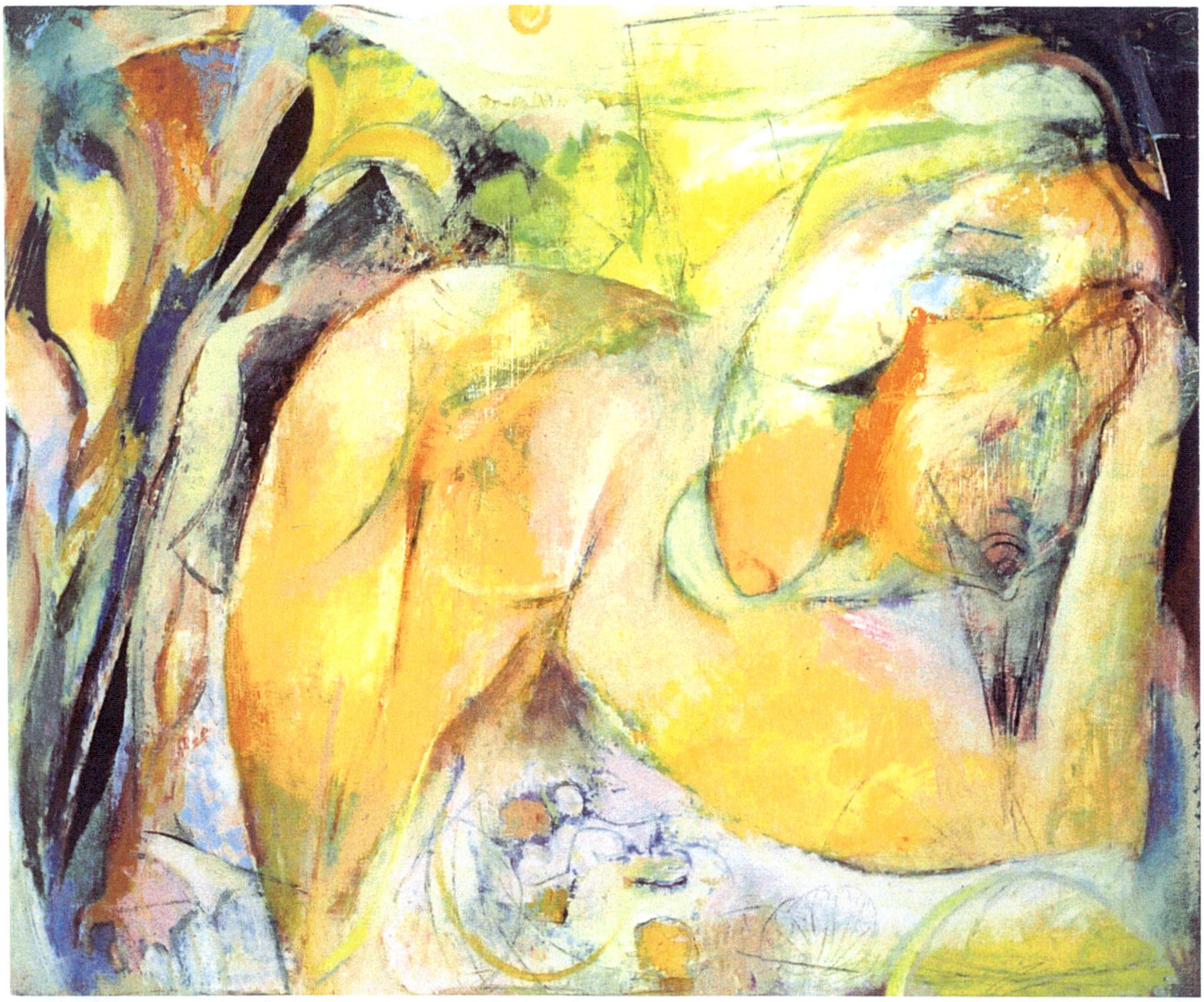

Fig. 531　Spring　2nd version　　　　　　　　　　　Oil on Board

4 THE STONE PIT

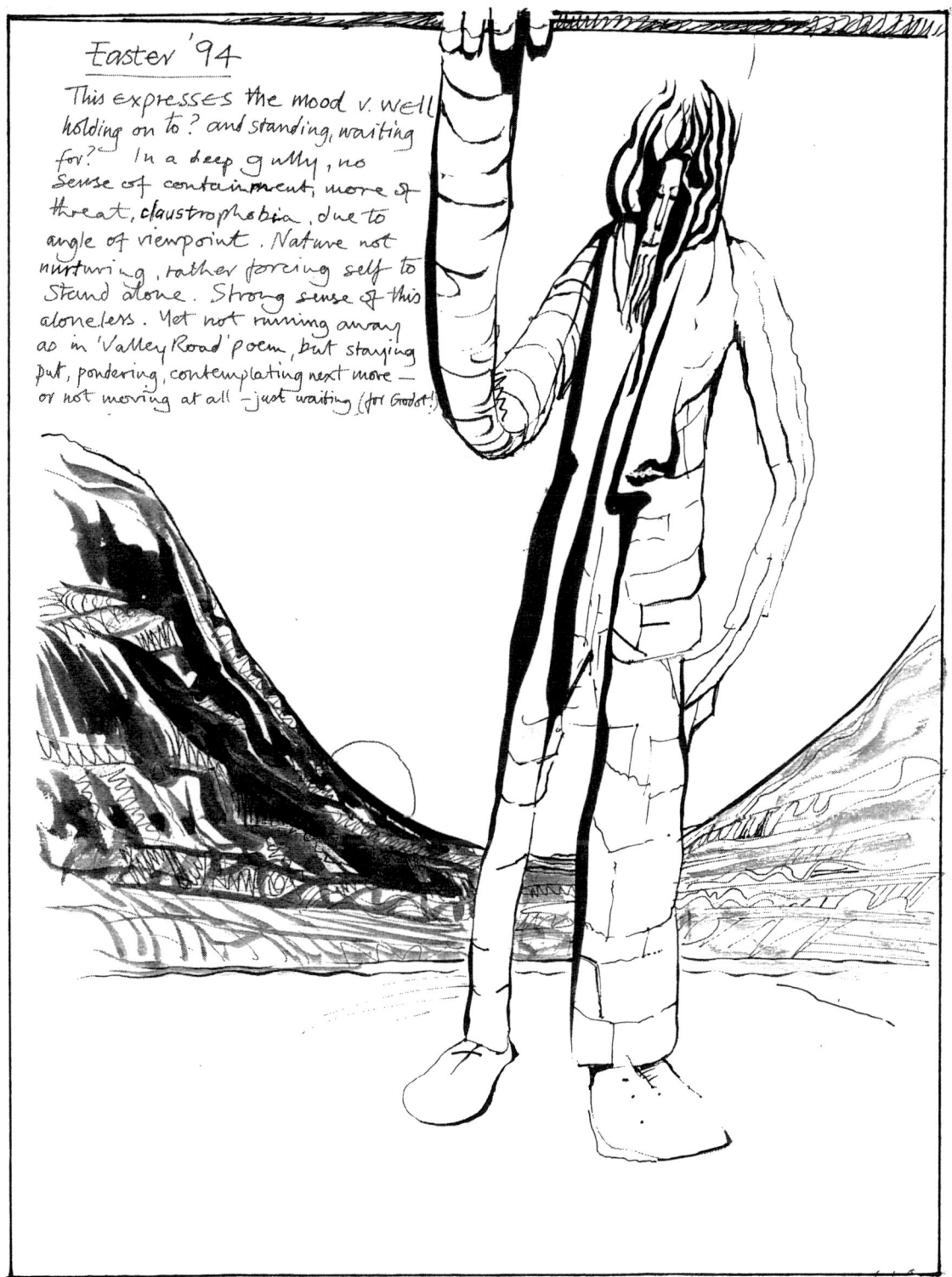

Easter '94
This expresses the mood v. well — holding on to? and standing, waiting for? In a deep gully, no sense of containment, more of threat, claustrophobia, due to angle of viewpoint. Nature not nurturing, rather forcing self to stand alone. Strong sense of this aloneness. Yet not running away as in 'Valley Road' poem, but staying put, pondering, contemplating next move — or not moving at all — just waiting (for Godot!)

Fig. 532   The Stone Figure   Pen & Ink

There was a free-style drawing and two significant dreams in 1994 which were to influence the imagery I was later to find in the rockface of the largest limestone quarry above Watery Bottom (a valley of springs which faces to the North of Cleeve Common). The drawing above shows a lonely standing figure holding onto something. He seems to be carved out of the quarry in which he stands, cracks separating the stone blocks of his body. To the left a text describes the mood of the day.

The first dream is dated 20th. May '94:
'The soldiers are going into battle along narrow passages. One side eventually wins because their leader sacrifices himself for his men. There is a vivid image of this 'Hero' being carried shoulder-high by the men who lead a procession of mourning followers through the lower end of the valley. His body is pierced with arrows and holed by bullets.' 'Were all the enemy weapons directed only at him,' I ask, 'and I wonder how this man was chosen' I receive no answer.

There had been a lively pen and chalk drawing illustrating this dream but it (along with forty others, including paintings) was destroyed in 1997 in an outpouring of negative thinking some months after the therapy with C.
It was one of the old problems - this one is 'good', that 'bad', or 'not good enough. in technique', so it got thrown away. Some of these losses impoverished these pages but this rejective nature is also part of this on-going therapeutic direction.

The second dream occurred on 1st July '94:
'In a market like the Casbah there are many interesting stalls, tents and appartments full of colour and shapes; also costumes of many cultures. I turn off this main thoroughfare into a small section devoted to a festival of native peoples. Here are a small group of 'savages' from a primitive tribe. All of them eye me suspiciously but don't stop me joining them.
In an attempt to communicate with them I embrace their leader who emits a strange smell of musty rotting flesh. He has open wounds which instead of bleeding look dry and dusty - almost 'cobwebby'. The tribe, also wounded, look at me with curiosity as I give the leader a pen and paper in the hope that he will communicate with me. I write on the paper 'This is for you - a gift. Keep in touch'. I then dash off.

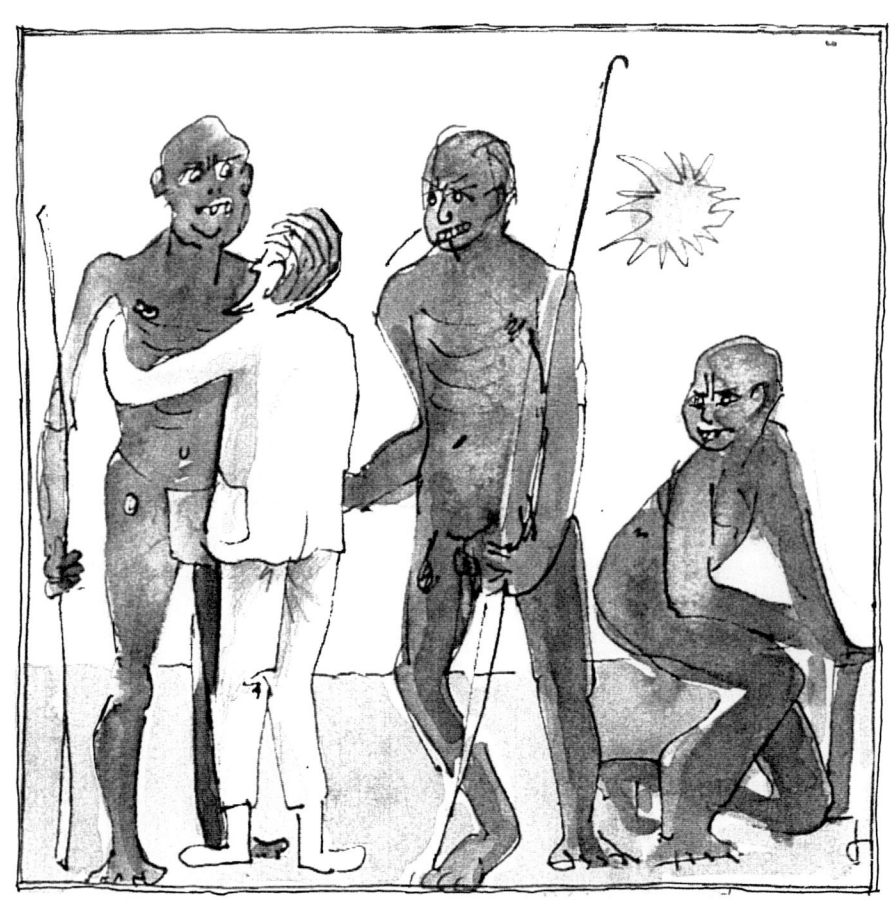

This illustration to the dream has affinities with the warriors I was later to find in the quarry rockface - they too were of giant size and three in number

Perhaps they had answered that request in the dream to communicate later.

Left: Fig. 533
The Primitive Tribe

Pen & Wash

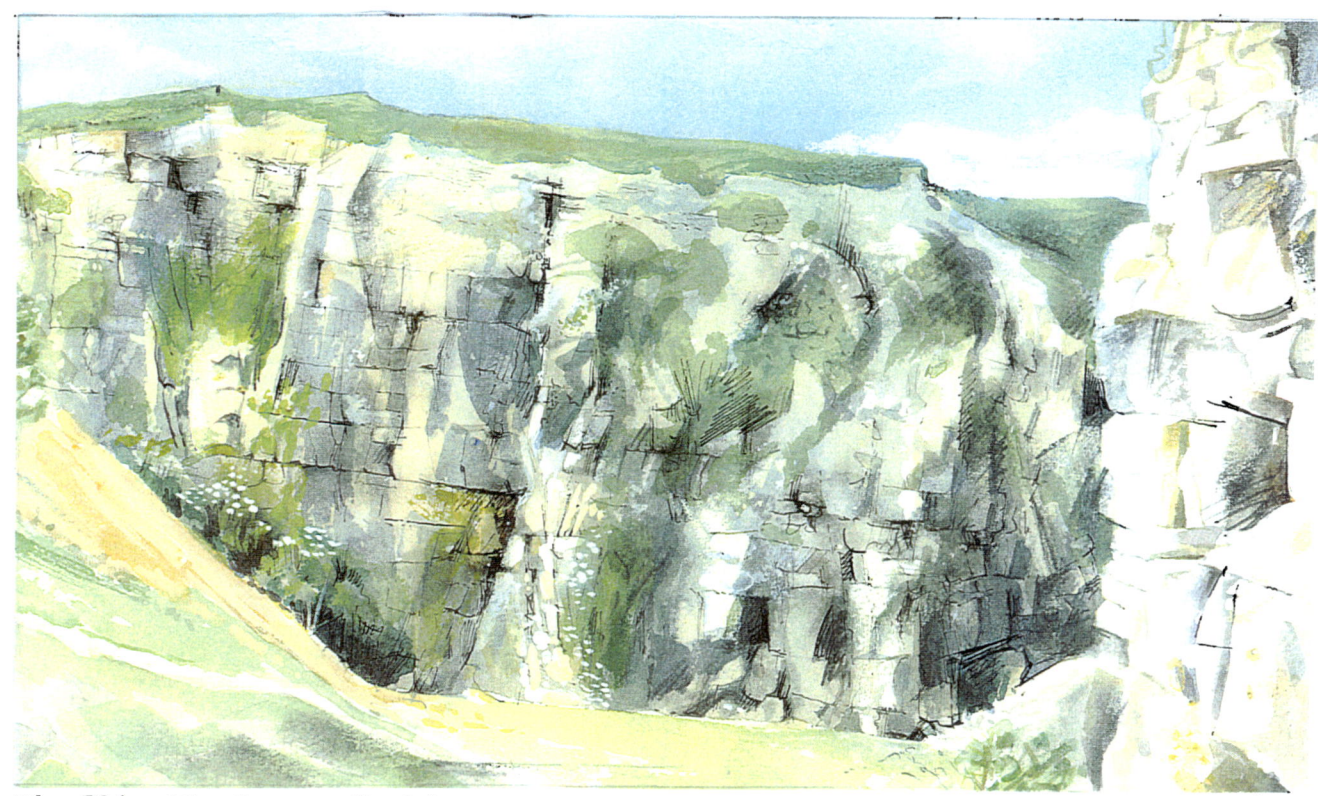

Fig 534   The Quarry Rockface   Pen, Ink & Watercolour

This area of disused quarrying had been of visual interest for many years and I used it for pictures of quarry scenes and studies of rock formations. These works tended to be straightforward studies, very realistic, of the effects of light and shade on rocky outcrops mixed with assorted plants, trees and screes (fig 534).

Following the first dream, however, the rockface started to yield something quite different. I had until then noticed a radiating set of what looked like blast lines from an explosive charge of dynamite and had registered only its fan-like arrangement. Within a week or so and on my next visit to the site I noticed a subtle shift in emphasis somewhere within these lines which intrigued me, yet I couldn't understand what was taking place.

Then a month later it swiftly crystallised. I was looking at an exultant warrior Hero, limbs (partially amputated) forming a Greek Cross. This caused me to complete a watercolour on the spot (fig 535) and write a poem 'Stone Pit' shortly afterwards

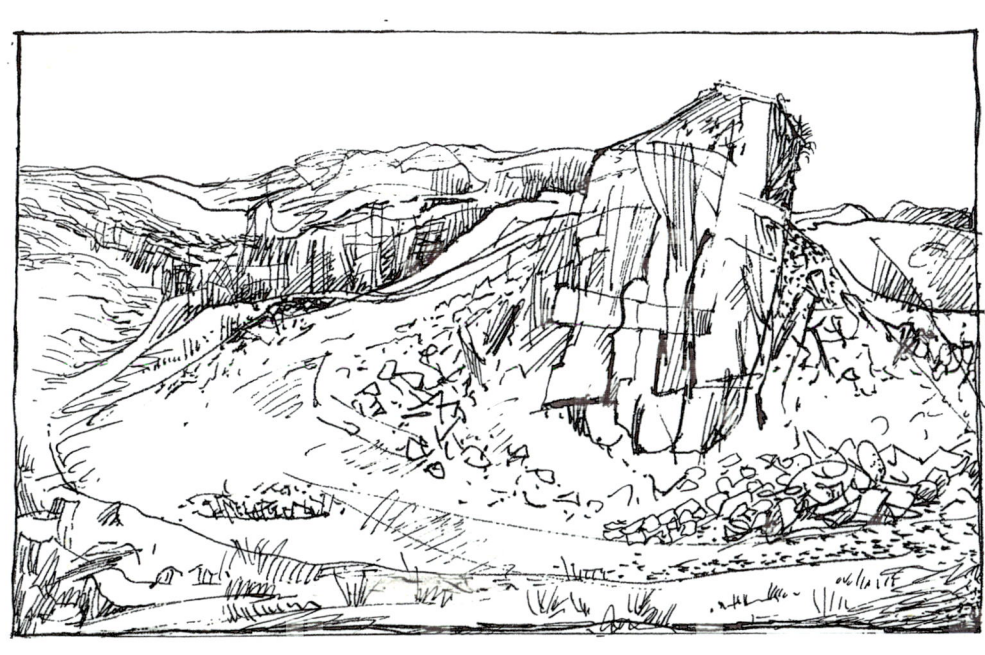

Left: Fig. 534A
Limestone Outcrop
Pen & Ink

Standing like a sentinel this outcrop guards the front of the quarry face.

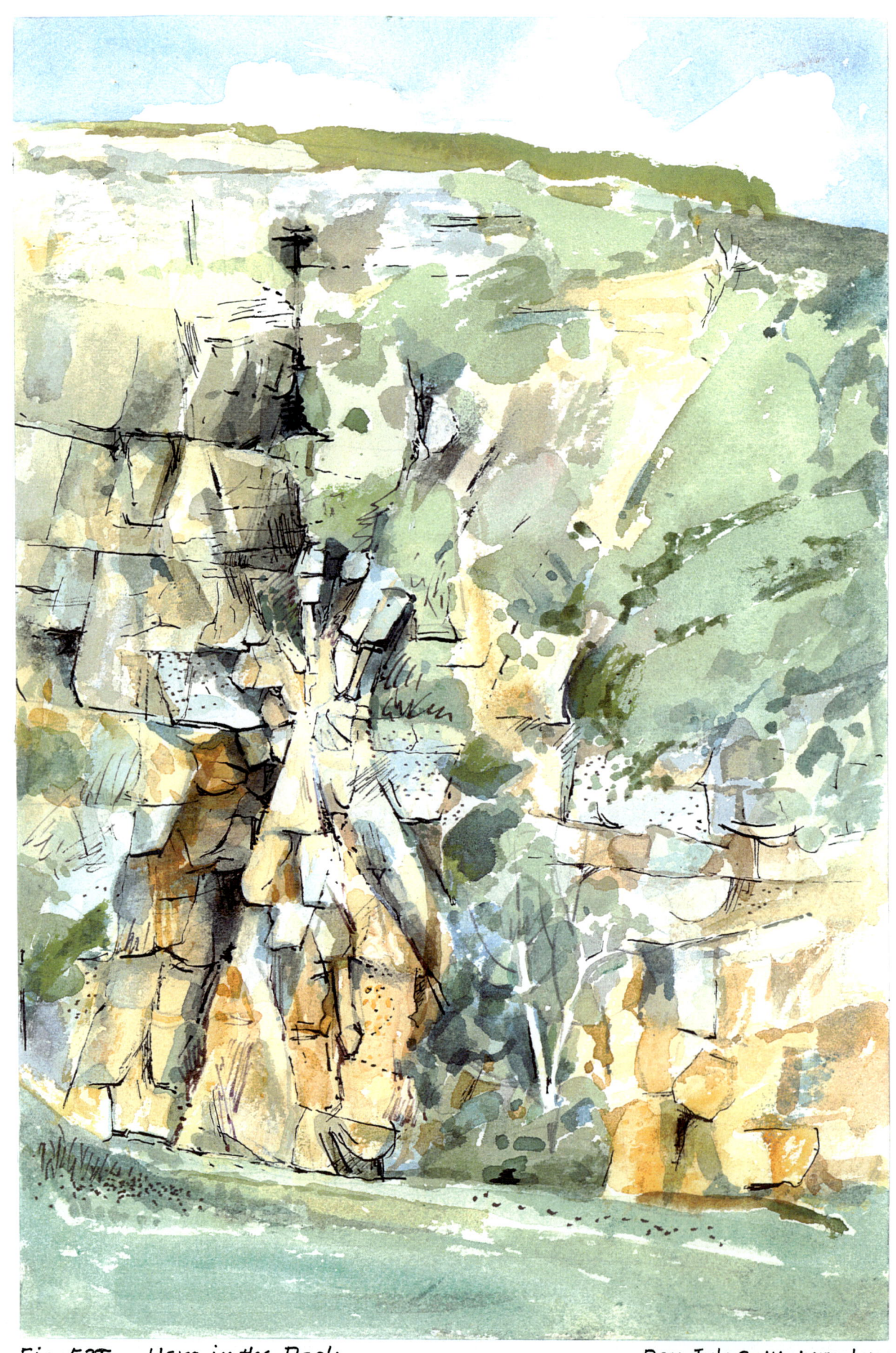

Fig. 535   Hero in the Rock   Pen, Ink & Watercolour
(Painted immediately following the 'apparition' in the rockface of the 'Stone Pit').

Stone Pit

Sudden whirr-winging skylarks lift off
From foot-firm shimmering grass
Then no place to step but down.

Inside this deep-dug place the
Rockface holds its fissured secrets.
Mum with stillness, heat.

Giants born in moments of illumination, stand
Stoic attendants to a huge sad head,
Wreathed in Emerald mystery.

In the radiant centre a
Warrior exultant, limbs akimbo,
Shouts victory from the cliff.

Proud, proper to his standing,
An Indian brave, hair blazing,
Wears an ochre-umbered face.

As stone echoes animate the heart
I hear crying in the wind.
Skylarks.

The Stone Pit poem, written during this period, attempts to convey the varied figures 'found' in the rockface.

The Stone Pit Giants

While I continued to draw the structure of the rockface, three more forms 'grew' out of the cliff above and to the left of the hero, much larger than him and with the odd hint of 'crusader' helmets. Later I made the rather tenuous connection to the aboriginal 'warriors' with their large bows, their giant size and three in number. They had answered my call for communication. (Fig. 533)

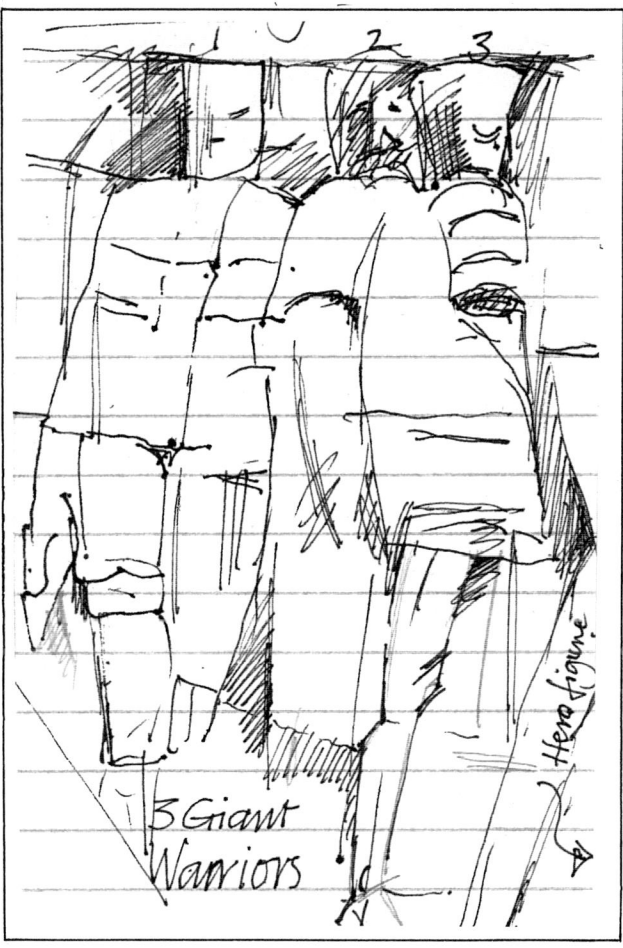

Fig. 537   Three Giant Warriors   Pen & Ink

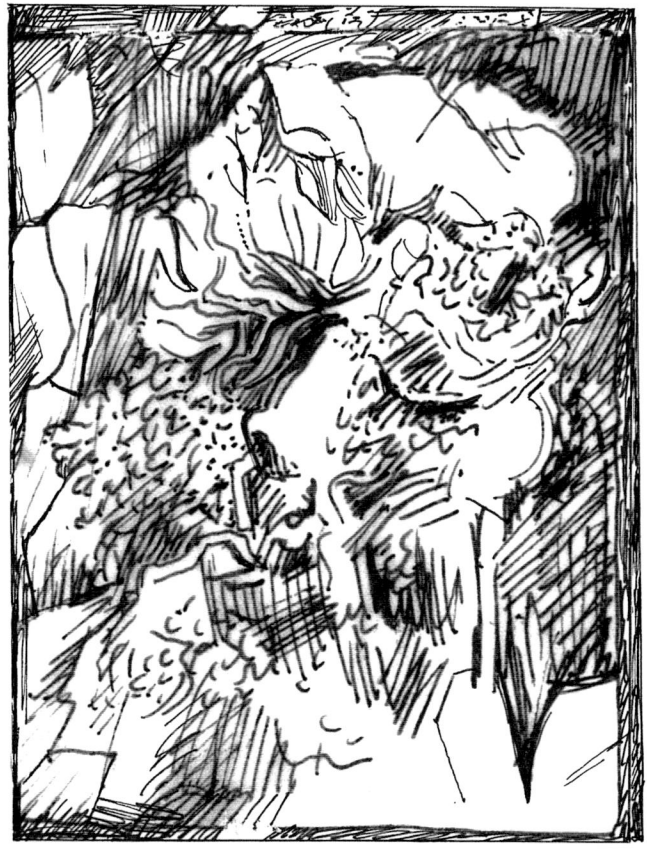

Fig. 536   Giant Head   Pen & Ink
(the 'huge sad head' in the Stone Pit poem)

Very soon afterwards (there were now frequent visits across the Common to the Stone Pit), a 'find' in the cliff of a giant head emerging out of a mix of creeper and cracked rock took me unawares. The more I looked, the stronger the impression — here a wreath across the forehead, an eye socket and a slight hint of a chin. An overall sense of a huge sad head, reflecting the mood of inner sadness — what my therapist, on seeing the drawing, thought was a head of suffering (fig. 536).

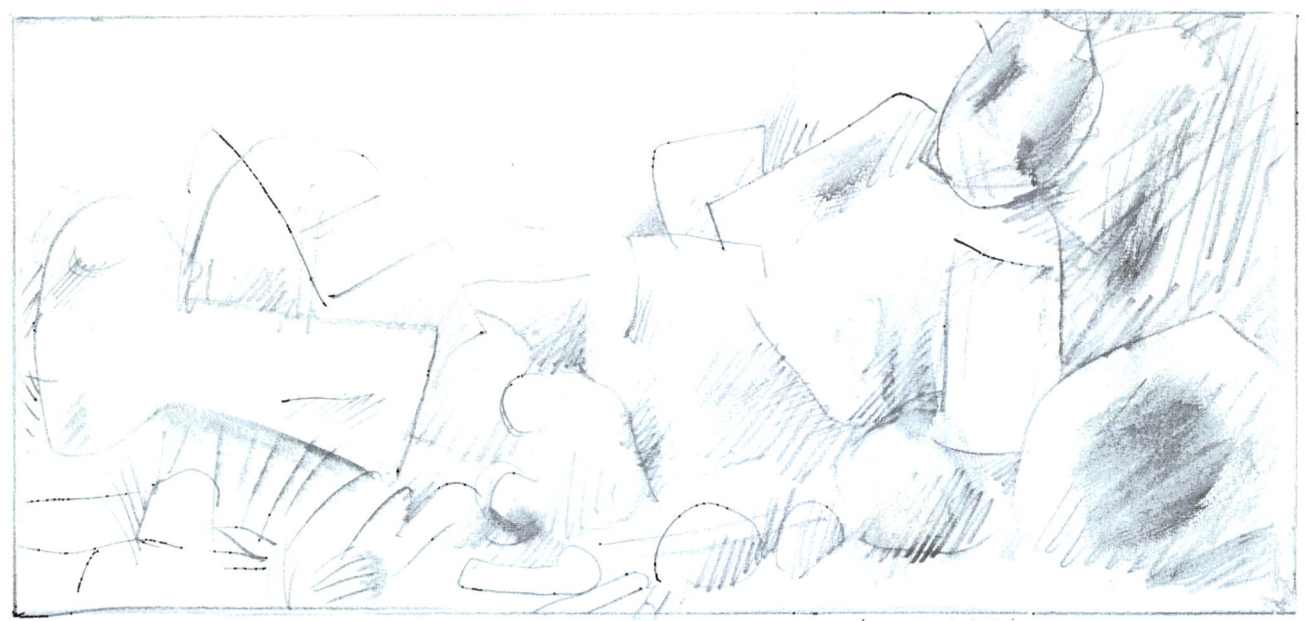

Fig. 538   Fragmented Stone Man   Aquarelle Pencil

At the base of the cliff lay many larger rocks which I re-arranged into a fragmented reclining figure (fig.538). This idea later figured in the 'Stone Pit' painting (fig. 540).

The Hero and his military support group represented an optimistic bright light into dark subterranean moods, but it was soon countered by another image of more sombre content.

'Moon with Fragmented Figure' allowed the darkness to dominate.

Painting in the freestyle method enabled the hand to roam freely across the surface and conjure up a hero fragmented under the influence of the moon.

C.'s admonitions to 'stay with it' (i.e. depressive feelings, hopelessness, pain, etc.) were beginning to prove beneficial, because the image now revealed the purpose of the inner conflict – that the challenge was with a chimera. Nothing less than the fear of fear itself, the constant rejection by the mother image I superimposed on every woman, the retreats from any form of conflict which evoked past patterns of rejection i.e. being fostered out, being sent like an orphan to boarding school – in a word, abandonment.

This recognition was all that was required to penetrate the chimera's mask.

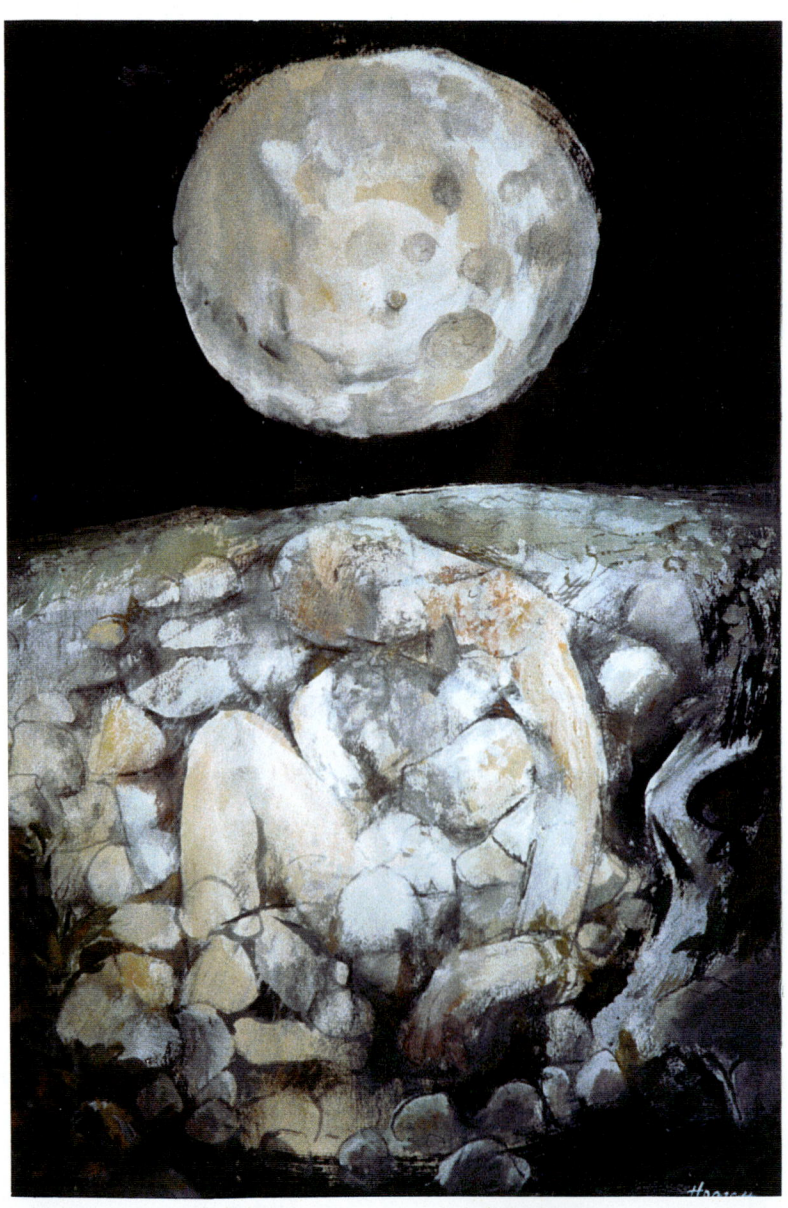

Fig. 539 Moon with Fragmented Figure   Gouache

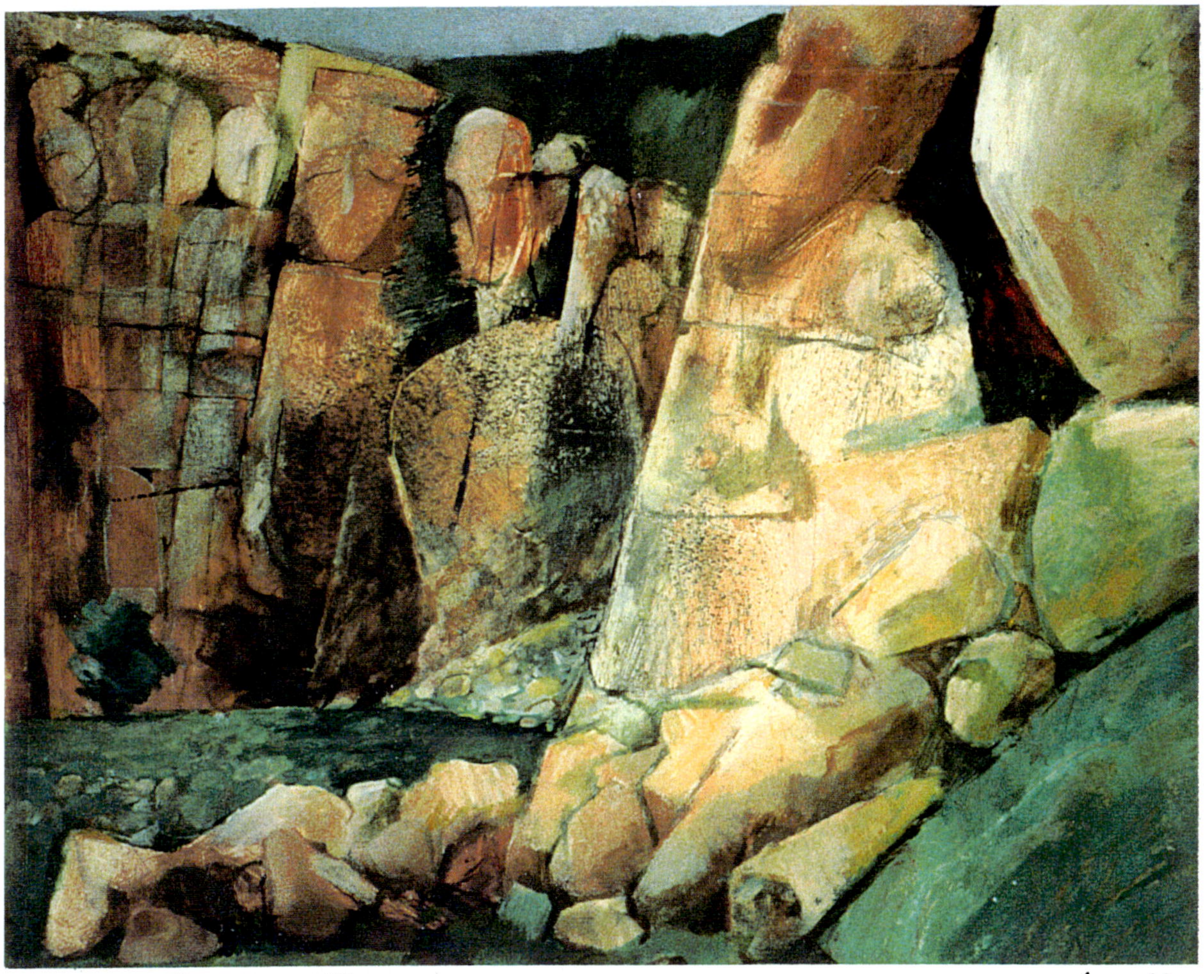

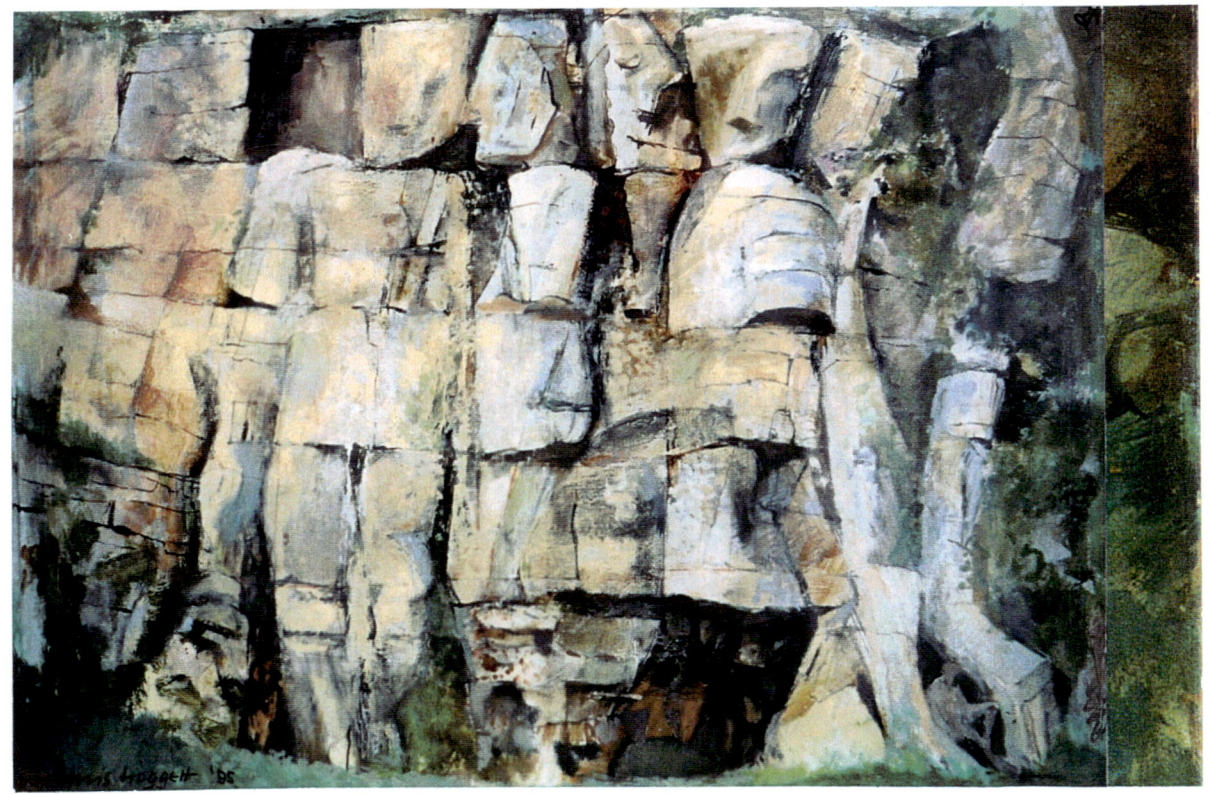

Fig. 540 The Stone Pit   Acrylic

The 'Stone Pit' attempts to fit most of the imagery into the quarry space. The 'Indian Brave' never reappeared - he vanished from the scene (see poem, page 319).

Fig. 541 Rockface Warriors (based on pen sketch, page 319).   Gouache

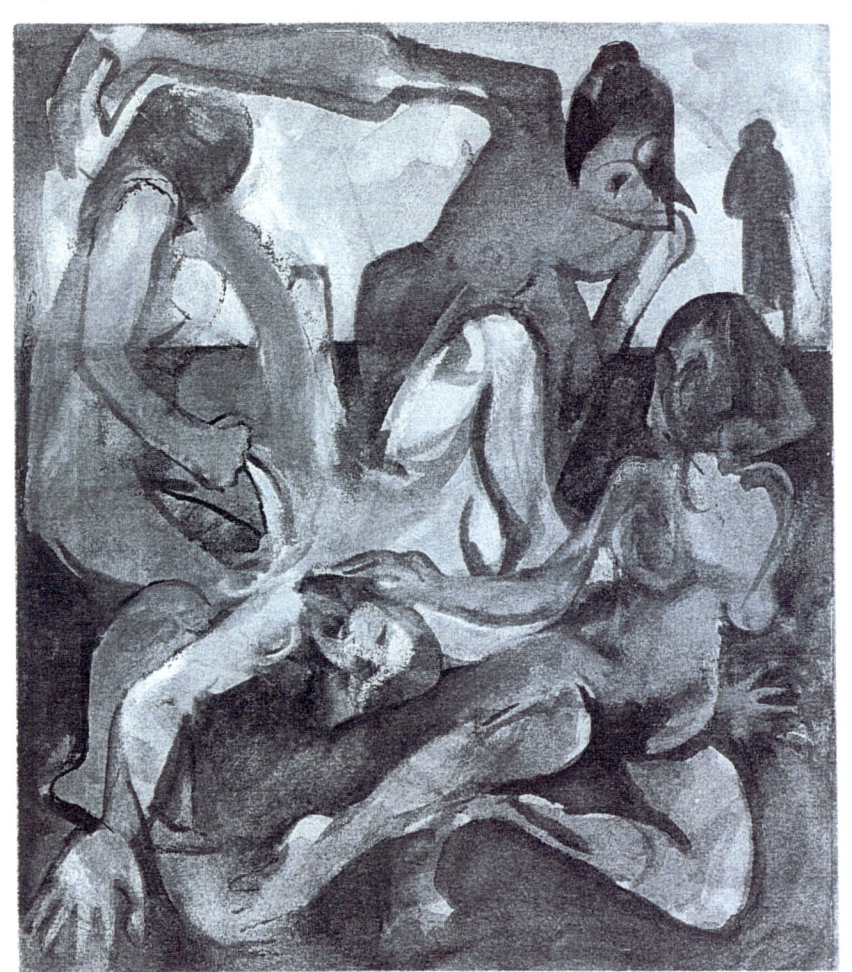

Untitled 1 1980s

Three women are giving a drubbing in one form or another to a spread-eagled male figure. Beyond stands a shadowy older woman. This small painting is the precursor of many retentive memories of childhood experiences of rejection.

Fig 542 Untitled I   Gouache

Untitled II (1996)

If 'Untitled I' was perhaps the first visualised acknowledgement of feelings of rejection by the woman, this more recent painting is confirmation of it. The protagonists are so close they can share a mouth and nostrils yet are so emotionally distant that the man is frozen with suspicion, his hands totally disengaged. He rejects because he has been rejected.

Fig 543 Untitled II   Acrylic

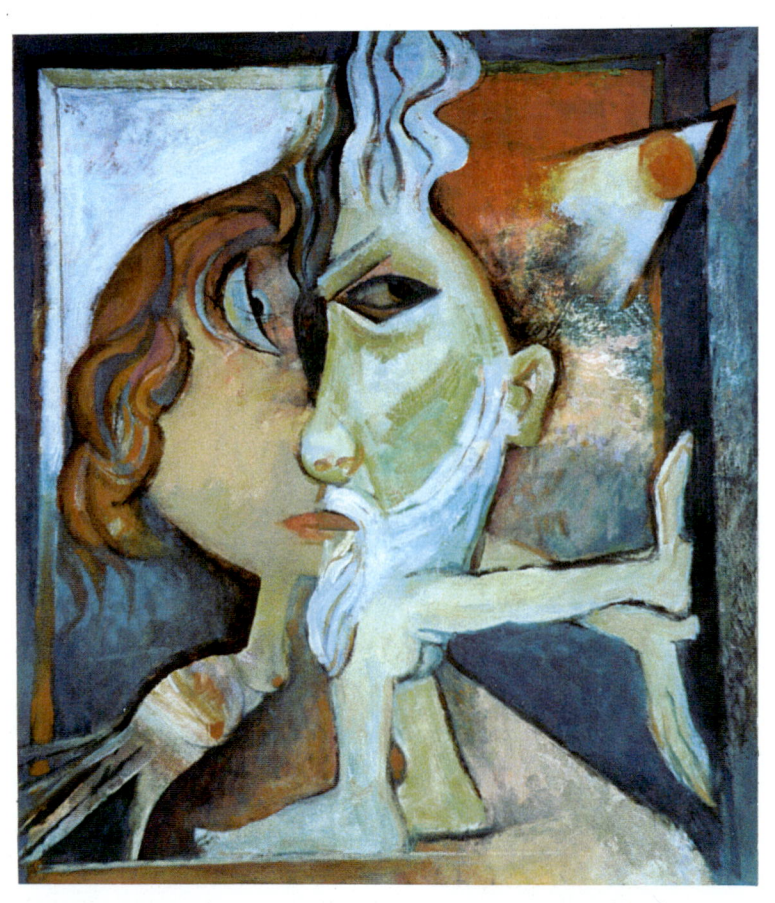

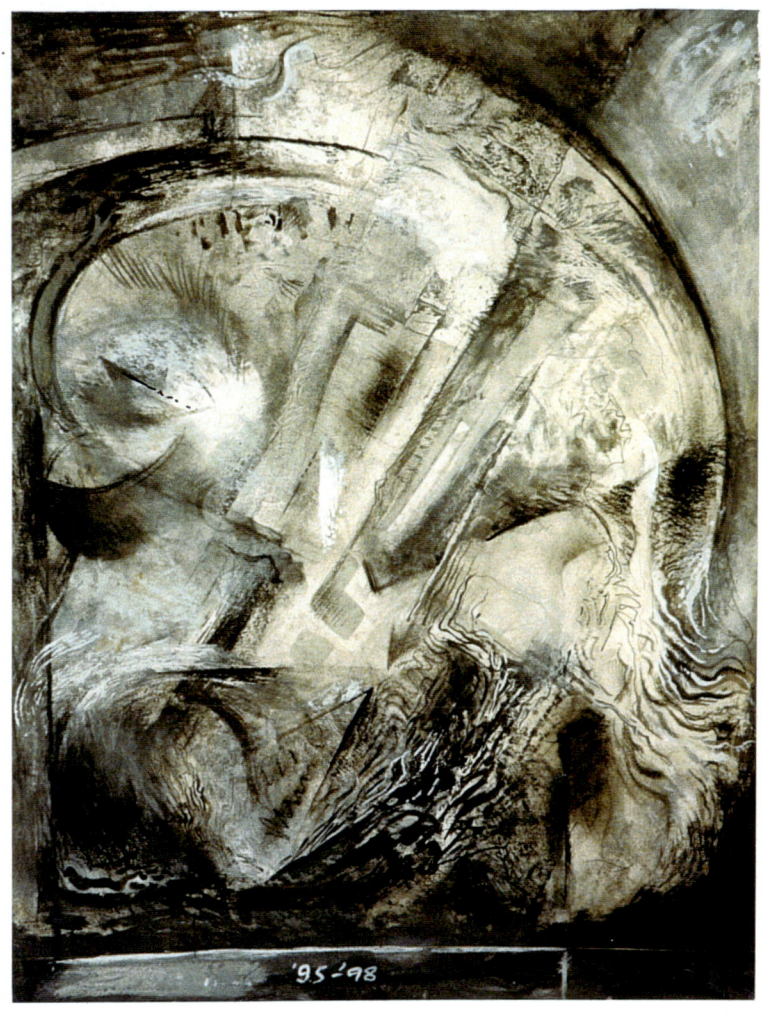

The Old Warrior 1995/1998

A re-working on top of an earlier free-style painting. On top of the confusion of lines and a conglomeration of textures I found the disgruntled warrior with his world-weary suspicious nature ready for confrontation.

He has risen again from the broken figure in the 'Moon' picture (fig. 539).

He was ready to meet the Goddess' challenge when next it came.

Fig.544 The Old Warrior
Mixed Media

In 1998 when this and the final sequence of these hero-Goddess myths were completed one more image was to appear on an earlier photograph of the rock-face. Sometimes one cannot see what is there, unless ready to receive it. On returning to the site to confirm whether the image in the rock matched that seen in the photo I found that it was indeed there - minus a mouth.

Perhaps the message was "You've said enough - it's time to move on".

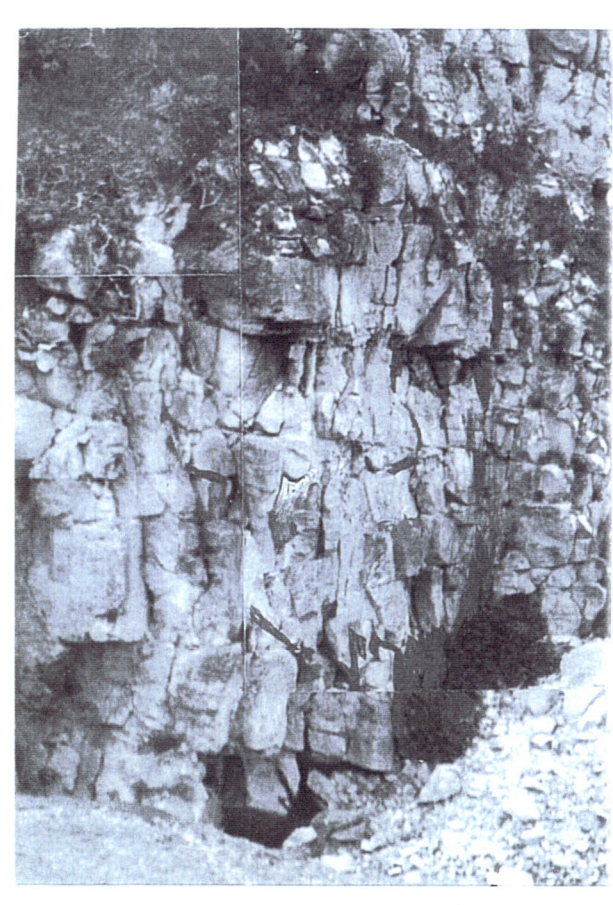

Fig. 545 Self portrait in the 'Stone Pit' - minus a mouth   photo.

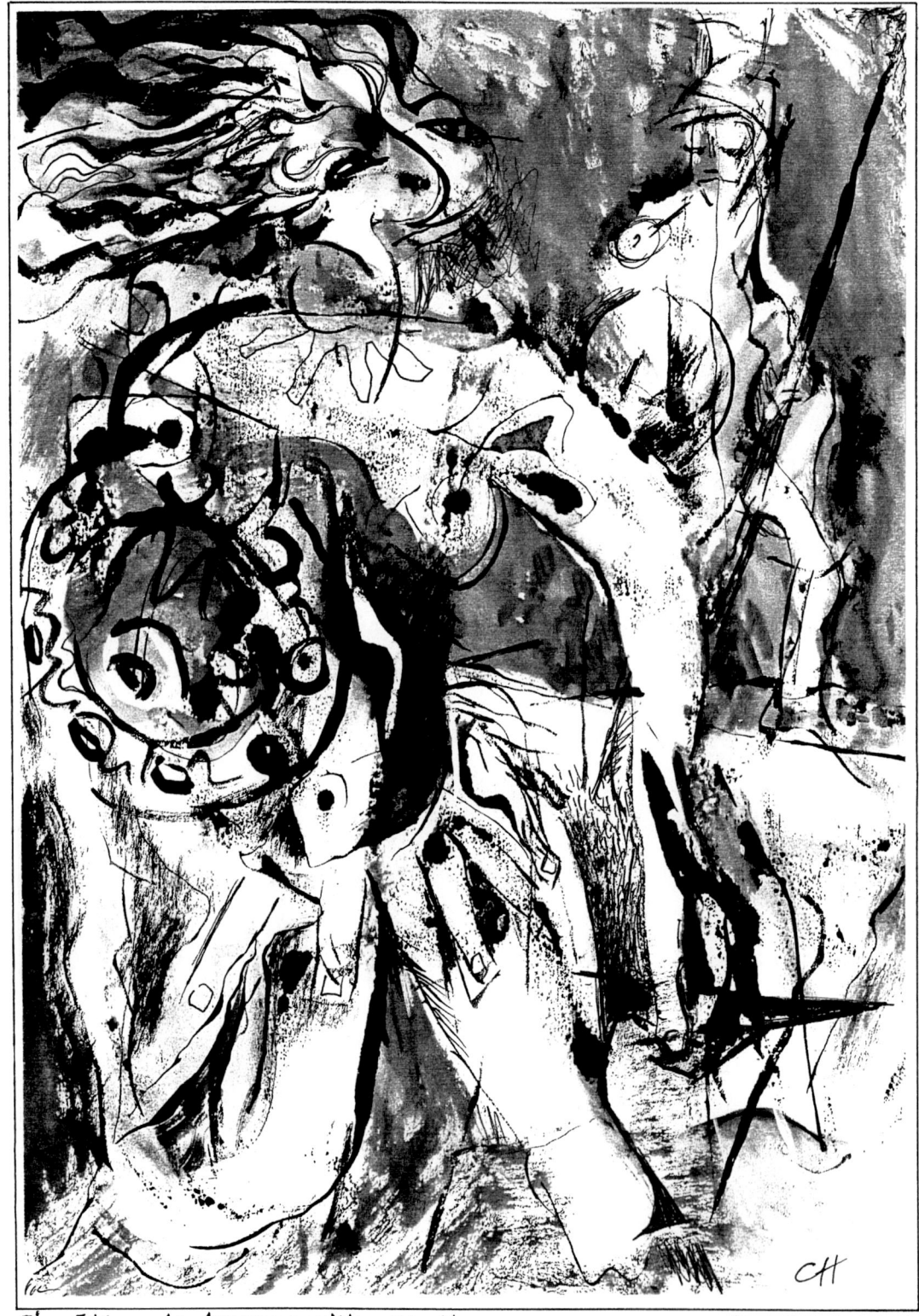

Fig. 546 An Amazon with a Challenger Pen, Ink & Wash

A postscript to the 'Stone Pit' sequence lay within this free-style brush drawing, completed shortly after finding the giant head (fig. 536).
'Amazon with a Challenger' felt like a skirmish before the conflict. The hero (for it is surely he) stands behind, in a moment of indecision — the moment before the challenge (fig. 546).

5 POSTLIP WARREN

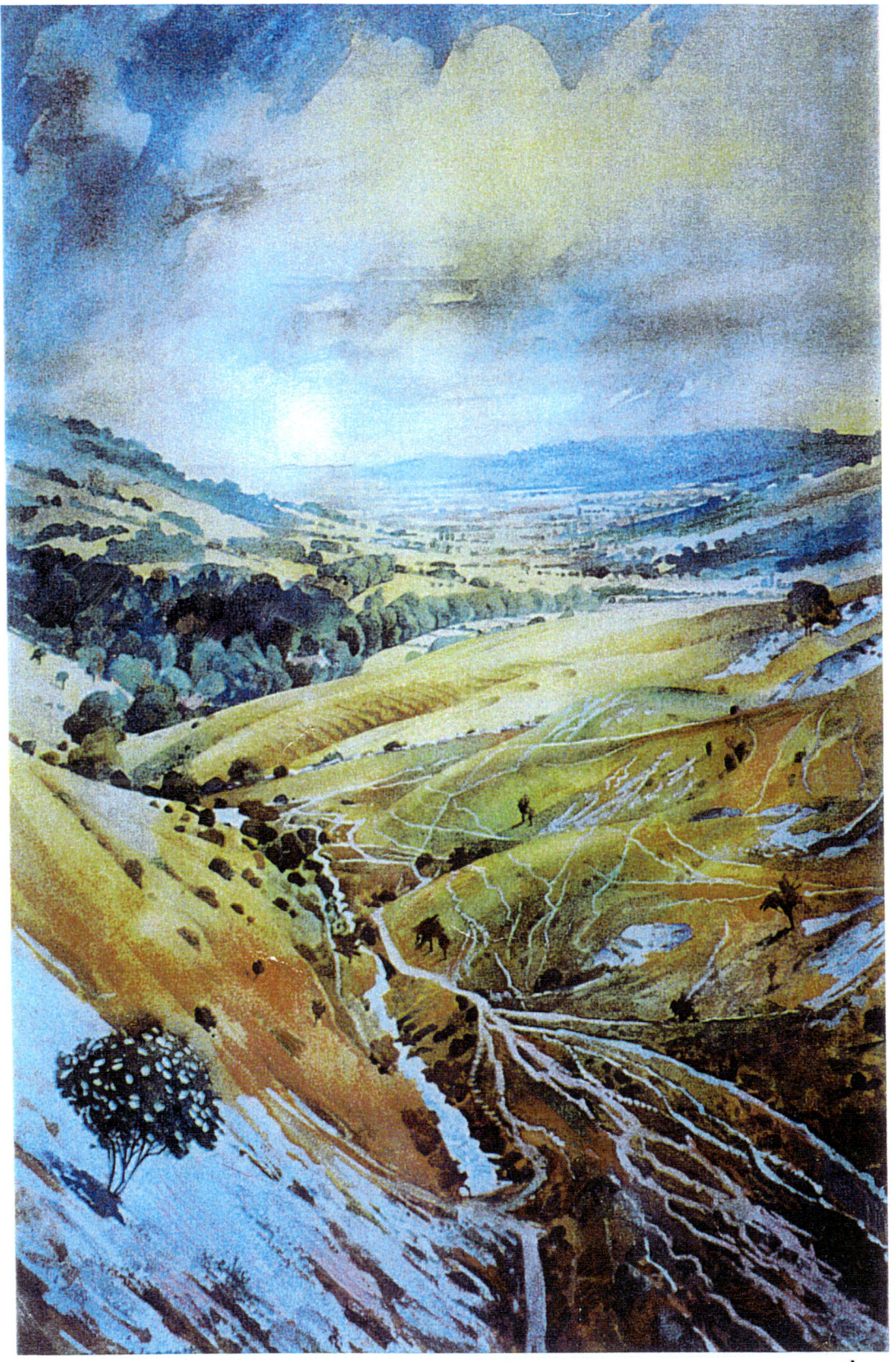

Fig.547 Summer - Postlip Warren and Watery Bottom, Cleeve Common   Watercolour

May 1997. From the scree top I look down into Watery Bottom valley. A small stream springs out from sources beneath the limestone, flows down to a pond, and meanders on towards Winchcombe. Behind the pool Postlip Hall, its great barn and a chapel stand in a wooded enclosure, while beyond lies the Vale of Evesham.

To the right of the stream, tufted grassland steeply rises to meet the crumbling boundary wall of the Common. This is the Warren, said to abound in rabbits – I've yet to spot one after years of painting here. Its undulating form is scarred with old quarry-workings with scattered elders amongst the stones.

Up until the Spring of 1997 this viewpoint had brought much visual delight, leading to a succession of naturalistic watercolours, until I ventured into new territory, including the 'Stone Pit' quarry.

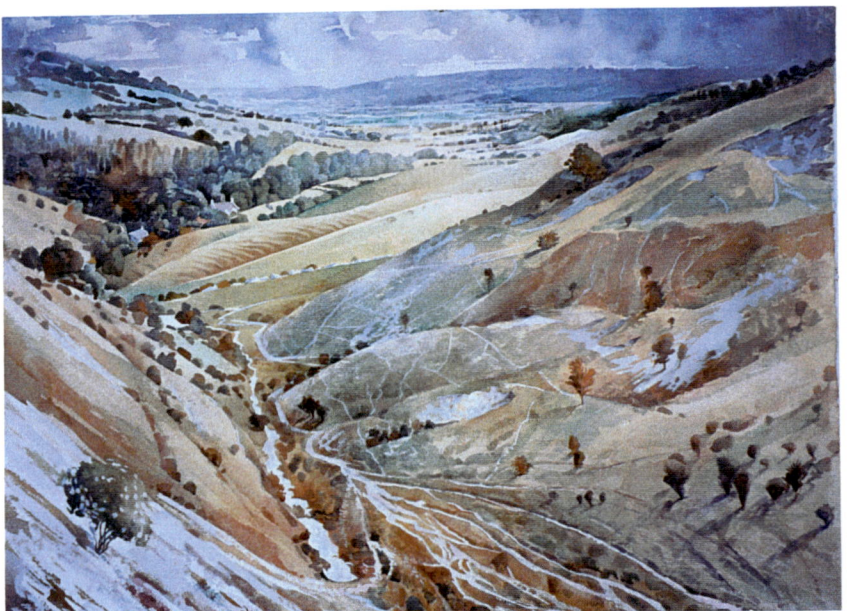

I painted the Warren and Watery Bottom at different seasons of the year:

Fig. 547 (previous page) Summer

Fig. 548 Early Autumn, the tufted grass bleached into pale umbers

Fig. 549 November, with cool blue-greys and rising mist

Fig. 548 Autumn, Watery Bottom   Watercolour

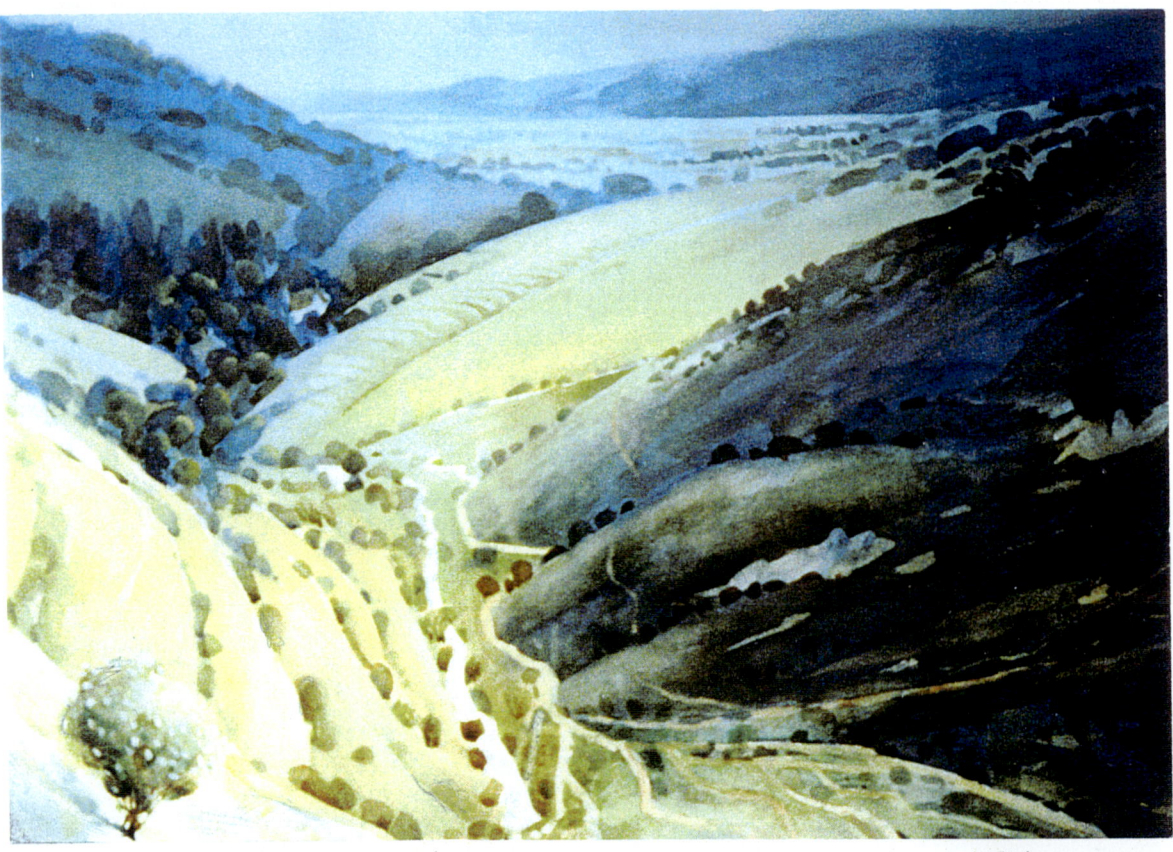

Fig. 549   November. Rising mist, Watery Bottom   Watercolour

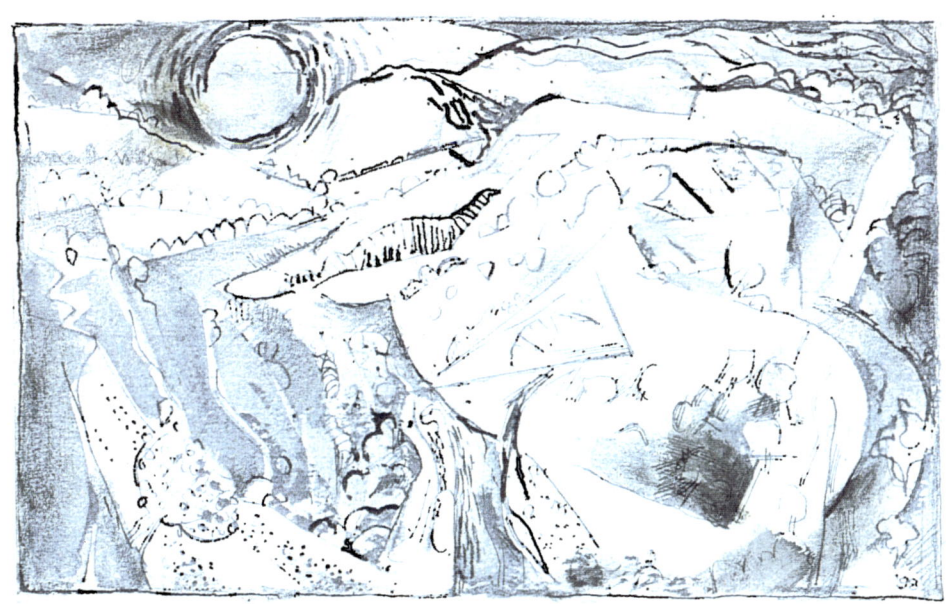

Left: Fig. 550
Postlip Maiden - I

Pen and wash sketch of Watery Bottom - the first of a sequence of new pictures of the valley

At foot: Fig 551
Postlip Yellow, Watery Bottom.

Pen and watercolour sketch using a much freer style of painting directly from nature.

I felt 'recalled' to the valley for entirely different reasons a year later following the experiences in the Stone Pit quarry. This once quiescent valley was responding to some new-found need. It held something erotic in its form and was even richer in sensory impressions than the quarry.

Very soon I'd worked on a number of pen and colour sketches which loosened up some of the rigid structures of the earlier paintings (figs 547-549).

One painting (fig. 555, from the New Zealand tour a few years previously) had a dramatic sky effect and was to influence later pictures of the Postlip area. The style of this new work (fig. 556) allowed me to be much freer in the handling of the brush. A sense of 'letting go', of taking risks, did at last seem possible.

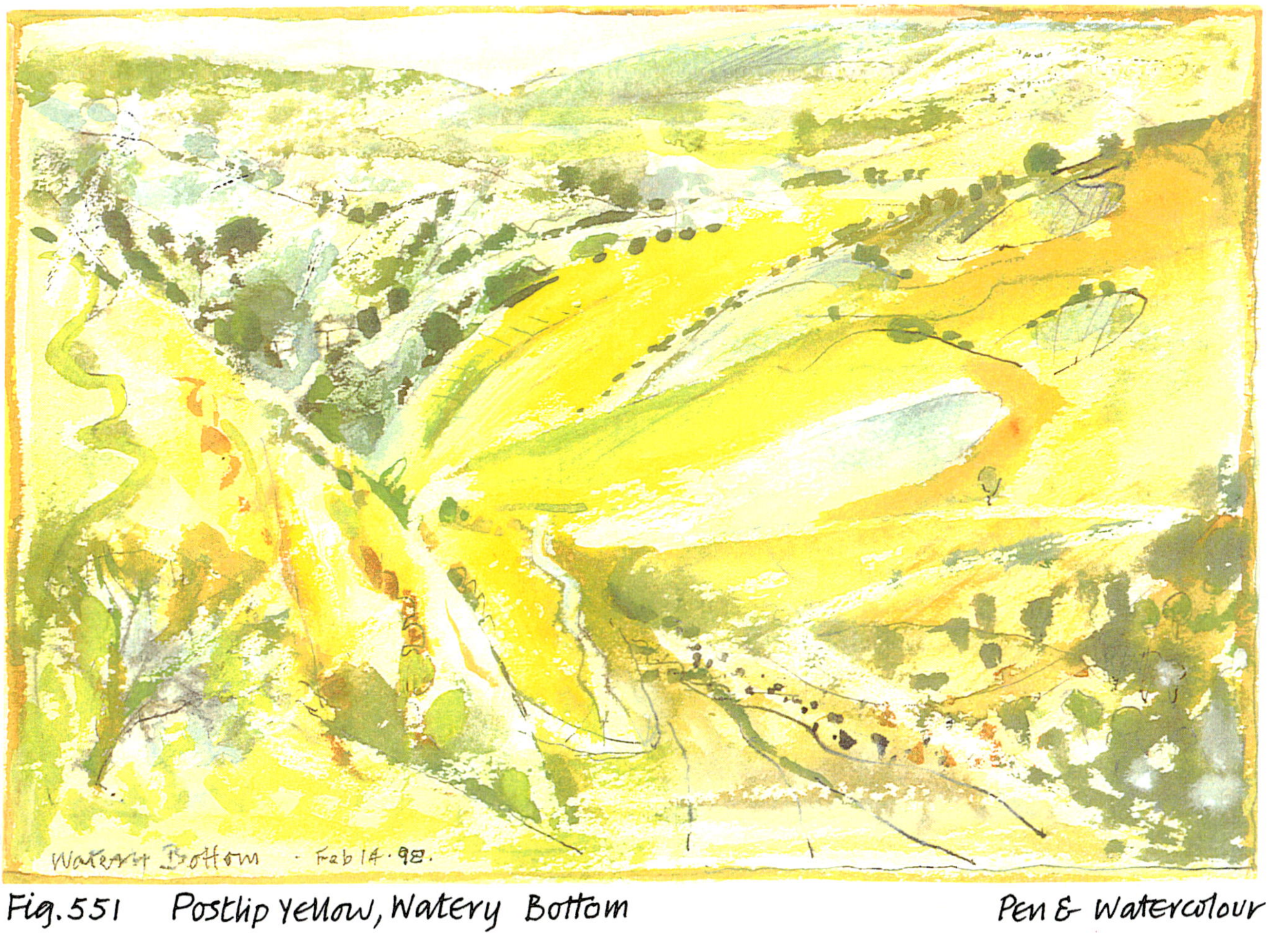

Fig. 551   Postlip Yellow, Watery Bottom   Pen & watercolour

327

Three examples of freestyle paintings of Watery Bottom

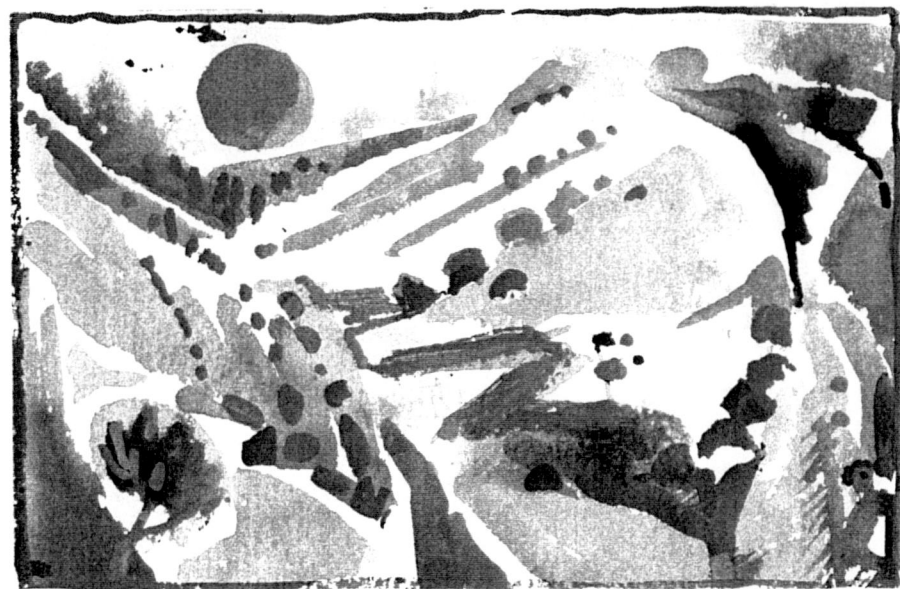

Fig.552 The Valley
Gouache & Watercolour

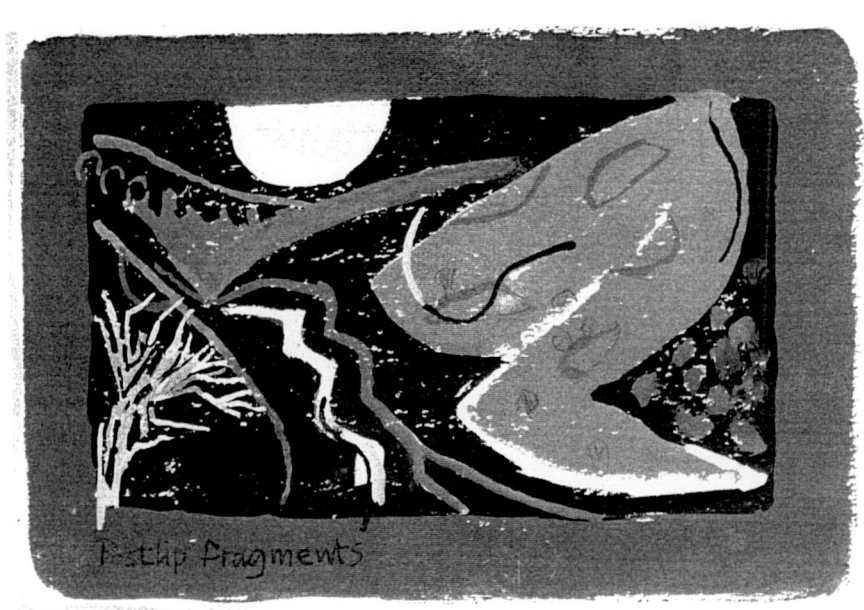

Fig.553 Postlip Fragments
Gouache

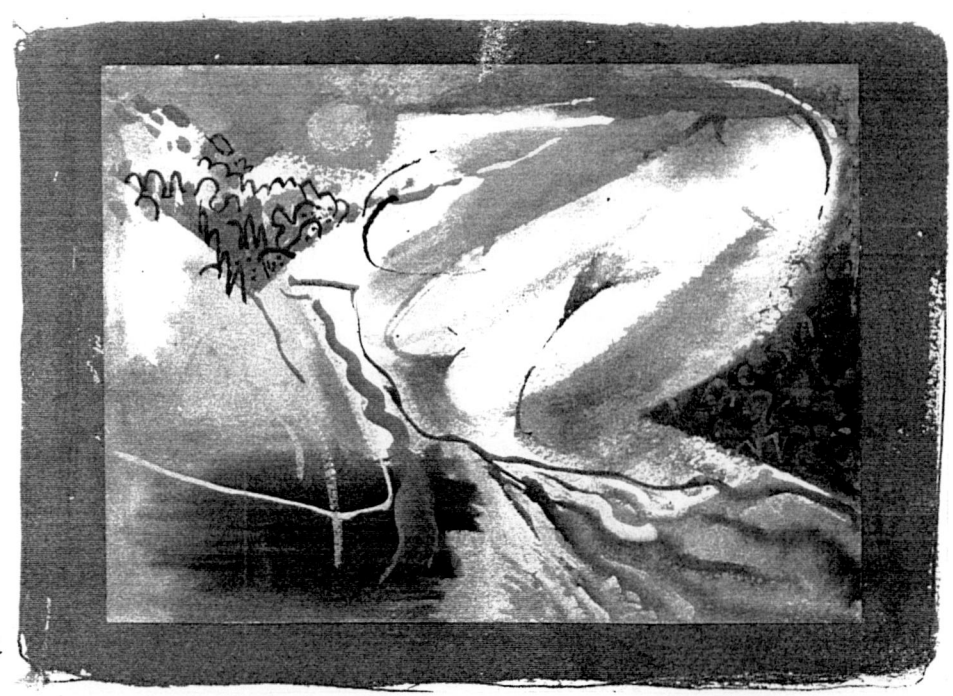

Fig.554 Postlip Maiden-2
Gouache

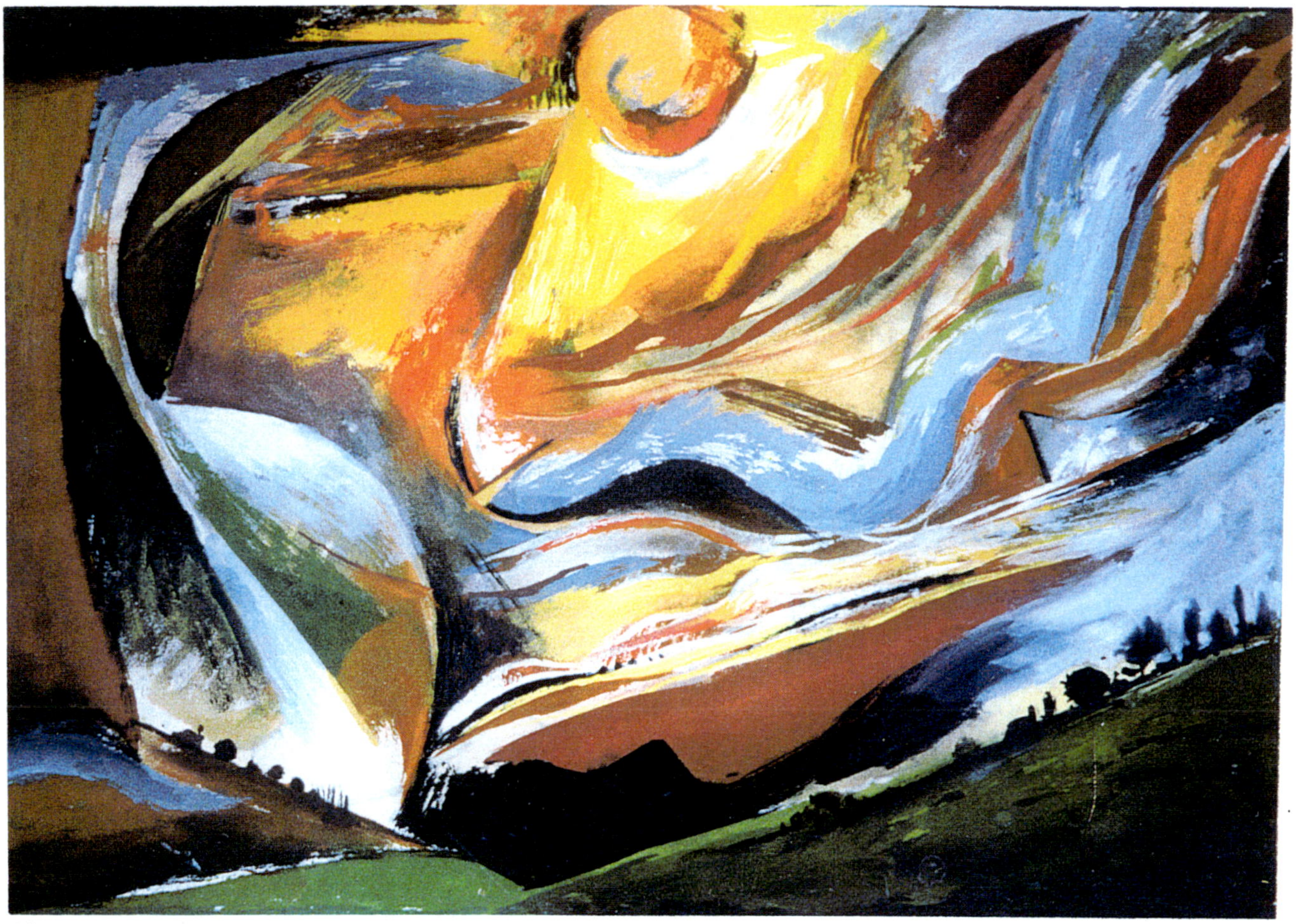

Fig. 555 Fiery Sky, Wanaka, New Zealand   Gouache

Above: An inflamed sky near Wanaka, South Island, New Zealand. A painting which later influenced a freer style of painting the valley

Right: More energetic and expressive brushwork — straight meets curve: zigzag meets flowing and spherical forms, night meets day.
A confrontational landscape.

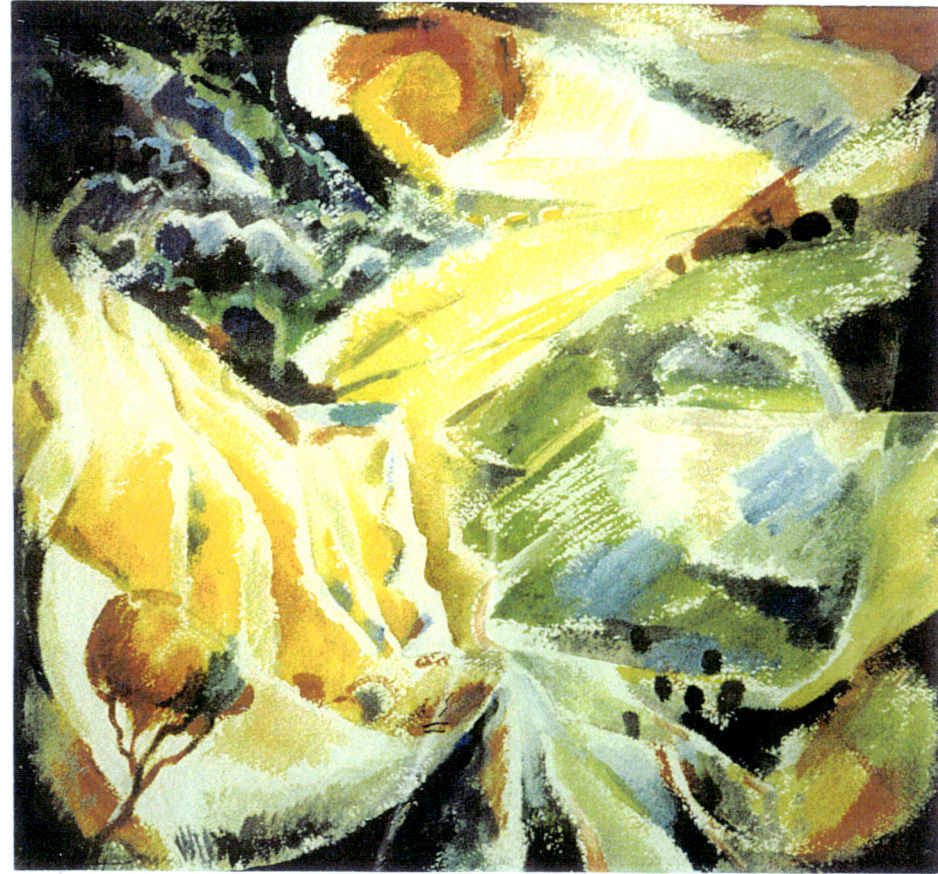

Fig. 556 Night and Day, Watery Bottom Gouache

329

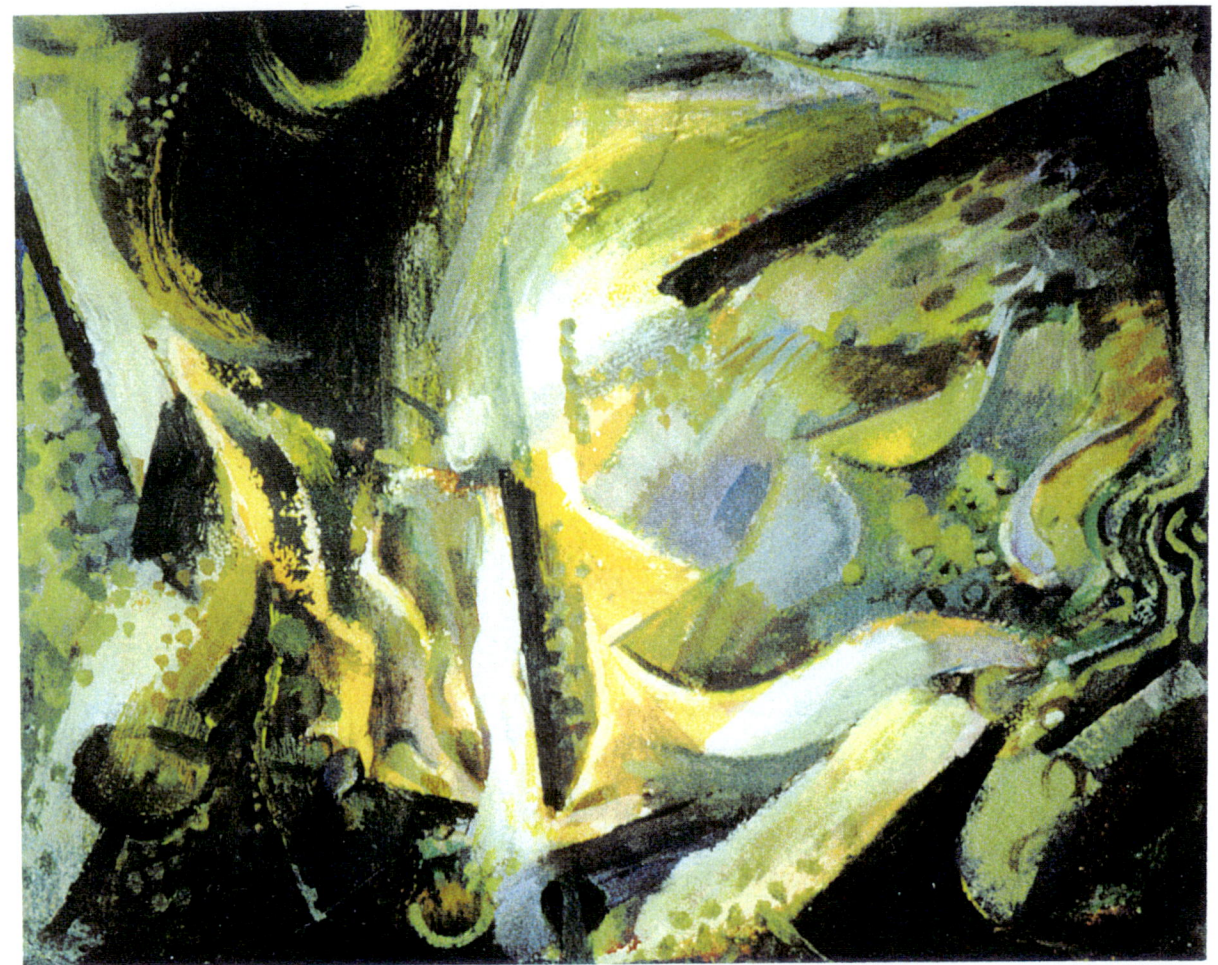

Fig. 557 Darkness at Noon, Postlip Warren, Watery Bottom   Oil on Board

Finally, on a wet afternoon in the studio I decided to overwork one of the earlier paintings of the place and started 'Darkness at Noon'. It began calmly enough, had a warm range of colour, then leaned towards the sentimental — not at all what I was aiming for. Suddenly enraged, I loaded a brush with black paint, working it vigorously across the surface in broad gestures, dragging and scumbling the work.

Pausing for a moment to consider the next stage I waited, and waited — and put down the brush. I knew it was complete, containing within itself the resolution I'd sought so long to achieve. The doubts and conflicts surrounding my feelings towards women, from early childhood onwards, were resolved.

CLEEVE COMMON AND UFFINGTON — A PERSONAL MYTHOLOGY

In attempting to express my fears, doubts, joys and emotional turmoil within these five landscapes, I've laid myself open to all sorts of charges of naivety, fantasising and so on. As I find myself unable to explain the phenomena in any rational way, other than to say that the 'visions' are the result of projections growing out of emotional needs, I would have to agree with any sceptics for whom it could all seem to be no more than the result of an over-active or extravagant imagination.

I can only counter this by saying that the process of drawing and painting at these particular sites, produced certain emotional responses which, in turn, resulted in feelings of growth and progress.

Through writing about this pictorial journal, many bits and pieces made over some twenty years, had to be correlated and edited — sense made from chaos. In the end it was about making connections between the past and the present — of allowing the conscious and unconscious to work together.

I found that the way out of the depression was to follow a kind of 'Pilgrims Progress' into my personal Black Hole, actually seeking a way down to where darkness reigns, into the creative centre. Paradoxically it was here where lightness was re-discovered — waiting in the womb's darkness before re-birth.

POSTSCRIPT
The Joker's Domain

THE JOKER'S DOMAIN	333
THE 'BIRTH' OF THE JOKER	335
THE CHILDHOOD OF THE JOKER	336
THE STAGE PERFORMER	338
THE CIRCUS – CLOWNS AND ACROBATS	340
QUEST OF THE JOKER	342
BACKSTAGE 1997	343
UPSIDE-DOWN FIGURE	344
HELLO, EVERYBODY!	345
THE MASKMAKER	346
LATER MANIFESTATIONS OF THE JOKER	347
FINAL CURTAIN?	348
A BACKSTAGE CONVERSATION	349
STRANGE MEETING	350
ZANY PRANCING	352

THE JOKER'S DOMAIN

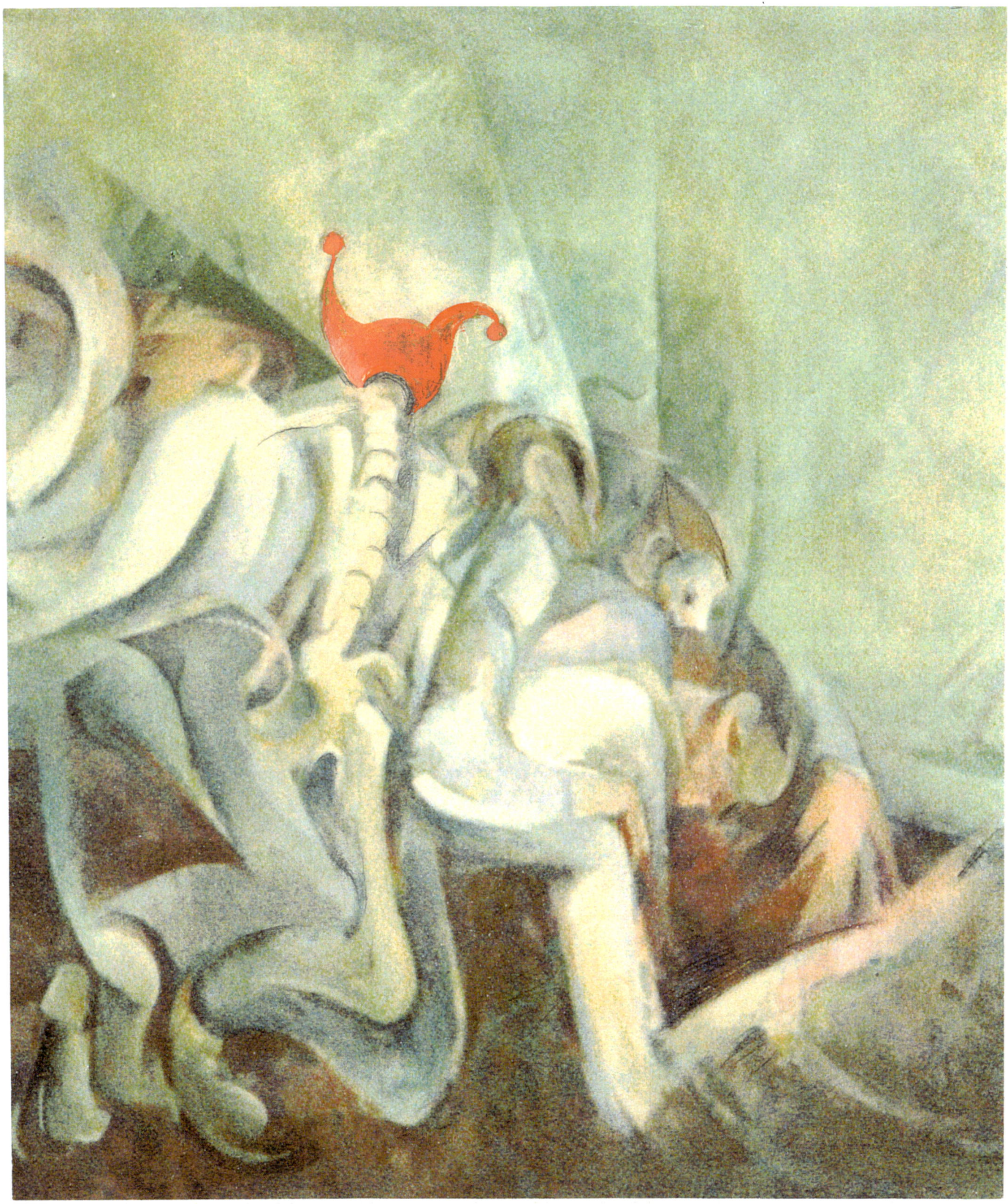

Fig. 558   Freefall - Falling (enlargement of Fig. 31, page 18).   Acrylic

Identified by his cap (highlighted in red) this enlargement of the illustration on page 18 was the first 'appearance' of the Joker. One other was hinted at in fig 29 on page 17. This was 'Spillage', where the cap took the form of a feather. (See text on next page).

Of all the characters I've recently discovered or re-discovered in the making of this book one has wormed his way into my consciousness as an essential component of my recovery. What surprised me so much was his late arrival. I was over halfway through the writing when he randomly appeared in this 'theatre of the absurd'.

So many questions needed answering :- Had I felt obliged to put a two-horned cap on top of a skeleton and if so, why? (fig. 558 previous page). What possible sense can be made of this picture and the two versions of the 'Joker's Birthplace' (figs. 559 and 560)?

There appeared to be no premeditation in their making. Because I could find no explanation, I felt compelled to call them psychic images - voices from elsewhere, leaving messages to be unravelled. Does a filtering occur, an osmosis through the wall between conscious and subconscious, until the essence of the imagery is made clear? One can't push this too far without getting into a quagmire of obscurity, but it does seem to explain how a personal mythology might develop towards an understanding.

How then was the image of the Joker recognised? Firstly the headgear, usually a 'horned' cap, occasionally a straw hat or even a crown of sorts (fig. 575); secondly, a physical attribute - his tendency to stand on one leg and hop or dance (for example, fig. 589); thirdly his stretching out (like the front cover illustration) or embracing with his arms. Given these attributes it was surprising how long it took to recognise his presence - perhaps certain things which are said to 'stare us in the face' are made invisible by their very closeness.

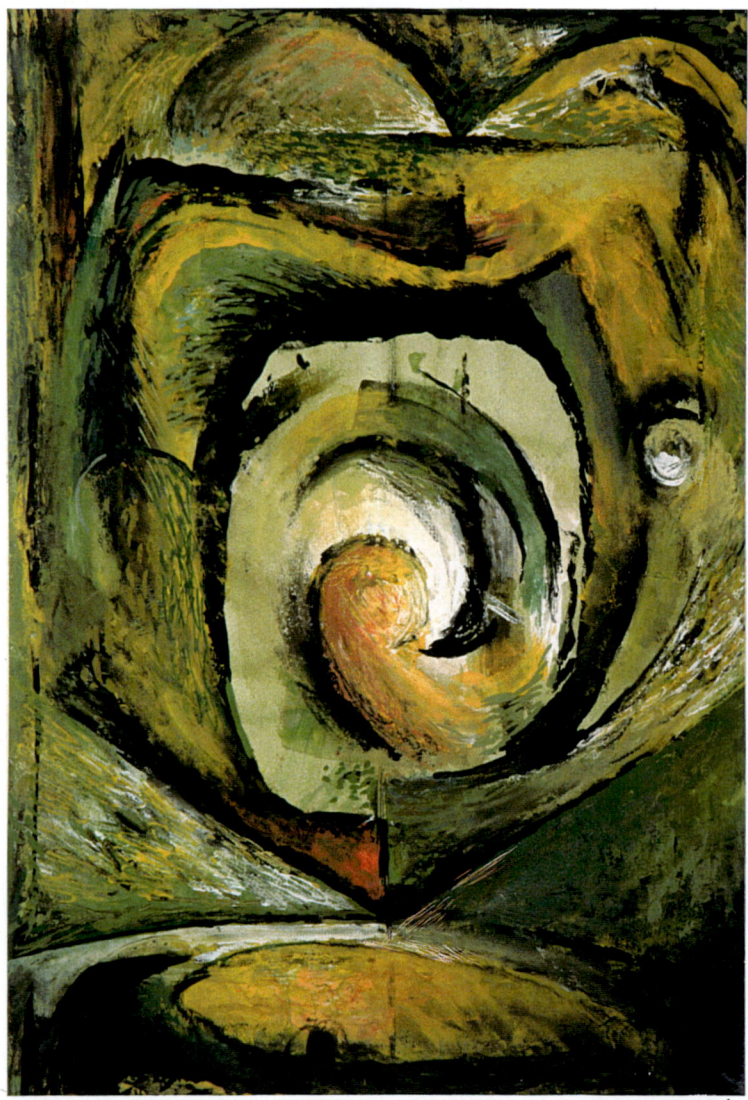

Above: Fig. 559   Regeneration   Gouache
The arrow points to the inspiration of the painting - Belas Knap Long Barrow (pages 297 to 306). The place for a rebirth of ideas, from old attitudes, beliefs and repressed emotions.

In the early appearances one idea did begin to predominate - the Joker invariably related to some element of mortality, of skeletal imagery.

Caught unawares during the final editing and checking through the images was a 'sighting' in 'Spillage' (fig. 29) - the smiling mask-head, long feathered ear and attached spinal column pointed to the prototype and precursor of all the later joker images.

When, however, he was identified then the gods and goddesses, heroes and warriors, the many peopled reveries and the array of creatures, angels and monsters all stood in the wings as the protagonist took his rightful place - centre stage in the Joker's drama.

He has many names as only a Joker can: Jester, merryfellow, trickster immediately come to mind. But also Jack-in-the-box, mask-maker, clown. Then, less obviously perhaps, companion, guardian (angel), maker (of images), helper - a seemingly infinite list.

This consistently inconsistent figure reflects, only too well, the many-sided swings of mood during manic, but mostly depressive, phases in the last twenty years or so.

THE BIRTH OF THE JOKER

I'm still curious as to what caused the two-horned headpiece to attach itself to a spinal column, for it related to nothing I'd experienced on that or any other day.
 The mere fact 'he' was there perhaps gave a hint of an optimistic nature behind all the trauma - for like a Jack-in-the-Box he struck me as one always capable of making a comeback. If the headpiece attached to a skeleton perhaps related to fears of mortality, could it also symbolise the 'dying of the Self' to effect a re-generation of the spirit?

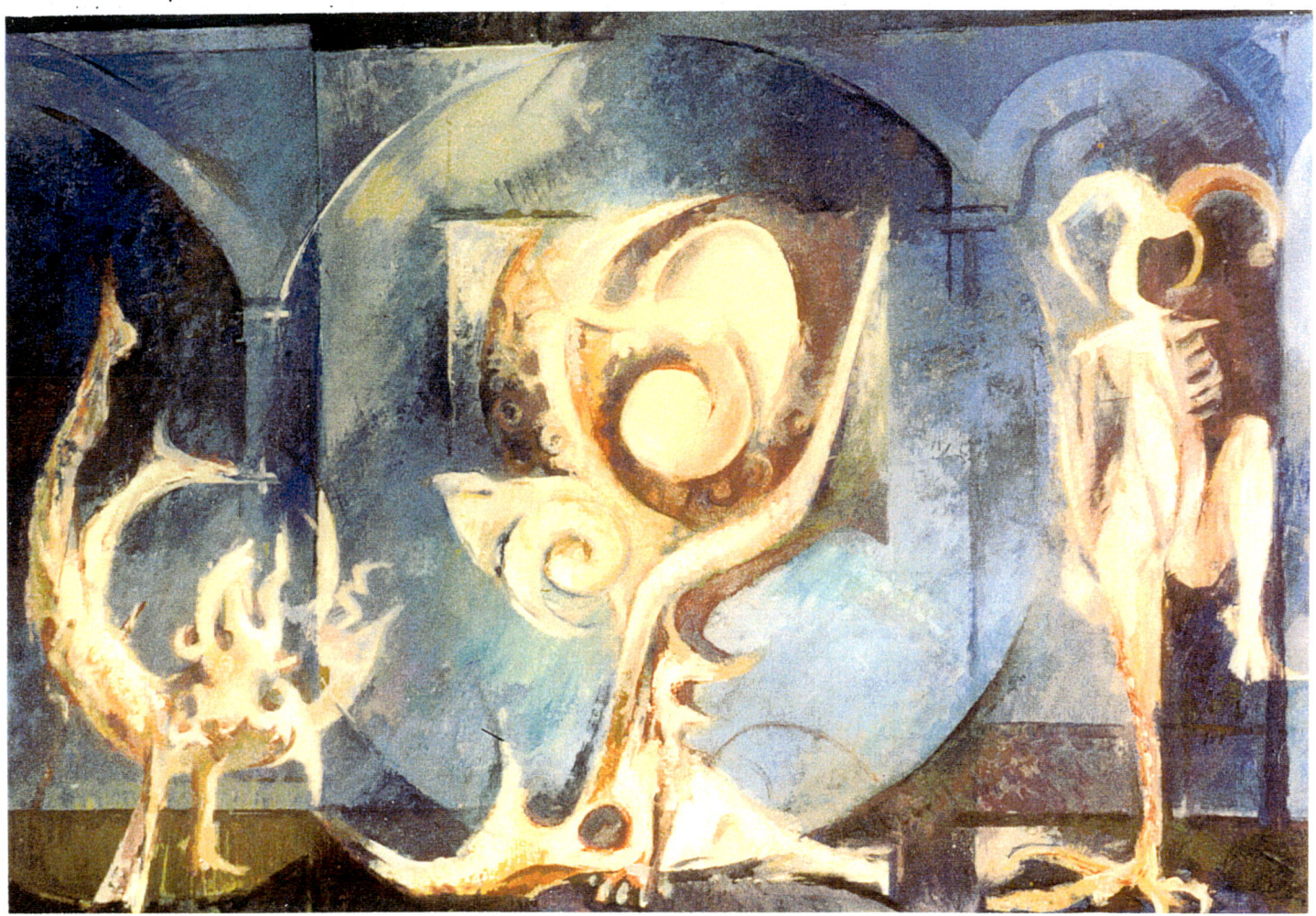

Fig 560   The Joker's Birthplace   Acrylic on Board

In 1985, a group of bone chalices evolved from various skeletal images (pages 52 and 53). From these sacrificial containers came symbols of rejection and suffering and redemption. A few paintings showed the chalice with an attendant (fig 103).
 One picture in particular interested me the moment it was completed - 'The Joker's Birthplace' above. Here was not only a chalice, but a foetus contained within, an acrobatic tree-root and, most importantly, a jester.
 This picture had seemed a mystery for years - now it began to make a kind of sense. Here was a scene of vaulted subterranean gloom, a fanciful concept, yet uncompromisingly bleak. It spoke to me of the subconscious nudging me to recognise the need for an actor companion, a jolly fellow who would compensate for the depressive aspects of the illness. He would be a temporary support system until I could deal with the situation myself.
 It was a bringing into the light what had been neglected or misunderstood. E M Forster's 'Only connect.... live in fragments no longer' could well be a defining comment on these images. This picture, a mystery for years is understood through the Joker.
 He is capable of constant transformation to meet all contingencies. Here he appears to be changing himself either into (or out of) a bird by stamping vigorously.
 And the spritely tree-root? Perhaps the midwife to a positive outcome.

THE CHILDHOOD OF THE JOKER

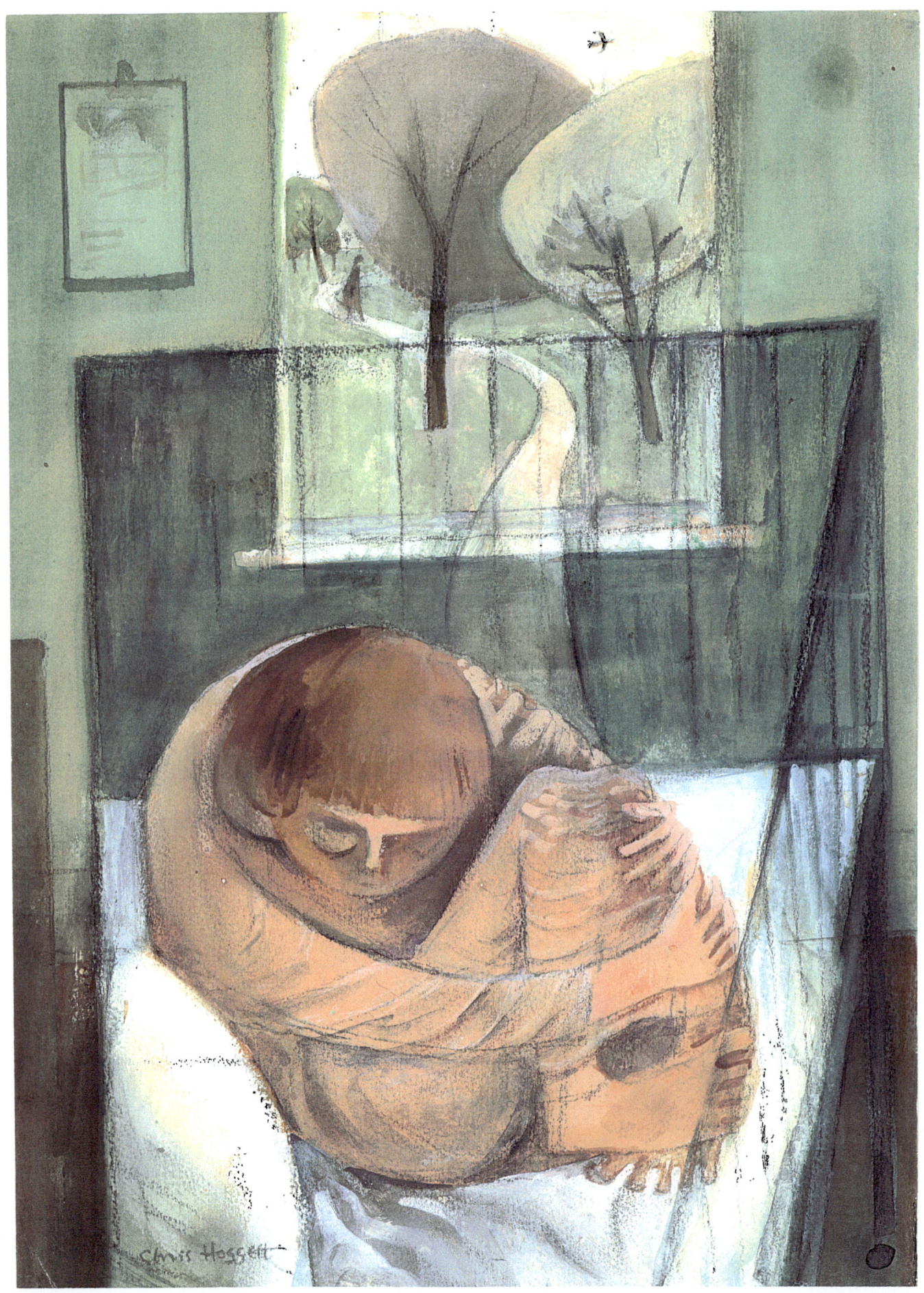

Fig 561 The High-railed Cot   Gouache

The High-railed Cot

The illustration opposite was the precursor of the 'Childhood of the Joker' below (see also the frontispiece).

Following the rage and resentment of the Incarceration sequence (pages 206 and 207) a more resigned mood emerged in this final painting.

The Childhood of the Joker

This retrospective painting relating to the 1930s hospital experience is a reverie or fantasy where inner feelings of rejection are transformed by this idea of a Joker who now becomes my protector, my defence or mask.

The various elements which make up the composition: rounded head and body, square frame of cot and window, various tree forms and path beyond — these are now rearranged to form the basis of the clown/joker head.

This progenitor of future emotional support is the mocker of those who might wish to probe too closely. He's here to strengthen one through depressive phases......

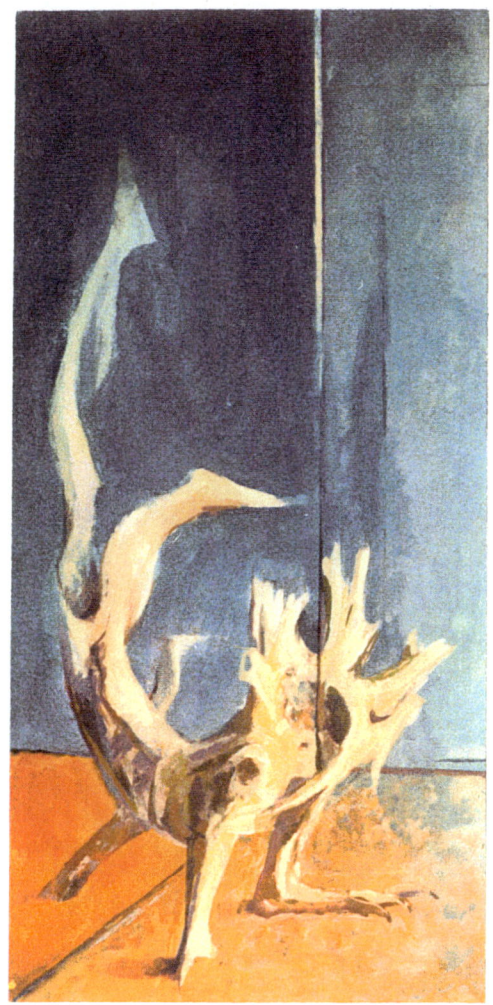

Fig. 563   Dancing Tree Root Acrylic

Dancing Tree Root

This acrobatic tree-root is a reworking of the dancing figure to the left of 'The Joker's Birthplace' (page 335).
(It is also the only record which remains of the painting, I having destroyed the original in a moment of disillusionment)

Following this painting came the realisation that this was yet another version of the circus figures on pages 340 and 341

The feeling now is of a transforming character — one who gives an inner strengthening to creative activities.

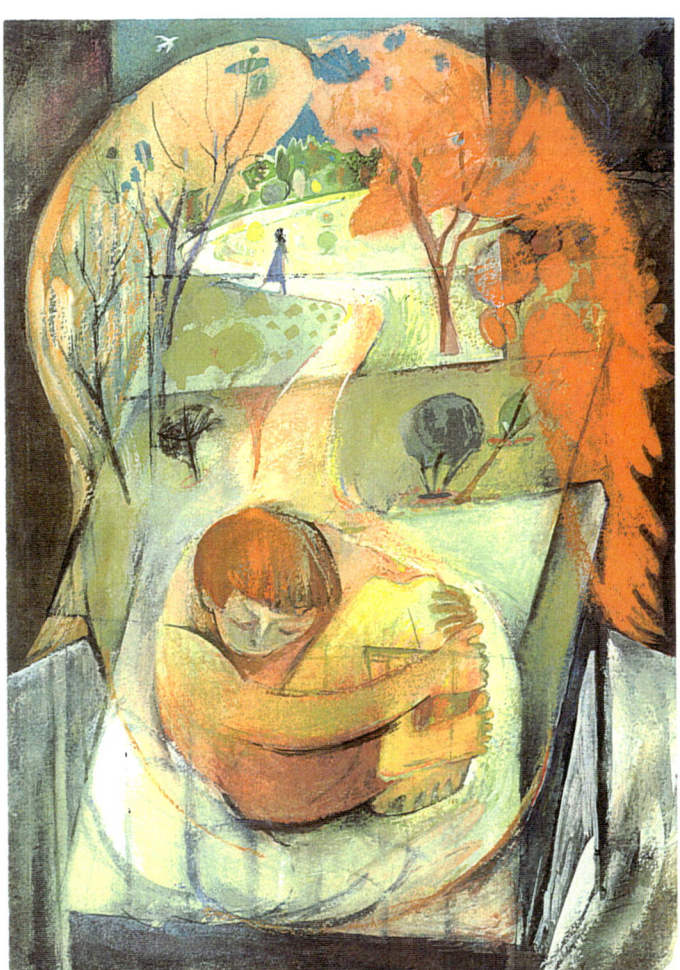

Fig. 562 Childhood of the Joker. Gouache

THE STAGE PERFORMER

All this speculation was conjured up when I looked more closely at the Joker's odd-man-out appearances, often in times of deepening depressions or loneliness — here he would be again in freestyle sketches as a compere, actor or a 'show off' as if to say, 'We can do it!' or 'Here I am, this is My Show!'

During the more vulnerable times the joker part of myself protected me like a suit of armour, turning me from a shy, depressed youth into the 'strong silent type', or putting on some social gloss when none existed, or covering up ineptitude with a grin — and finding ways of making excuses to avoid embarrassment.

Probably there was nothing unique about these reactions to life's opportunities and challenges, just an average response for any shy or sensitive person. The problem was how to deal with the consequences of self-imposed 'protectionism' when circumstances changed — when the once impregnable suit of armour is found to be a prison instead of a fortress.

Right: Fig. 564 Sketch for front cover
Brush & Paint

Below: Fig. 565 Neither Fish nor Fowl
Pen, Brush & Ink

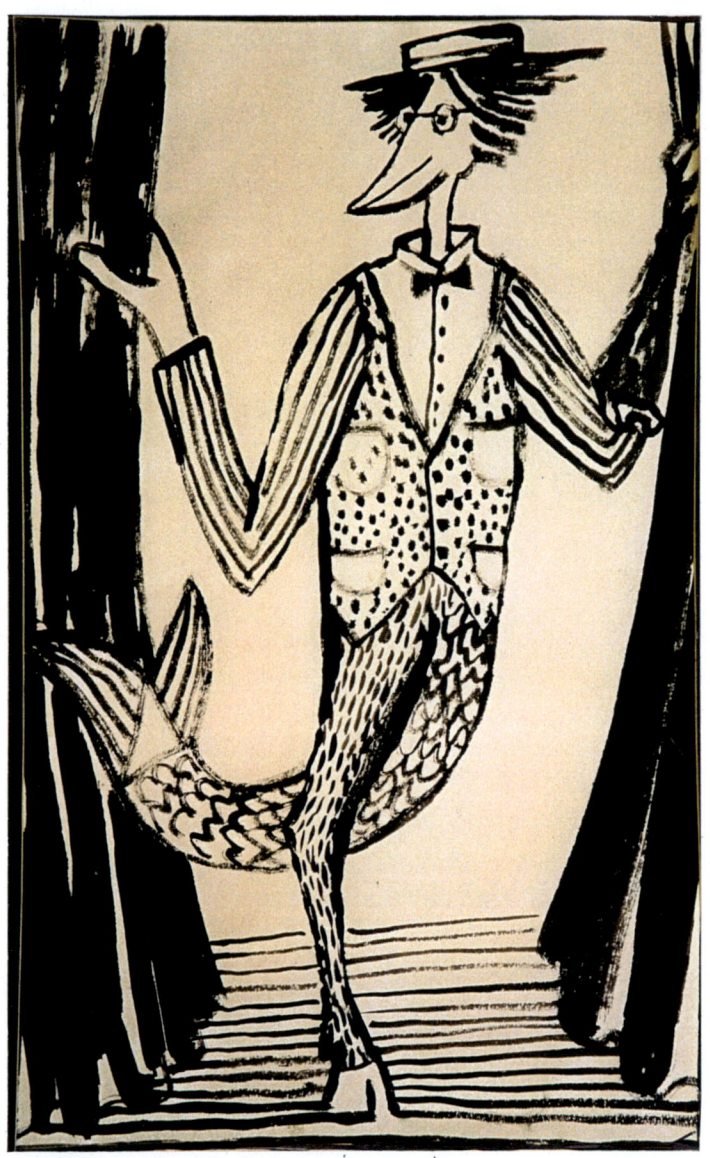

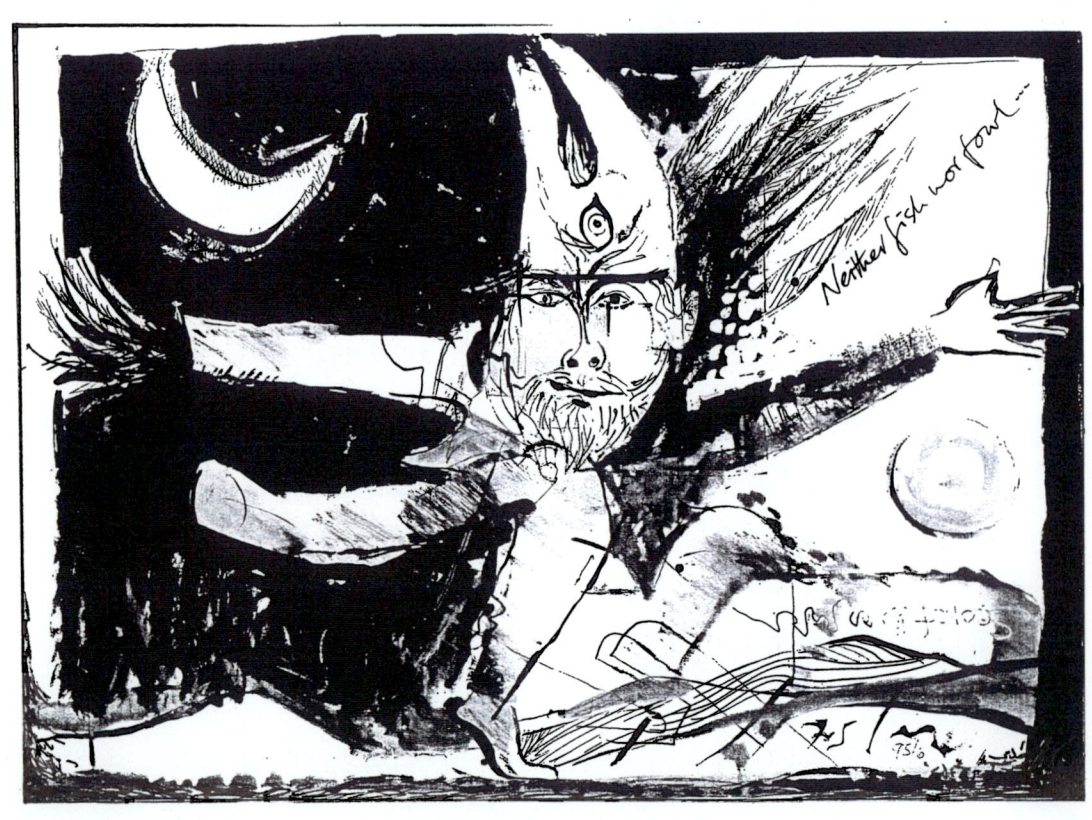

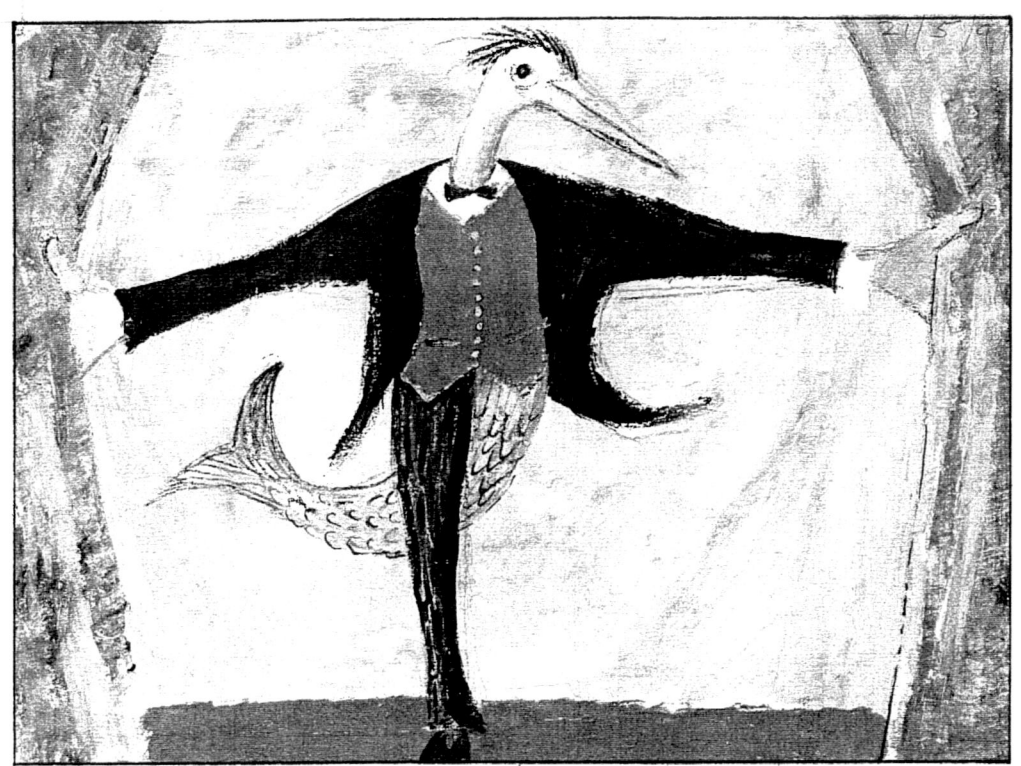

Left: Fig 566
The Compere
Gouache

Below: Fig 568
Woman & Joker
Pencil

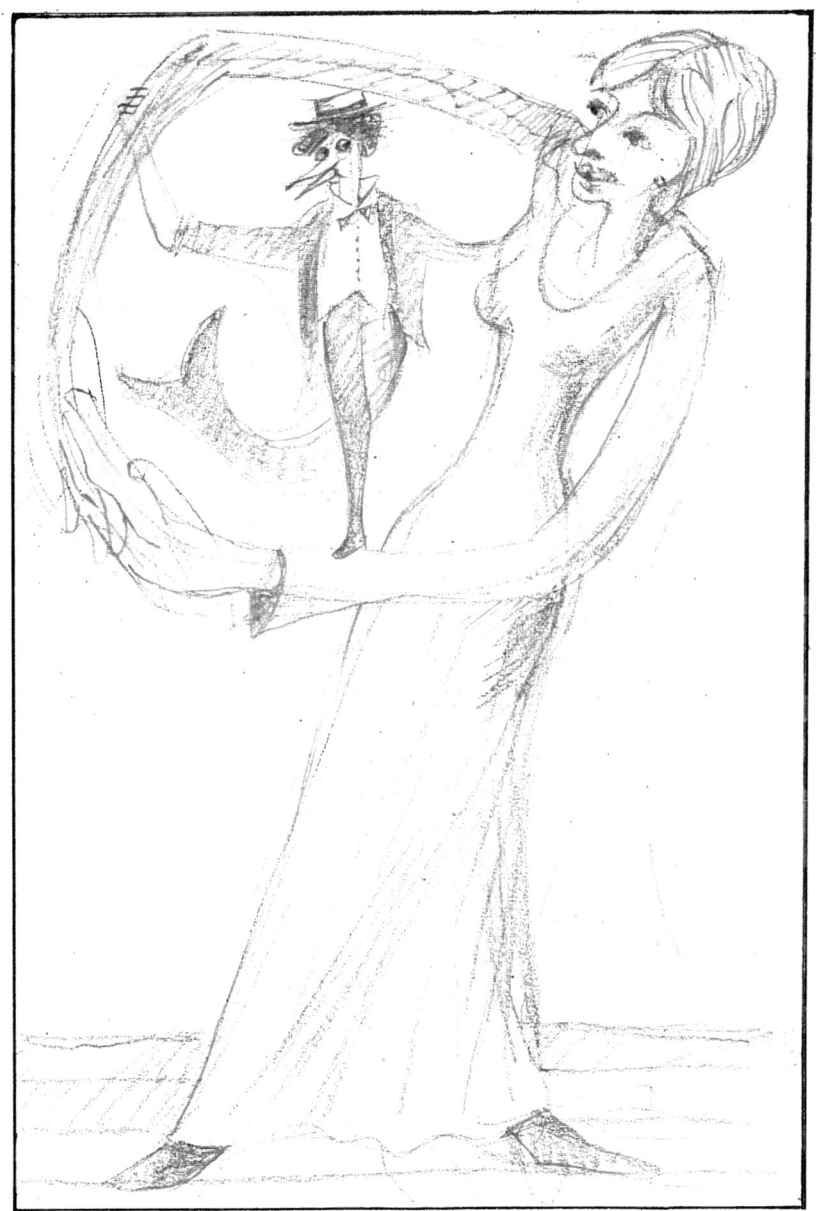

Above: As compere, the wide expressive gesture of open arms.

Right: The Joker as 'Trickster', performing to pacify 'the woman-as-house', a sort of Thurberesque variation.

Below: The traditional Music Hall trouper with straw hat and cane (yet still retaining a fishtail!)

Fig. 567 Dancing Joker
Pen & Pencil

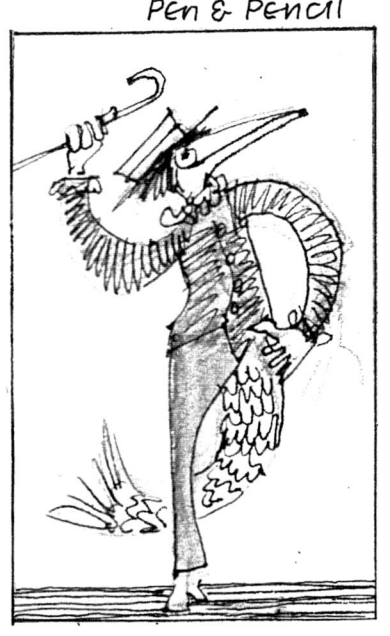

THE CIRCUS - CLOWNS AND ACROBATS

Just as a number of found drawings related to the theatre, others hinted at circus environments, suggested by a costume or the ambience. The painting 'Tightrope Walker' (fig. 570, right) includes the sawdust ring - a painting which concluded the Swivel Chair section (page 46).

Top Right: Fig. 570 This is a repeat of Fig. 94 on page 46 which concluded the 'Swivel Chair' section. The painting tries to maintain an equilibrium between opposites: highs and lows, light and shade, depression and elation.

Top, Far Right: Fig. 571 'The Old Clown'. A very downbeat, angry mood backstage either before or after facing the public. As a child I recall being manically happy at a clown's antics in the ring but when glancing behind the scenes I saw the looks of weariness and sadness.

Bottom Right: Fig. 572 'Clown with a Bull's Horn'. Some empathy reflected here with the Gilgamesh Epic - strong animal, human connections. (see pages 298 to 301).

Below: Fig. 569 'The Jester and his Partner'. A freestyle drawing which grew out of a fog of greyness, the two figures gradually appearing out of the gloom. The jester seems to be seeking reassurance to face his public by placing his hand on his partner's breast - as the youthful 'odd-man-out' he needs constant support.

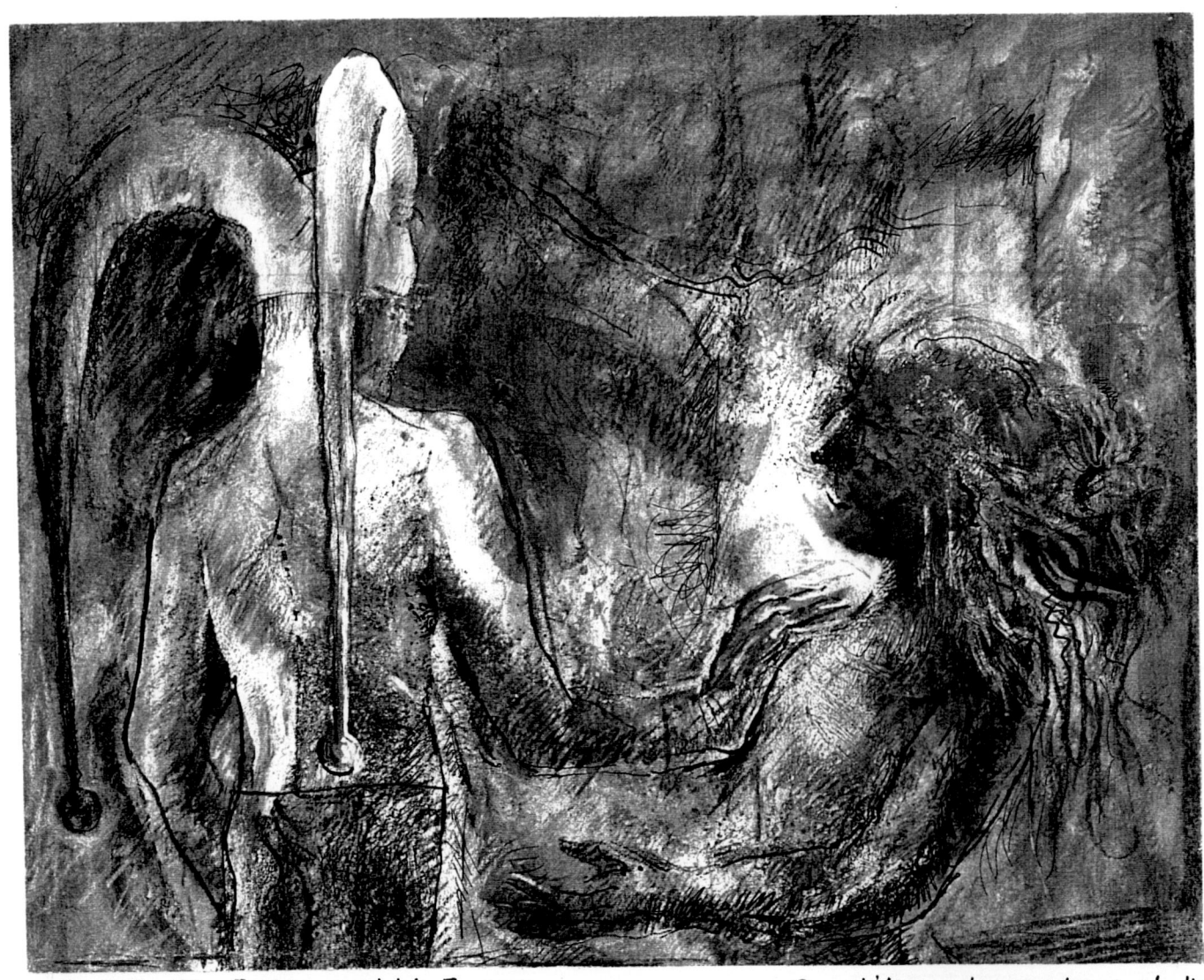

Fig. 569 The Jester and his Partner   Graphite powder, pen, brush, chalk

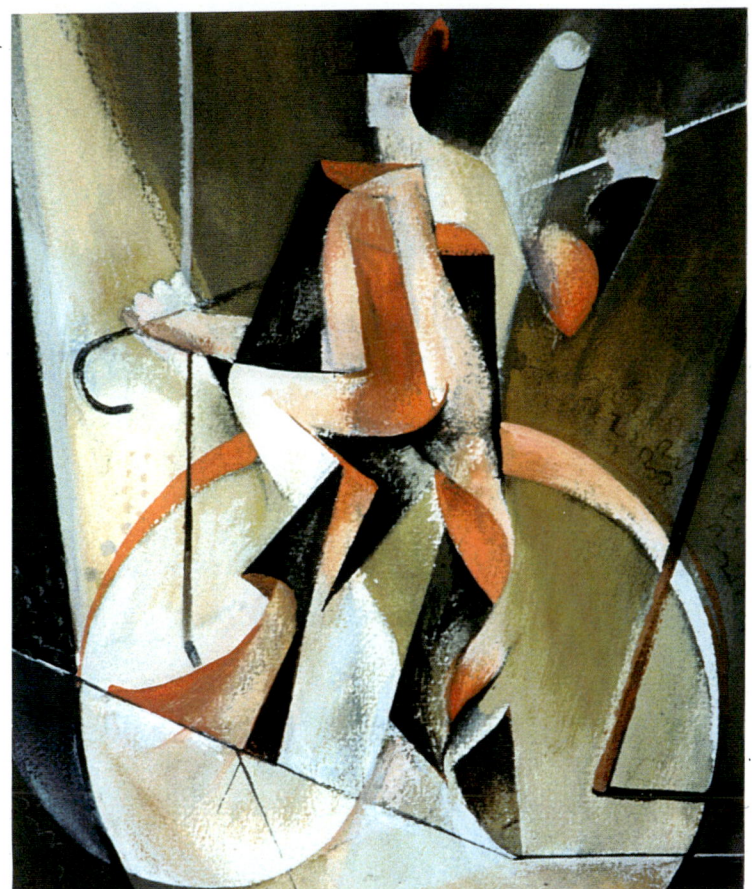

Fig. 570   Tightrope Walker   Gouache

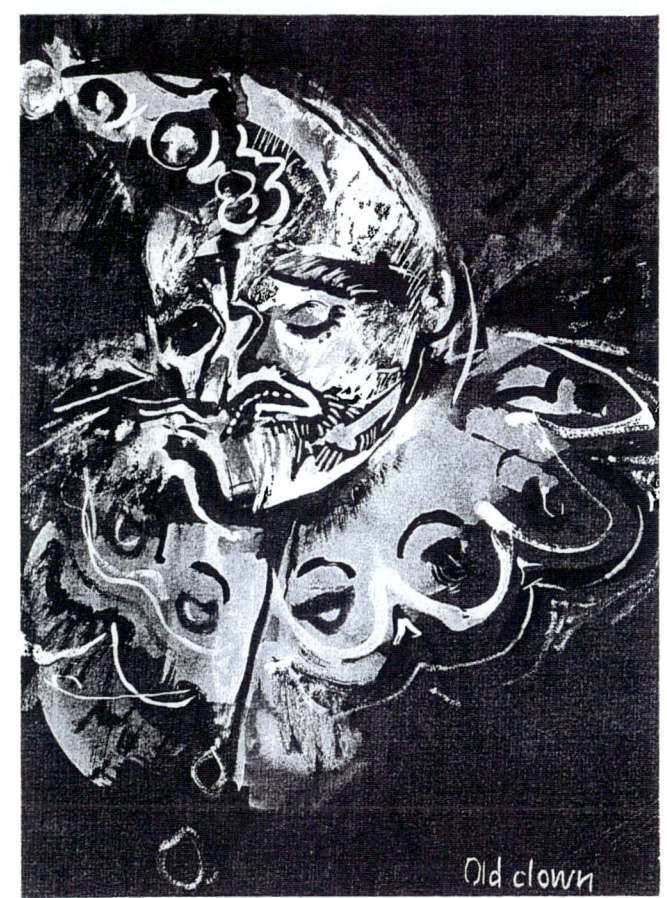

Fig. 571   The Old Clown   Gouache

Fig. 572   Clown with a Bull's Horn   Use of child's Finger Paints — some brushwork

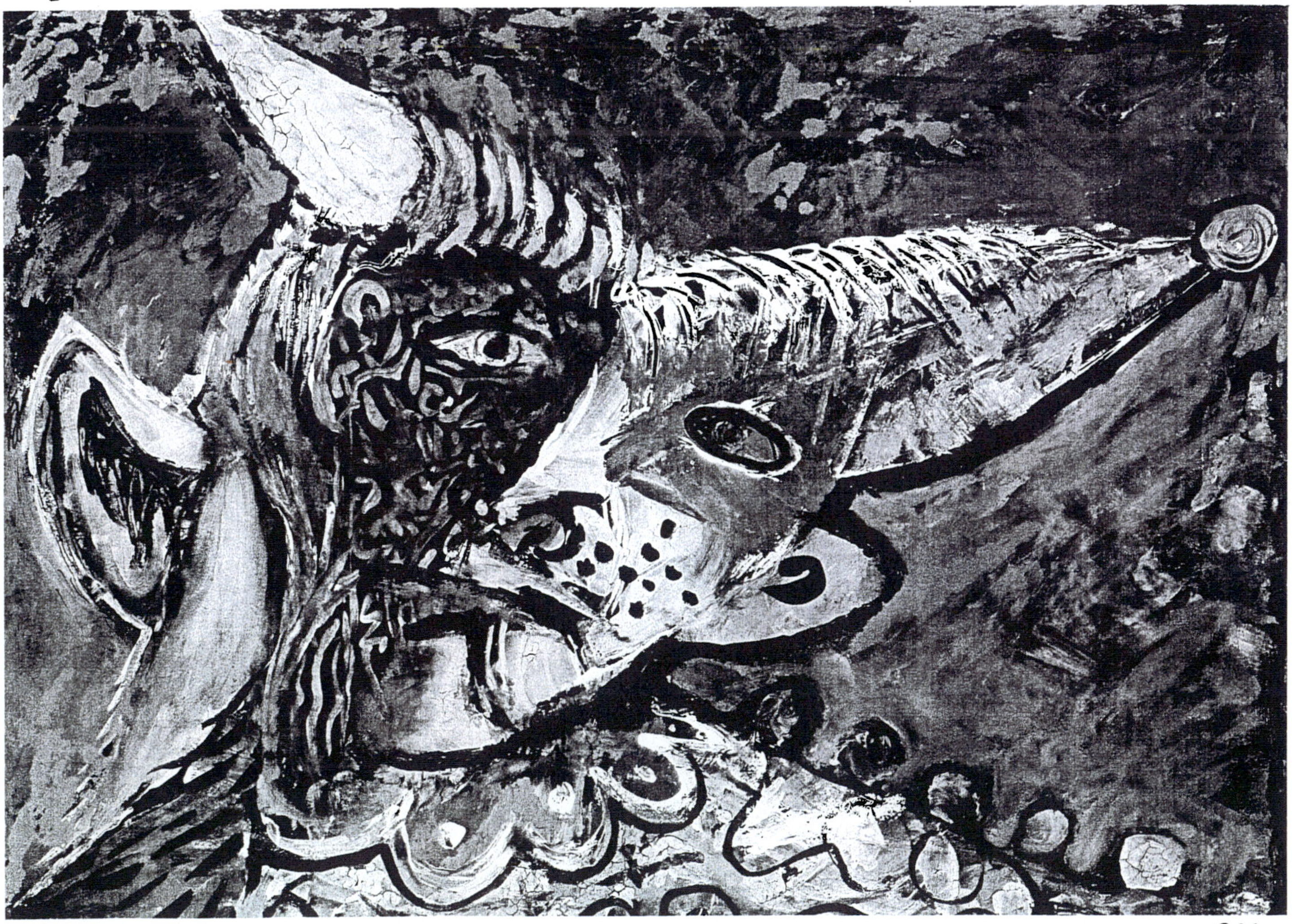

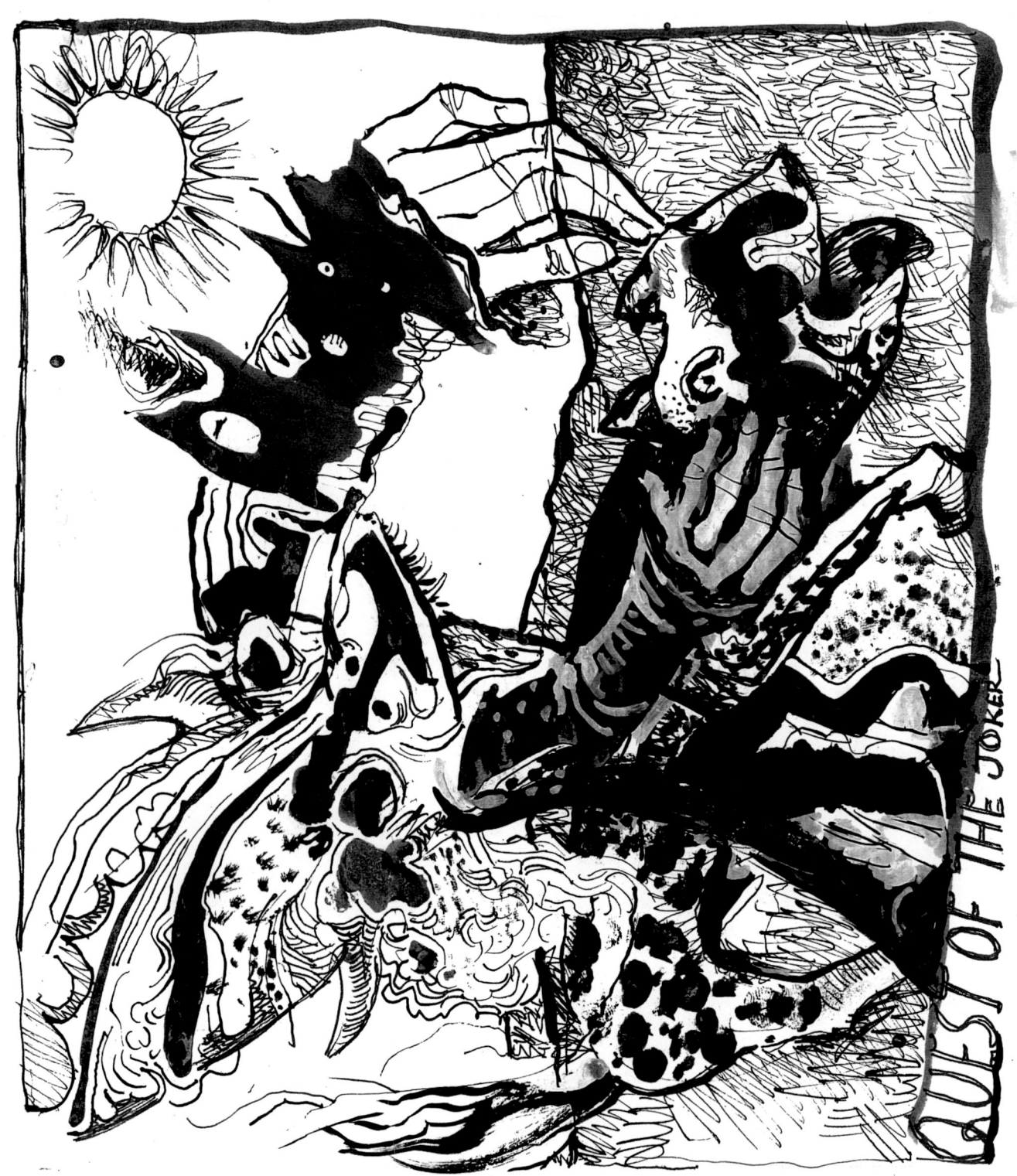

QUEST OF THE JOKER

The joker seeking down to his animalistic roots, his fingers lightly touching the instinctive nature of his dog. Both receive an exchange of energy — a re-charge.

Fig 573 Brush,
Quest of the Joker Pen & Ink

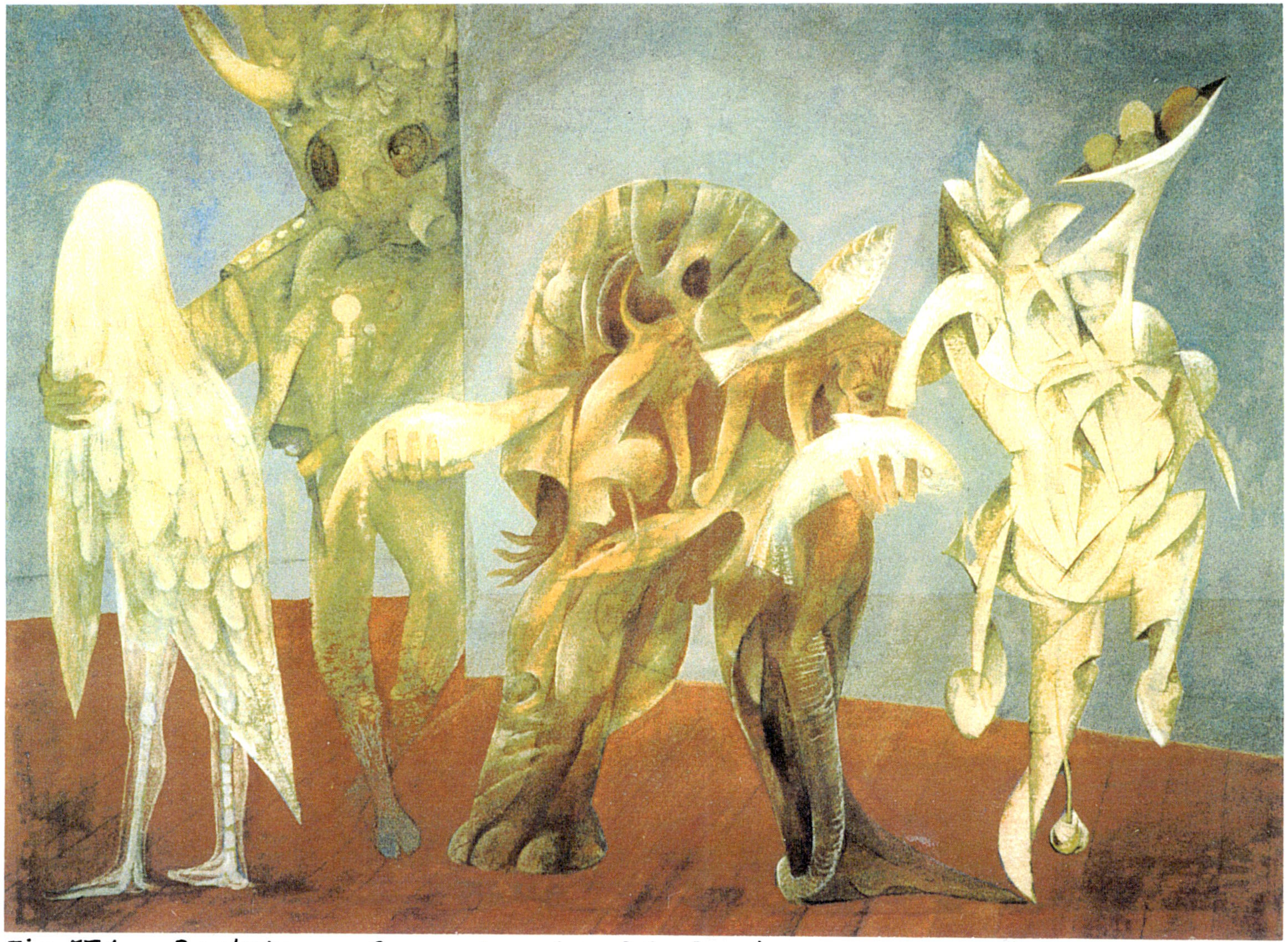

BACKSTAGE 1997

At this point the psychic joker starts to re-invent himself. Comes up with a 'new look', a 'front man', to carry me through to the next stage. The emperor's clothes have to be exchanged for a degree of open vulnerability.

Here the joker becomes a set of abstract shapes and trips forward in a joyous dance step. His fellow actors backstage are a bird victim (the anima?), a control freak/warlord and an insatiable glutton who, in a moment of generosity, offers the joker some food.

Fig. 574 Backstage – Some Aspects of the Psyche   Acrylic

UPSIDE-DOWN FIGURE

Asked to design a millennium poster (misspelt on the rough!), I found the joker character now in another guise, wearing a paper crown and letting rip at the party to end the old and to welcome in the new.....

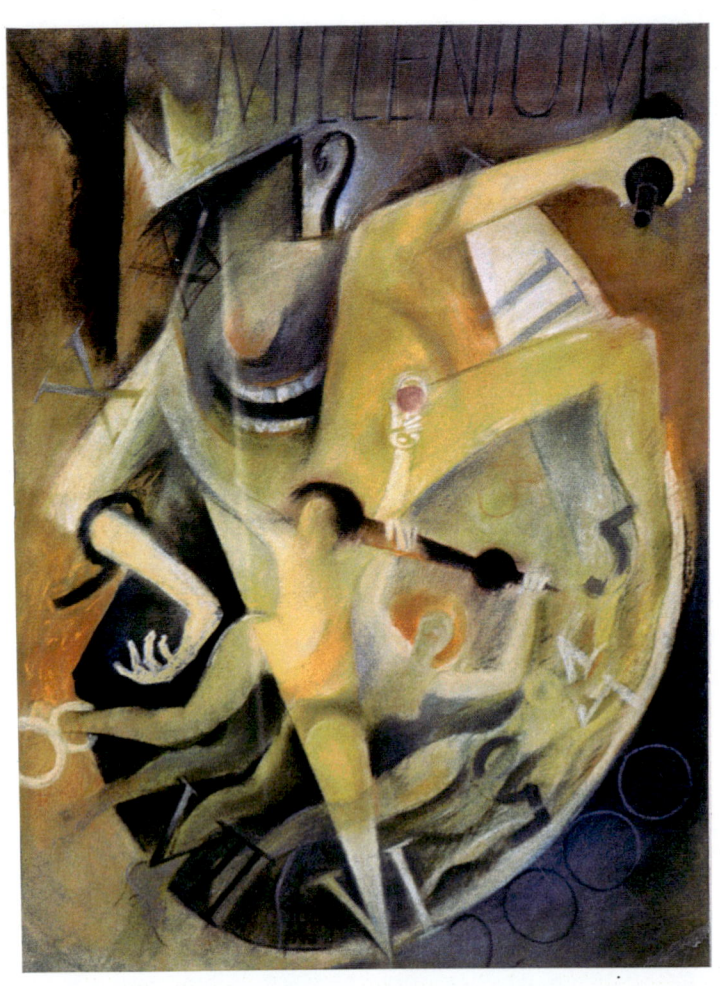

Fig. 575 Millennium Poster   Pastel

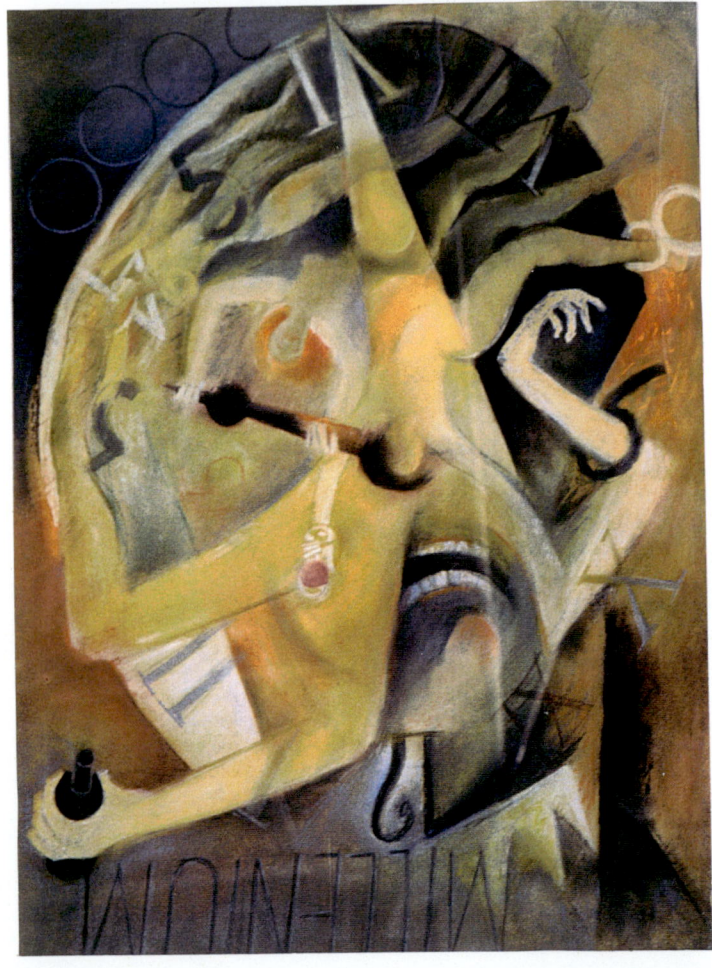

.... only to find an anxiety-laden face when the poster design was accidentally turned upside down. Behind all the merriment blackness loomed; on the other hand, if reversed again......

Fig. 576 Design Upside Down   Pastel

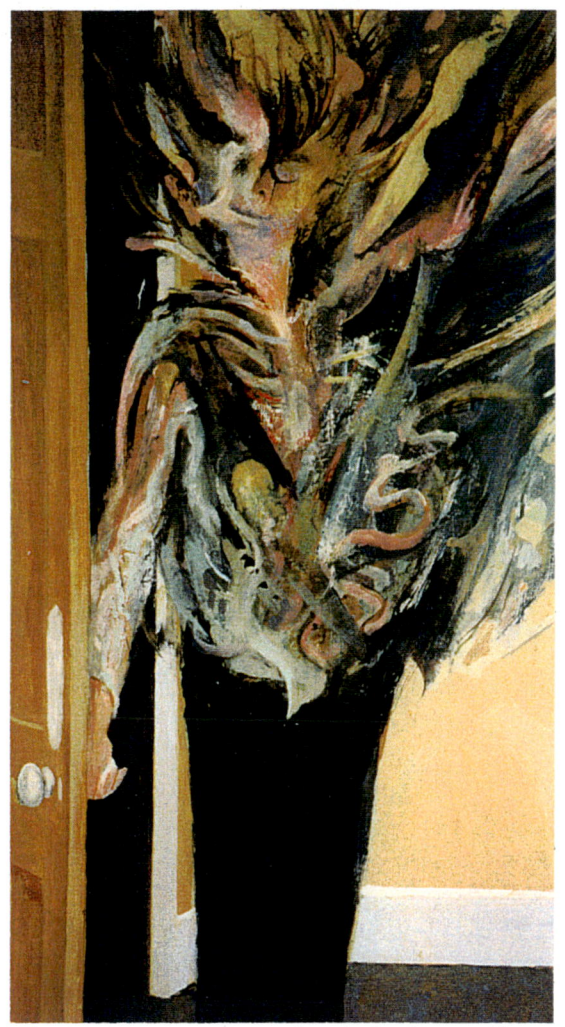

Fig. 577 Hello, Everybody! (detail). Oil on Board

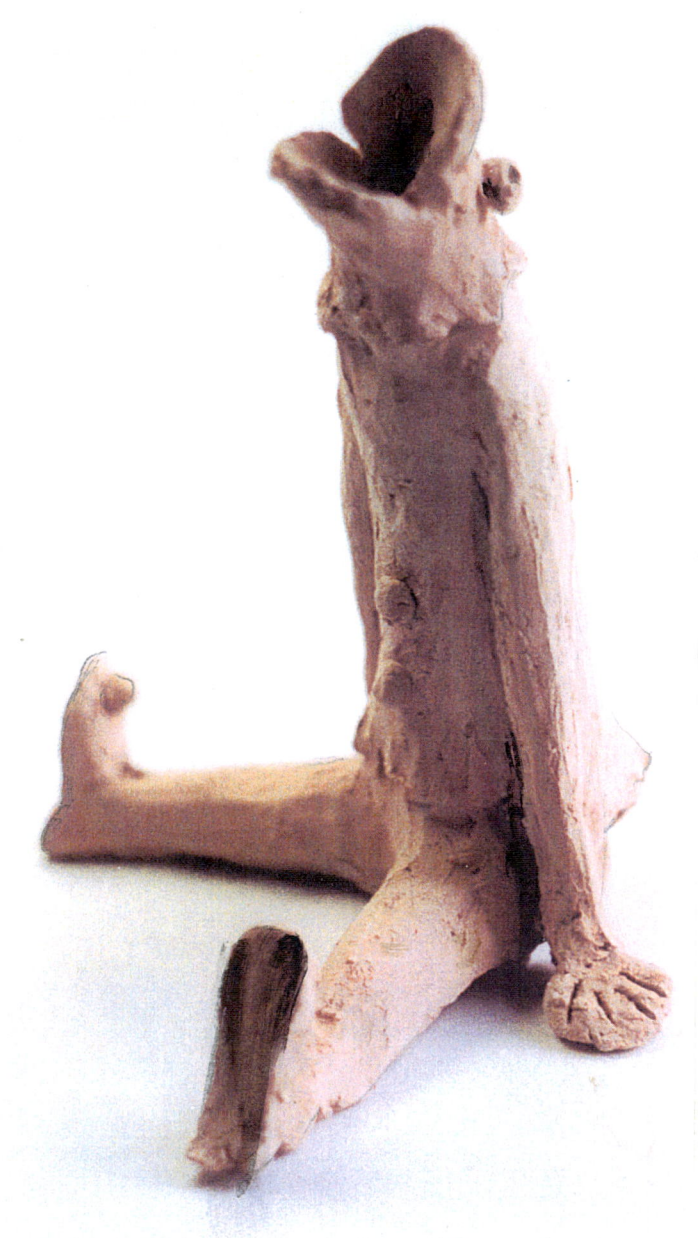

Fig. 578 Joker as Frog Prince   Ceramic

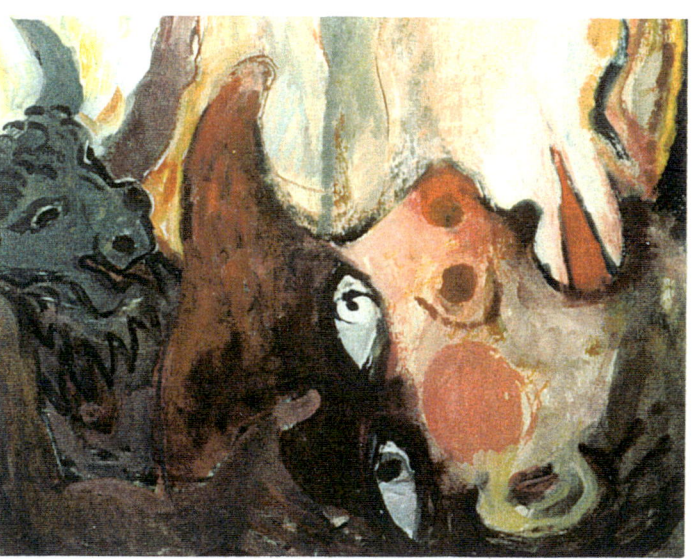

Fig. 579 Joker plays Enkidu (detail). Gouache

HELLO, EVERYBODY!

Fig. 577 An explosive moment of self-esteem after years of self-doubt.
  The character vents his expressive nature with a show of anger and creativity.
  Perhaps the turning point of the Joker's role-playing – a prophetic visual comment on what one hoped might lie ahead (see page 94, fig. 178).

Fig. 578 Another example of the Joker dressed up as a clown (see page 117 for origins of this clay figure).

Fig. 579 Another example of the influence of the Gilamesh epic. (see page 288, fig. 500).

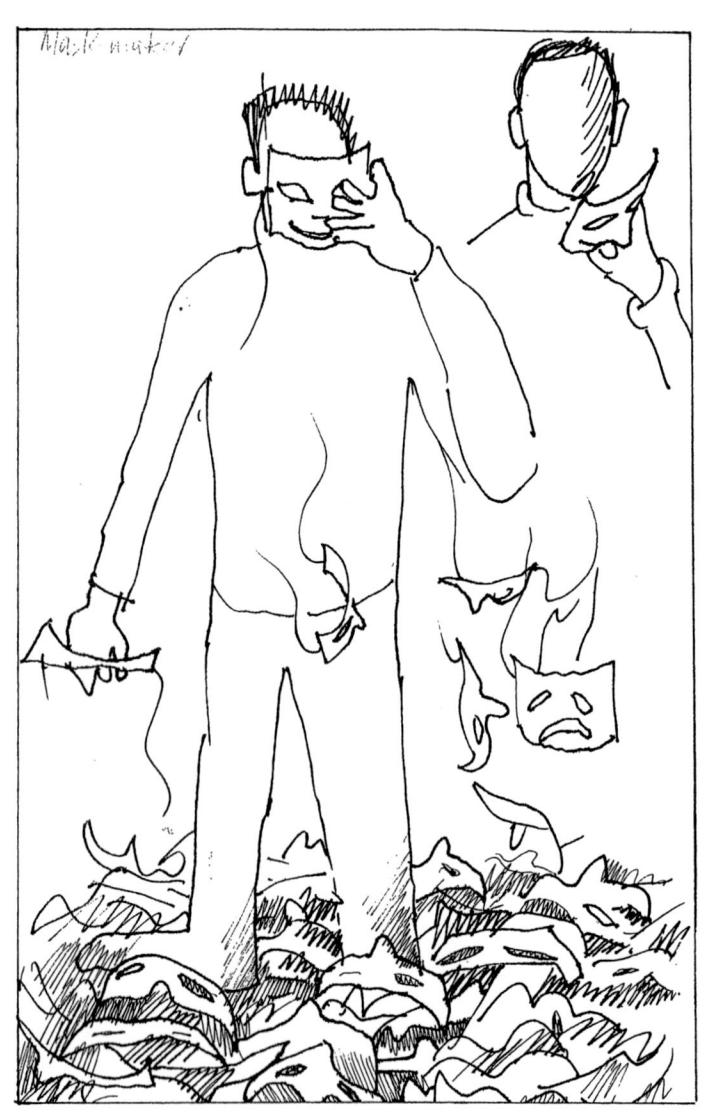

THE MASKMAKER

When the armour begins to screech with rust, the masks of comedy melt into tragedy - then the 'strong silent type' collapses into noisy tears. The 'breakout' is well under way.

The joker can ease himself out of mask-making - can hang up the horned cap.

This drawing shows him reaching frustration point, no mask seems to fit. Finally when he takes one more away he realises he's lost even his temporary identity.

(SEE also 'The Maskmaker-1 fig 332 page 188).

Fig. 580 The Maskmaker-2   Pen & Ink

The Maskmaker's Choices

Another version of above. Having relied so heavily on the use of the mask, he realises subterfuge no longer is effective. Here he is in the last throes of despair before finally letting go.

Fig 581 The Maskmaker's Choices. Pen, Chalk

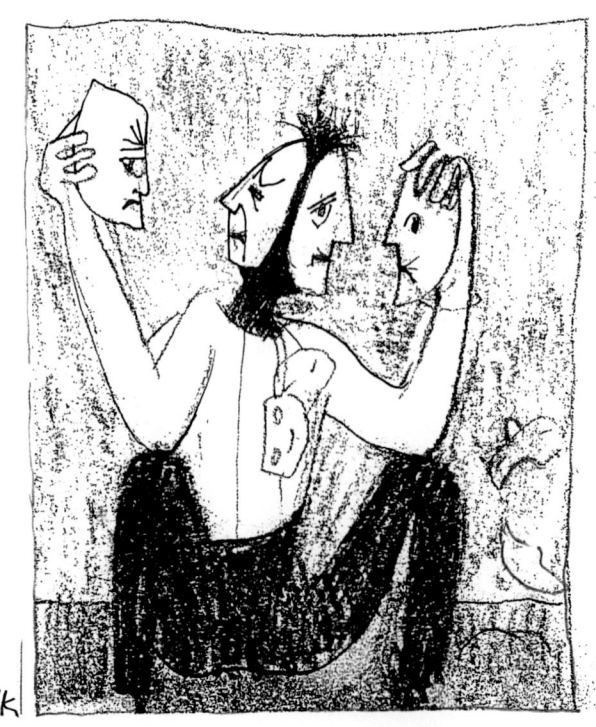

LATER MANIFESTATIONS OF THE JOKER

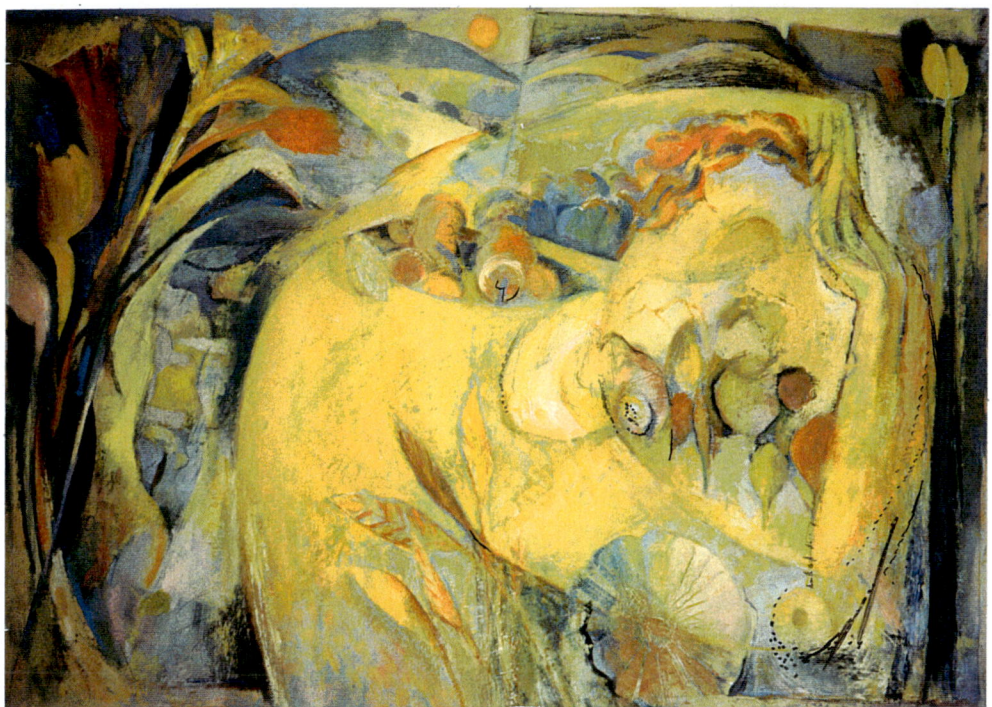

Fig. 582   Spring – 1st version (Fig. 530), amended   Oil on Board

The Joker now makes his presence felt in the early version of 'Spring' (see page 314). A few changes to the landscape reveal eyes, mouth and a floppy horned cap on his reclining head.

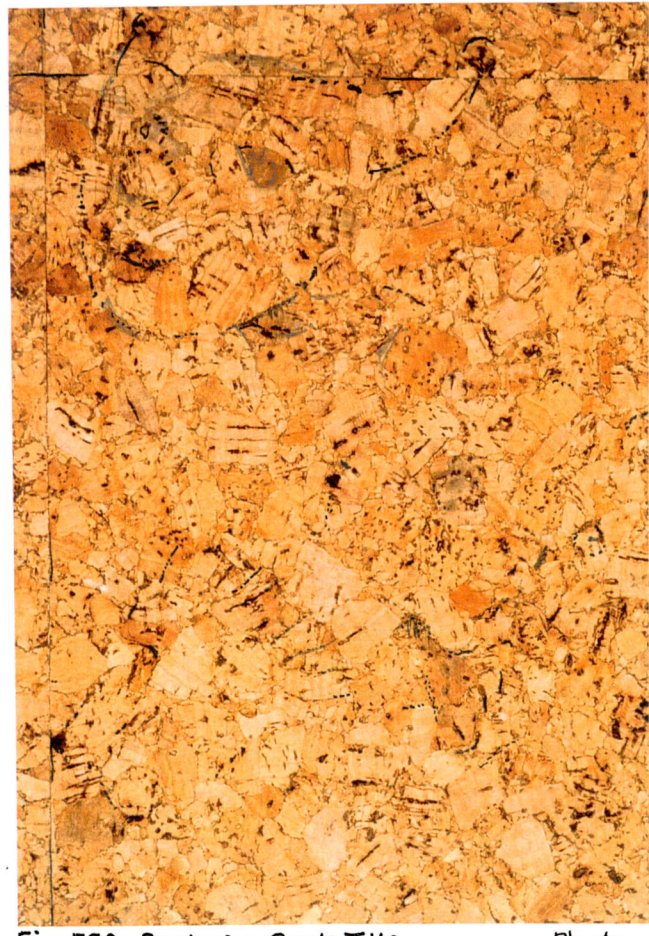

Fig. 583 Part of a Cork Tile   Photo

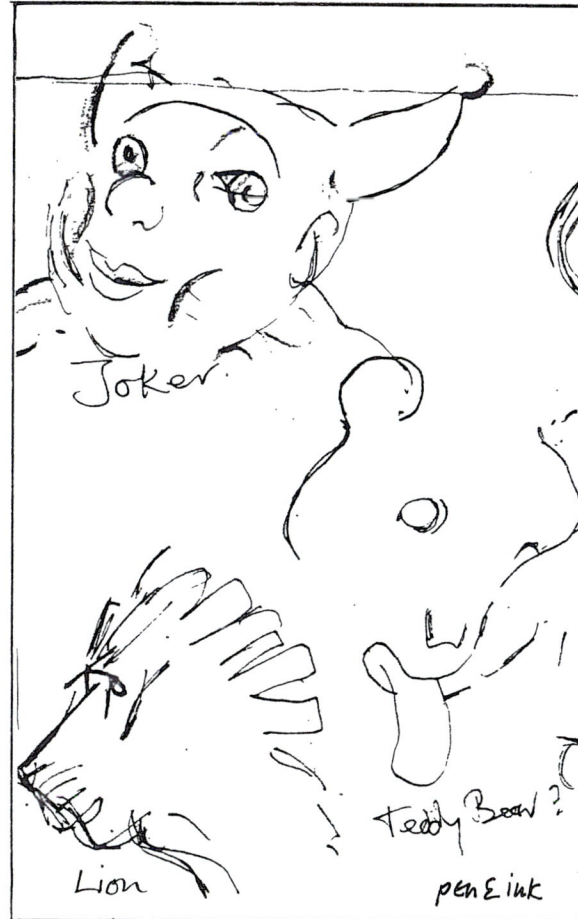

Fig. 584 Facial Features in Cork Tile

Another reappearance occurred in a reverie, when I was looking at wall tiles. One of the tiles suggested the heads of creatures, including a head with two-horned cap.

347

Final Curtain?

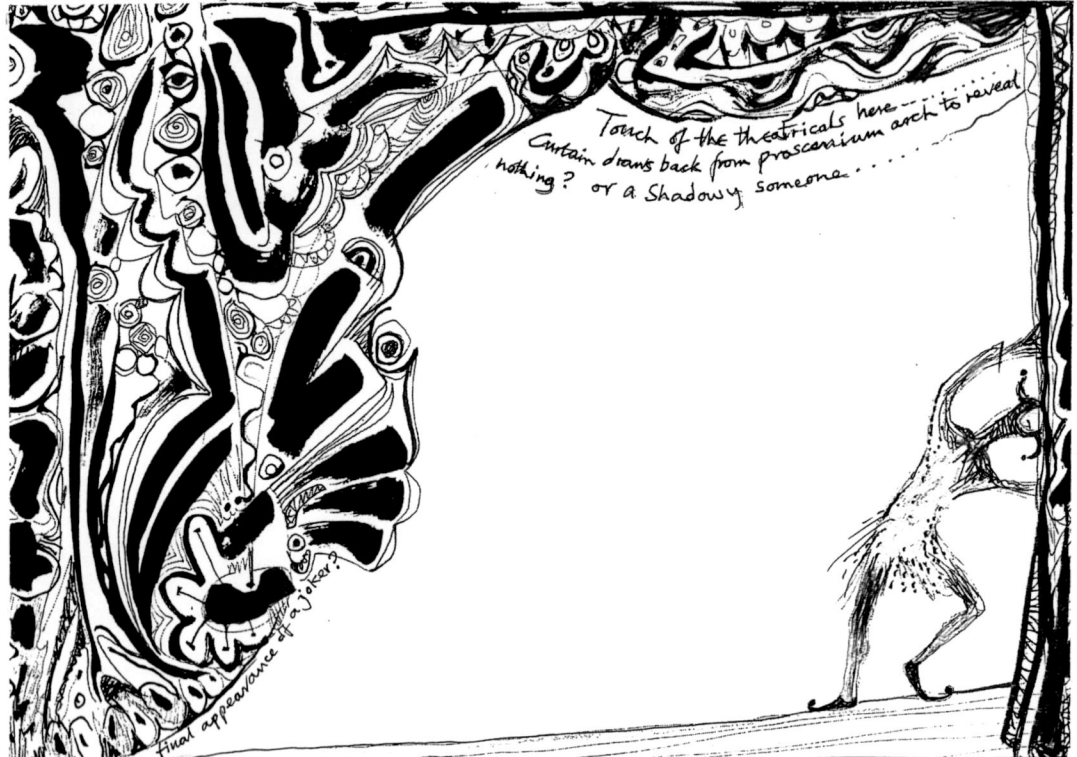

Fig. 585   Final Appearance   Pen, Brush & Ink

The feeling that the Joker hadn't made an appearance for some time may have prompted these two pen and brush drawings.
In 'Final Appearance' he is edging himself off-stage. In 'Curtain Call' below he takes a final bow. Perhaps, in my ignorance, I imagine there's no further need? Yet this 'final curtain' is more apparent than real.
The continuing construction of the self still needs his support as the new manifestations robustly display on the final few pages......

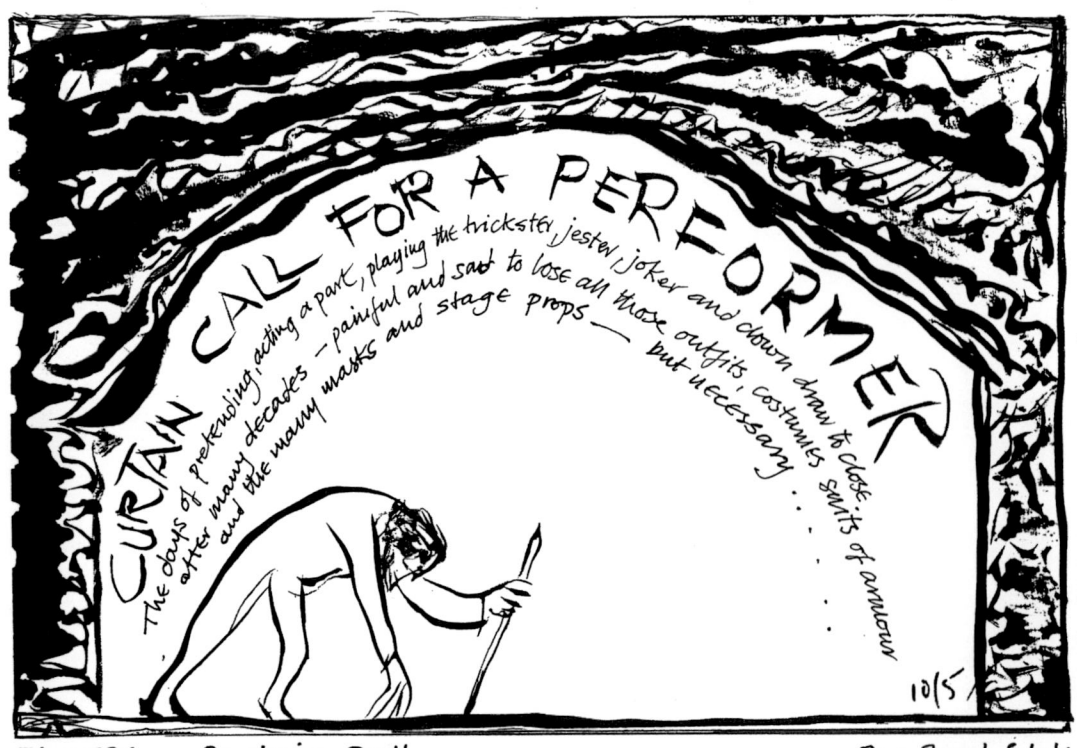

Fig. 586   Curtain Call   Pen, Brush & Ink

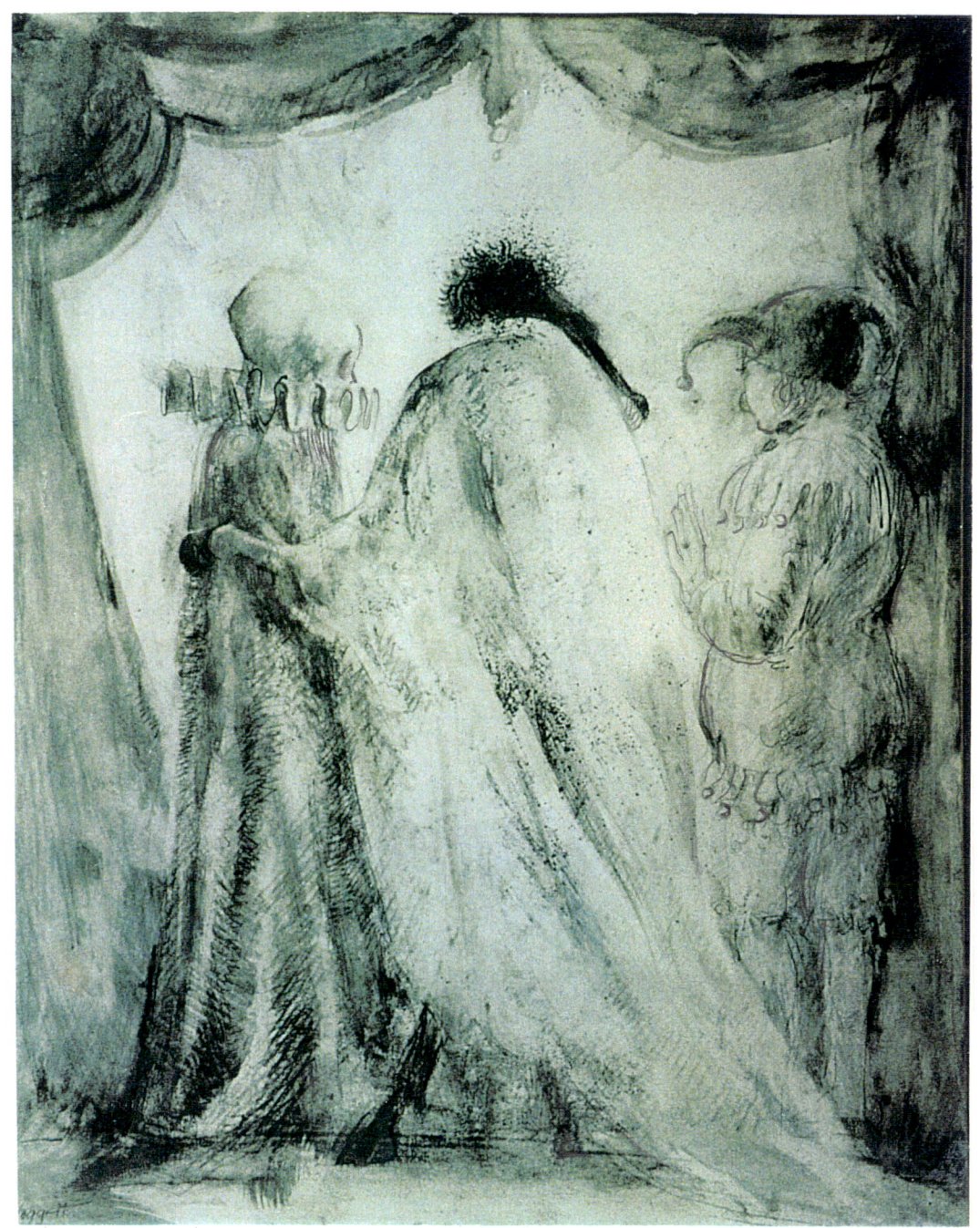

Fig. 587   A Backstage Conversation.   Pencil & Graphite Powder

A Backstage Conversation

The 'odd-man-out' puts his cap back on, comes out of retirement and returns on a part-time basis. I seem to have brought him back as a free-lance negotiator.

Looking more corpulent, relaxed and wiser, he chats to Old Nick, Prince of Darkness who in turn brings the Reaper into the centre stage. Perhaps they are rehearsing their 'lines' backstage.

On the other hand the curtains are drawn back and the protagonists may be performing before the public whilst I view them from backstage.....

So the Joker is back where he started, relating to the skeletal form, not now as a cap only, but as a future companion.

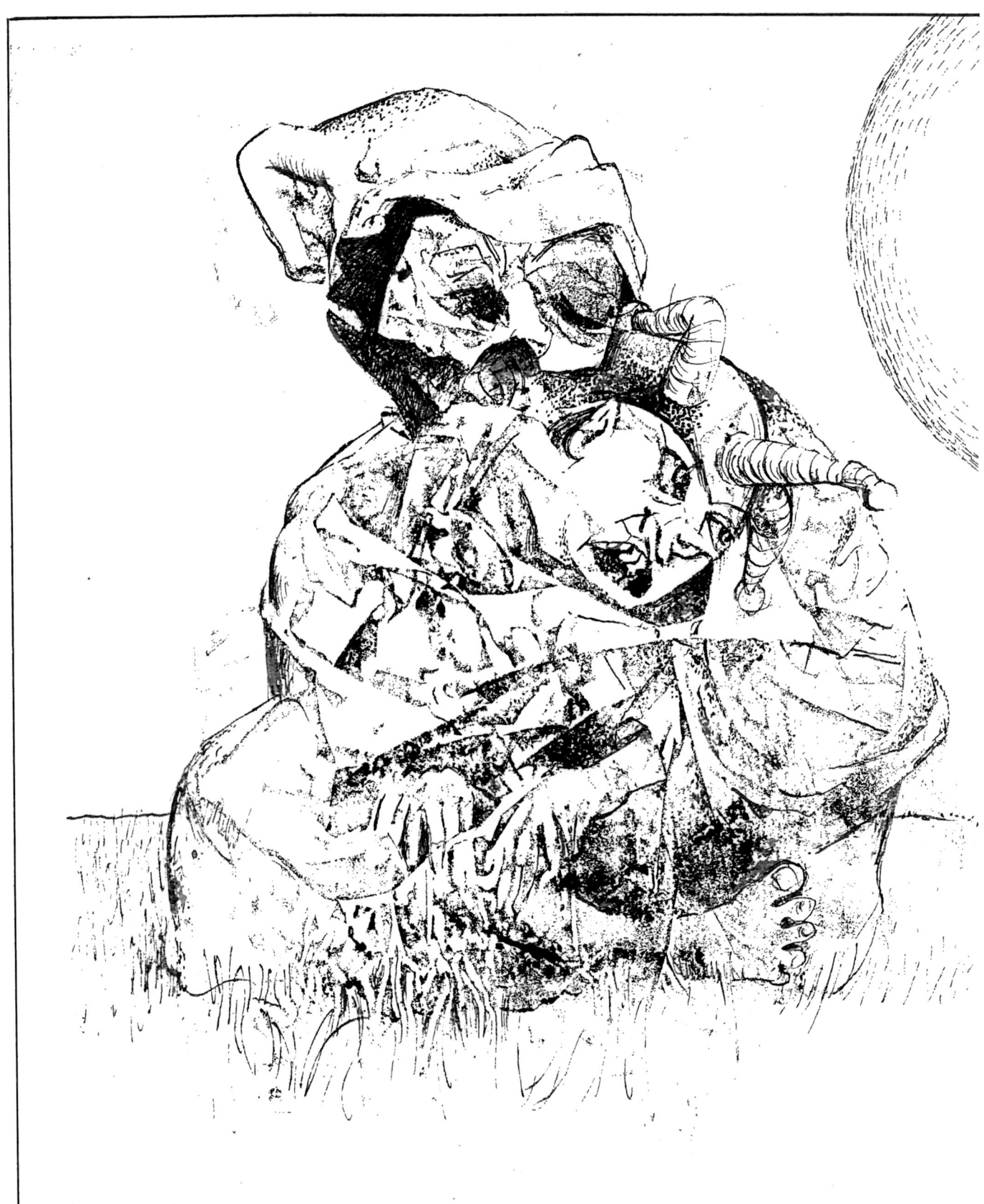

Fig. 588 Strange Meeting — (The Cripple meets the Joker)

Strange Meeting

On a barren heathland, against a low setting sun, an elderly cripple struggling along is surprised by a new manifestation of the Joker. Caught at a moment of transformation, he is elbowing his way out from under his previous character, now in deep shadow between a crumpled cap and a mask.
From the cripple's viewpoint this appears as an act of defiance and a show of independence

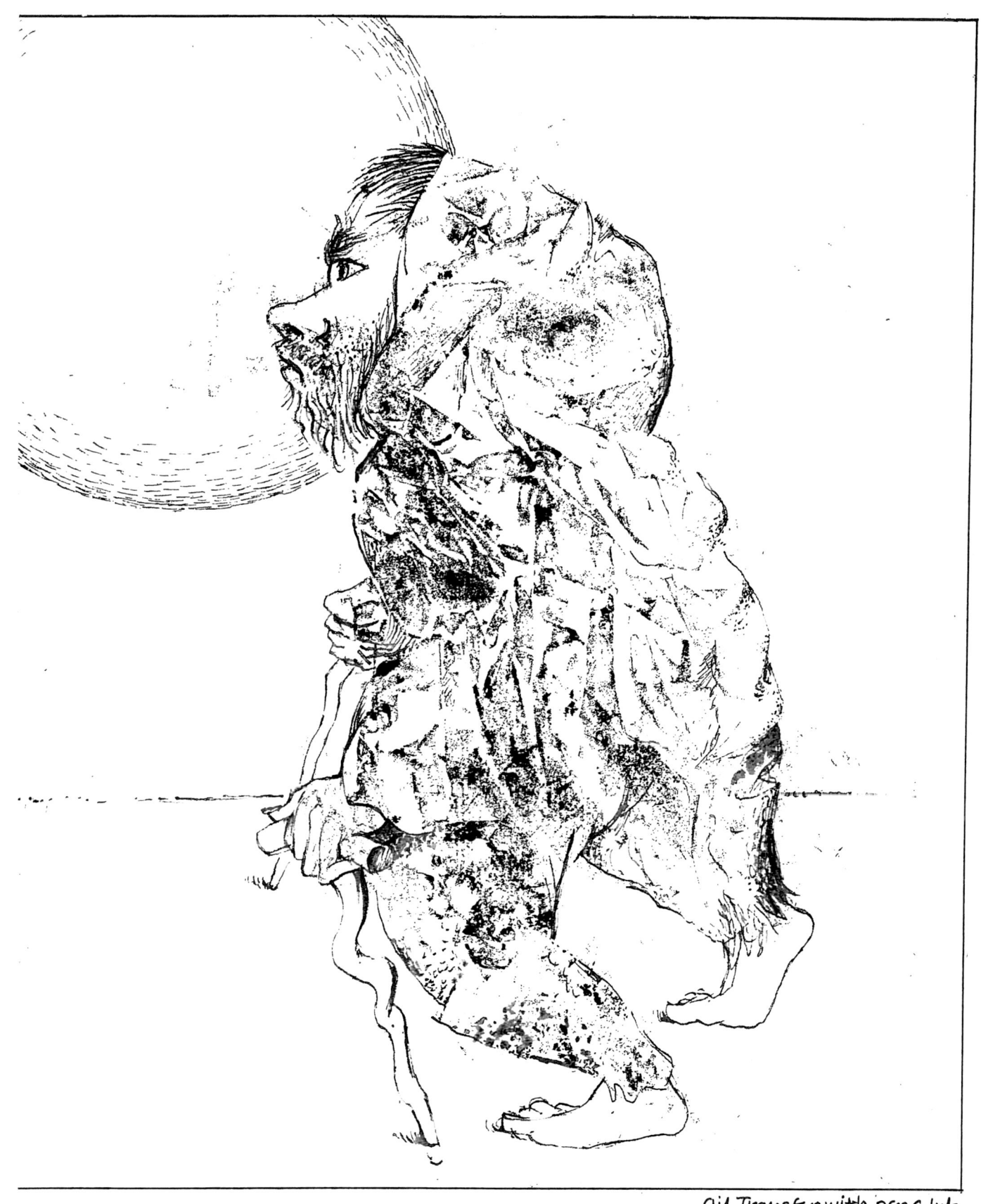

Oil Transfer with pen & Ink

which he finds difficult to cope with. Before he had been able, as a 'player', to dictate the rules - to control this changeling in the pack.
 There is this ability to effect a real transformation from within. Yet the moment is filled with with ambiguity. Is the Joker on the defensive, anxious to disguise his misdemeanour - or is his attitude one of malignancy and aggressiveness?

 Everything seems finely balanced, awaiting a choice or decision.............

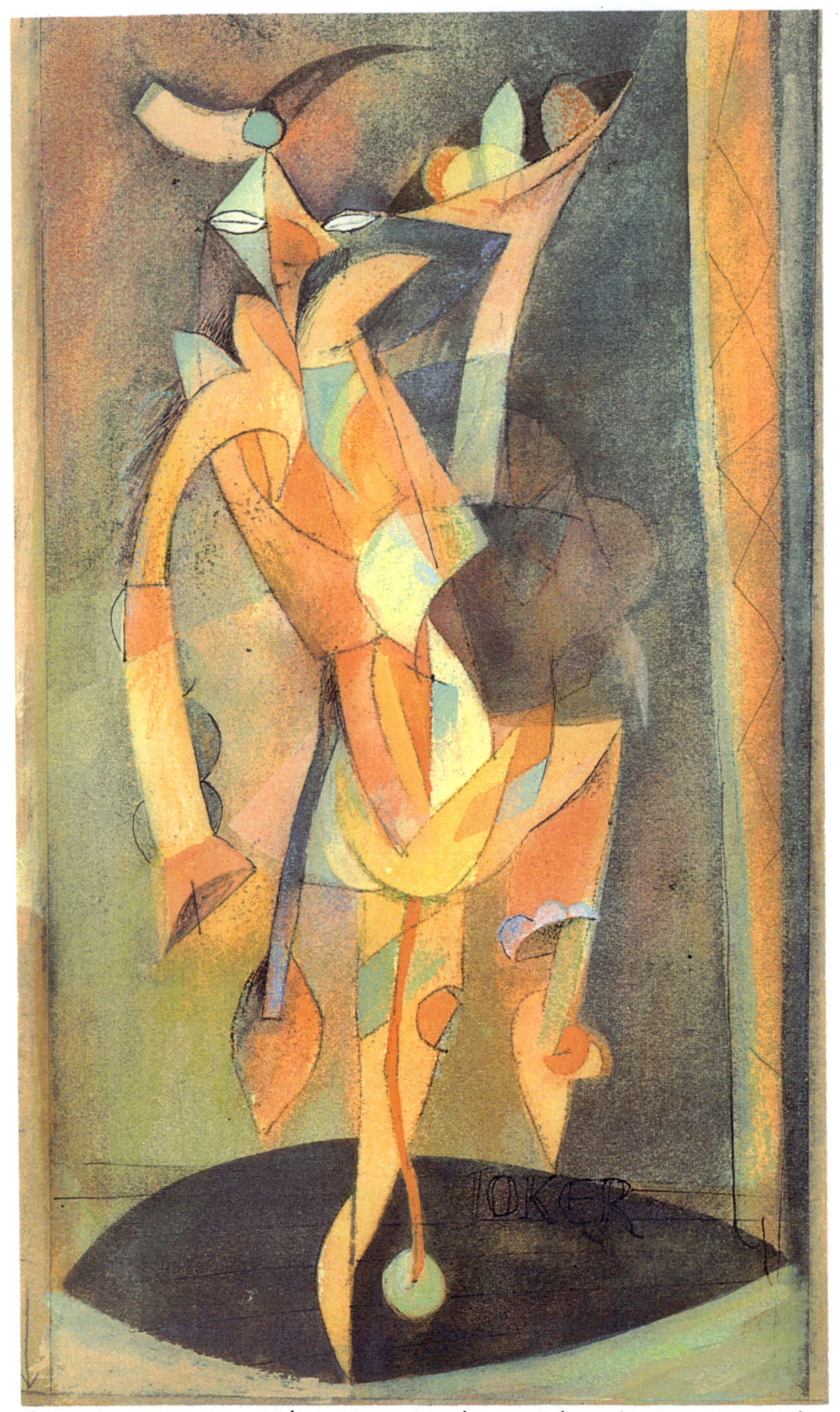

Fig. 589 Zany Prancing – 2nd. version of Joker, Fig. 574 Gouache

'Zany Prancing' encapsulates the essence of this book, countering the ambiguities of 'Strange Meeting' (overleaf). The prancing movement, the fragmentary structure of the figure, bearer of the Earth's fruit, the warmth of the colours – all these attributes symbolise the optimistic nature of the continuing fantasy of dream and reverie inherent in Joker. Out of the fears and incomprehensions of the pictorial story of a 'Breakdown – Breakout' personal history grew a defensive system which clarified this confrontational material .... the story continues........

First published 2006 by Clover Cliff Press
112 Winchcombe Street
Cheltenham
Gloucestershire
GL52 2NW

ISBN-10: 0-9552736-0-9
ISBN-13: 978-0-9552736-0-5

Copyright © 2006 Chris Hoggett

A CIP catalogue record for this book
is available from the British Library.

Chris Hoggett has asserted his right under
the Copyright, Design and Patents Act, 1988,
to be identified as the author of this work.

All rights reserved. No part of this publication
may be reproduced in any form or by any means –
graphic, electronic or mechanical, including
photocopying, recording, taping or information
storage and retrieval systems - without the prior
permission in writing from the publishers.

Printed and bound in the UK by Printwyze, Cheltenham